W0259657

the herb book

THE STORIES, SCIENCE, AND HISTORY OF HERBS

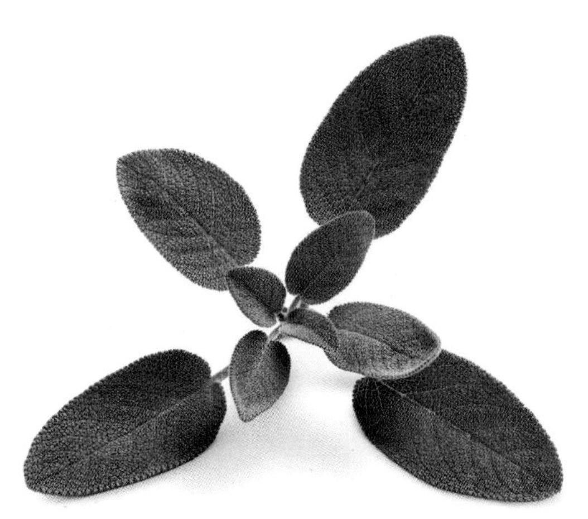

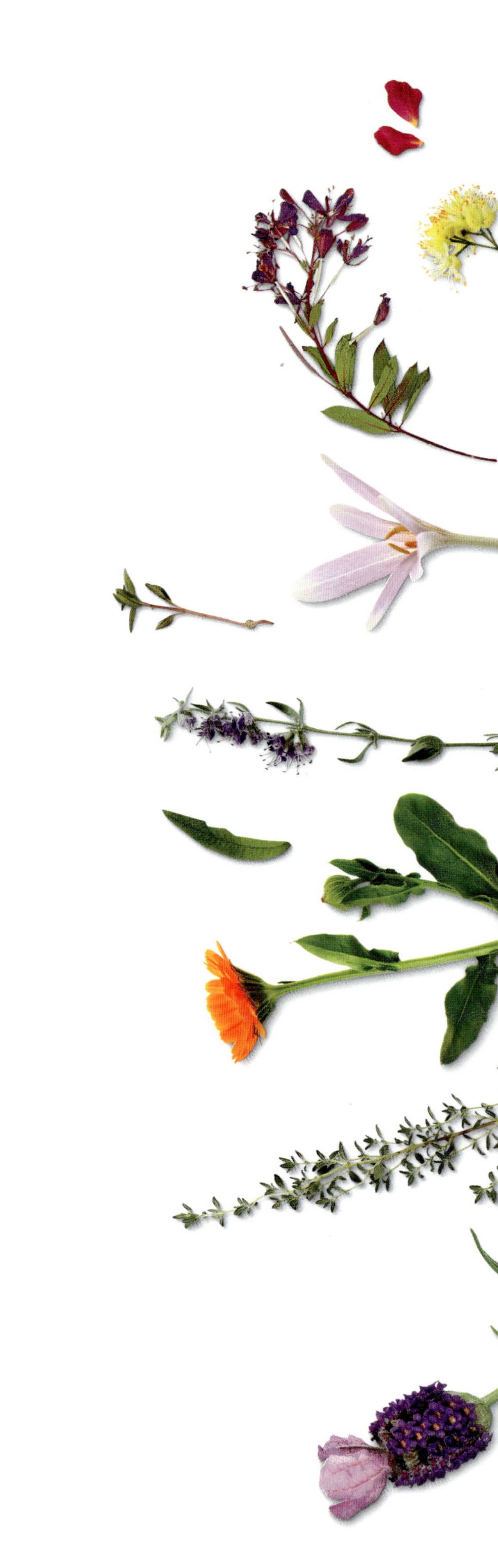

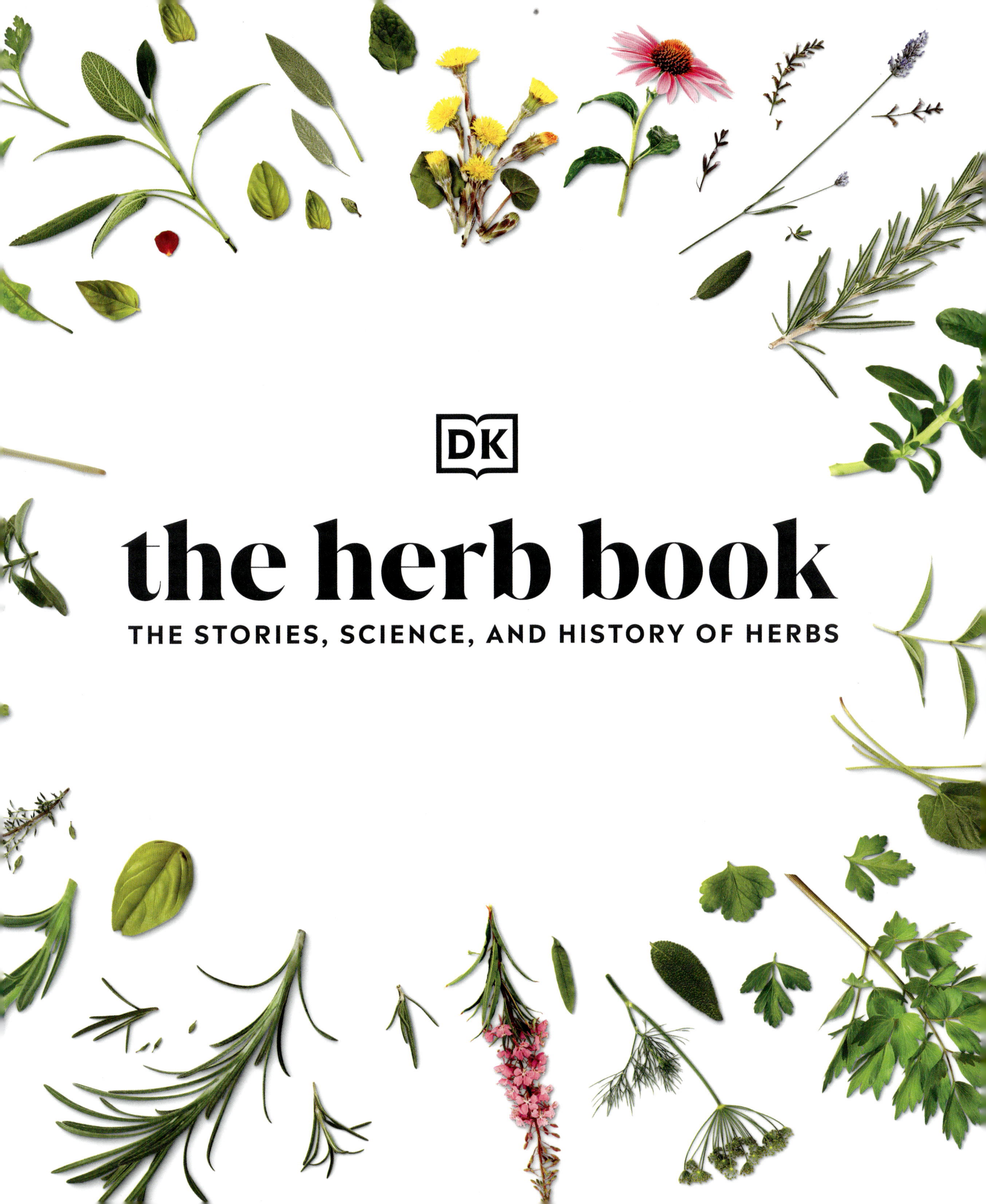
DK
the herb book
THE STORIES, SCIENCE, AND HISTORY OF HERBS

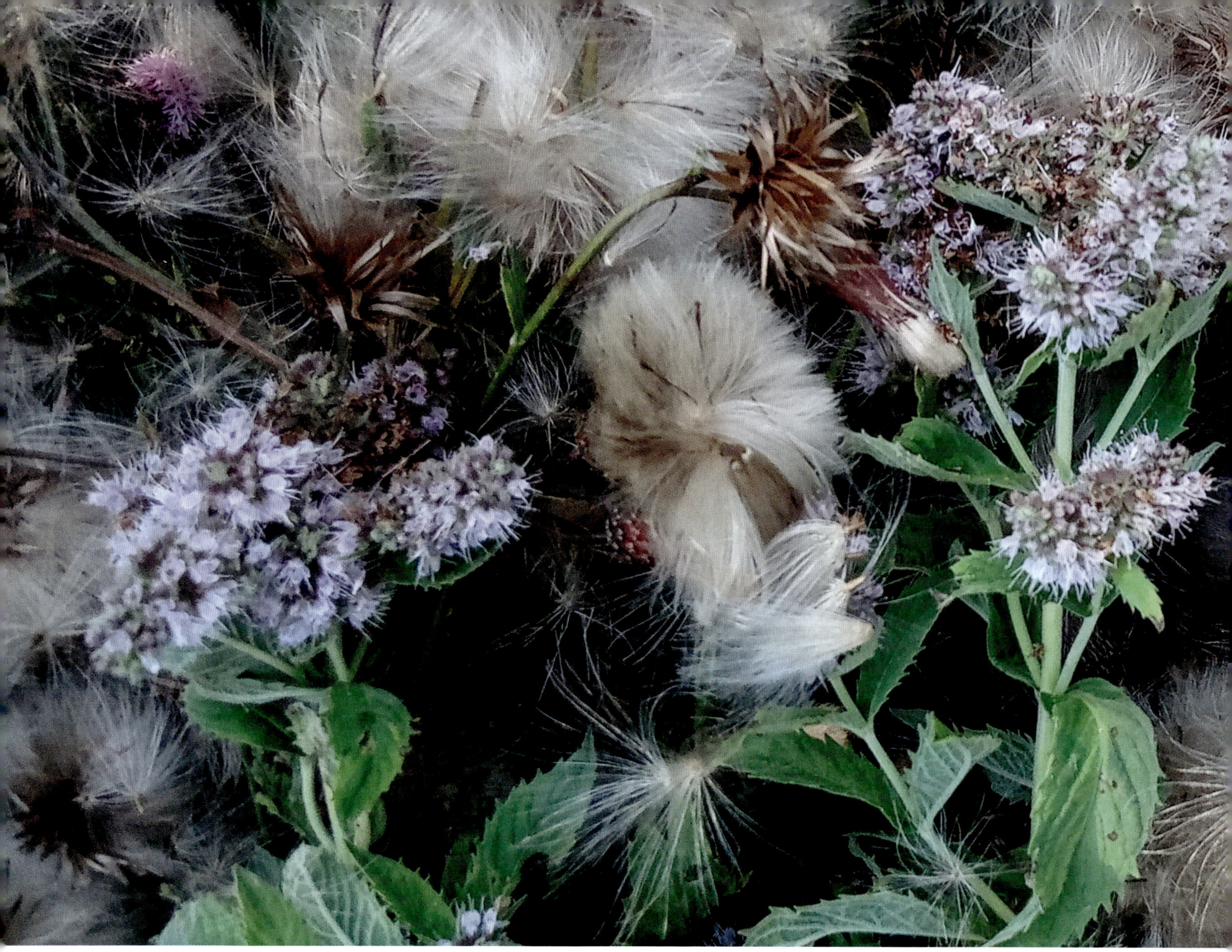

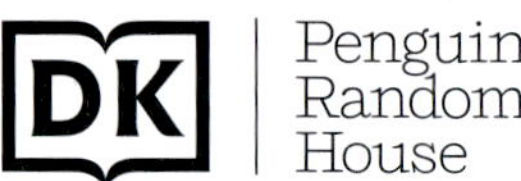

DK LONDON

Senior Editor Hugo Wilkinson
Editors Annelise Evans, Becky Gee, Annie Moss
Production Editor Rob Dunn
Senior Production Controller Meskerem Berhane
Managing Editor Angeles Gavira Guerrero
Associate Publishing Director Liz Wheeler
Publishing Director Jonathan Metcalf

Senior Art Editor Sharon Spencer
Design Assistant Clarisse Hassan
Senior Jackets Designer Surabhi Wadhwa-Gandhi
Jackets Design Development Manager Sophia MTT
Picture Researcher Sarah Smithies
Managing Art Editor Michael Duffy
Art Director Karen Self
Design Director Phil Ormerod

DK DELHI

Senior Editor Anita Kakar
Editor Ekta Chadha
Jacket Designer and Illustrator Vidushi Chaudhry
Senior Jacket Designer Suhita Dharamjit
Senior Jackets Coordinator Priyanka Sharma Saddi
Senior Managing Editor Rohan Sinha
Pre-production Manager Balwant Singh
Editorial Head Glenda R Fernandes

Senior Art Editor Vaibhav Rastogi
Art Editors Arshti Narang, Sonakshi Singh
DTP Designers Rakesh Kumar, Mohammad Rizwan, Anita Yadav
Production Editor Anita Yadav
Illustrator Priyal Mote
Managing Art Editor Sudakshina Basu
Production Manager Pankaj Sharma
Design Head Malavika Talukder

First published in Great Britain in 2023 by
Dorling Kindersley Limited
DK, One Embassy Gardens, 8 Viaduct Gardens, London SW11 7BW

The authorized representative in the EEA is Dorling Kindersley Verlag GmbH.
Arnulfstr. 124, 80636 Munich, Germany

10 9 8 7 6 5 4 3 2
003–331843–Apr/2023

A CIP catalogue record for this book is available from the British Library.
ISBN: 9-780-2415-6950-4

Printed and bound in China

For the curious
www.dk.com

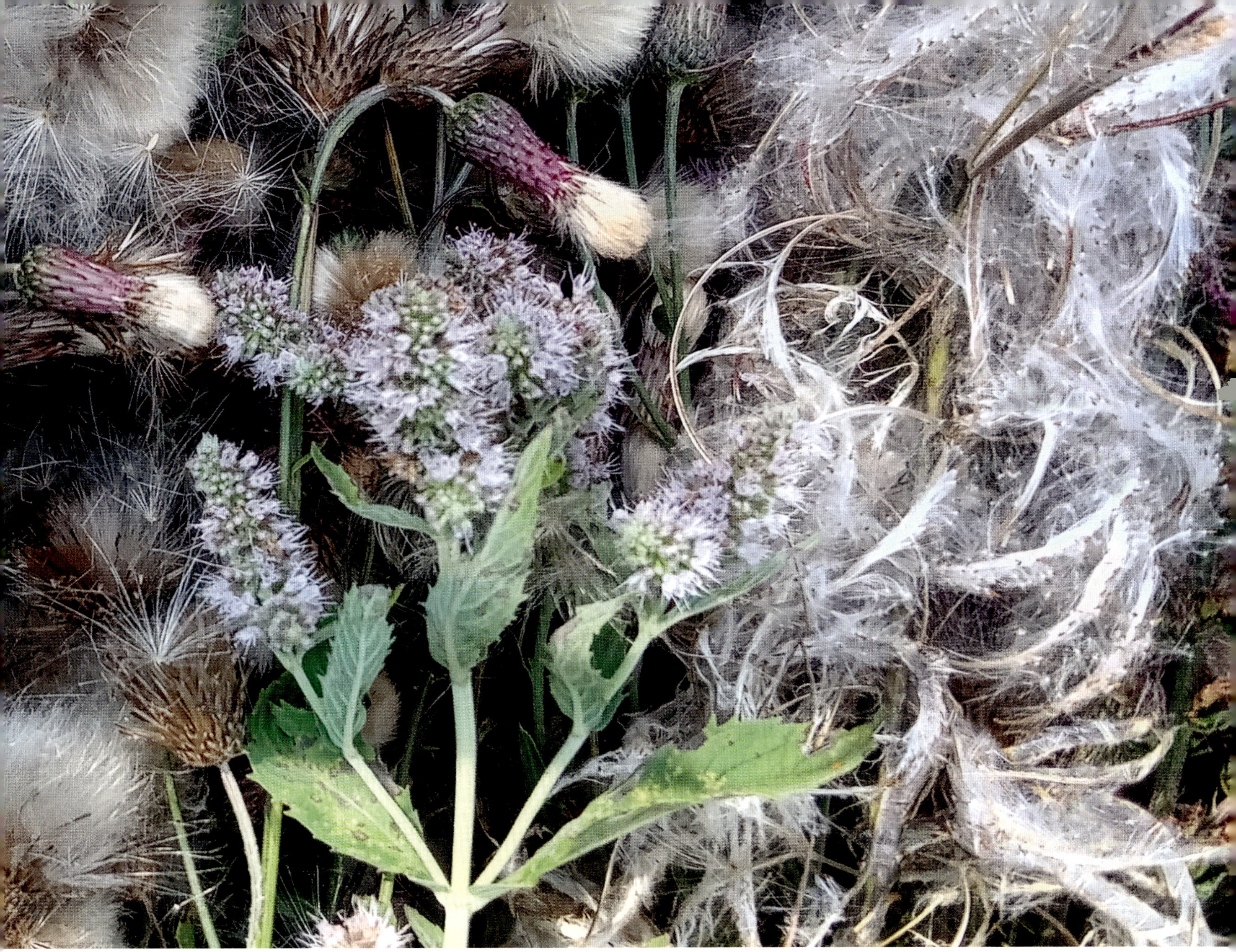

Contributors

Dr Ross Bayton is Assistant Director of the Heronswood Garden, Washington, US. Trained in plant taxonomy at the Royal Botanic Gardens, Kew, he is author of several books on botany and horticulture, including *The Gardener's Botanical*. He also contributed to DK's *Flora*.

Peter Marren is a wildlife writer, journalist, and authority on invertebrate folklore and names. His books include *Rainbow Dust; The New Naturalists*, which won the Society for the History of Natural History's *Thackray Medal*; and *Britain's Rare Flowers*, which won the Botanical Society of the British Isles' Presidents' Award.

Sonya Patel Ellis is a writer, editor, and artist exploring interconnections in nature through the prism of a botanical world. This includes the history and healing power of herbs. Her books include *Collins Botanical Bible*, *The Heritage Herbal*, and *The Modern Gardener*.

Michael Scott OBE has a degree in botany and is a natural history writer, broadcaster, and conservationist. Now largely retired, he is travelling the world as a natural history speaker on cruise ships. His books include *Scottish Wild Flowers* and *Mountain Flowers*.

Consultant

Dr Elizabeth Dauncey is a poisonous and medicinal plant scientist with a background in botany and plant taxonomy. For the past 30 years she has worked for organizations including the London Poisons Unit, the Royal Botanic Gardens, Kew, the Horticultural Trades Association, and the Veterinary Poisons Information Service. She is author of several books and publications on poisonous and medicinal plants, including *Plants that Kill*, *Plants that Cure*, and the *HTA Guide to Potentially Harmful Plants*.

Half Title page Sage, *Salvia officinalis*
Title page Circle of herbs
Imprint page Wild herbs and flowers
Contents page Apothecary's rose, *Rosa gallica* var. *officinalis*

DISCLAIMER: see p.302

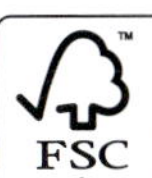

MIX
Paper | Supporting responsible forestry
FSC™ C018179

This book was made with Forest Stewardship Council™ certified paper – one small step in DK's commitment to a sustainable future.
For more information go to www.dk.com/our-green-pledge

CHAPTER 1

Herbs and their Uses

CHAPTER 2

Trees and Shrubs

CHAPTER 3

Perennial Flowering Herbs

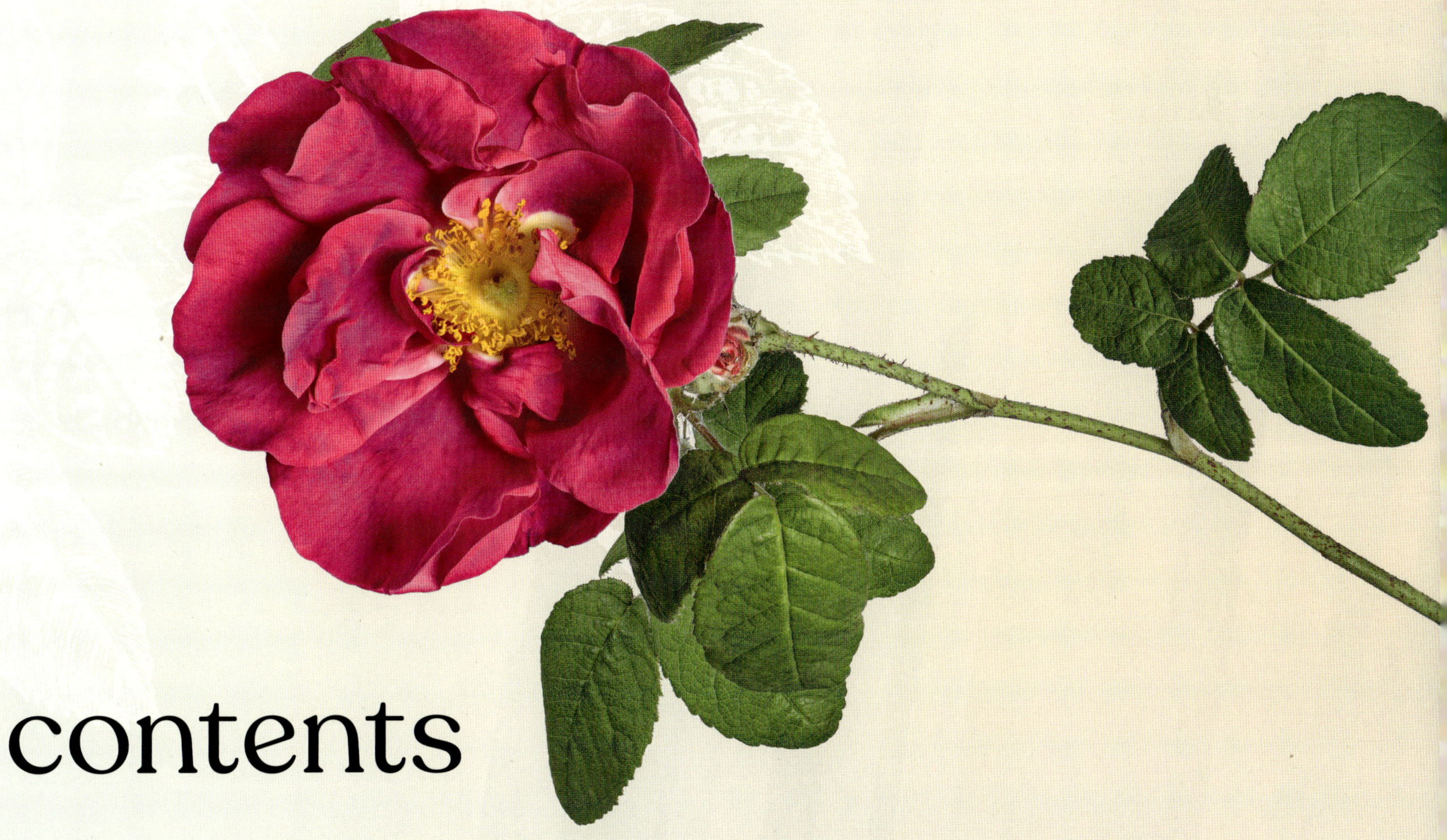

contents

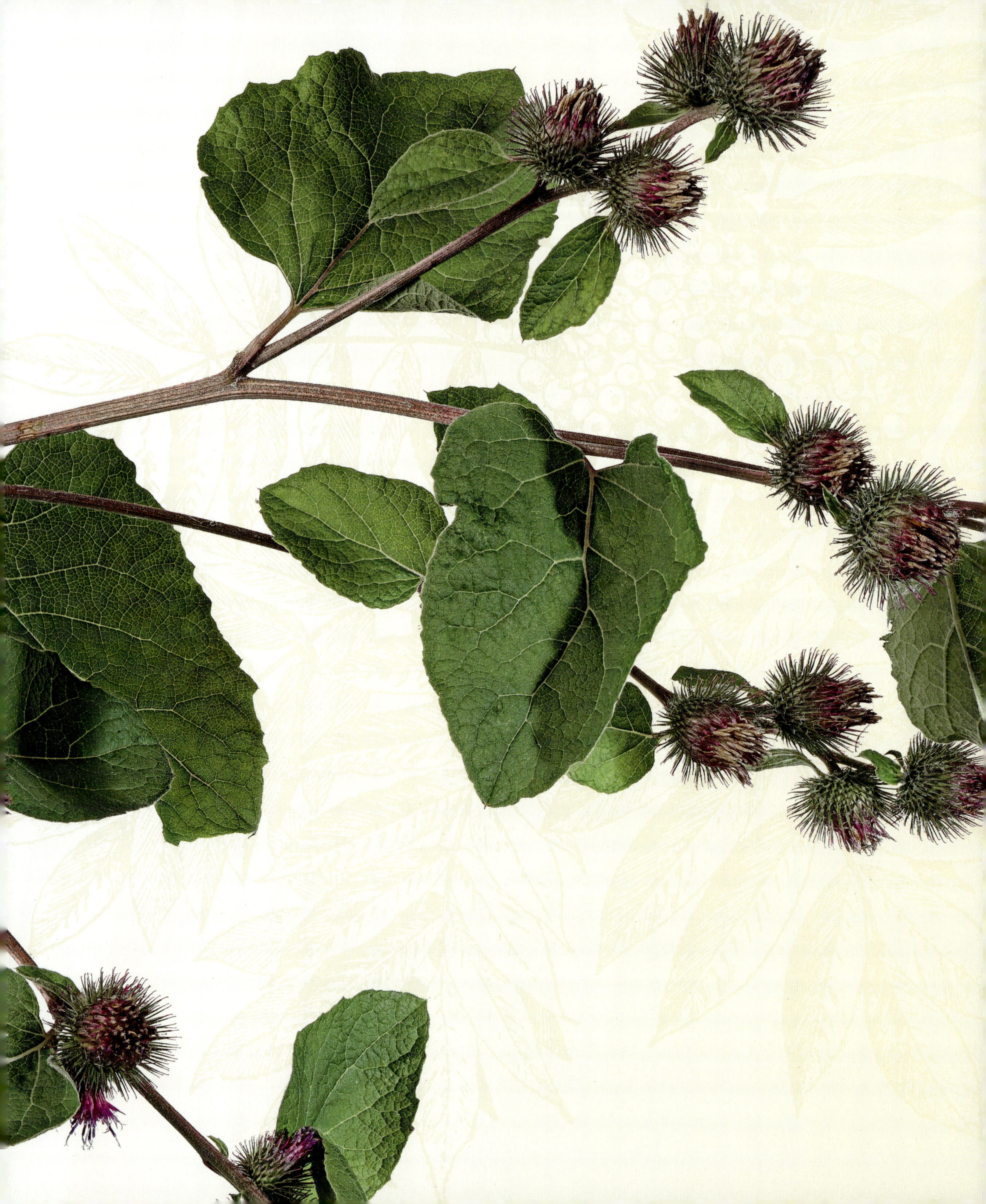

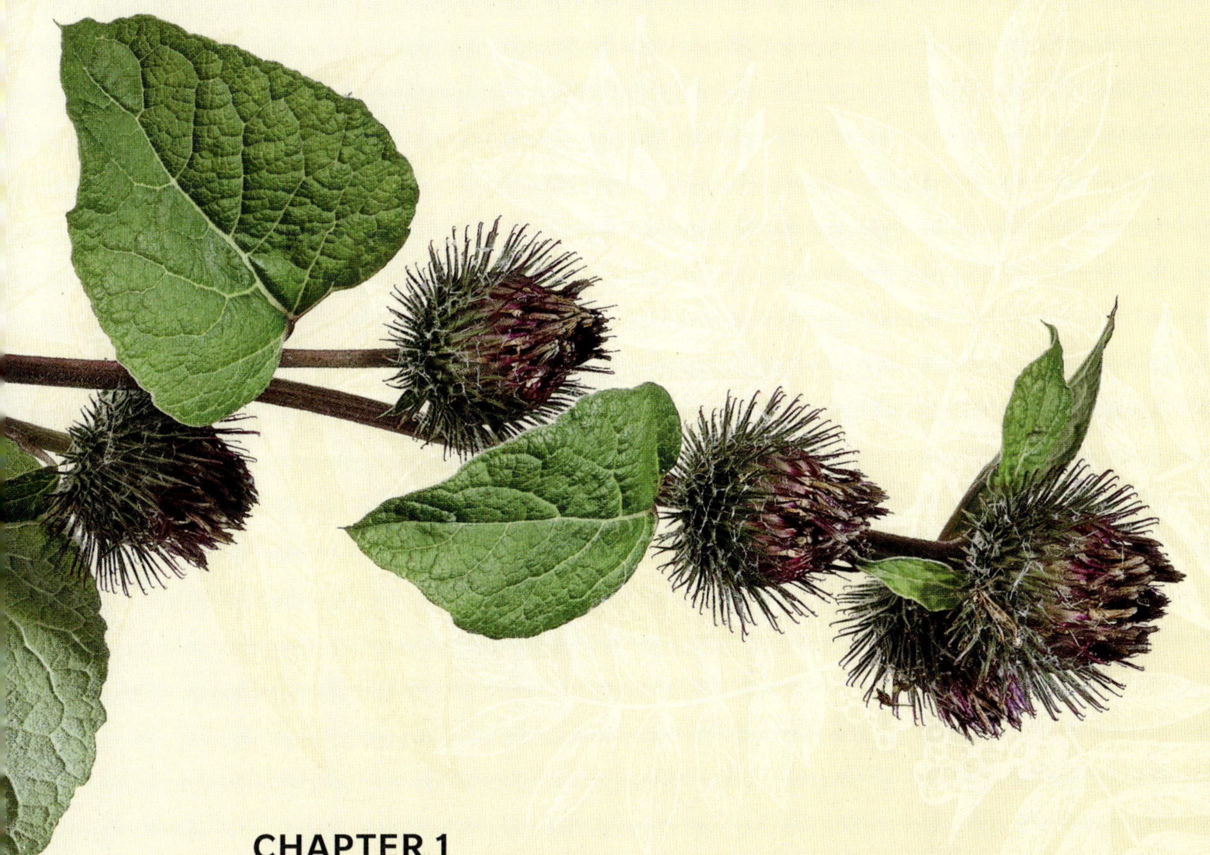

CHAPTER 1

Herbs and their Uses

Humans have been using plants for thousands of years for purposes that go far beyond food. In this book we define a herb as a plant that has medicinal, culinary, or cosmetic uses.

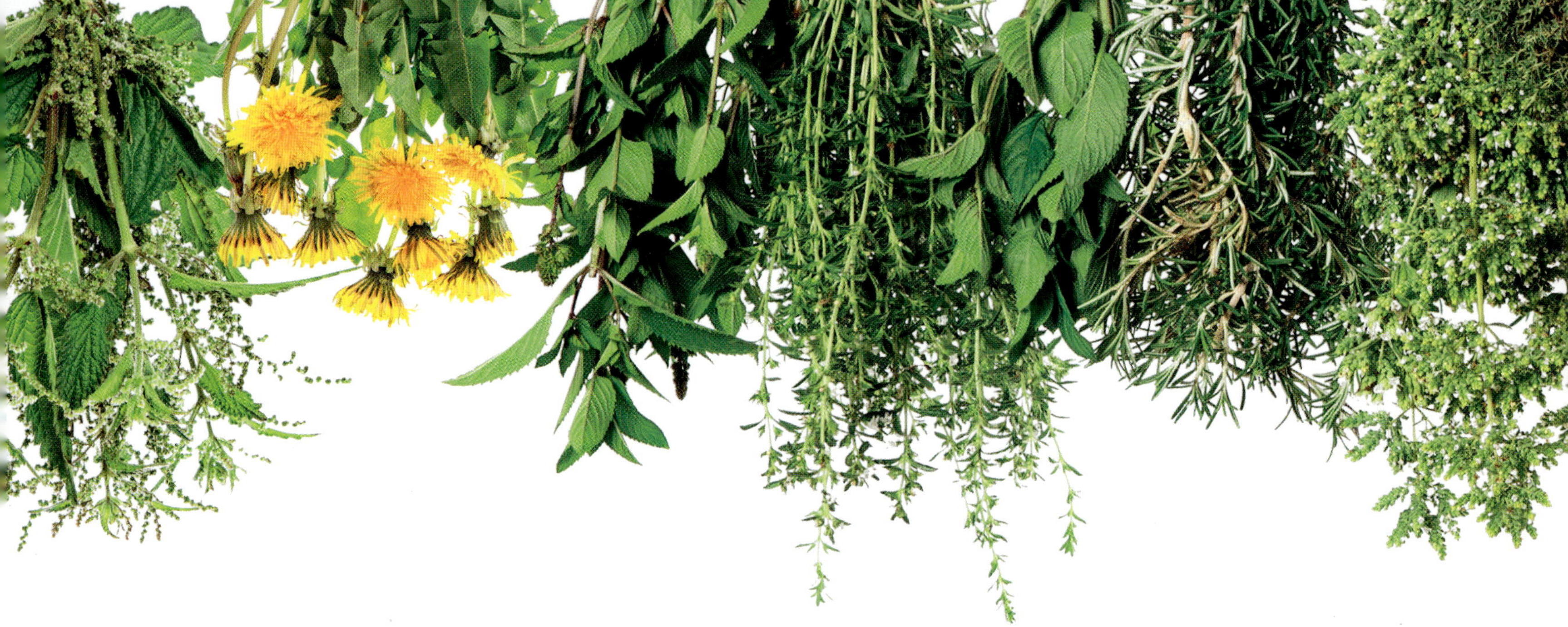

Introducing Herbs

Herb is a term with several, overlapping meanings, but in this book it refers to any plant that humans cultivate or collect for use in cooking, medicine, cosmetics, perfumery, dyes, and other applications.

HERBS OR SPICES?

In cooking, "herb" describes the herbaceous, aromatic leaves, stems, and flowers that are best used fresh and confer subtle flavours to food, for example thyme (see pp.100–103). "Spices" are the more strongly flavoured, pungent, or bitter, often dried products, usually made from seeds, roots, or bark that are richer in essential oils. However, all are herbs in the broader sense of a useful plant.

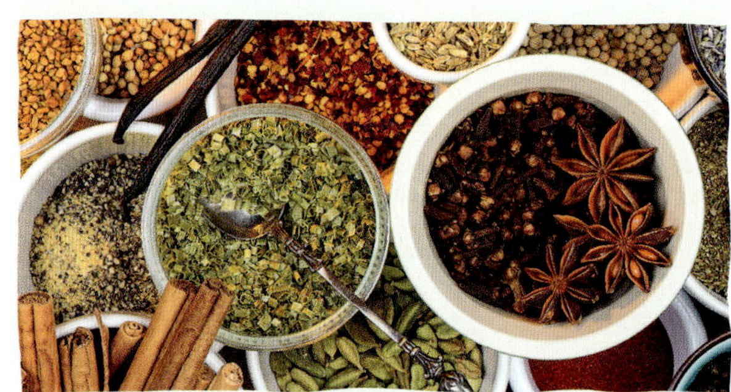

DRIED HERBS AND SPICES

The definition of a herb

To a botanist, a herb (or herbaceous plant) is a non-woody plant that dies back to the ground at the end of the growing season, as opposed to a tree or shrub, which has one or more perennial, woody stems. An alternative definition of a herb, and one that is used in this book, is a plant which has leaves, flowers, seeds, fruits, shoots, sap, or roots – tasting or smelling sweet, bitter, aromatic, or pungent – that in limited quantity make food more flavoursome, aid human health, or produced pleasing fragrances. These useful plants make life better, healthier, or sweeter-smelling.

Herbs as medicines

Egyptians planted the first herb gardens around 4,000 years ago. They cultivated culinary herbs mostly, but other herbs had medicinal uses. By trial and error, humans had learnt that many plants have health benefits, reducing symptoms of disease or helping wounds to heal. Herbalists collected this knowledge and then advised on treatments for specific ailments. This tradition continued to modern times (see pp.18–19 and 22–23).

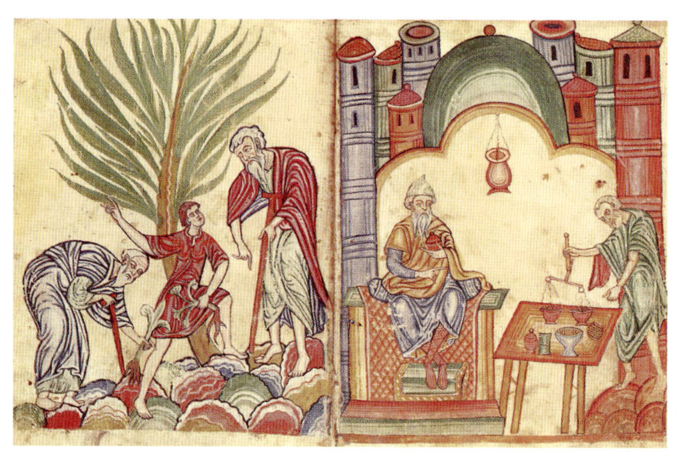

◄ The art of the herbal Apothecaries gathered, prepared, prescribed, and sold medicinal herbs. One of the earliest, the Greek Dioscorides, wrote a classic reference work, or herbal, called *De Materia Medica*, in 50–70 CE, which described many herbs and their uses.

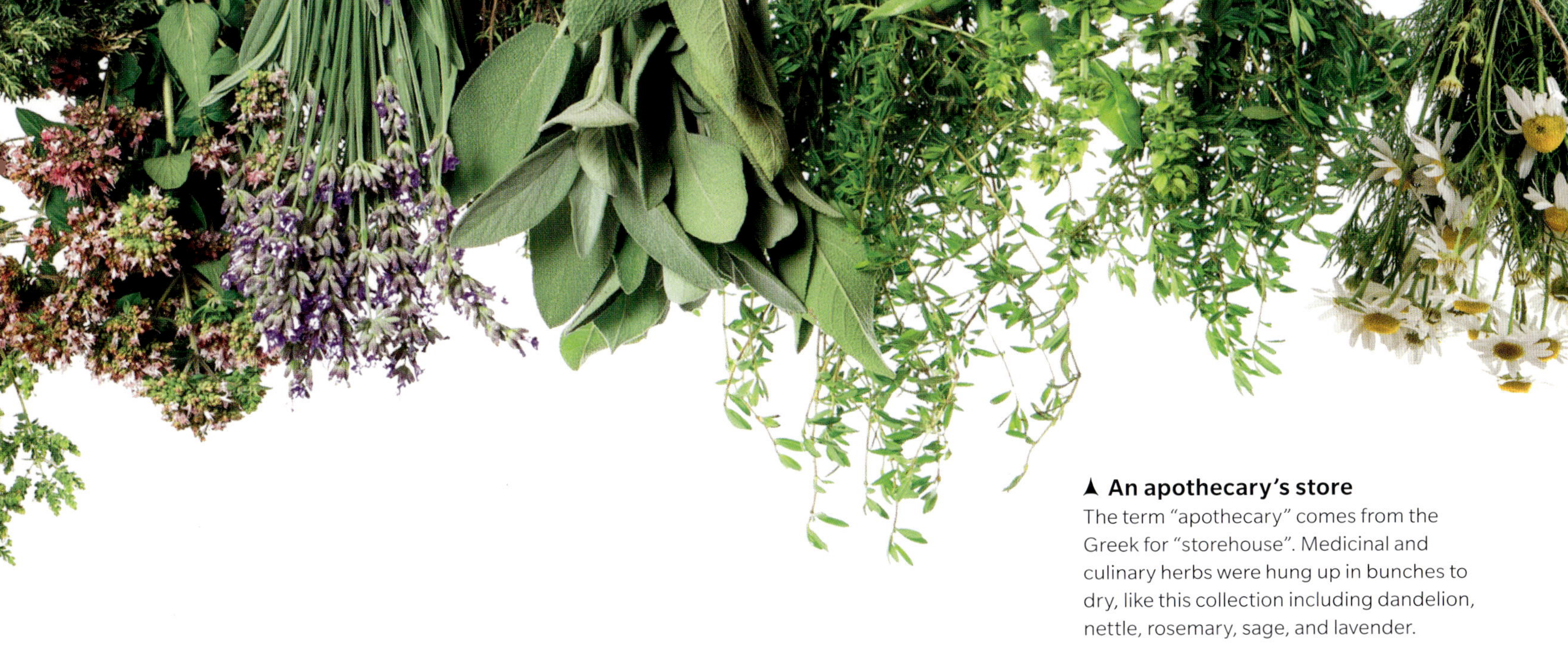

▲ An apothecary's store
The term "apothecary" comes from the Greek for "storehouse". Medicinal and culinary herbs were hung up in bunches to dry, like this collection including dandelion, nettle, rosemary, sage, and lavender.

Plant classification

Plant names in ancient herbals are often unfamiliar, and the many common names can also be confusing and vary considerably. Scientific names, in botanical Latin and based on Carl Linnaeus's 18th-century system, offer a consistent, international system of nomenclature that helps to describe relationships between species. For each species, there is a "type specimen" held somewhere in a herbarium collection, against which other plants can be compared.

HOW CLASSIFICATION WORKS

The relationship between plants is determined by comparing their key physical features, especially of flower forms, although the plant cell's chemistry and genetic material (DNA) are now also considered.

▼ **FAMILY** Group, like Papaveraceae, of one or more genera, which share some characteristics and probably a common ancestor.

▼ **GENUS** Group, within a family, of species that are closely alike in structure. The genus is the first word in the plant name, as in *Papaver*.

▼ **SPECIES** Genus subgroup of broadly identical plants that produce fertile offspring. Species names have two words, as in *Papaver rhoeas*.

▼ **CULTIVAR** A cultivated variety of a species, selectively bred by humans to enhance desirable traits, as in *Papaver rhoeas* 'Flanders'.

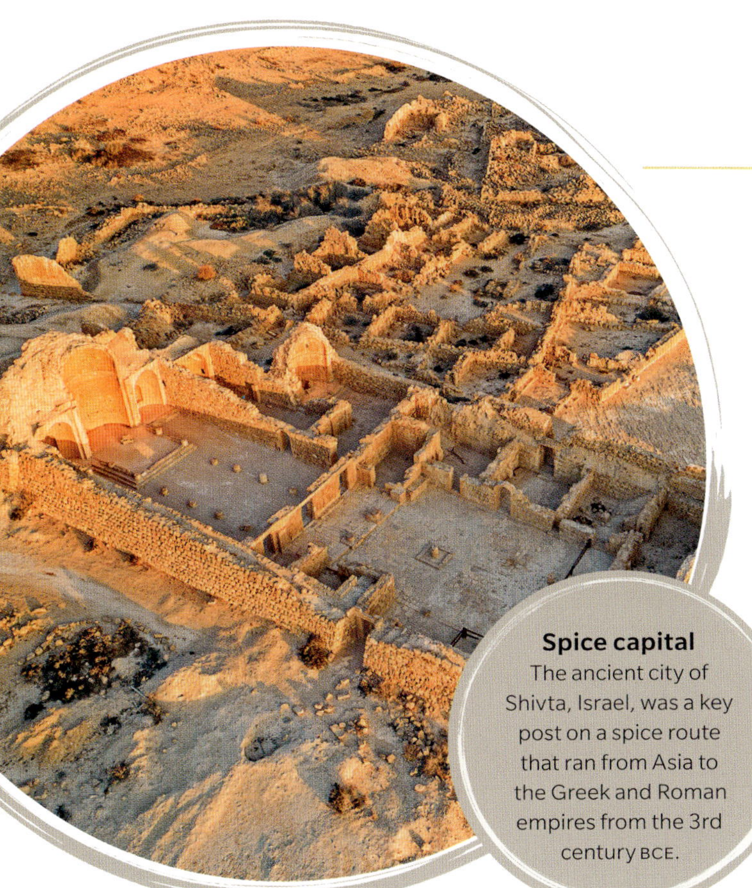

Spice capital
The ancient city of Shivta, Israel, was a key post on a spice route that ran from Asia to the Greek and Roman empires from the 3rd century BCE.

Herbs and human history

As humans began moving around the world, they took their precious herbal plants with them, so that today it is difficult to discern the natural range of many species. For example, ginger (see pp.170–73) was spread by human migrations that began 6,000 years ago. Over the millenia, various spice routes, by sea and over land, were established to trade herbs and spices and then waned. For example, two thousand years ago, Alexandria in Egypt had become the greatest commercial centre of the world, trading spices from India around the Roman empire. The European voyages beginning in the 15th century were also inspired in part by the search for new spices to trade.

> " Over the centuries, bloody battles were fought to win control of [the spice trade]. "
>
> UNESCO Silk Roads Programme, 1988—

Types of Herb

The term "herb" is sometimes used loosely for plants whose leaves or soft stems add flavour to cooked food. However, the world of herbs encompasses multiple uses for all kinds of species across the plant kingdom (Plantae) and other plant-like groups.

Trees and shrubs

Perennial woody plants are described as shrubs, which are multi-stemmed from the base, or trees, usually with one main woody stem or trunk supporting a crown of branches. Many of the most cherished culinary herbs come from shrubs, including rosemary and lavender, and some trees add equally vivid flavourings to cooking – for example bay leaves, tamarind, and cloves. As well as yielding leaves, flowers, fruits, and seeds, trees and shrubs offer bark, sap, and resin from their woody parts, all of which may have herbal uses in medicine, cosmetics, and perfumery.

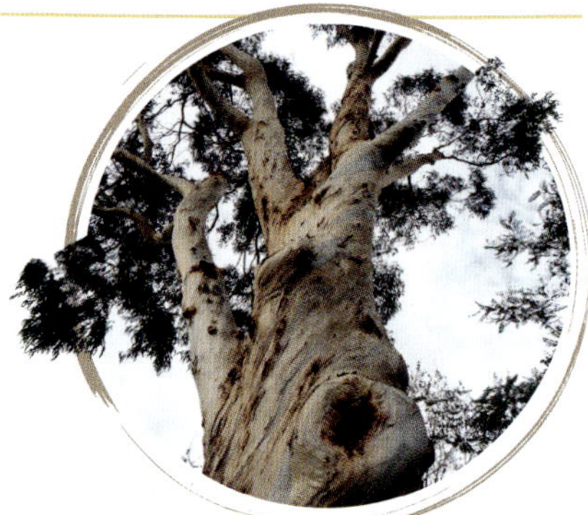

▲ Tree
Southern blue gum (*Eucalyptus globulus*) is the main source of eucalyptus oil, valued for its therapeutic and perfumery uses.

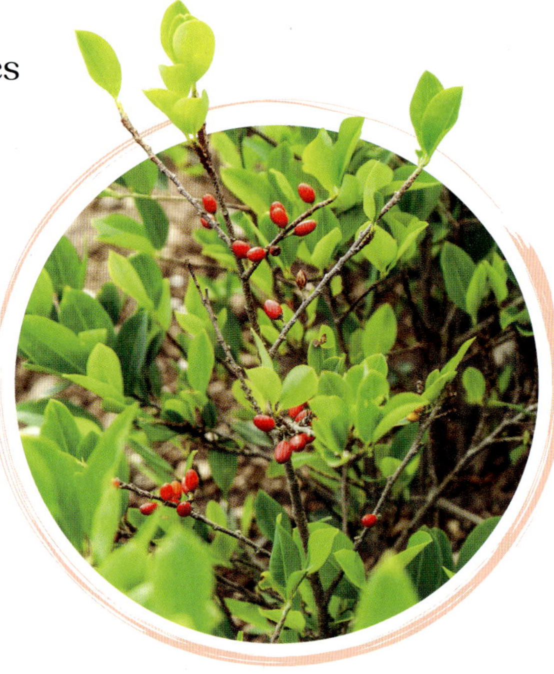

▲ Shrub
The leaves of coca (*Erythroxylum* spp.) are chewed or made into a tea to mitigate altitude sickness. Coca is also the source of cocaine.

Flowering herbs

In this book, herbaceous (non-woody) flowering herbs are divided into either perennial or annual and biennial herbs. Most of these herbs die down to ground level at the end of the growing season in temperate regions. However, some non-woody perennials are evergreen, especially in warmer climates. In cooler climates, some tender perennials are treated as annuals or biennials.

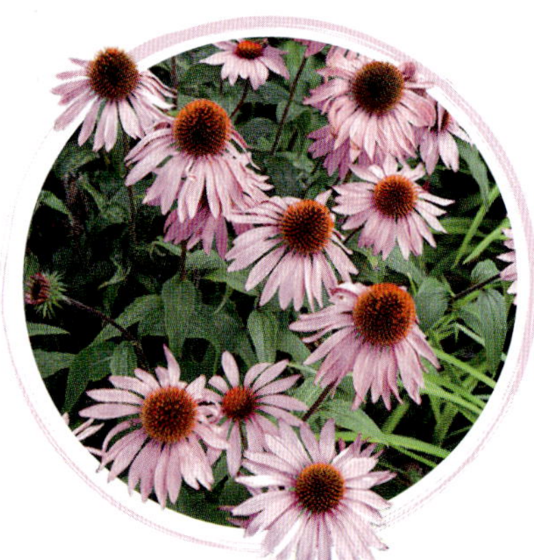

▲ Perennials
The top growth of herbaceous perennials, which live and flower for several years, like *Echinacea purpurea*, dies down in winter.

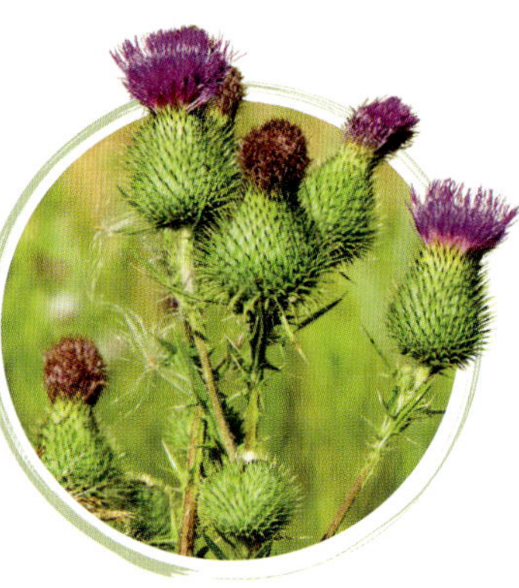

▲ Annuals and biennials
A plant that completes its life cycle in one year is an annual. Biennials flower and die in the second year. Both include some thistle species.

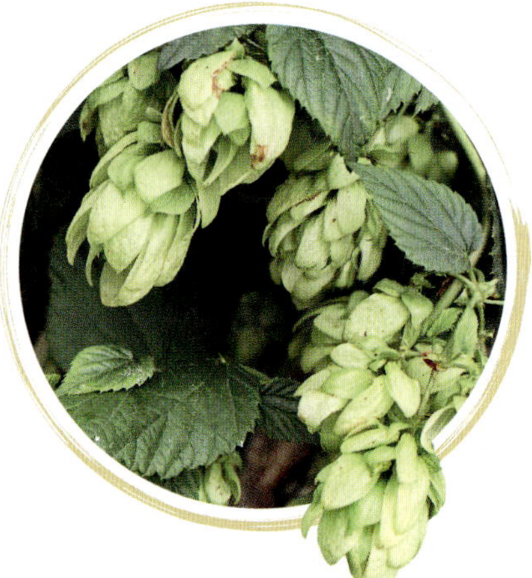

▲ Climbers
Some annuals or perennials such as hop (*Humulus lupulus*) climb up other plants or supports by twining stems, tendrils, or aerial roots.

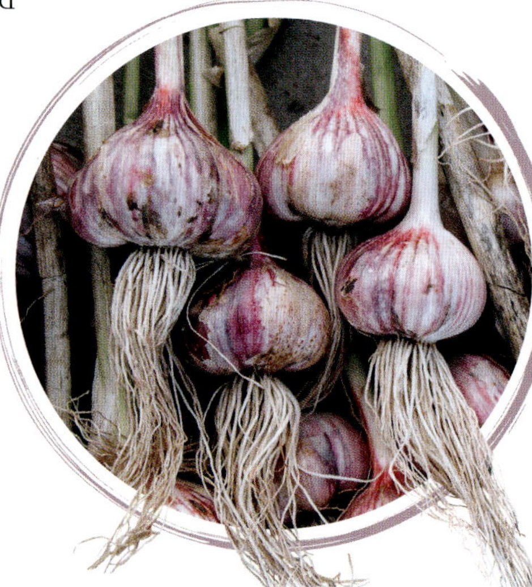

▲ Bulbs
A bulbous plant has a swollen underground organ; it could be a corm, rhizome, tuber, or true bulb, as in garlic (*Allium sativum*).

Other herbs

Non-flowering plants include conifers, which form seeds in cones, as well as ferns, mosses, and liverworts, which reproduce by spores. Algae are plant-like organisms, and some green algae may be related to plants. Red and brown algae, including most seaweeds, belong to Protoctista, a separate kingdom to Plantae. This book includes ferns, as well as red and brown algae, that are used as herbs.

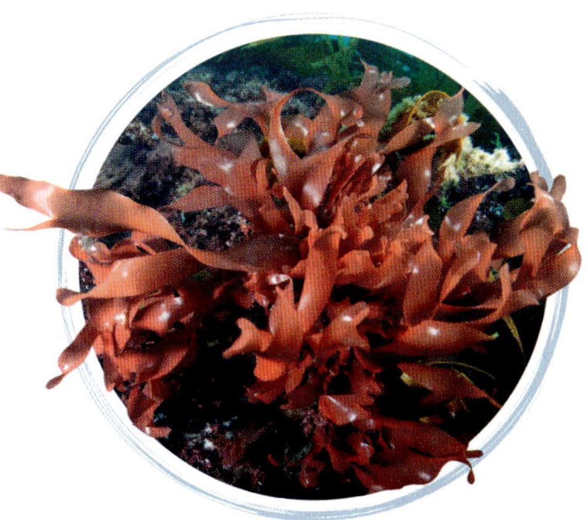

▲ Seaweed
Dulse (*Palmaria palmata*) is a marine red algae that is edible, with a high fibre and protein content. It is also used in skincare products.

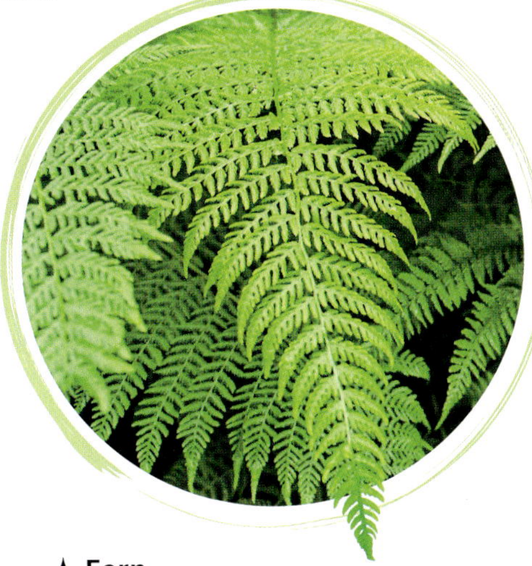

▲ Fern
The young shoots of certain species of fern are eaten and used in traditional medicine. Parts of the plant may also be used in soap.

BREEDING BETTER

Some herb species tend naturally to breed with other species from the same, or a closely related, genus. The resulting hybrid may over time become a species in its own right. Humans have exploited this propensity to breed more useful herbs. For instance, citrus fruits such as the lemon (see pp.52–53) have a complex ancestry, but they have been selectively bred to produce bigger fruits that are rich in vitamin C, used to fight colds.

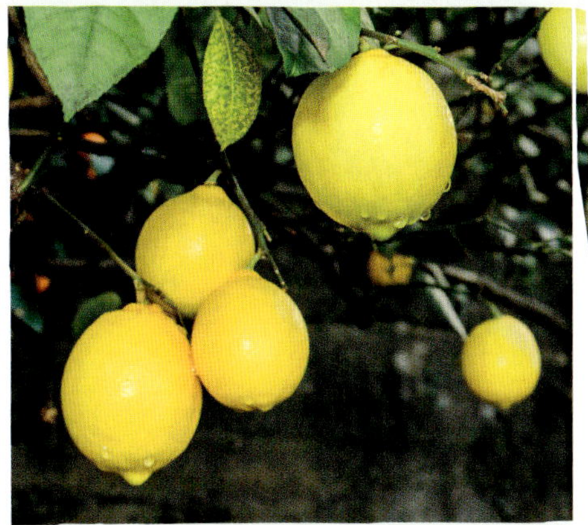

LEMON (*Citrus x limon*)

Fungi

Mushrooms and toadstools are the fruiting bodies of fungi, which form their own kingdom. Some mushrooms are toxic, but many are edible. *Ganoderma lingzhi* (see p.288) is not used in cooking, but for more than 2,000 years in the Far East has been a prized traditional medicine.

Some fungi are moulds and have been crucial since ancient times to food processes such as production of some cheeses, leavening of bread, and fermenting of wine and beer. Another group of moulds, including penicillin, gave us antibiotics and a revolution in modern medicine.

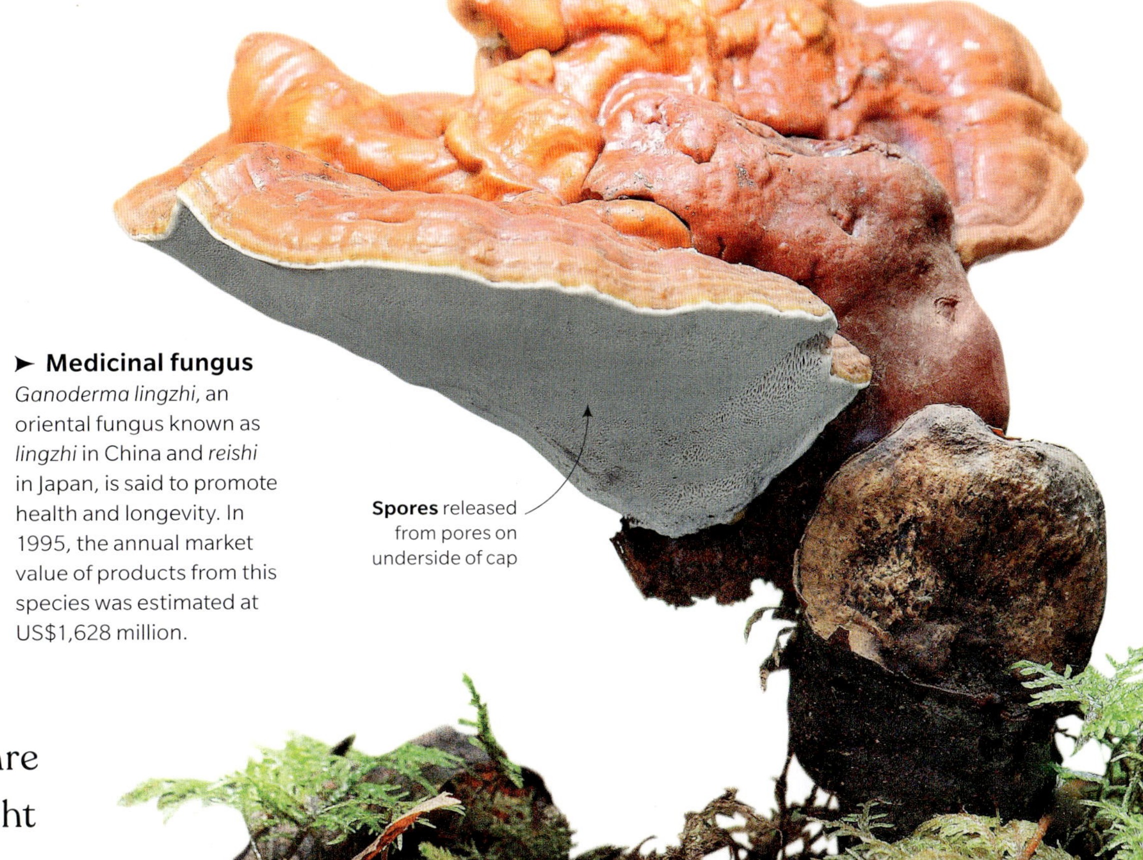

► Medicinal fungus
Ganoderma lingzhi, an oriental fungus known as *lingzhi* in China and *reishi* in Japan, is said to promote health and longevity. In 1995, the annual market value of products from this species was estimated at US$1,628 million.

Most mushrooms are 90 per cent water by weight

Useful Parts of a Herb

Any part of a plant can have herbal uses, and in some especially valued herbs, different parts from the same plant may have different uses. Most of the parts require some form of preparation to release their full potency.

Which parts to use?

In the Middle Ages, it was thought that the appearance of a part of a plant or where it grew, indicated its use in herbal medicine (see below). English botanist William Coles wrote in 1684: "The mercy of God maketh herbs for use of man, and hath not only stamped upon them a distinct form, but also given particular Signatures, whereby man may read the use of them". In the modern era, the function in nature of useful chemicals in plants is better understood. For example, some substances in leaves deter grazers, while perfumes in flowers serve to attract pollinating insects. This understanding can offer clues to their properties and uses.

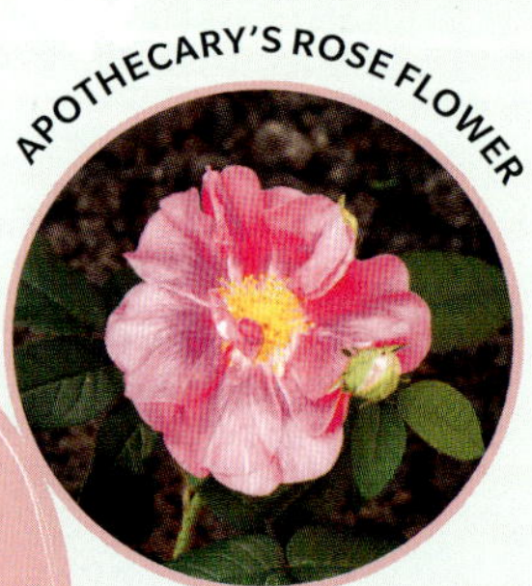

APOTHECARY'S ROSE FLOWER

FLOWERS

Flowers
Sweet-scented flowers are valued in perfumery, and herbal uses. Marigold (*Calendula*) flowers, for example, are used to soothe inflamed skin.

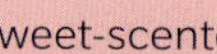

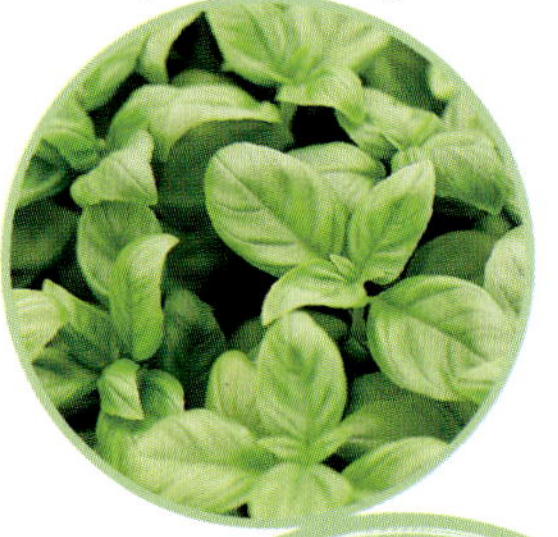

BASIL LEAVES

LEAVES

Leaves
Many plants' foliage contains bitter or pungent chemicals to discourage grazers. These can be used for flavouring, as antibacterial agents, and more.

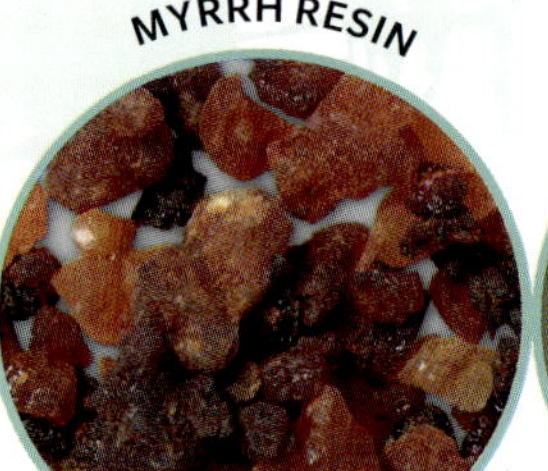

MYRRH RESIN

OPIUM POPPY LATEX

RESINS AND LATEX

Resins and latex
These viscous substances help to deter wood-boring animals. In human use, resins such as myrhh are valued for their scent.

STRIKING RESEMBLANCE

According to the medieval "Doctrine of Signatures", plants that resembled part of the human body could be used to treat ailments affecting it. For example, daisy-type flowers (right), which look like eyes, were believed to be a treatment against eye infections.

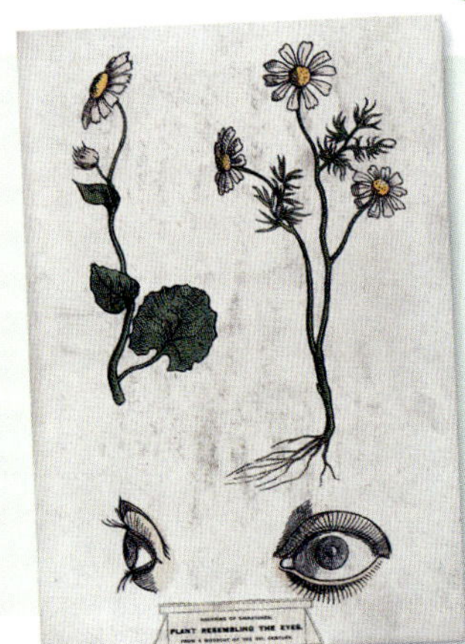

DOCTRINE OF SIGNATURES

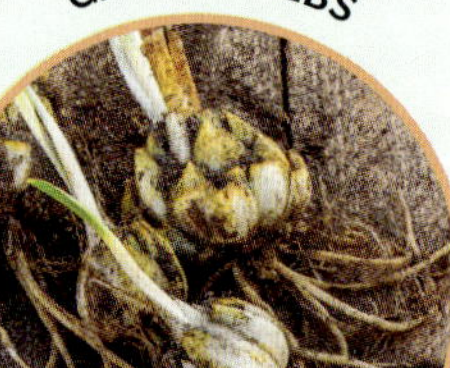

GARLIC BULBS

BULBS AND CORMS

Bulbs and corms
These storage organs are rich in sugars and starch. Some have strong flavours valued in cooking; others are toxic.

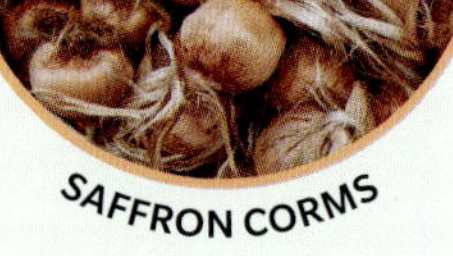

SAFFRON CORMS

Saffron spice comes from the stigmas and styles of crocus flowers

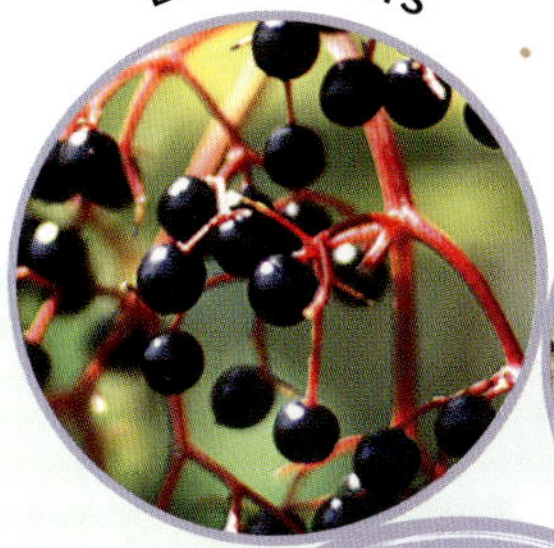

ELDER FRUITS

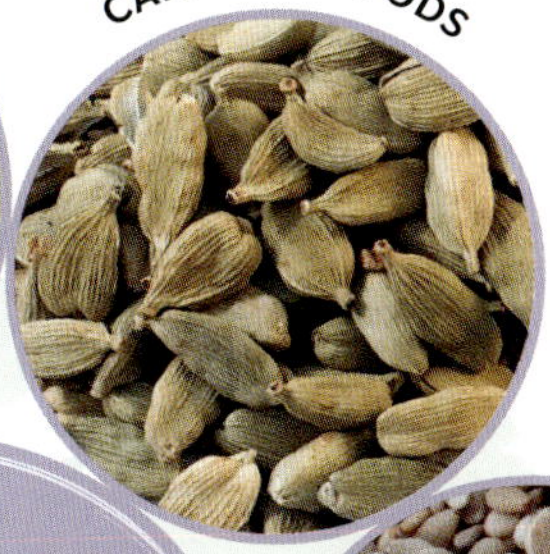

CARDAMOM PODS

FRUITS AND SEEDS

Fruits and seeds
Seeds, often encased in fruits, fuel the initlal growth of a plant. They are sources of nutrients and antioxidants.

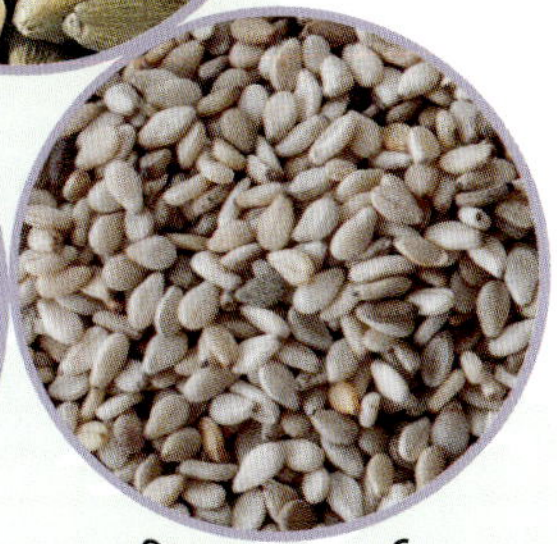

SESAME SEEDS

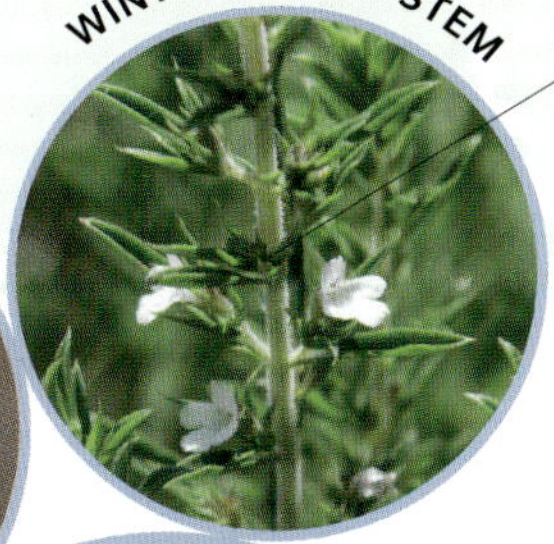

WINTER SAVORY STEM

Leafy stem

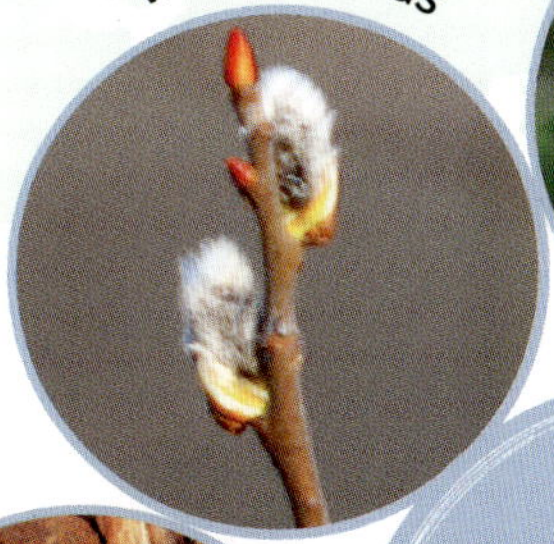

WILLOW TWIGS

STEMS, TWIGS, AND BARK

Stems, twigs, and bark
Stems and twigs support leaves and flowers. They may be ground to powder to release their active ingredients.

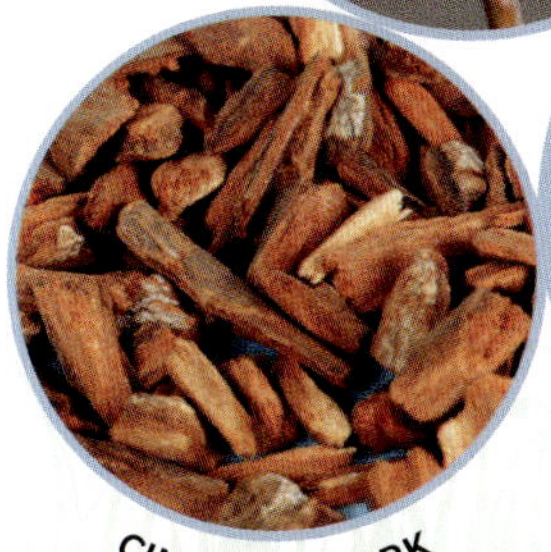

CINCHONA BARK

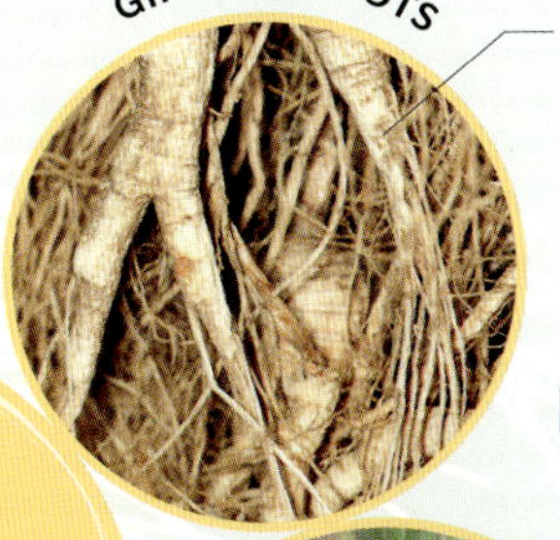

GINSENG ROOTS

Fleshy roots

ROOTS AND RHIZOMES

Roots and rhizomes
Roots and rhizomes supply water and minerals to growing plants. In herbal usage, some contain key health-giving chemicals.

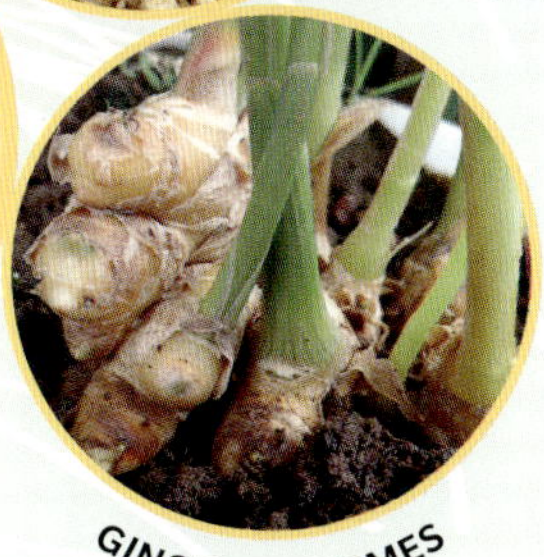

GINGER RHIZOMES

Harvesting herbs

Traditional herb harvests are artisanal, using small-scale collection by hand from the countryside or herb gardens. Some highly valued or popular herbs are grown and harvested on an industrial scale. Collection of herbs is increasingly mechanized using specially adapted combine harvesters.

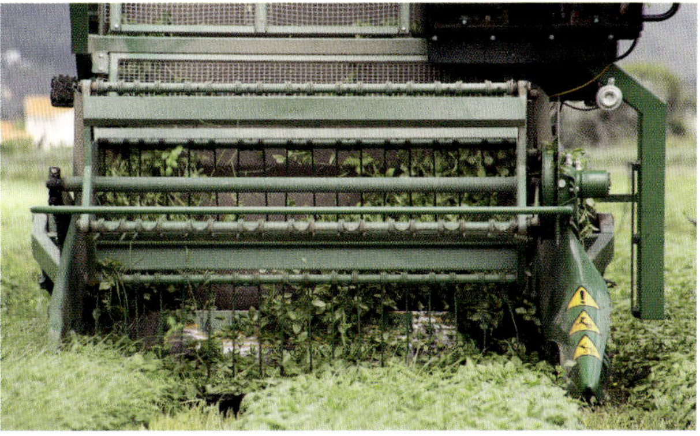

▲ Basil harvesting
Basil is sold fresh or dried. The expanding market for pesto sauce containing basil has made it worthwhile to grow on a field scale, gathered by mechanical harvesters.

Processing herbs

Processing can be as simple as air-drying fresh leaves, then steeping or pulverizing them to make infusions or tinctures (see pp.20–21), or roasting and grinding nuts and seeds. More involved methods involve distillation and extraction of oils. On an industrial scale, active ingredients are extracted in complex biochemical processes.

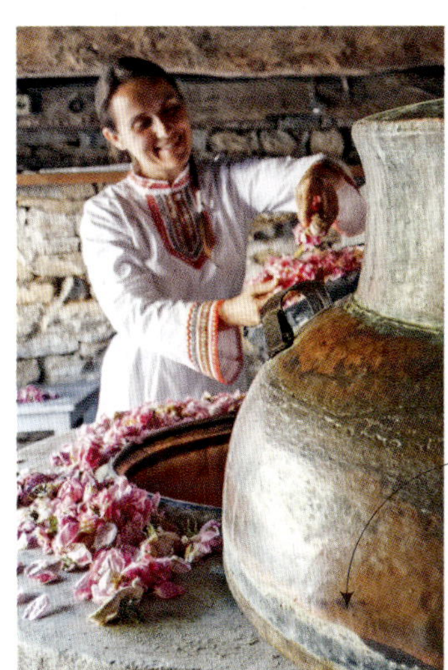

◄ Extracting rose oil
Rose petals are harvested by hand before sunrise, and the fragrant oil is prepared the same day by steam distillation or solvent extraction.

Still uses steam to extract oil from fresh petals

Active Ingredients

Chemicals in plants that have a physiological effect on humans are known as active ingredients. The characteristic tastes or scents of herbs depend on the subtle combinations of these chemicals, and the efficacy of medicinal herbs may result from individual, isolatable ingredients or complex interactions.

Using active ingredients

The organic chemicals that give herbs their flavours, scents, and medicinal and cosmetic properties have important biological functions in the plant. Often, these chemicals attract pollinators to the herb by creating an aromatic scent or bright colours, or they repel pests with a bitter taste. Some of these chemicals can be isolated for human use, with scientific analysis leading to some being synthesized. Salicylic acid, for example, is the metabolic product of salicylates found in willow (see pp.40–41) and meadowsweet (see p.195) and a synthesized version is used in aspirin.

➤ Attracting pollinators
Lavender (*Lavandula officinalis*) contains a range of chemicals, known as volatile oils, that create a scent attractive to pollinating bees and butterflies.

Pollen dusted onto the legs of bees is carried between flowers, enabling pollination

➤ Different forms

There are a number of ways active ingredients are used by humans. Herbs can be eaten in their natural form, or the active ingredient can be extracted and either consumed in a concentrated form or applied topically. Turmeric (*Curcuma longa*) contains curcumin, a polyphenol. Polyphenols are compounds containing more than one phenol (a type of active ingredient).

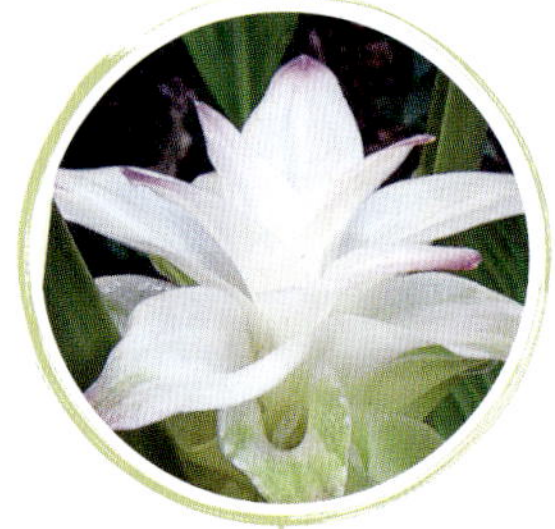

Tapping into turmeric
Turmeric is used in many ways, from flavouring curries to treating pain through traditional Chinese medicines.

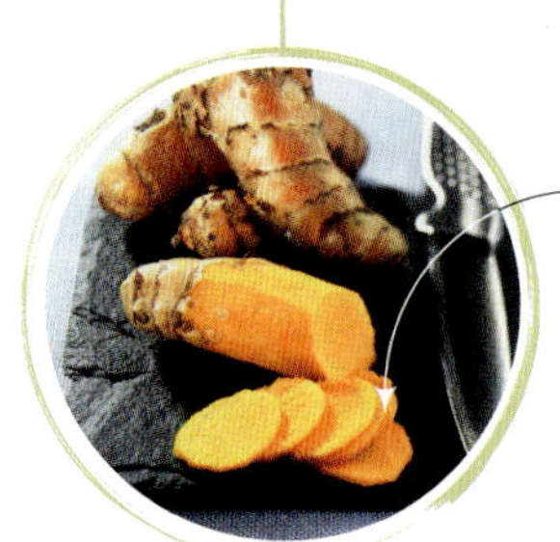

Rhizomes can be boiled, steamed, and ground

Eaten in natural form
Rhizomes add flavour and colour to food dishes, and are anti-inflammatory.

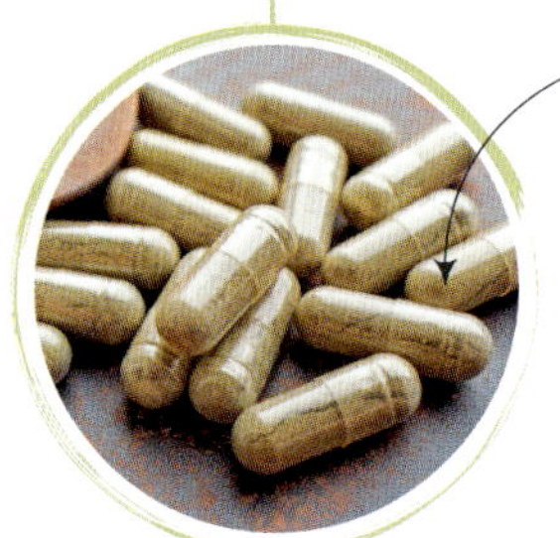

Capsules are densely packed with powder or dried extracts

Taken in concentrated form
Powdered rhizome is used in traditional medicine and dietary supplements.

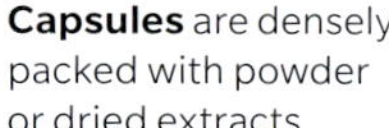

Topical creams and ointments mix extracts with oils, fats, or water

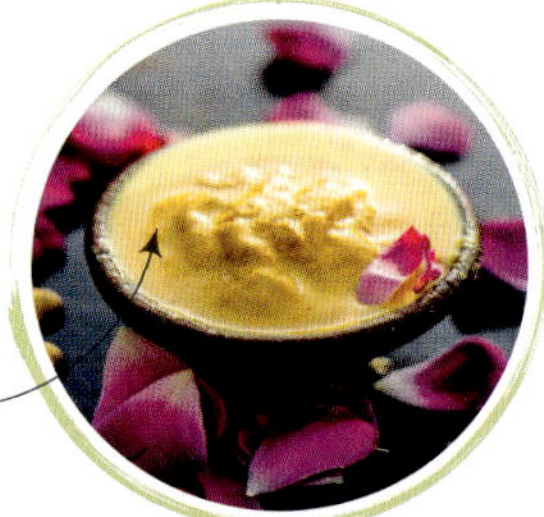

Applied topically
Turmeric paste is applied to the skin to ensure skin health and heal wounds.

TYPES OF ACTIVE INGREDIENTS

The organic chemicals that form living tissue are based around carbon, hydrogen, and other atoms, but are built into a wide range of complex structures. These chemical structures can be grouped into broad classes, which relate to their properties or roles within plants. For example, all alkaloids contain nitrogen and react when they come into contact with acids, creating salts, while some glycosides also contain nitrogen but do not react with acids. Herbs contain many different types of active ingredient, below are some.

ALKALOIDS
Among the most active compounds; often poisonous to animals, but small quantities can be used medicinally, as in morphine.

BITTERS
This miscellaneous group of bitter-tasting compounds from varied plants may stimulate the digestive system and improve appetite.

CARDIAC GLYCOSIDES
These glycosides, found in various plants such as foxglove, act on the heart to increase its strength and slow its beat.

CYANOGENIC GLYCOSIDES
These glucose-based chemicals are plant defence compounds. They release cyanide, which is poisonous.

FLAVONOIDS
With functions including plant pigmentation and chemical messaging, flavonoids are anti-inflammatory and aid circulation.

PHENOLS
Related to alcohol but dissolving readily in water, phenols have antibacterial properties and include blood-clotting agents.

POLYSACCHARIDES
Said to have anti-ageing properties, these insoluble carbohydrates include energy-storing starch and the cellulose in cell walls.

PROANTHOCYANIDINS
Found in various flowers, fruits, and seeds, these bitter chemicals deter pathogens. They can ease joint pain and improve circulation.

SAPONINS
Toxic, especially to fish, this group of glycosides can foam and are used in detergents. Some are also cough medicines.

TANNINS
Bitter tannins make bark and leaves unpalatable to animals, give tea its taste, and have anti-bacterial properties.

VOLATILE OILS
Readily evaporating into the air, these oils discourage competing plants and grazers. They are valued in perfumes and flavourings.

TERPENOIDS
These very prevalent organic chemicals, contribute to the scent of roses, flavour of cinnamon, and colour of tomatoes.

How active ingredients are extracted

The medicinal, culinary, and cosmetic values of many herbs depend on the holistic mix of chemicals within their parts. These can be accessed through simple traditional processes, such as drying and crushing leaves (see pp.20–21). However, it may be useful to extract specific components that have been individually identified as being responsible for a particular benefit. These can be separated out at industrial scale, by steam extraction or using chemical solvents.

▼ Distillation process
Steam is passed into a chamber containing plant material. This releases compounds from the plant cells, which are then condensed and collected in a container, where they separate.

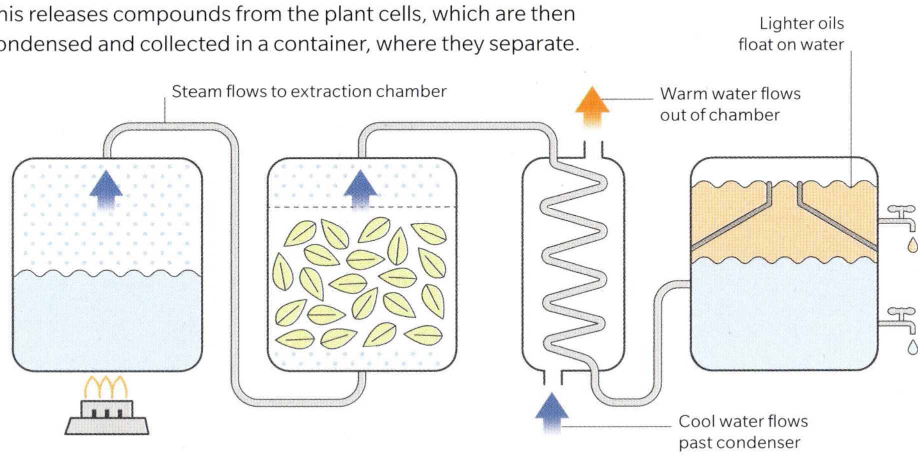

DISCOVERY OF MORPHINE

First cultivated more than 5,000 years ago around the Mediterranean, opium from opium poppy (*Papaver somniferum*, see pp.228–33) became known as a panacea, curing pain and easing sleep. Its most active ingredient, morphine, was first isolated from its latex around 1804 and marketed commercially by 1827. Codeine is also obtained from the plant.

SEED CAPSULE EXUDING LATEX

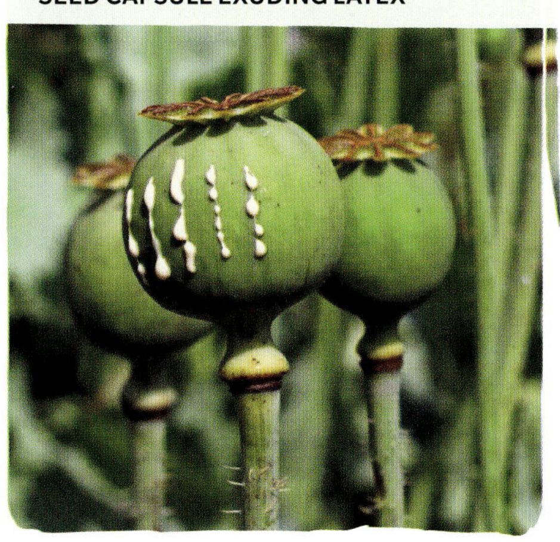

Healing Traditions

Developed over thousands of years to combat illness and promote wellbeing, herbal healing traditions exist all over the world. These have paved the way for breakthroughs in modern medicine, and continue to be used to treat illnesses.

TRADITIONAL CHINESE MEDICINE

Traditional Chinese Medicine (TCM) is an ancient system of medicine that has been used to prevent, diagnose, and treat illness for thousands of years. The earliest written record of it is the *Huang Di Nei Jing* (*Yellow Emperor's Classic of Medicine*), dating back at least 2,000 years, which includes theories about the body and mind; yin and yang; the five elements; acupuncture; nutrition; and herbal remedies.

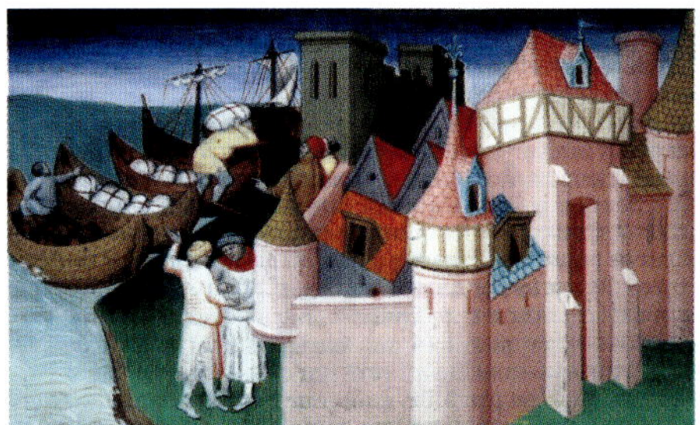

SILK ROUTE

3rd–2nd centuries BCE
Trade routes between Europe, the Middle East, and Asia introduced many medicinal and culinary herbs and spices, such as aromatic, antiseptic cloves (*Syzygium aromaticum*).

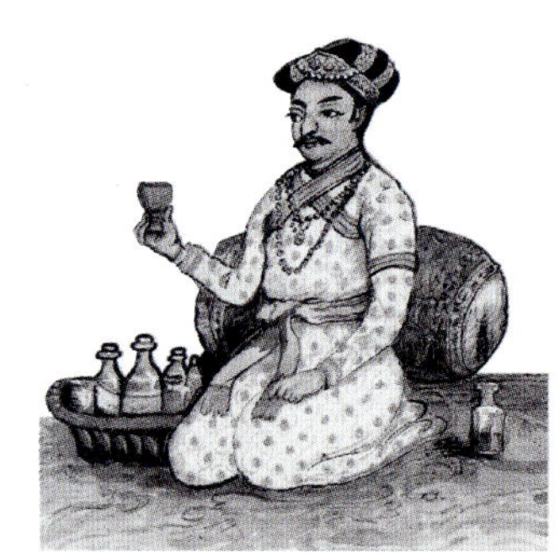

CHARAKA

c.400 BCE
In the Indian medical treatise *Charaka Samhita*, Charaka described about 350 herbal medicines, including wound-healing gotu kola (*Centella asiatica*) and the anti-asthmatic toothpick plant (*Visnaga daucoides*).

1st century CE
The Perso-Arabic healing tradition Unani detailed medicines derived from herbal, mineral, and animal sources. It was later built upon by 11th-century polymath Ibn Sina.

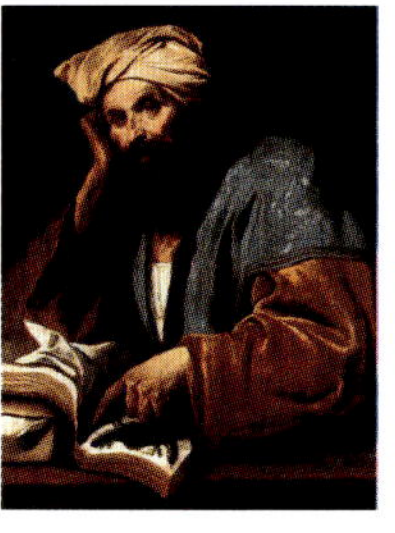

IBN SINA

c.10th century
Evidence has been found from around this time of the South American psychoactive drink ayahuasca, made from local plants.

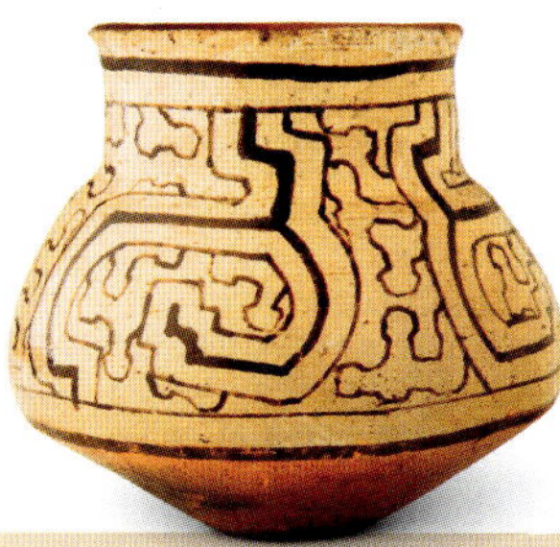

PERUVIAN POT DEPICTING AYAHUASCA VISIONS

1838
Italian chemist Raffaele Piria isolated salicylic acid from salicin, found in white willow bark (*Salix alba*). The finding inspired the late 19th-century creation of the anti-inflammatory drug Aspirin.

Corked glass vials

HOMEOPATHIC MEDICINE CHEST

1807
German physician Samuel Hahnemann conceived the alternative therapy known as homeopathy, based on the "like cures like" use of highly diluted animal, plant, mineral, and synthetic substances.

1913
French physician Henri Leclerc popularized the term "phytotherapy" to describe the evidence-based use of plant-derived medications (as opposed to using received wisdom).

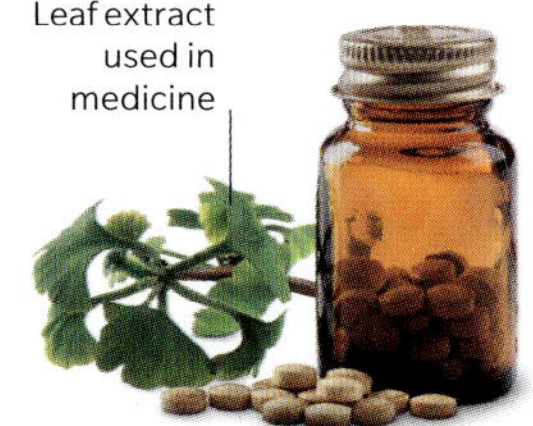

Leaf extract used in medicine

GINKGO-DERIVED MEDICINE

1914–18
Healing herbs, such as naturally antibiotic garlic and potentially antiseptic sphagnum moss (*Sphagnum* spp.), were used in World War I to treat wounds and infections.

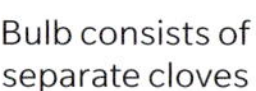

Bulb consists of separate cloves

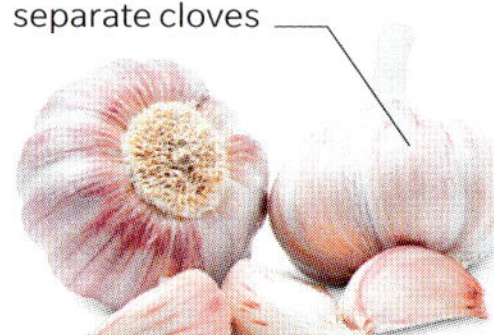

GARLIC

1953
The South African Medical Association banned traditional medicine. This act was just one example of the fear-based outlawing of ancient or indigenous healing practices in the 20th century.

" The art of healing comes from nature, not from the physician. "

PARACELSUS, physician and alchemist, c.1493–1541

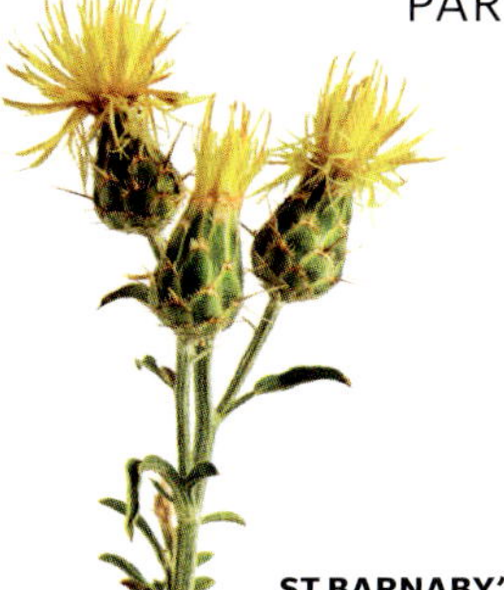

ST BARNABY'S THISTLE

60,000 years ago
Neanderthal remains found at Shanidar Cave, northern Iraq, reveal evidence of a "flower burial" that included several species of healing herb, such as St Barnaby's thistle (*Centaurea solstitialis*).

49,000 years ago
The dental plaque of a Neanderthal skeleton found at El Sidrón, Spain, includes microfossils of potentially medicinal yarrow (*Achillea* spp.) and chamomile (*Matricaria chamomilla*).

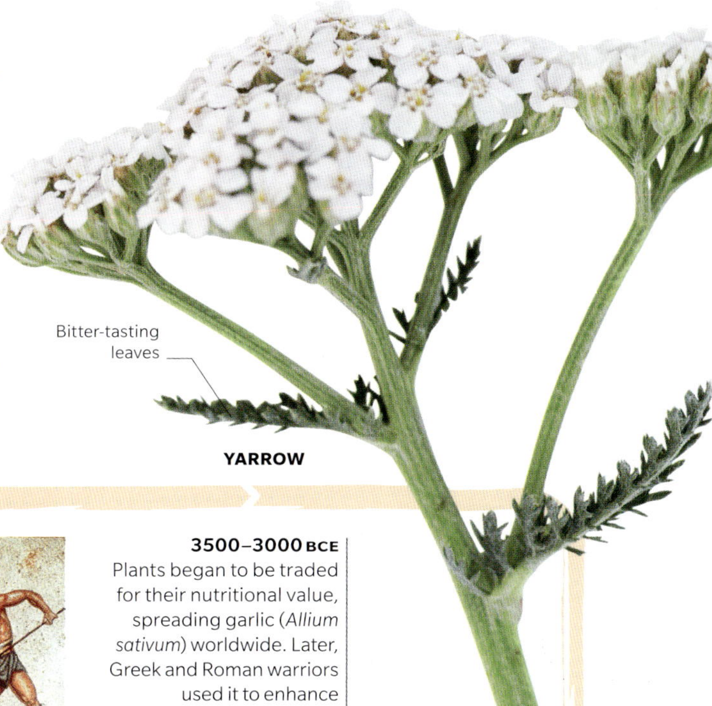

YARROW

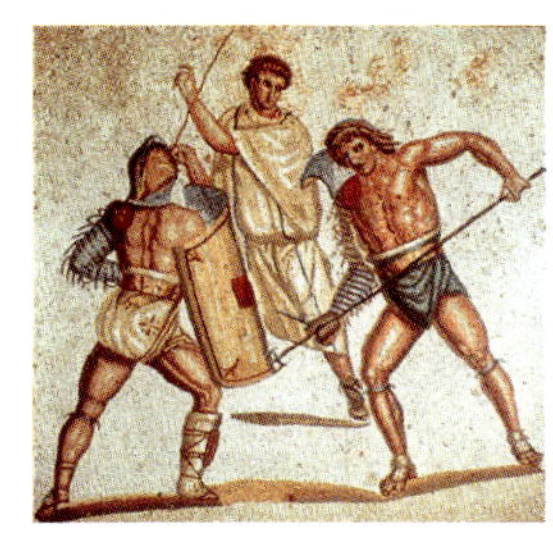

EBERS PAPYRUS

c.1550 BCE
The most extensive and best-preserved record of ancient Egyptian medicine, the Ebers Papyrus, compiled lists of medicinal plants and related spells and remedies.

ROMAN GLADIATORS

3500–3000 BCE
Plants began to be traded for their nutritional value, spreading garlic (*Allium sativum*) worldwide. Later, Greek and Roman warriors used it to enhance performance in battle.

Medieval period
Widespread use of healing herbs prompted further research and theories regarding medicinal properties, including the "doctrine of signatures", which claimed that a plant's appearance indicates which diseases it may cure or relieve.

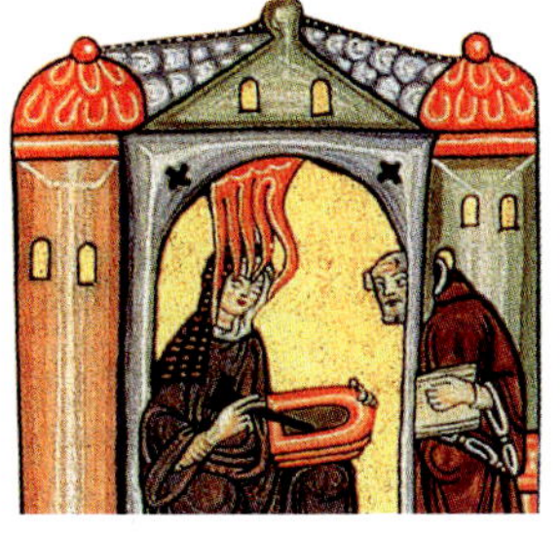

HILDEGARD OF BINGEN

12th century
German healer, Hildegard of Bingen, wrote about the healing properties of herbs, including Asian galangal (*Alpinia officinarum*), reflecting the world trade in herbs.

1492
Christopher Columbus arrived in the Caribbean, kickstarting centuries of colonization of the Americas and contributing to the first botanical and physic gardens designed to investigate new species of useful plants.

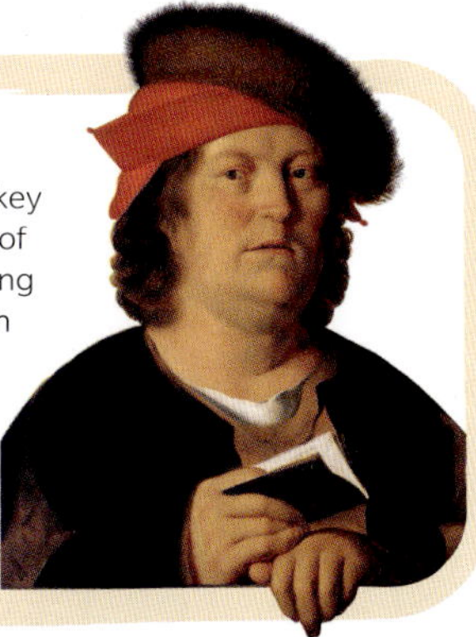

PARACELSUS

16th century
Paracelsus became a key figure in the evolution of modern medicine, taking a holistic approach with specific uses and doses of herbs to fight disease.

Early 19th century
Isolating active ingredients from plants enabled single compounds to be used as medicines, such as morphine from the opium poppy (*Papaver somniferum*).

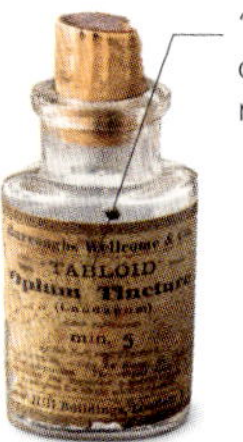

OPIUM TINCTURE

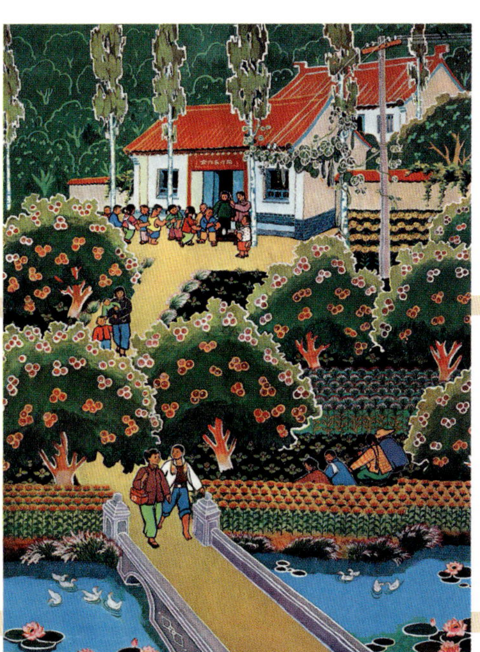

BAREFOOT DOCTOR

1960s
In China, the "barefoot doctors" system linked traditional and modern practices, offering a blend of acupuncture, herbal medicine, and Western approaches.

1971
The Indian Medical Council officially recognized traditional healing such as Ayurveda, Unani, and Siddha from India's history of alternative practices.

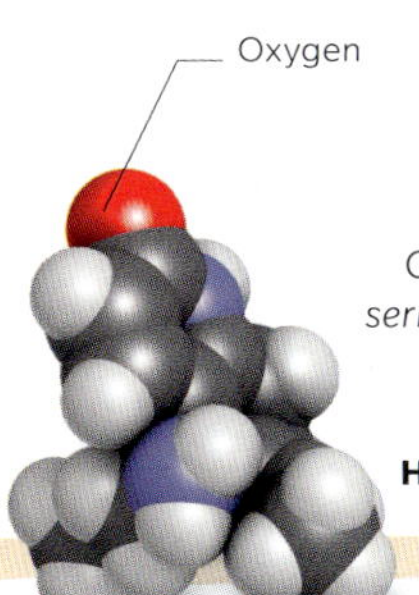

HUPERZINE A MOLECULE

Present day
Scientists continue to investigate compounds in plants to treat or cure illnesses. Examples include Chinese clubmoss (*Huperzia serrata*), a source of huperzine A, used to treat epilepsy.

Herbal Preparations

There are numerous ways to access the benefits of plants, from the topical application of oils, compresses, poultices, and balms to ingestible infusions, decoctions, syrups, and tinctures. These preparation methods are used to extract ingredients for health and wellbeing.

Herbal wine was used in **ancient Egyptian, Greek, Roman,** and **medieval** times

What is a herbal preparation?

The useful compounds from a plant can be extracted or isolated for medicinal or therapeutic purposes using a variety of methods. These were employed by many ancient civilizations. The earliest written records date back to around 5,000 years ago, and outline 12 recipes for herbal preparations, referring to more than 250 plants. Before using herbal preparations, it is important to consult health experts for advice. Herbs can have harmful side effects and some can adversely react with other medications.

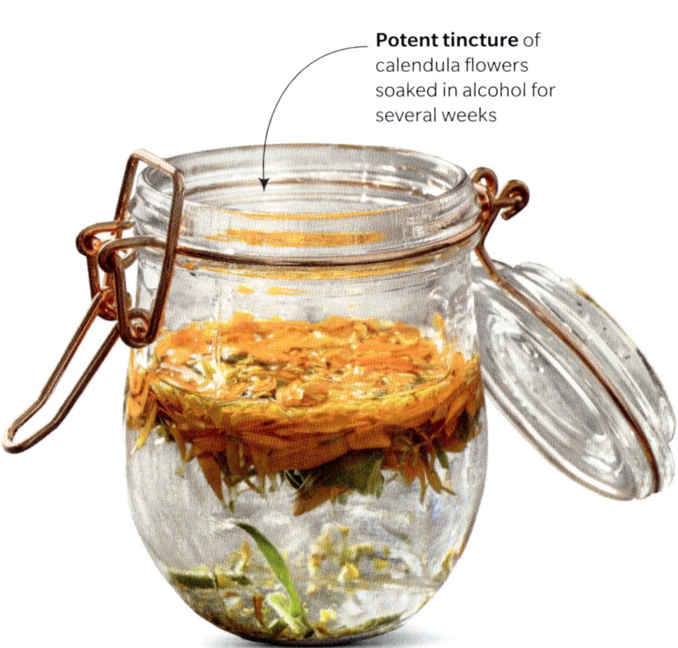

Potent tincture of calendula flowers soaked in alcohol for several weeks

▲ **Calendula tincture**
A tincture of *Calendula officinalis* flowers is the strongest and longest-lasting way to harness this herb's antimicrobial and anti-inflammatory powers. It is useful in healing wounds, sore throats, and skin conditions.

TYPES OF HERBAL PREPARATIONS

The simple preparation of herbs – or "simples" – include traditional ways of delivering herbal properties, passed down over thousands of years, then adapted through the ages to reflect newfound knowledge and changing lifestyles. While many recipes have changed, methods of preparation have remained remarkably constant for centuries and include the following examples:

INFUSIONS
Infusions are herbal teas or water-soluble extractions of tender leaves, stems, flowers, or buds steeped in just-boiled water.

DECOCTIONS
Like infusions but heated more vigorously, decoctions are the woody roots, stems, berries, seeds, or nuts of a plant simmered in boiling water.

TINCTURES
Tinctures take the form of a concentrated herbal extract in an alcohol solution, such as 80–90 per cent proof vodka.

GLYCERITES
A non-alcoholic alternative to tinctures, glycerites consist of a vegetable glycerine base infused with parts of a plant.

VINEGARS
Delicate herbs are preserved in wine vinegar, and stronger-flavoured plant parts in apple cider vinegar, for medicinal or culinary use.

STEAM INHALATIONS
The infused water vapour from herbs steeped in just-boiled water is inhaled to relieve respiratory congestion or soothe the skin.

SYRUPS
Sweet medicinal or culinary syrups are based on herbal infusions or decoctions cooked down with honey or sugar.

ROBS
Similar to syrups, robs are sweet preparations that consist of concentrated fruit or vegetable juices with water or honey.

ELECTUARIES/HONEYS
Useful for less palatable medicinal plants, electuaries and herbal honeys are powdered dried herbs in sweet substances such as syrup or honey.

BATHS
Therapeutic bath soaks often feature muslin bags or pots of mineral salts with skin-soothing, decongesting, or relaxing herbs.

COMPRESSES AND POULTICES
Applied to the skin, poultices consist of mashed-up plant parts held between two bandages, while compresses are made from infusion-soaked cloth.

OILS
Plant oils can be infused with herbs for external use, while essential oils (see top right) are extracted from plants' oil glands.

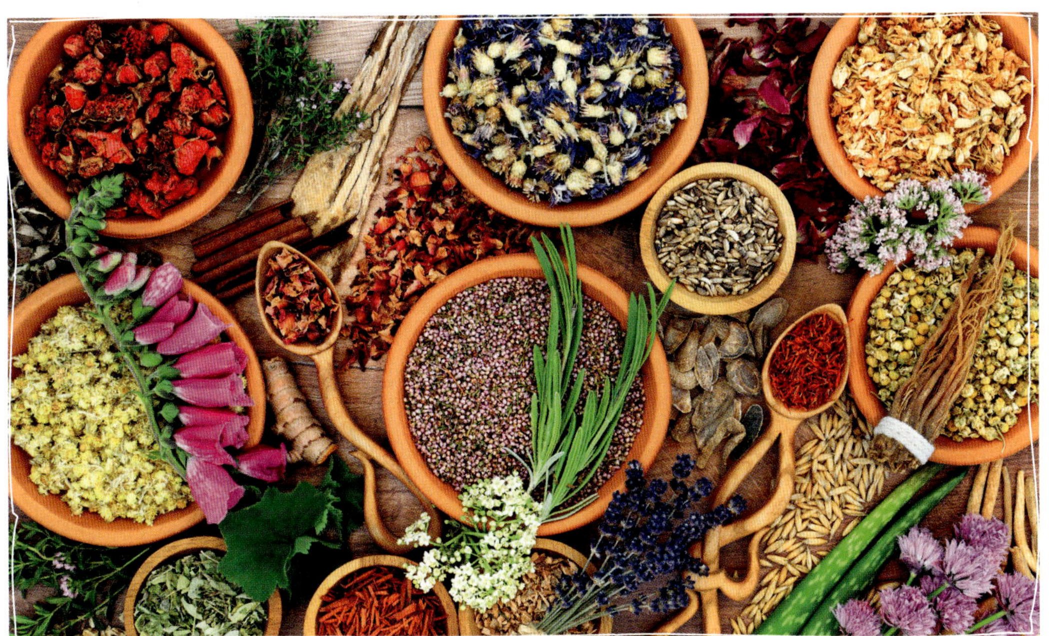

▲ **Dried herbs**
One of the simplest ways to prepare many types of herbs is to dry them. All parts from flowers and buds to leaves, roots, and fruits can be dried.

Nature's remedy

Some herbal preparations are almost ready-made in nature, such as the fragrant, medicinal resin of plants such as myrrh (see pp.84–87) and frankincense (see pp.82–83). Known historically as balsam or balm, such soothing resins include the Balm of Gilead as mentioned in the King James Bible (1611) and the medieval panacea Balsam of Matariyya (both thought to be *Commiphora gileadensis*).

ESSENTIAL OILS

Essential oils are volatile substances – evaporating quickly at normal temperatures – that are stored in small droplets in oil glands in plants. They have a strong scent and antimicrobial properties to protect the plant from disease. In herbal use, they can be used for fragrance, hygiene, medical and therapeutic purposes. They are extracted by distillation (see p.17), or other methods such as pressing and solvent extraction.

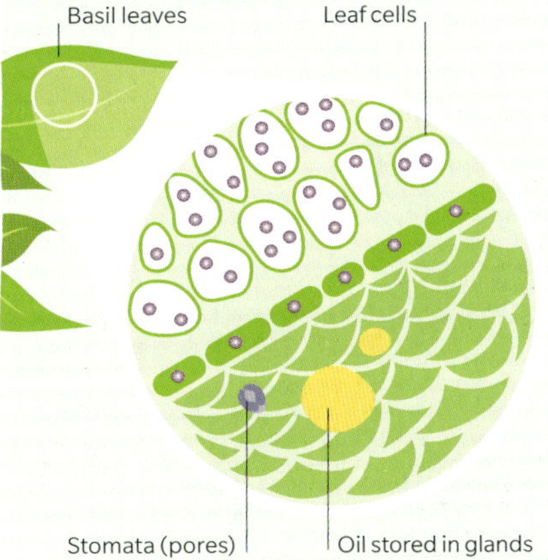

OIL GLANDS IN A BASIL LEAF

Preparation methods

Some of the processes used to unlock a herb's active ingredients may include, singly or in combination, the application of heat, extracting in liquids, and crushing or grinding. This creates health-giving, sometimes flavourful products that may be ingested, either alone or as ingredients in other food or beverages, or applied topically and in other therapeutic ways. Explained here are four popular methods of making herbal preparations for medicinal and culinary use, all of which can be done in the home. Some of the tools and equipment used to make these preparations, such as jars, bottles, or stirrers, are sterilized beforehand to avoid contamination. In some cases, dark glass containers may be used to protect the preparations from breaking down and losing their potency in storage due to the effects of sunlight.

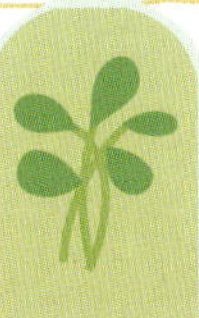

Tinctures
The herb is placed in a sterilized glass jar with a lid and covered completely with alcohol. It is sealed for 4–6 weeks, shaken regularly, then strained.

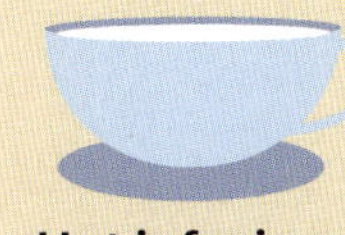

Hot infusions
The plant parts are steeped in just-boiled water for around 5–40 minutes, depending on the herb.

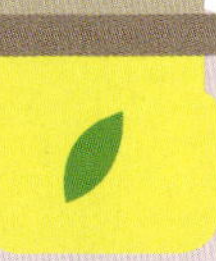

Syrups
A herbal infusion or decoction is simmered until reduced by half, then strained. Honey is then stirred in over heat.

Poultices
Herbs are mashed to form a paste, with extra water if necessary. The paste is then placed in a cloth container and applied to the skin.

Herbs and Modern Medicines

While many modern drugs are based on synthesized ingredients, natural herbs remain an invaluable part of medicine. Various widely-used drugs are based on natural products, and chemicals derived from plants continue to be researched in the development of new medicines.

Plants pharmacy

Natural chemicals found inside plants perform a varied set of functions in their hosts; for example, many are anti-microbial, defending plants against the effects of invasive bacteria. In some instances, these chemicals can have a similar, or other, beneficial effect on human health. Salicylic acid, for example, is a hormone present in willow and other plants. In these plants, it helps defend against microbes and other environmental stresses, as well as regulating growth. In medicines, salicylic acid is used to treat skin conditions such as corns. It is also a precursor to aspirin (see opposite).

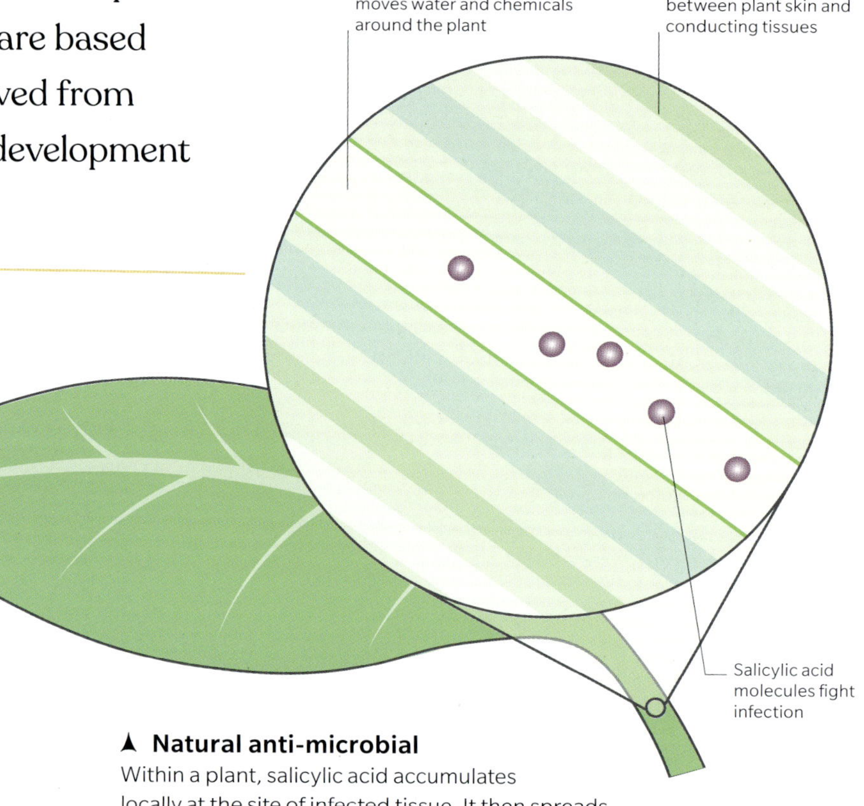

▲ **Natural anti-microbial**
Within a plant, salicylic acid accumulates locally at the site of infected tissue. It then spreads throughout the rest of the plant via the phloem to aid resistance to infection.

RAINFOREST TREATMENTS

Tropical rainforests contain thousands of plant species, many of which have evolved specialized survival mechanisms. Medical science has only recently begun to tap into rainforest plants for their active ingredients, and many modern cancer treatments now come from rainforest plants. However, deforestation risks eliminating potential future medicines as habitats are destroyed and plant species become extinct.

RAINFOREST IN PRASLIN, SEYCHELLES

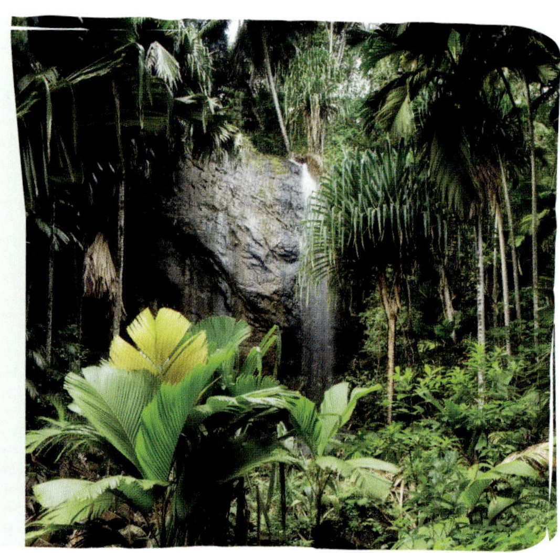

Plant-based drugs form **11 per cent** of those considered **essential** by the World Health Organization (WHO)

Herb-based drugs in the modern age

The arrival of the now-ubiquitous aspirin and morphine heralded the modern era of medicine, and they were also among the first highly successful modern drugs to be created from herbs. In both cases, their early uses in traditional medicine prefigured their later pharmaceutical usage.

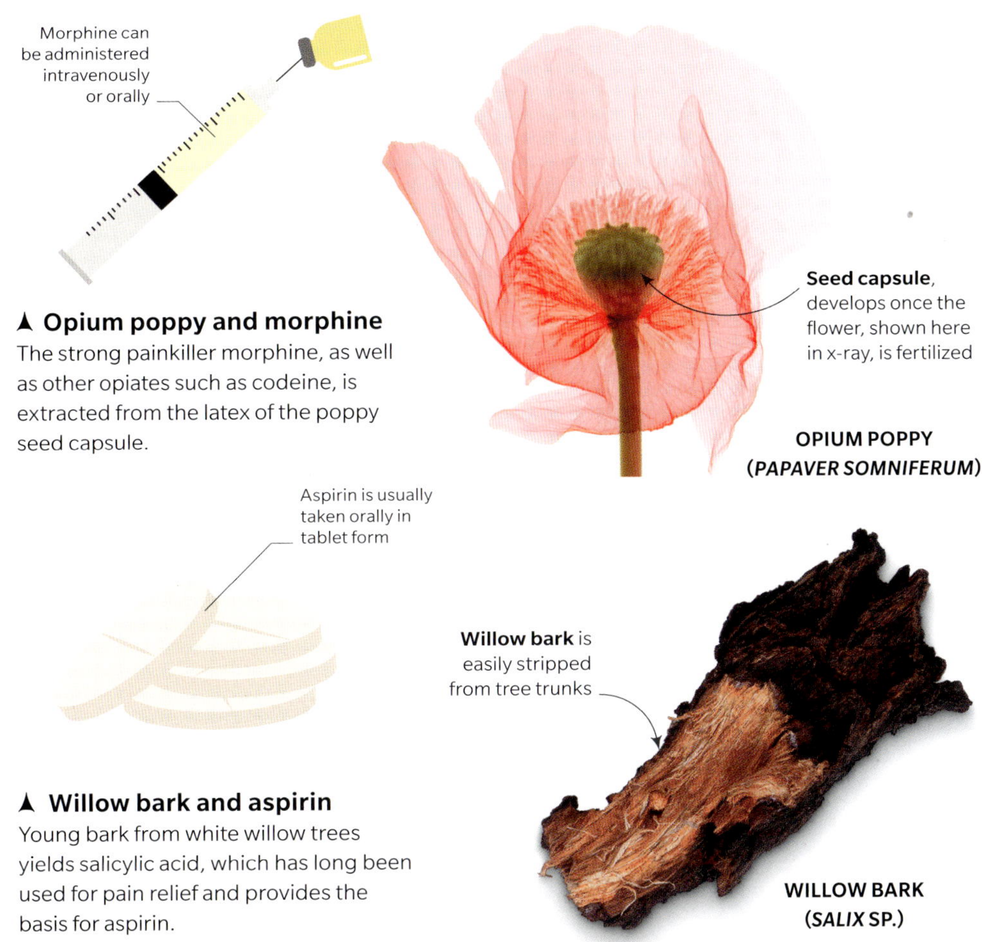

▲ Opium poppy and morphine
The strong painkiller morphine, as well as other opiates such as codeine, is extracted from the latex of the poppy seed capsule.

▲ Willow bark and aspirin
Young bark from white willow trees yields salicylic acid, which has long been used for pain relief and provides the basis for aspirin.

Genetically modified plants and medicines

Genetically modified (GM) plants are used in the development of new medicines. For example, in South Africa maize has been genetically engineered to grow anti-HIV antibodies. Some plants can be engineered to enhance their beneficial traits, while others may be used as "edible vaccines", in which an antigen is introduced into a consumable part of a plant and absorbed into the human body.

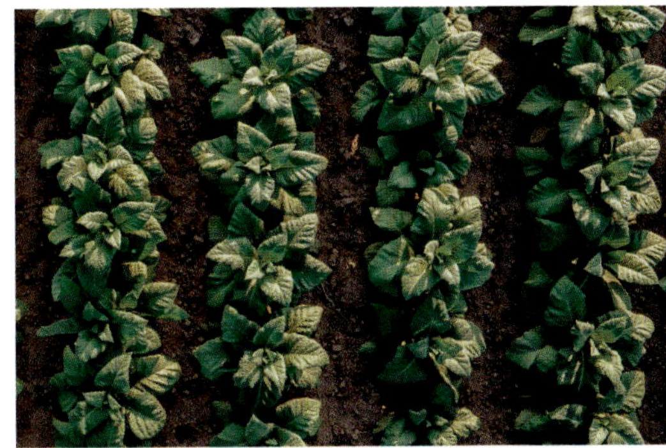

▲ Disease-fighting tobacco
A modified form of tobacco is used as a bioreactor for the production of pharmaceutically useful proteins such as antibodies and vaccines. Th plant is also used to host a modified virus used for medicine.

Looking to the future

Research into new plant-based medicines is ongoing, and there are already naturally-derived treatments for some of the leading causes of death including heart and lung diseases, strokes, and forms of dementia. Plants with existing palliative qualities are being researched, as are new species. Some plant-based drugs have even originated through observations of animal behaviour: for example, anti-malarial molecules found in the plant *Trichilia rubescens* were discovered after chimpanzees in Uganda were observed using the plant to treat themselves.

► Water hyssop
This tropical aquatic, *Bacopa monnieri*, has long been used in traditional medicine to support brain function. It may help to protect the brain from decline in old age.

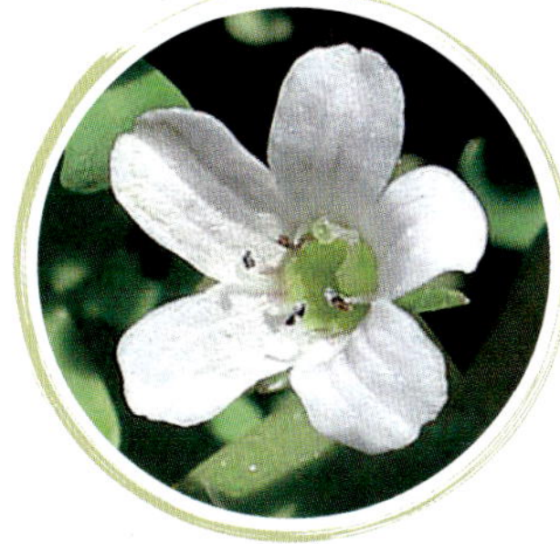

► Snowdrop
Although poisonous if eaten, the bulb of this perennial flowering plant, *Galanthus nivalis*, yields an alkaloid that can slow the progression of Alzheimer's disease.

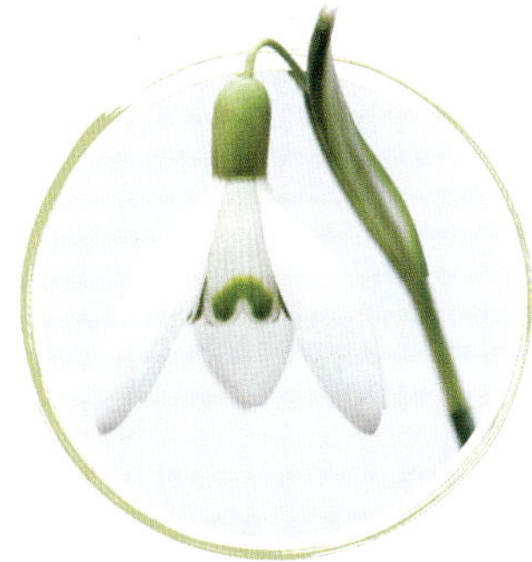

► Madagascar periwinkle
Two closely related drugs, vincristine and vinblastine, are derived from *Catharanthus roseus*, and are now used to treat leukaemia and lymphoma.

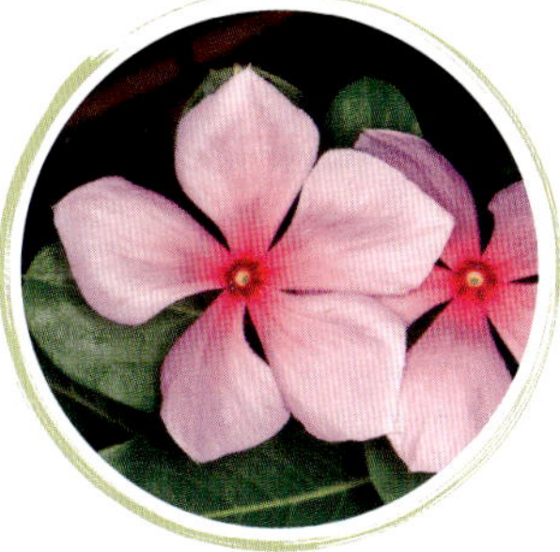

Herbs in Cosmetics

The application of cosmetics to rejuvenate, beautify, or otherwise enhance the user's appearance goes back at least 4,000 years. Many familiar modern-day cosmetic formulations, from lipstick to skincare, are based on ancient herbal practices and ideas.

Cosmetic box known as *pyxis*, with a ring handle

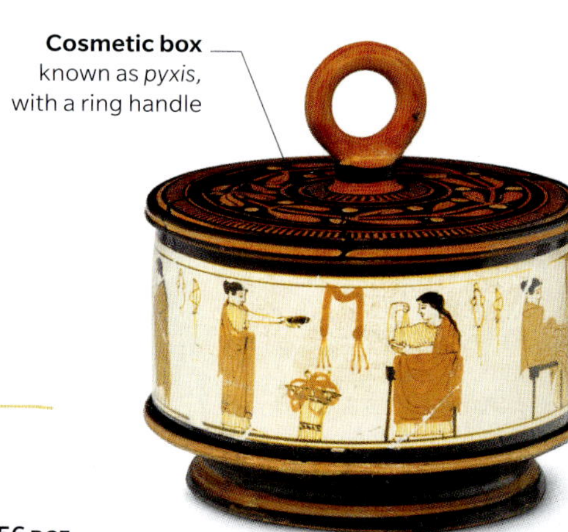

GREEK POWDER POT

EYEBROW PAINTING

c.700 BCE
Ovid's *The Art of Love* described ancient Roman cosmetics, including tubes of pre-mixed face masks made from olive oil, rosewater, animal fat, rocket, cucumber, almond oil, and eggs.

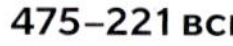

COSMETIC TUBE

1046–256 BCE
During the Chinese Zou Dynasty, eyebrow, lip, and face makeup, facial cream, and fragrance were produced. *Kouzhi* ("oil for lips") was made from plant oil and cinnabar.

1200–323 BCE
Flushed cheeks were prized by the ancient Greeks, who used crushed mulberries to add blush onto whitened faces to show social status.

475–221 BCE
During the Warring States period, Chinese women created strong eyebrow shapes – believed to be related to their fate – by painting them with the soot from burned willow branches, or a blue mineral known as *dai*.

Symbolic designs

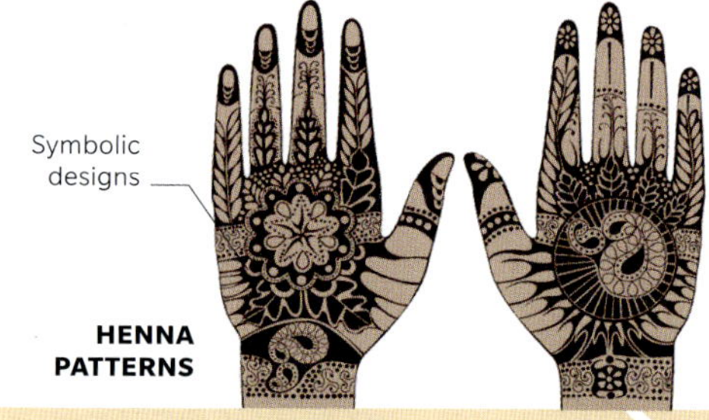

HENNA PATTERNS

c.300–400 CE
Evidence from this time shows that henna, from the dried leaves of the *Lawsonia inermis* tree, was used to dye skin, hair, and fingernails, and create symbolic mehndi designs at Hindu weddings and other rituals and festivities.

Early 1800s
Flaxseed became popular as a crop and was used to make a cosmetic balm for inflamed skin, including boils; it was also used to make an edible oil, fuel, and fibre for fabric.

Oil may be yellow or colourless

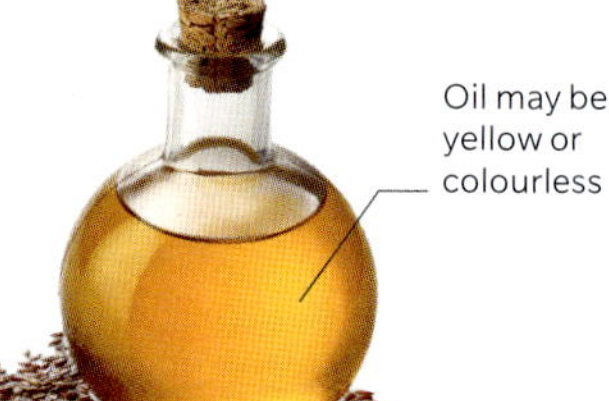

FLAXSEED OIL

1800s
European makeup styles evolved to create more defined contrast around facial features, using rice powder as a base and beetroot juice to stain cheeks a deep, crimson red.

LA DIAPHANE
Poudre de Riz
SARAH BERNHARDT
32 Avenue de l'Opéra PARIS

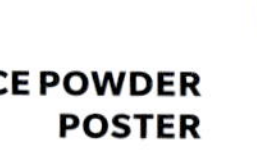

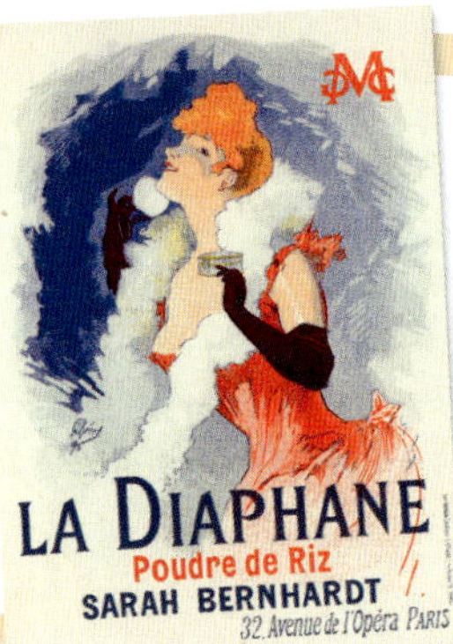

RICE POWDER POSTER

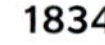

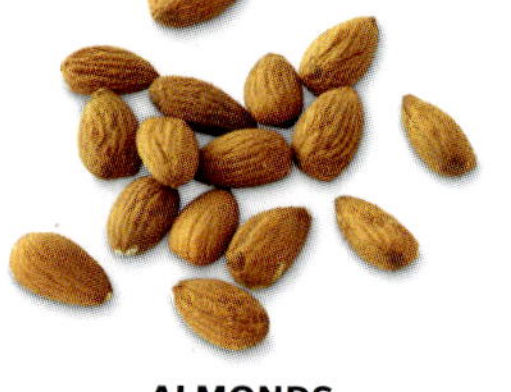

ALMONDS

1834
The Toilette of Health, Beauty, and Fashion included "directions on the use of most safe and salutary cosmetics", including recipes of bitter almonds, green pineapples, cucumbers, spinach flowers, and strawberries.

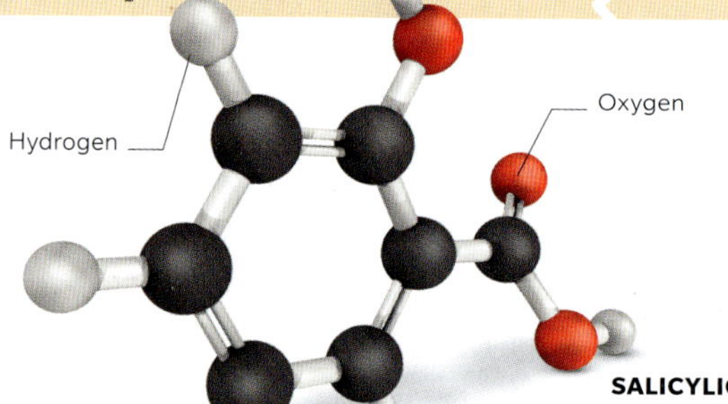

SALICYLIC ACID

1852
Salicylic acid, the active derivative of salicin from willow bark (*Salix alba*) and precursor to Aspirin, was synthesized. It also provided a pore-penetrating, exfoliating ingredient for acne-prone skin.

Mineral-based red ochre was used to adorn the bodies of early *Homo sapiens*

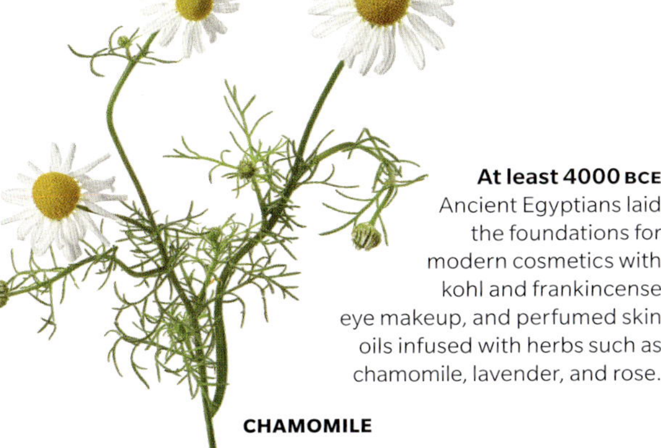

CHAMOMILE

At least 4000 BCE
Ancient Egyptians laid the foundations for modern cosmetics with kohl and frankincense eye makeup, and perfumed skin oils infused with herbs such as chamomile, lavender, and rose.

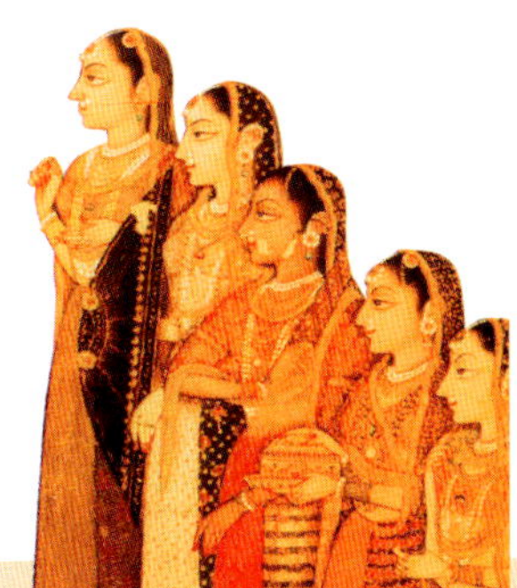

CEREMONY WITH TURMERIC

c.3500 BCE
Turmeric was used in India to boost immunity and beautify skin. It is now known to have powerful anti-inflammatory and antioxidant properties due to the polyphenol curcumin.

3000 BCE
In ancient China, early nail varnishes, enamels, and lacquers were made by experimenting with gum Arabic, beeswax, egg whites, gelatine, and coloured vegetable dyes.

c.1600–1046 BCE
Early cosmetics makers in the Chinese Shang Dynasty manufactured lip and cheek rouge – or *yanzhi* – from the petals of safflower (*Carthanus tinctorius*).

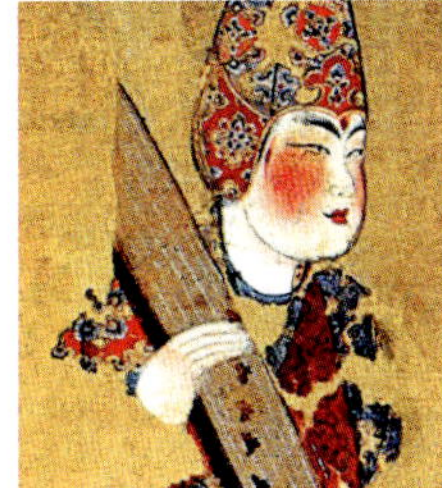

MUSICIAN WITH ROUGED CHEEKS

2nd millennium BCE
The ancient Egyptians pioneered skincare using herbs, tree resins, minerals, and animal derivatives such as honey and fat to create sunblock, scar-fading cream, resinous perfume, deodorant, and skin-softening oil.

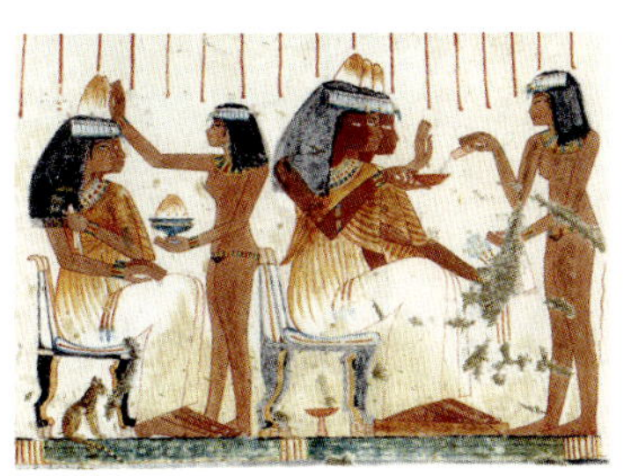

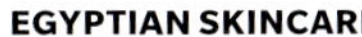

EGYPTIAN SKINCARE

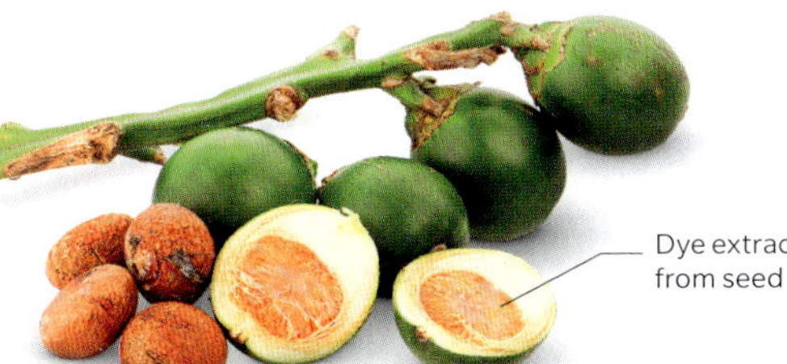

Dye extracted from seed

BETEL NUT

c.400–1100 CE
Indian cosmetic routines around this time included a dye from the betel nut (*Areca catechu*), used to darken lips and teeth, almond paste to soften skin, mineral pigments and wax to paint faces, and aromatics for scent.

11th century
Called Picts ("painted ones") by the Roman invaders, ancient British Celtic peoples used crushed, dried, and fermented leaves of woad (*Isatis tinctoria*) to dye their hair and make war paint.

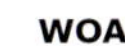

WOAD

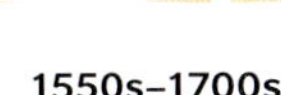

1550s–1700s
Lipstick made from herbal and other plant-based dyes became popular in Europe, especially in red tones. Plant-based dyes were also used to transform hair and eyebrows.

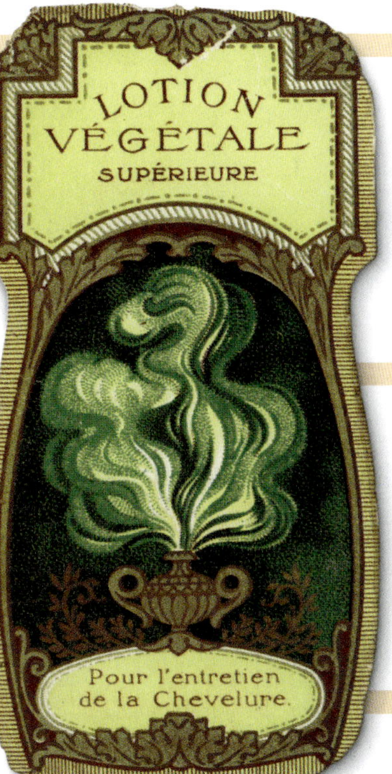

1300s
Zhenzhu powder extracted from the fruit of the of purple flowering Mirabilis jasmine (*Mirabilis jalapa*) became a popular form of Chinese Ming Dynasty makeup.

MIRABILIS JASMINE

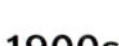

1900s
Hydrating emulsions and lotions, made with plant-based "vegetal" ingredients such as coconut, palm, or olive oil, provide new foundations for a range of facial and body-based skincare.

VEGETAL LOTION

20th century
"Natural skin care" became fashionable, using the soothing, antioxidant, anti-inflammatory, hydrating, and astringent properties of plants such as chamomile, calendula, witch hazel, and aloe vera.

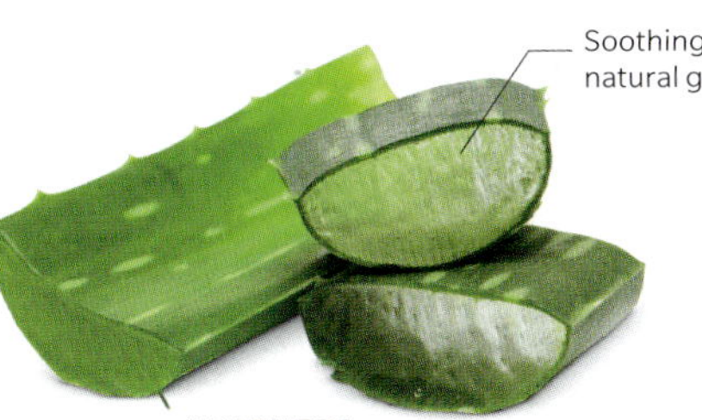

Soothing natural gel

ALOE VERA

Culinary Herbs

Herbs are widely used to enhance the flavour of food. They may be used raw in salads or as a garnish to a cooked dish, and may release different flavours depending on how they are used. Some herbs are well suited to both sweet and savoury dishes.

CHILLI "BURN"

The heat that is experienced when eating or handling chillis (see pp.106–111) is due to the alkaloid capsaicin. This chemical irritant, which occurs in chilli plants, produces a sensation of burning in some tissues with which it comes into contact. Capsaicin stimulates heat-sensing nerve cells so that the brain and body responds as if has been burned, even though there is no tissue damage.

Herbs and flavours

The chemical constituents of food released by chewing and dissolved in saliva wash over taste buds on the tongue and are experienced as flavour. There are five main flavour groups, which are commonly found in herbs and other foods: sweet, sour, salty, bitter, and pungent. As well as these, there are tastes that are more subtle and less easily analyzed, such as earthy, fruity, or fragrant. Many herbs have flavours that are palatable to humans in their raw state; others are tempered by cooking, during which they undergo subtle changes. As well as adding flavour, many herbs contribute vitamins and minerals to dishes – thyme, for example, is high in vitamin C – and some are added to aid digestion.

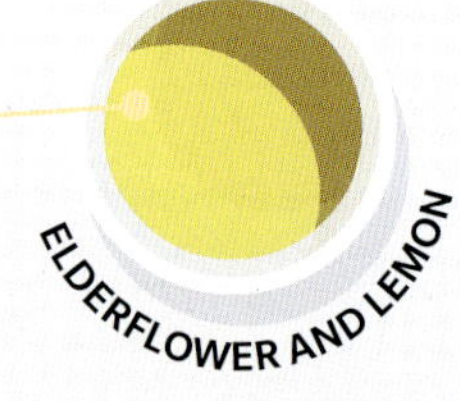

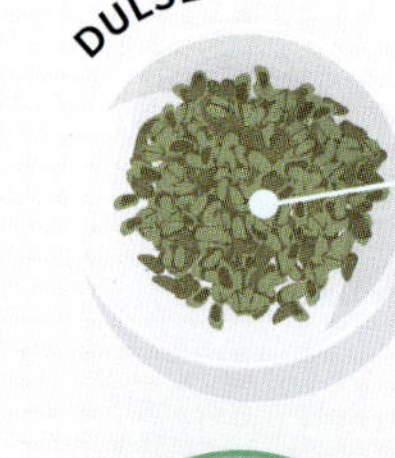

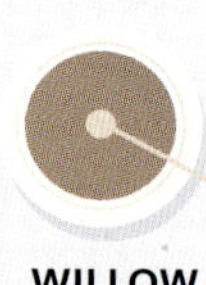

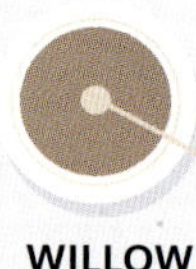

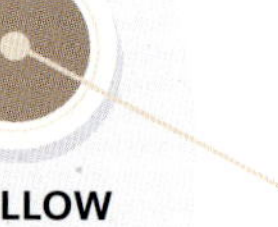

Sour
Certain acids in herbs are perceived as sour and can be pleasant in small quantities; this flavour can also signal underripe or spoilt foods.

Salty
Saltiness, in moderation, can enhance other flavours. Salt itself is a mineral, not a herb, but certain herbs have a salt-like flavour.

Bitter
Although it can be experienced as unpleasant, a bitter taste can be desirable, as it stimulates the liver and gall bladder, improving digestion.

Sweet
Sweetness in herbs and other foods can signal the presence of carbohydrates, which have a high calorie count and raise energy levels when eaten.

Pungent
Usually created by the presence of aromatic volatile oils and resins in herbs, hot or spicy, pungent flavours are typically strong and stimulating.

▲ **Flavour profiles**
Herbs can create a complex balance of flavours in a meal, enhancing and complementing flavours, and some can provide an alternative flavour to salt.

Cooking with herbs and spices

It is important to consider the type of herb in order to get the best flavour. Garlic, spices, and woody herbs (see below) are robust, releasing flavour more slowly, and can be added near the beginning of cooking. The flavour of fresh, delicate herbs, such as basil and coriander, evaporates quickly, so these are usually added towards the end of cooking. Spices (see p.10) release their aromatic oils when heated, especially in oil.

▼ Heating in oil

Many recipes recommend heating spices in oil first. The flavour molecules dissolve in the oil much better than in water, carrying the flavour through the food.

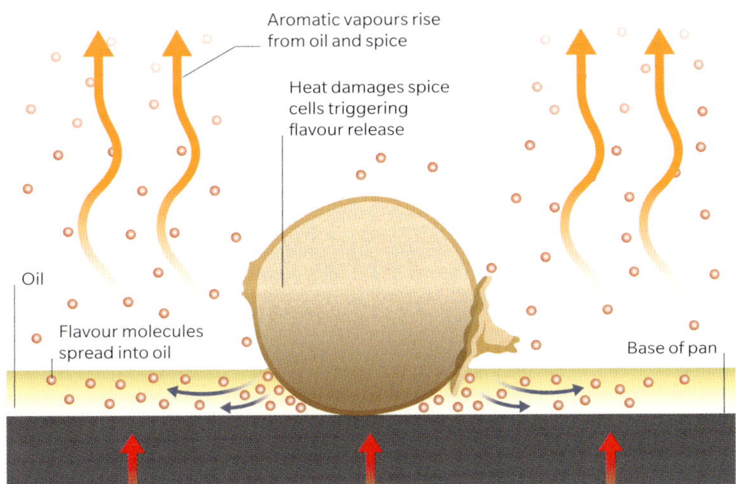

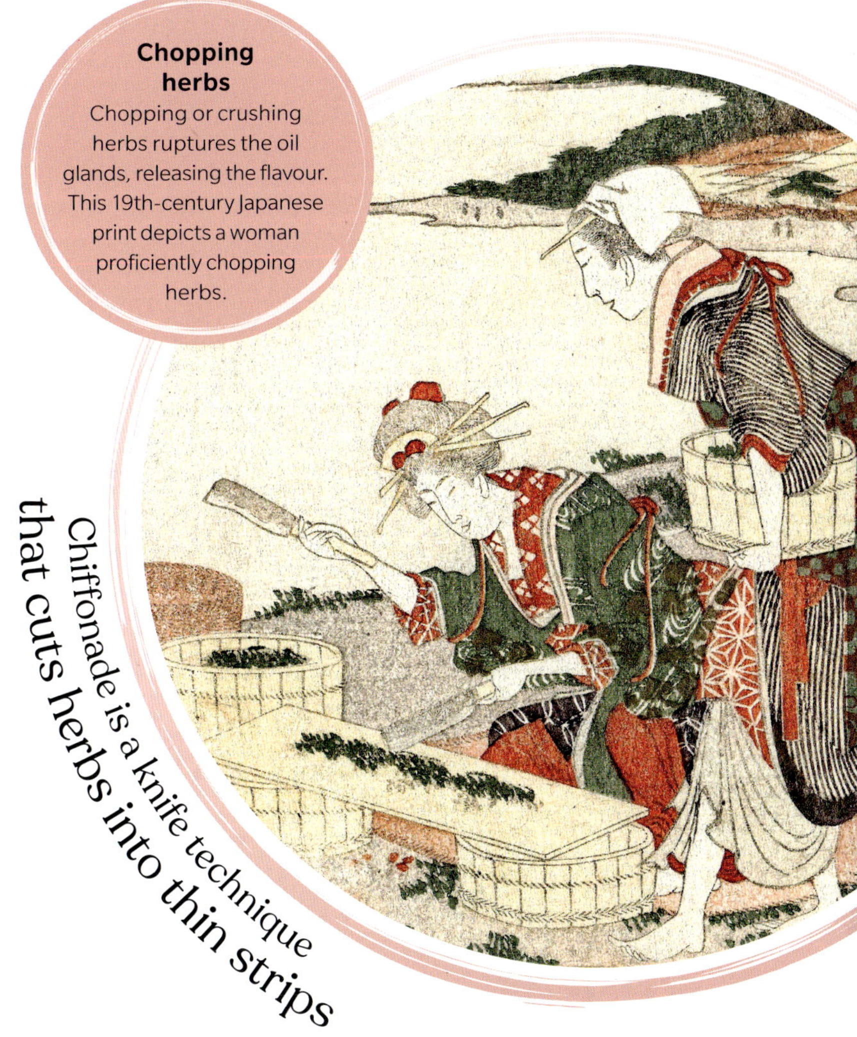

Chopping herbs
Chopping or crushing herbs ruptures the oil glands, releasing the flavour. This 19th-century Japanese print depicts a woman proficiently chopping herbs.

Chiffonade is a knife technique that cuts herbs into thin strips

WOODY HERBS AND SOFT HERBS

Woody herbs have woody stems, while soft herbs have a delicate structure. Leaves on woody-stemmed plants can be tougher and stronger in flavour; they are often stripped from the stems prior to use or sprigs are discarded before serving. Soft herbs' stems are often chopped and used alongside the leaves.

Woody
Woody-stemmed plants such as rosemary (see pp.92–93) have a permanent framework of stems and are often evergreen. Stems are woodier towards the base of the plant and only the softer, younger shoot tips are harvested, as these have the best flavour.

Soft
Soft-stemmed herbs such as peppermint (see pp.180–85) are susceptible to wilting, and so are best used as fresh as possible, ideally straight from the plant. Leaves towards the stem tip are usually smaller but often have the sweetest flavour.

ROSEMARY

PEPPERMINT

FRESH AND DRIED HERBS

Many herbs can be dried for use out of season, with some loss or change of flavour. This is often used as a way of preserving annuals or other plants that die back. The stems can be dried in a well-ventilated place or in a low oven. Once brittle, the leaves can be stripped from the stems for storage.

Dried herbs are more robust in cooking
Fresh herbs can be fragrant and sweet

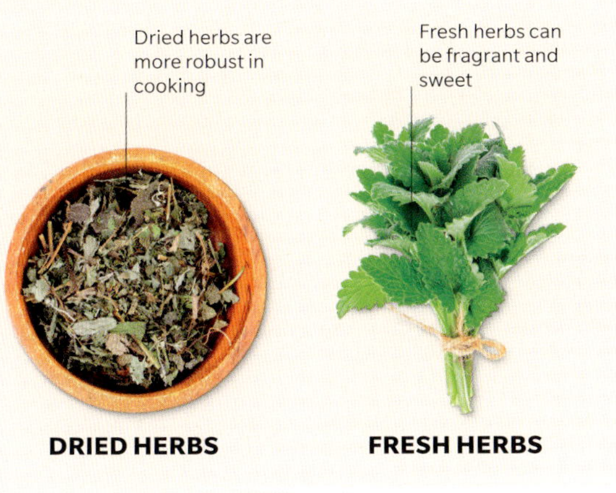

DRIED HERBS

FRESH HERBS

Herbs in Cuisines

Herbs and spices are vital components of cuisines around the world, and common combinations from each country or region are used in signature dishes. Shown here is a small selection of popular cuisines and some of their key herbs and spices.

NORTH AFRICAN

CARDAMOM, CUMIN, PAPRIKA, TURMERIC, GINGER, CINNAMON, RAS EL HANOUT

North Africa is well known for its spice-laden bazaars, and its cuisine is rich in earthy flavours. Shakshuka, harira (soup), and tagines rely on herbs and spices.

Spices such as turmeric were grown in India, where they are native, from at least the 8th century BCE

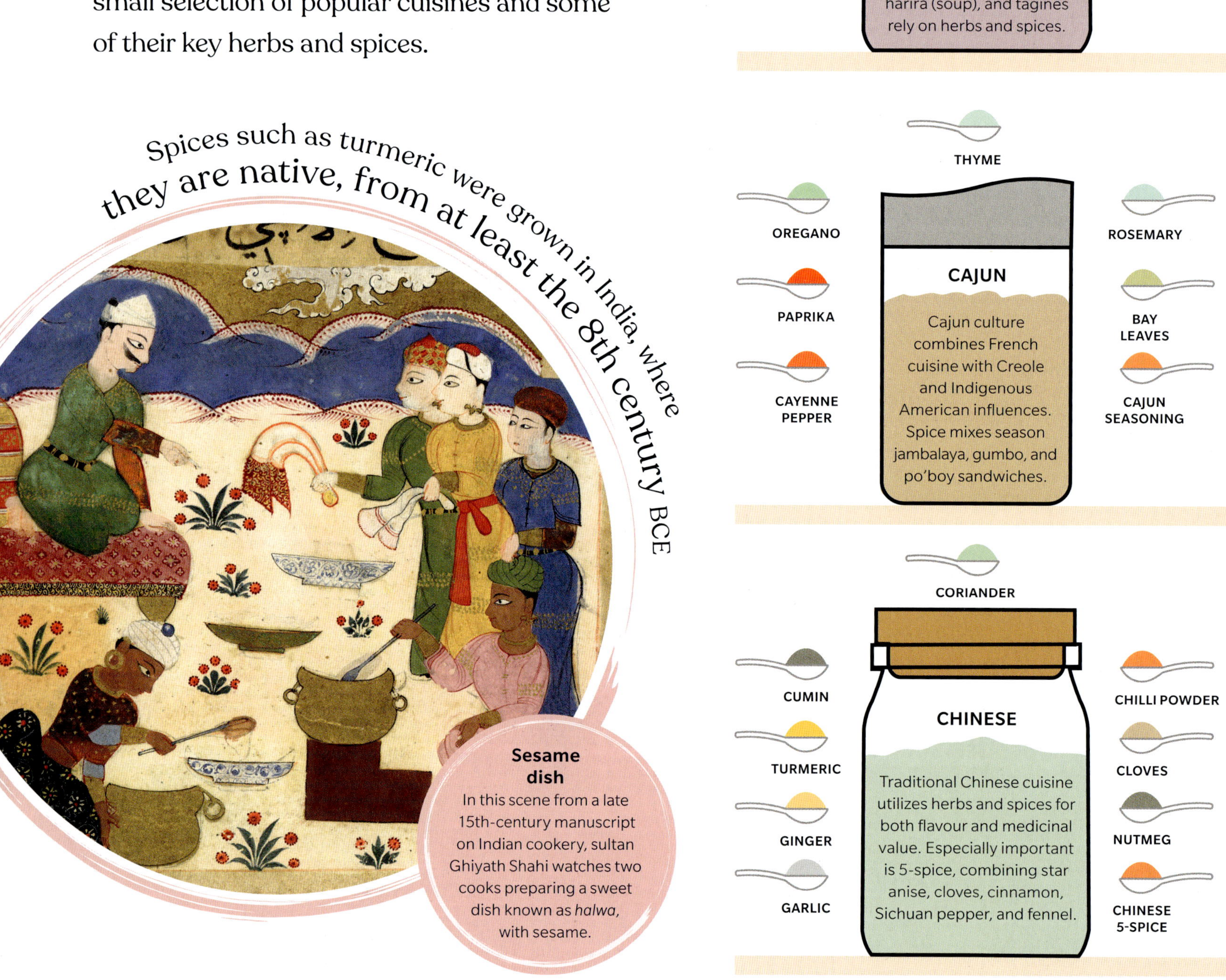

Sesame dish
In this scene from a late 15th-century manuscript on Indian cookery, sultan Ghiyath Shahi watches two cooks preparing a sweet dish known as *halwa*, with sesame.

CAJUN

THYME, OREGANO, PAPRIKA, CAYENNE PEPPER, ROSEMARY, BAY LEAVES, CAJUN SEASONING

Cajun culture combines French cuisine with Creole and Indigenous American influences. Spice mixes season jambalaya, gumbo, and po'boy sandwiches.

CHINESE

CORIANDER, CUMIN, TURMERIC, GINGER, GARLIC, CHILLI POWDER, CLOVES, NUTMEG, CHINESE 5-SPICE

Traditional Chinese cuisine utilizes herbs and spices for both flavour and medicinal value. Especially important is 5-spice, combining star anise, cloves, cinnamon, Sichuan pepper, and fennel.

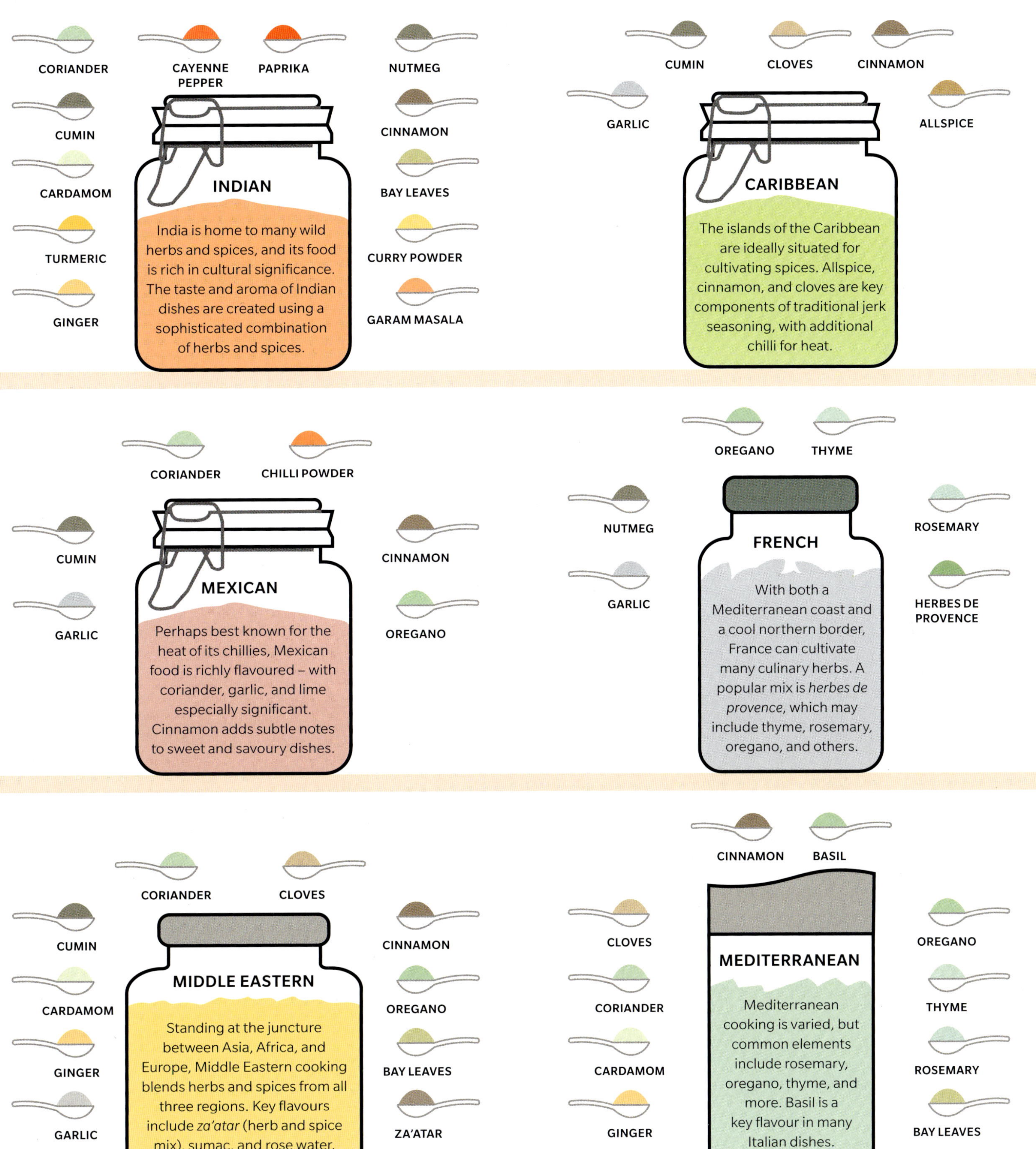
CORIANDER
CAYENNE PEPPER
PAPRIKA
NUTMEG
CUMIN
CINNAMON
CARDAMOM
BAY LEAVES
TURMERIC
CURRY POWDER
GINGER
GARAM MASALA
INDIAN
India is home to many wild herbs and spices, and its food is rich in cultural significance. The taste and aroma of Indian dishes are created using a sophisticated combination of herbs and spices.
CUMIN
CLOVES
CINNAMON
GARLIC
ALLSPICE
CARIBBEAN
The islands of the Caribbean are ideally situated for cultivating spices. Allspice, cinnamon, and cloves are key components of traditional jerk seasoning, with additional chilli for heat.
CORIANDER
CHILLI POWDER
CUMIN
CINNAMON
GARLIC
OREGANO
MEXICAN
Perhaps best known for the heat of its chillies, Mexican food is richly flavoured – with coriander, garlic, and lime especially significant. Cinnamon adds subtle notes to sweet and savoury dishes.
OREGANO
THYME
NUTMEG
ROSEMARY
GARLIC
HERBES DE PROVENCE
FRENCH
With both a Mediterranean coast and a cool northern border, France can cultivate many culinary herbs. A popular mix is *herbes de provence*, which may include thyme, rosemary, oregano, and others.
CORIANDER
CLOVES
CUMIN
CINNAMON
CARDAMOM
OREGANO
GINGER
BAY LEAVES
GARLIC
ZA'ATAR
MIDDLE EASTERN
Standing at the juncture between Asia, Africa, and Europe, Middle Eastern cooking blends herbs and spices from all three regions. Key flavours include *za'atar* (herb and spice mix), sumac, and rose water.
CINNAMON
BASIL
CLOVES
OREGANO
CORIANDER
THYME
CARDAMOM
ROSEMARY
GINGER
BAY LEAVES
MEDITERRANEAN
Mediterranean cooking is varied, but common elements include rosemary, oregano, thyme, and more. Basil is a key flavour in many Italian dishes.

The Symbolism of Herbs

Herbs are largely defined by their practical uses, but can also symbolize many things, including spiritual beliefs, emotions, and more. Some of these may be linked to a herb's scent or taste, and others to a traditional use or property.

Spiritual symbolism

From ancient times, in cultures around the world, herbs have been used in religious or spiritual ceremonies – sometimes for their fragrance or psychoactive properties, but often for other, less tangible associations rooted in a culture or belief. Some herbs have themselves been considered sacred, including Aztec marigold in Central America, vervain in ancient Egypt and Europe, and meadowsweet by Druids. In ancient religions of south Asia, the juice of "soma", a still-unidentified plant, was used in ritual offerings, while in Buddhism, the lotus, an aquatic plant, is associated with purity because it arises clean and bright from murky waters. In China, some plants are considered particularly auspicious, including orchids, chrysanthemum, pine, and bamboo.

PASSOVER HERBS

By Jewish tradition, a meal with herbs called the seder is eaten on the night of the Passover, the holiday that celebrates the escape of the Israelites from slavery in Egypt. Roasted lamb and unleaved bread, or matzo, are accompanied by bitter herbs, representing the bitterness of slavery. These usually include lettuce (chazeret) and horseradish (maror). Also included are parsley (karpas), and charoset, a paste of fruit and nuts representing mortar used by the enslaved people, and a roasted egg symbolizing a temple offering.

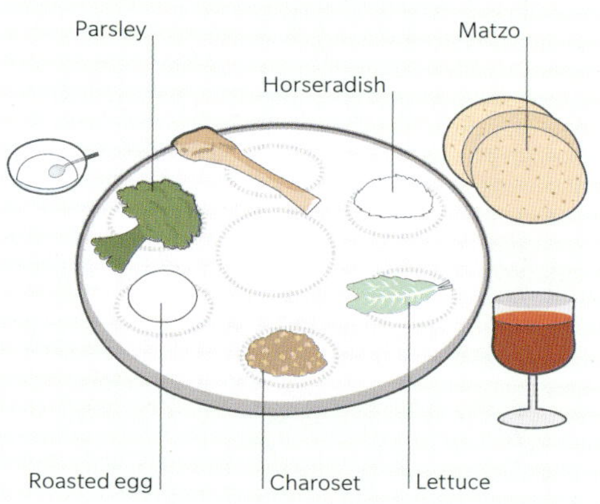

SEDER PLATE WITH BITTER HERBS

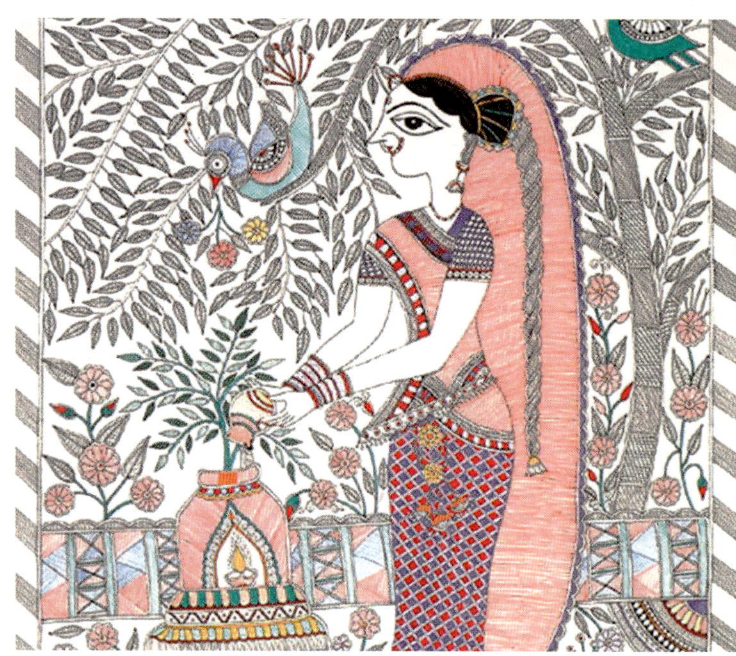

▲ Tulsi worship
Holy basil, known as the tulsi plant (see pp.256–61), is sacred in Hinduism and is believed to be the earthly form of the goddess Tulsi.

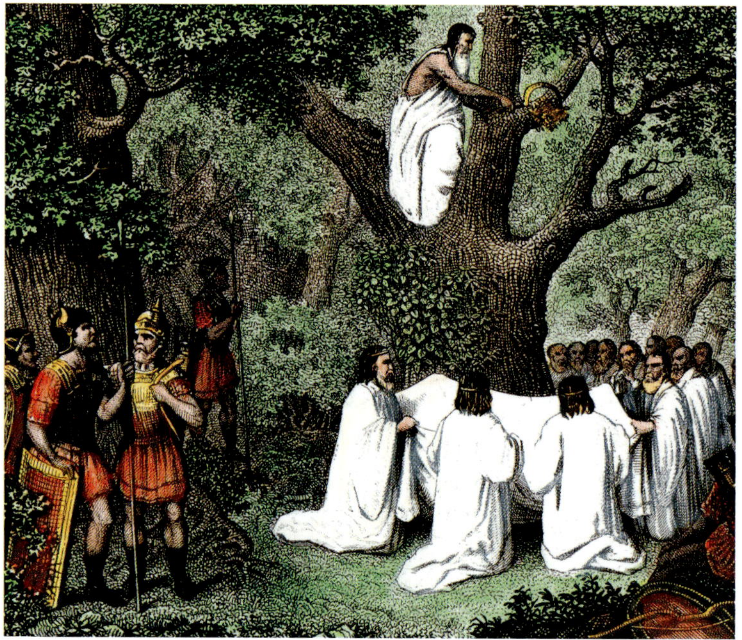

▲ Druids and mistletoe
Druids harvested mistletoe (see pp.66–69) with great ceremony, especially if found on an oak. A symbol of vitality, it was said to restore fertility in animals and humans.

Herbs in art

The oldest depictions of plants are in herbals (see p.10) describing the properties and "virtues" of medicinal plants, developed in Islamic art. The Western tradition of plant symbolism in art began with Dutch painter Jan Van Eyck in the 15th century, who depicted plants with religious qualities such as Madonna lilies (purity), columbine (humility), and the rose, which stood for love. In his painting *Primavera*, Sandro Botticelli included early blooming plants such as strawberry, cornflower, hyacinth, and orange blossom, symbolizing spring and ideals of love. In 19th-century Britain, Pre-Raphaelite artists often included flowers with symbolic connections, such as the red poppy and fritillary in *Ophelia* by John Everard Millais (see p.93), both of which symbolized sorrow.

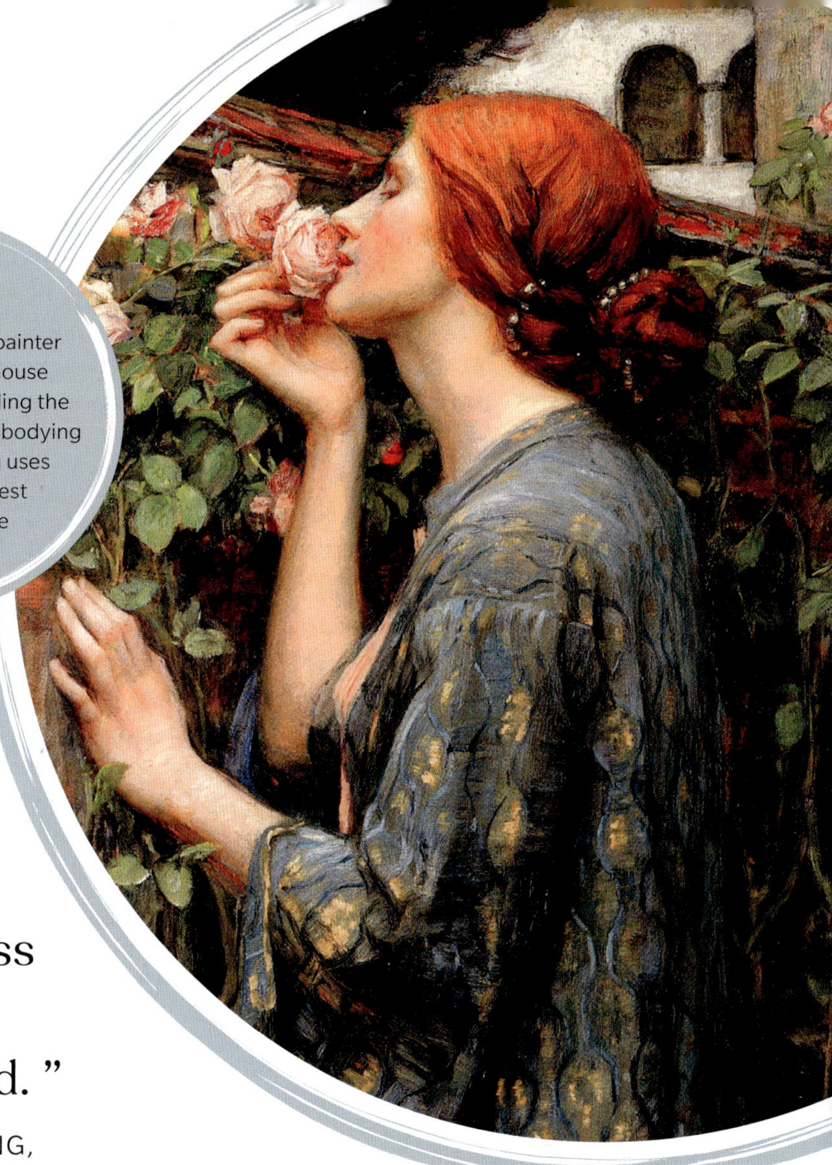

***Soul of the Rose*, 1908**
This work by English painter John William Waterhouse depicts a woman inhaling the scent of a rose, here embodying beauty. The painting uses the scene to suggest ideas of romance and courtship.

> " A plant or root is thought to possess virtue, not only when swallowed... but when carried in the hand. "
>
> ANDREW LANG,
> Scottish author and historian, *Custom and Myth*, 1885

CULTURAL ASSOCIATIONS

Traditions around the world have a rich history of herbal symbolism, and connections can arise for myriad reasons. Fragrances often evoke emotions, associating herbs with feelings such as joy, love, or sadness. Bold scents, such as that of thyme, can embody qualities such as strength and courage. Flavour can also build associations, with bitter herbs often being associated with suffering or repentance. Beliefs can also echo a plant's appearance: under the "doctrine of signatures" (see p.14), herbs that resemble parts of the body were thought to cure ailments in those areas. For example, eyebright, whose flowers resemble the human eye, was used as eyedrops.

BASIL
Basil has been considered both a talisman of strength and a symbol of dread and suspicion, as well as a holy herb.

CINNAMON
The phoenix was said to have used cinnamon for its funeral pyre, and so the spice became a symbol of renewal at Christmas.

SAFFRON
In Hinduism, saffron symbolizes sacrifice, light, and salvation. It is also a colour of the Indian flag, signifying strength and courage.

FENNEL
Fennel has long symbolized courage. Roman gladiators ate its seeds, while the Anglo-Saxons used it to ward against witchcraft.

GINSENG
An adaptogen in traditional Chinese medicine, this sacred herb is said to bring wealth, prosperity, and long life.

YARROW
Long associated with healing, yarrow is named from the Greek *hiera*, or holy herb. It is said to be a cure for a broken heart.

PATCHOULI
This native of south-east Asia is cultivated for its scented oil. Reputed to be an aphrodisiac, it represents love and fertility.

SAGE
Species of sage have been used in religious rites around the world. In Mexico, it is associated with the Virgin Mary.

BETEL NUT
An important herb in some Asian and Pacific cultures, betel nut is a symbol of love and marriage in Vietnamese tradition.

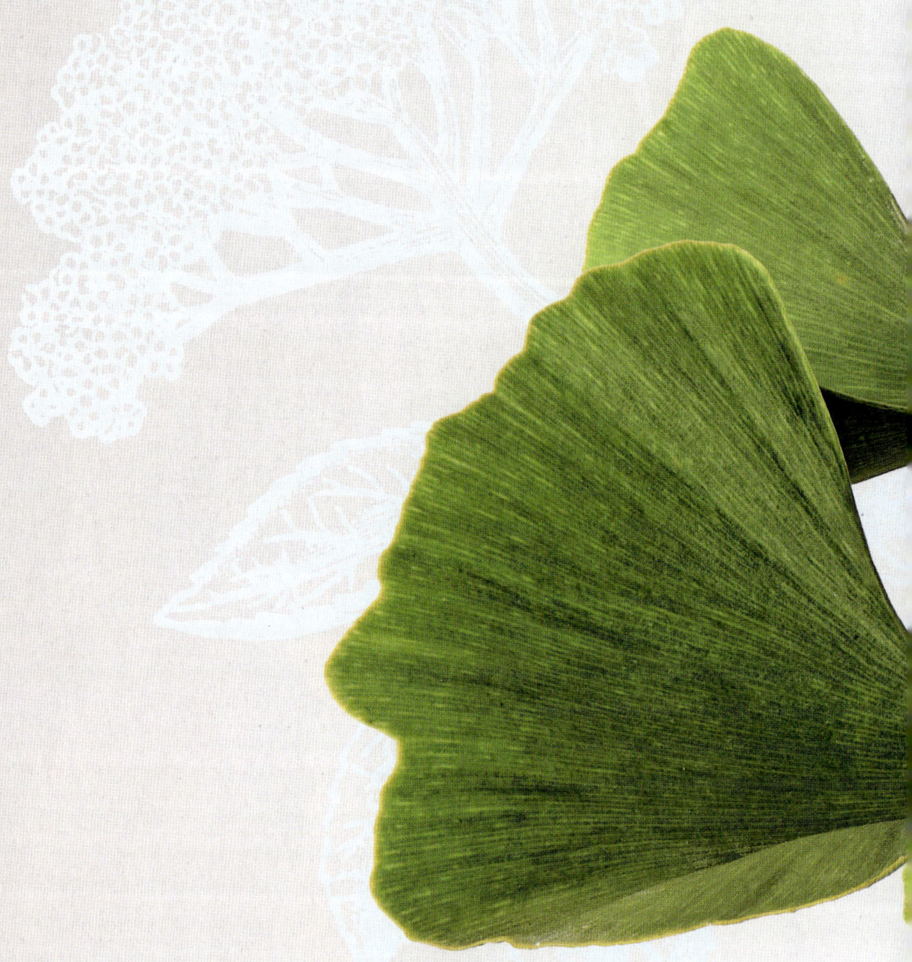

CHAPTER 2

Trees and Shrubs

Many parts of trees and shrubs, such as leaves, fruits, and bark, are widely used as herbs. Trees have a single woody stem, or trunk, while shrubs are also woody and have several branching stems arising from or near the base.

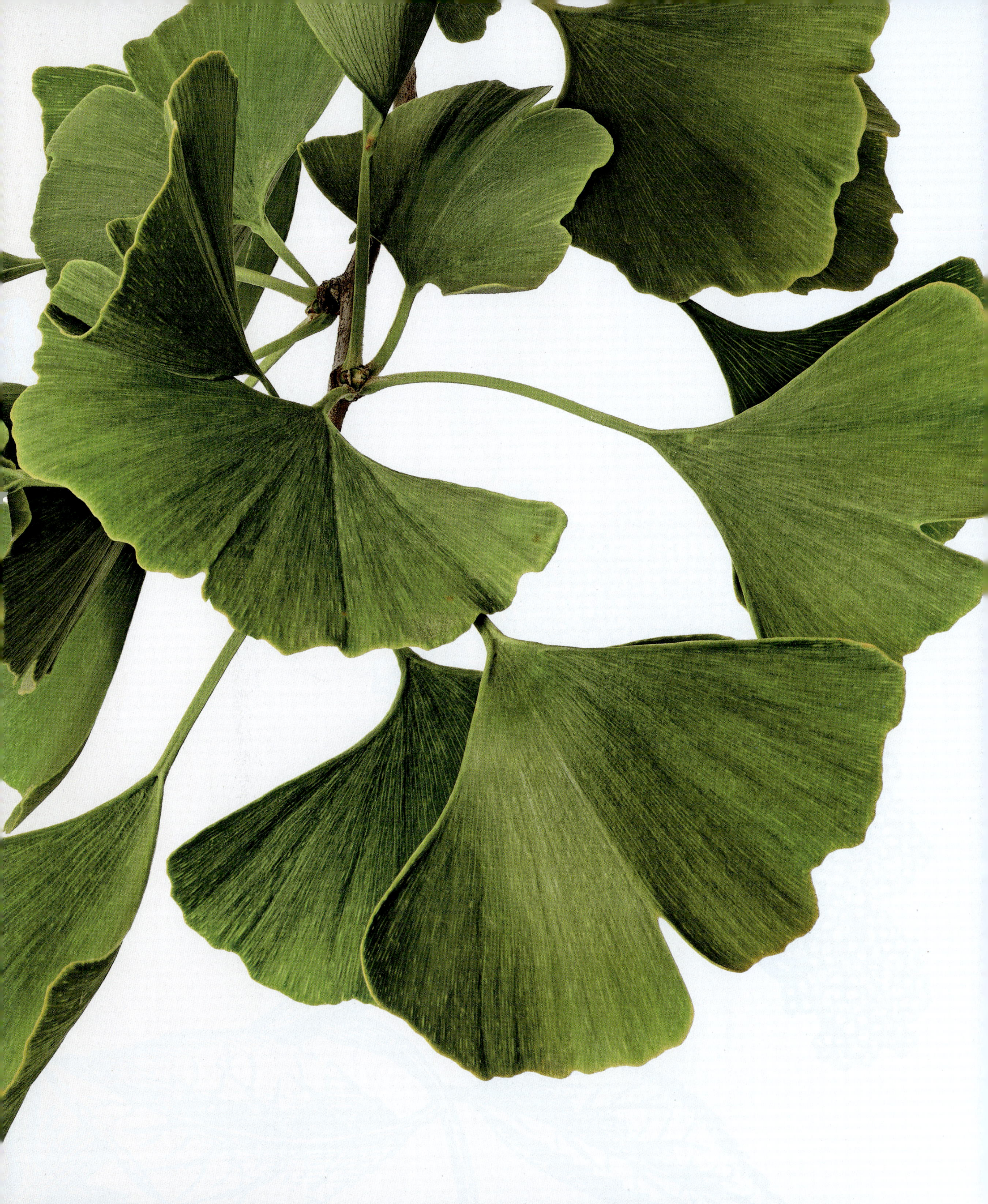

Uses Medicines for fever, varicose veins, leg cramps, increasing appetite

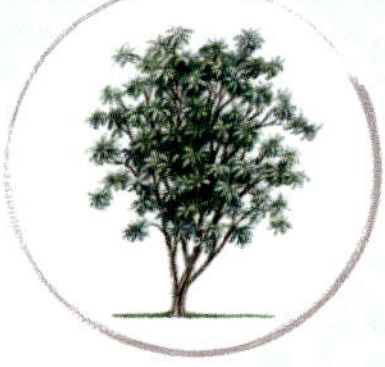

Parts used Bark

Active ingredients Quinine, quinidine, cinchonine, cinchonidine

Habitat Tropical montane rainforests

➤ Valuable quinine
Historically, cinchona bark was dried, ground, and mixed with alcohol. Today, quinine can be extracted from the bark or produced synthetically.

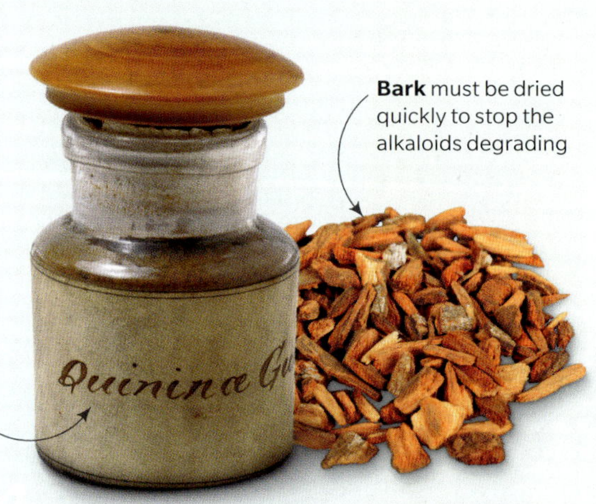

Bark must be dried quickly to stop the alkaloids degrading

Powdered quinine was often mixed with wine

Cinchona

Cinchona calisaya

Native to remote rainforests in Peru and Bolivia, cinchona was once an obscure tropical tree. It is now known worldwide, and its bark is used as an effective treatment for malaria fevers.

Quinine is used to treat the common disease **white spot** (or ich) in aquarium **fish**

Cinchona was named after the Countess of Chinchón, wife of the Viceroy of Peru, following a story, now known not to be true, that she was cured of fever in around 1630 using cinchona bark. The story may be fictitious, but cinchona bark (also known as fever tree, Jesuit's bark, and Peruvian bark) was used to treat fever by Indigenous people in South America long before colonization.

Cinchona bark contains a cocktail of drugs, particularly quinoline alkaloids, important in the prevention and treatment of malaria. This disease is caused by *Plasmodium*, a parasitic microorganism spread by mosquitoes. In infected humans, *Plasmodium* destroys red blood cells and causes cycles of fever and other symptoms. Quinine kills the *Plasmodium* by interfering with its ability to safely digest haemoglobin.

A tonic for tropical travellers

As European countries established colonies across tropical Africa, Asia, and the Americas, it became apparent that malaria brought considerable human and economic costs. The revelation that quinine could provide an effective treatment led to increased interest in the plant. By the mid-1850s, cinchona seeds were being exported to numerous countries, of which India and Java became by far the most productive. During World War II, when Japan captured and, therefore, controlled quinine supplies from Java, research turned to the production of synthetic alternatives, such as chloroquine.

Cinchona calisaya is one of a few species that are still used medicinally. Due to its high levels of quinine, it is also widely cultivated for commercial quinine production.

BITTERSWEET FAVOURITES

Cinchona bark is known for its bitter flavour, so various sweeteners, herbs, and spices were added to improve its palatability and to encourage its medicinal use. Cinchona is also an ingredient in several popular drinks. Known as the favourite tipple of Elizabeth II, the late British monarch, Dubonnet is an aperitif based on red wine, with added herbs and quinine. Quinine is also a bitter flavouring in tonic water and Scotland's much-loved soft drink Irn-Bru.

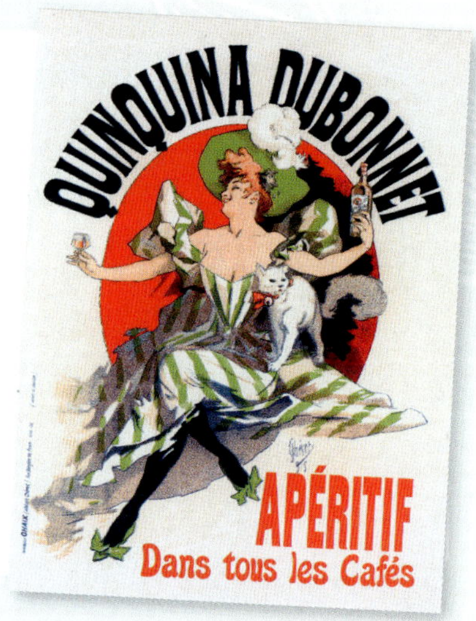

DUBONNET POSTER

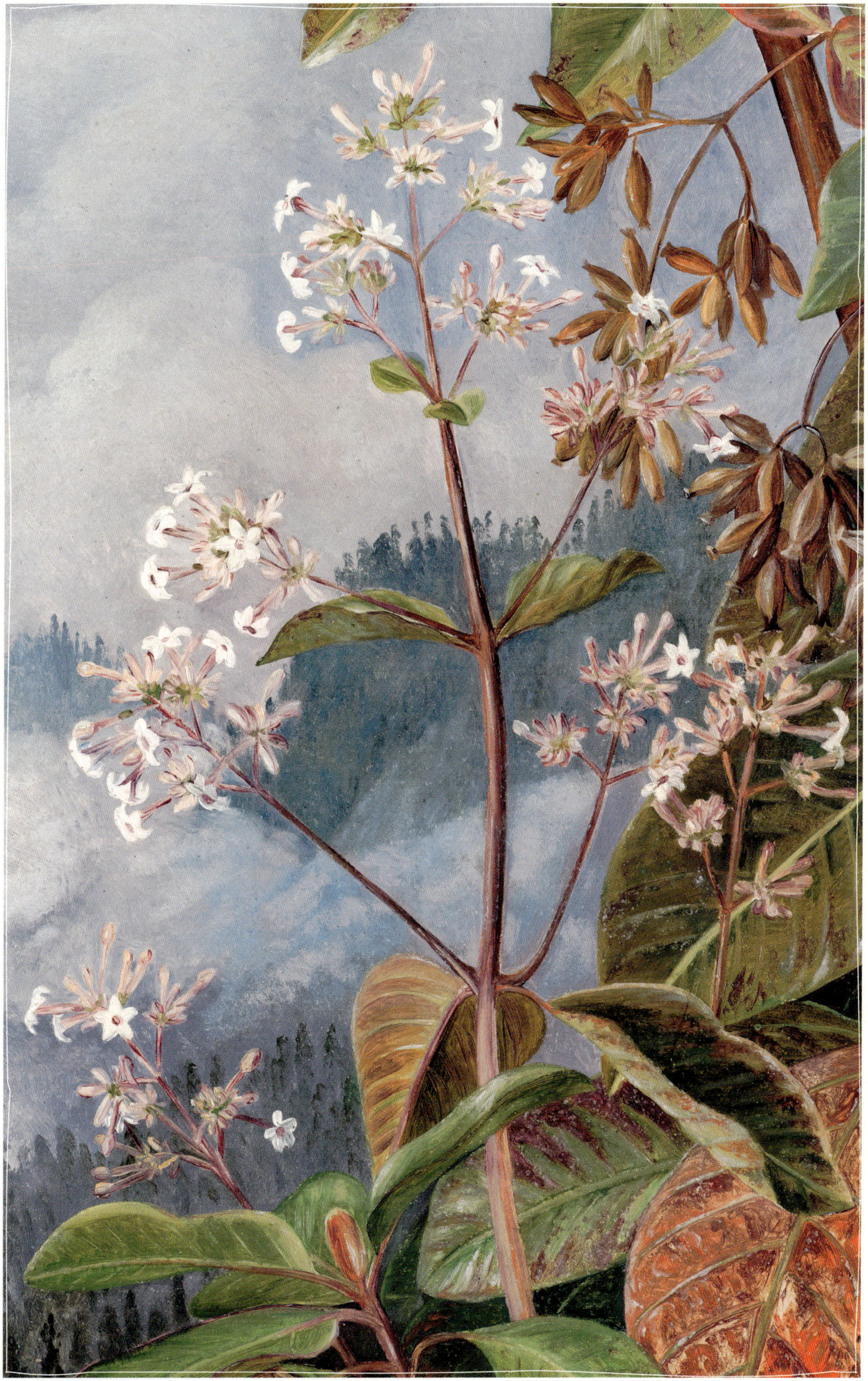

◄ Delicate blooms
Painted by biologist Marianne North in 1870, this image shows the cinchona flowers and seed capsules (right). The bark of this valuable plant was transported beyond South America from the 1640s.

Similar herbs

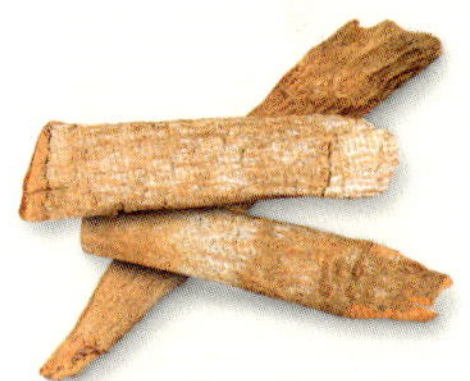

RED BARK
Cinchona pubescens
Red cinchona, another important source of quinine, originates in Costa Rica to Bolivia and is now an invasive species on a few small tropical islands.

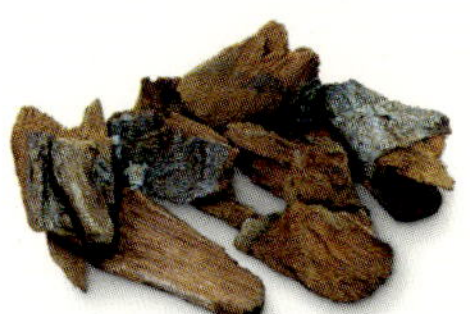

FEVER TREE
Cinchona officinalis
Restricted to Southern Ecuador, this species was one of the first to be grown in Indian plantations as a source of quinoline alkaloids.

Uses Medicines for dementia, cooking

Parts used Seeds, leaves

Active ingredients Ginkgo flavone glycosides (for example, ginkgetin, bilobetin), ginkgolides

Habitat Temperate deciduous forest

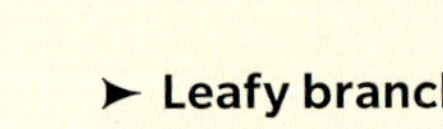

➤ Leafy branch
Ginkgo leaves are unique among trees, making fossil leaves easy to identify. The cleft in the centre, which divides the leaf into two lobes, is reflected in the word *"biloba"* in the scientific name.

Leaves resemble the frond divisions (pinnules) of maidenhair ferns

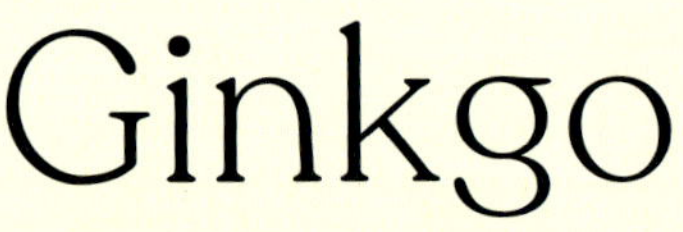

Ginkgo

Ginkgo biloba

With a fossil history dating back to the Jurassic and a lifespan of more than 1,000 years, ginkgo symbolizes longevity in China. Leaf-based medicines may also provide relief from age-related dementia in humans.

Ginkgo is native to China, although fossils suggest it was once far more widespread and could be found in Europe, North America, and elsewhere. Changes in climate and the rise of flowering plants may have led to its retreat, but it is unclear why it survived only in Asia. In Japan, ginkgo is a *hibakujumoku* (a tree that survived the atomic bombings of 1945), and its seedlings have since been planted around the world to promote peace.

Physicians, prayers, and pollution

Ginkgo has been an important component of Chinese traditional medicine for at least 2,000 years. The tree is dioecious (having distinct male and female plants) and only females produce seeds. Wrapped in an oily outer coating, each seed resembles an unshelled pistachio. Ginkgo seeds are still used in treatments for lung conditions such as asthma and tuberculosis, although they must be prepared first because they contain ginkgotoxins, which are poisonous in high doses. Seeds are also popular in Chinese, Japanese, and Korean cuisines, in which they are typically boiled, roasted, or fried. Chinese traditional medicine favours the seeds (*bai guo*), although the leaves (*yin xing ye*) are also used. More recently, ginkgo leaves have been utilized as a source of complementary medicines. Such medicines are primarily used for cognitive and memory decline in people with dementia, and this application is supported by some scientific studies.

Older ginkgo trees are revered in many Asian religious traditions, especially in Buddhism, Daoism, and Confucianism in China, and they

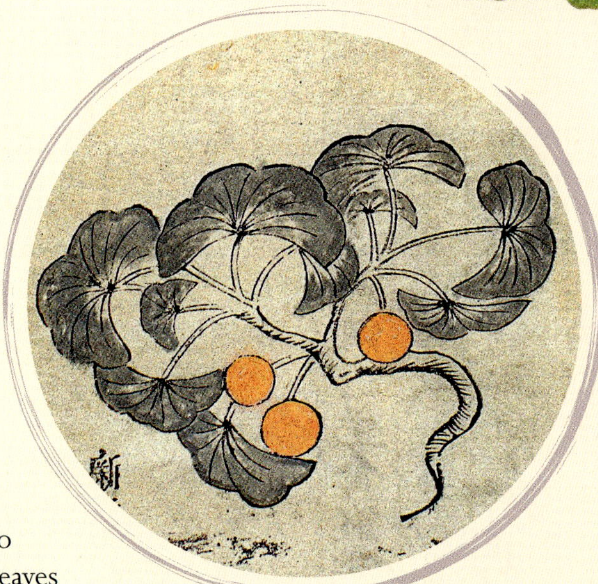

▲ Plum-like fruits
Ginkgo fruits have pungent orange flesh. They can be eaten in moderation, but the seed within is far more desirable, known in Japan, Korea, and China as a "silver apricot nut".

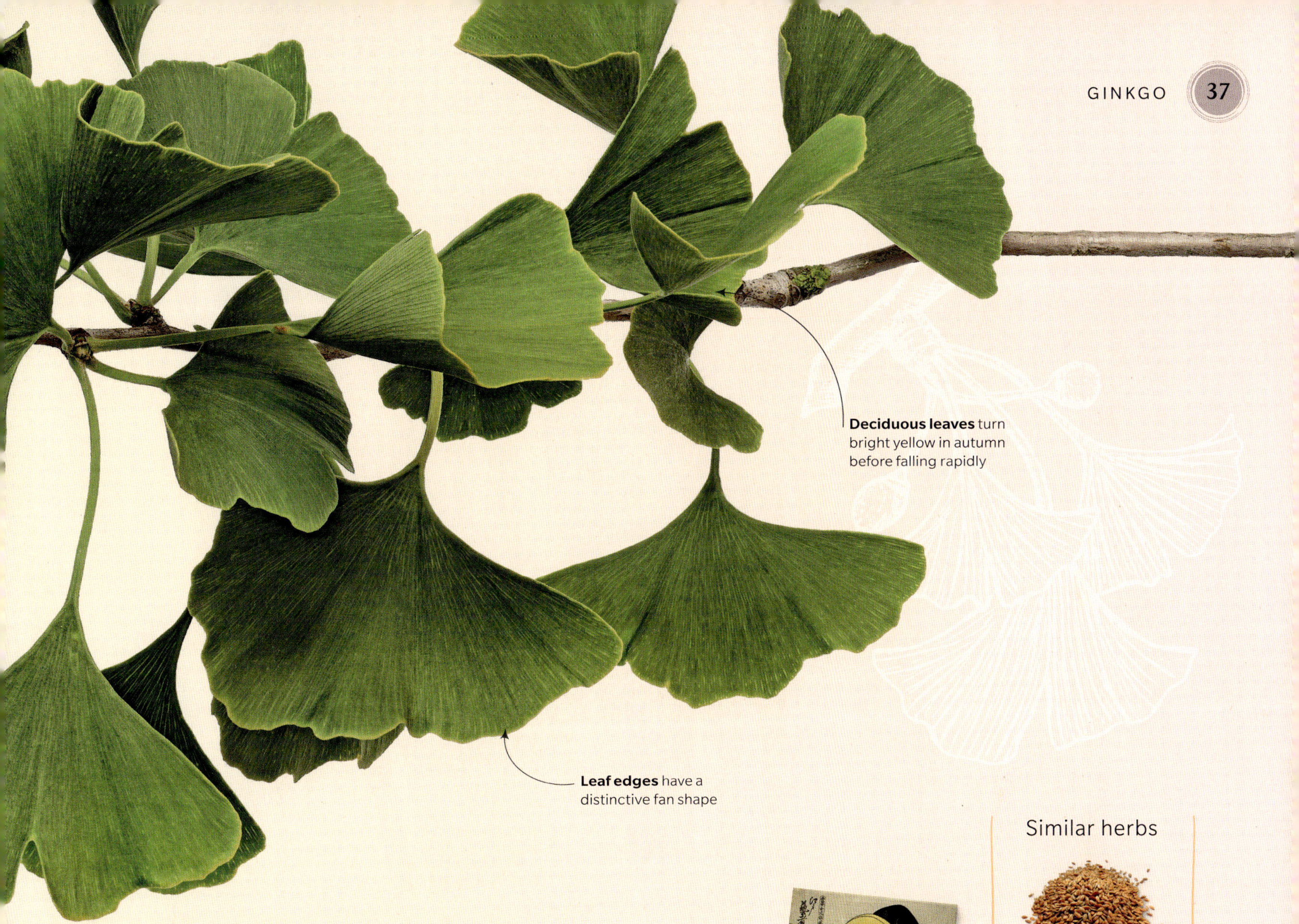

Deciduous leaves turn bright yellow in autumn before falling rapidly

Leaf edges have a distinctive fan shape

are nurtured in the grounds around temples. Ginkgo wood is used to carve idols, while prayer ribbons are attached to stems and trunk. Ginkgo is commonly planted, which complicates efforts to understand the natural distribution of this iconic species. Given the tree's narrow native range, it might be concluded that ginkgo has rather specialized habitat requirements, but this is not the case. Also known as a maidenhair tree, it thrives in temperate areas outside of China and is particularly tolerant of pollution. New York City alone is home to almost 60,000 ginkgo trees.

GINKGO IN ART

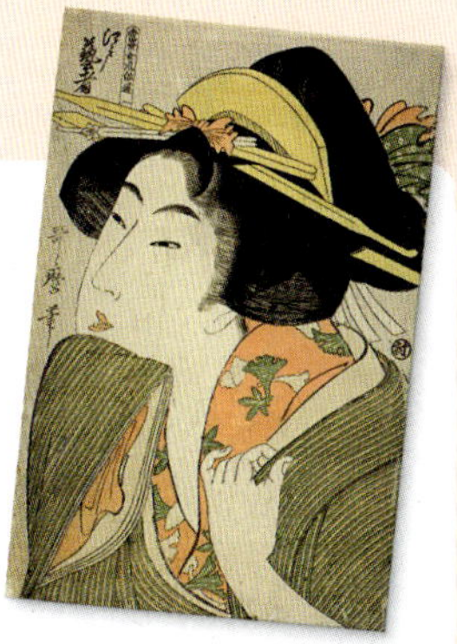

The great age attained by some ginkgo trees, together with their distinctive leaf shape, has given this plant huge significance in many Asian cultural traditions. The ginkgo leaf is widely reproduced in art, as seen in this Japanese woodblock print by Kitagawa Utamaro, from the series *A Guide to Women's Contemporary Styles* (c.1801–02). A stylized version of the ginkgo leaf is also the official symbol (*shinboru*) of Tokyo city.

GINKGO LEAF MOTIF

"From the East this tree's leaf shows
Secret sense for us to savour."

JOHANN WOLFGANG VON GOETHE, "Ginkgo biloba" in *West-östlicher Divan*, 1819

Similar herbs

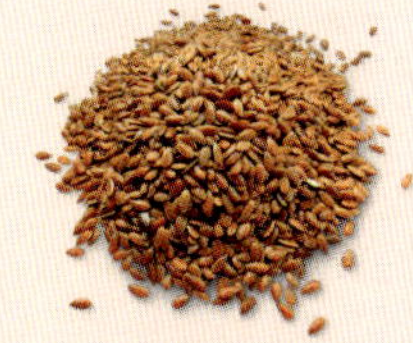

FLAX
Linum usitatissimum
The source of linseed oil, this Central Asian annual herb helps to lower dietary cholesterol. It can also moderate symptoms of menopause.

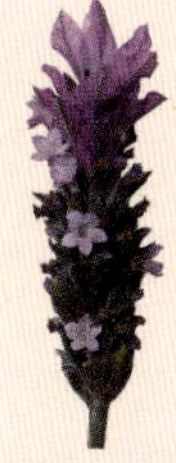

LAVENDER
Lavandula dentata
Spanish lavender occurs in Spain and parts of North Africa and the Middle East. It is used to treat headaches, rheumatism, and colds.

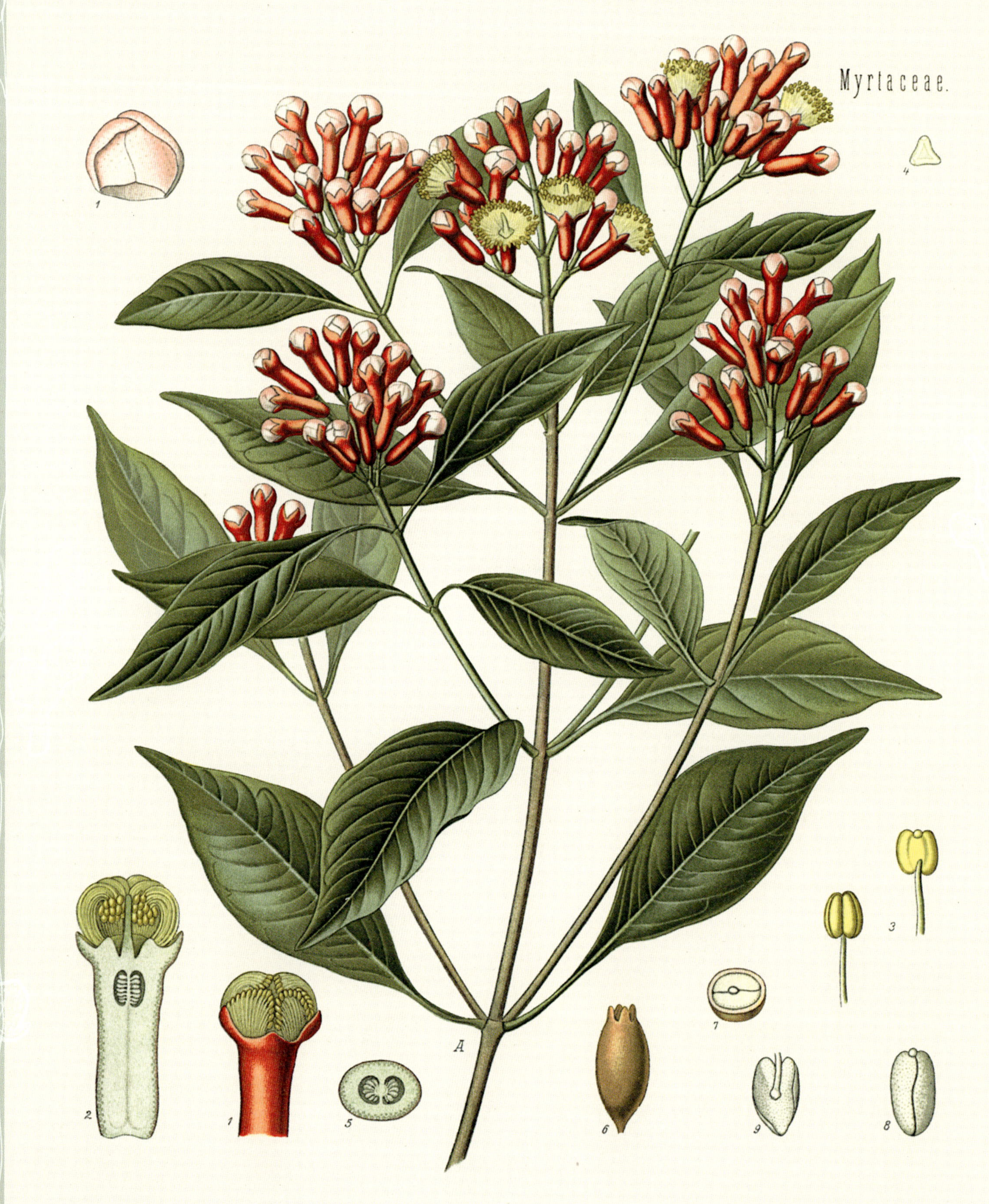
Myrtaceae.
1
4
3
7
A
2
1
5
6
9
8

Uses Medicines for infected wounds, spice, perfumery

Parts used Dried flowers, oil extracted from leaves and stalks

Active ingredients Eugenol and other volatile oils

Habitat Mixed forest at lower elevations on tropical mountains

Developing clove flower buds were picked twice a year, then dried in the sun

Clove harvesting
By the 19th century, cloves were grown for commercial harvest on plantations in Zanzibar. Enslaved people brought from mainland Africa were forced to work on these plantations.

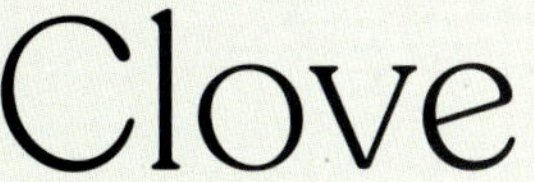

Clove

Syzygium aromaticum

This spice, used to flavour foods including ham, pickles, and fruit cakes, and for its scent in perfumery and potpourris, is produced from the dried, unopened flower buds of a tropical tree.

Standing around 20 m (82 ft) tall, clove trees are native to the Maluku Islands of Indonesia. Their dried flower buds were one of the earliest spices to be traded in China and India, and by the Middle Ages cloves were also known throughout Europe. They were a major element in the spice trade that led to conflict between colonial nations in the 17th century. The Dutch-owned East India Company established a monopoly in clove production, which they held until the late 18th century when plantations were established elsewhere from smuggled seeds and plants. Today, Indonesia is the main clove producer – more than 110,000 tons (130,000 metric tons) a year – followed by Madagascar, Tanzania, Comoros, and Kenya. India, Pakistan, and Sri Lanka are also important producers. The spice is widely used in sauces and pickles, and as flavouring in some cigarettes.

Dried in the sun

The flower buds are picked before they open, and turn brown as they are dried in the sun. When squeezed or crushed, the dried buds exude an oil with the characteristic clove aroma. This oil contains up to 85 per cent eugenol, a volatile ingredient used in a variety of household products, such as pesticides, insect repellents, laundry and cleaning materials, in perfumery, and in the drinks industry as a flavouring for vermouth. The strongly anaesthetic oil is valued for pain relief in dentistry and toothpastes.

◄ **Flowering clove tree**
Clove trees have bright green, glossy leaves and their flower buds have a rather fleshy appearance. The buds develop in small clusters at the stem tips.

► **Ready to spice**
The spice marketed as "whole cloves" consists of complete, dried flower buds from the clove tree. It is also sold in powdered form.

Round ball of developing flower, enwrapped in petals, with ovary below

Similar herbs

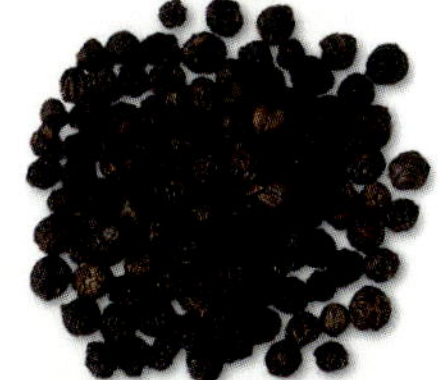

BLACK PEPPER
Piper nigrum
This climbing Indian vine has been cultivated for over 3,000 years. Its unripe, dried fruits (peppercorns) are widely used to season food.

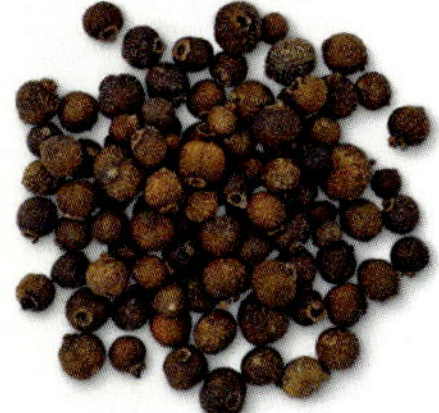

ALLSPICE
Pimenta dioica
The unripe, dried berries of this tropical tree get the name "allspice" because they seem to combine the flavours of cloves, cinnamon, and nutmeg.

Short-stalked, slender, lance-shaped leaves with toothed edges
Upper surface is covered with whitish hairs
Lower surface is greyish with dense, silvery hairs

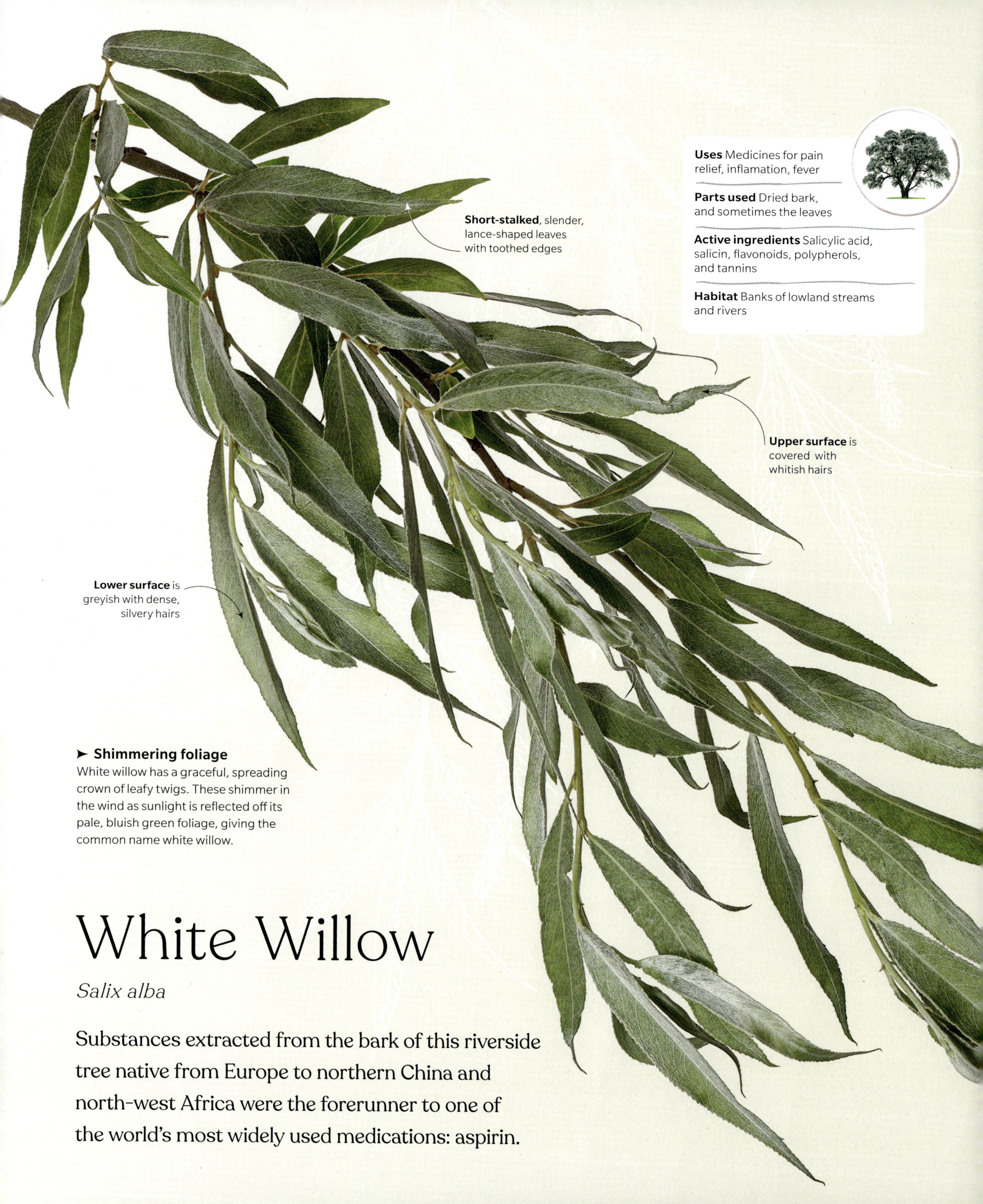

Uses Medicines for pain relief, inflamation, fever

Parts used Dried bark, and sometimes the leaves

Active ingredients Salicylic acid, salicin, flavonoids, polypherols, and tannins

Habitat Banks of lowland streams and rivers

➤ **Shimmering foliage**
White willow has a graceful, spreading crown of leafy twigs. These shimmer in the wind as sunlight is reflected off its pale, bluish green foliage, giving the common name white willow.

White Willow

Salix alba

Substances extracted from the bark of this riverside tree native from Europe to northern China and north-west Africa were the forerunner to one of the world's most widely used medications: aspirin.

Herbal preparations from willow trees may have been used to treat fever and inflammatory conditions for more than 3,000 years. The ancient Egyptians used willow leaves to treat inflamed wounds. In China, willow has been used to remedy fever for more than 2,000 years, while the 1st-century Greek physician Dioscorides recommended mashed willow leaves as a treatment for gout and back pain.

Key discovery

Around 1757, the Reverend Edward Stone, a chaplain from Oxfordshire, England, suffered a bout of fever. He knew the value of cinchona in treating malaria (see p.34) and believed that the remedies for many illnesses "lie not far from their causes". Thinking his illness might be waterborne, he wondered whether the bitter bark of white willows along local rivers might have similar properties to cinchona. He chewed a piece of the bark and later dried it in an oven then pulverized it into a powder. He was delighted to observe that "the ague was removed".

From ancient to modern

Stone tested this dried powder cure on around 50 people suffering fevers. When the health of most improved almost immediately, he reported his findings in a letter to the Royal Society in London.

THE WILLOW IN SONG

Several species of willow had a cherished place in the European landscape and culture, long before their medicinal values were known. This traditional folk song is the lament of a jilted lover sitting under a willow tree.

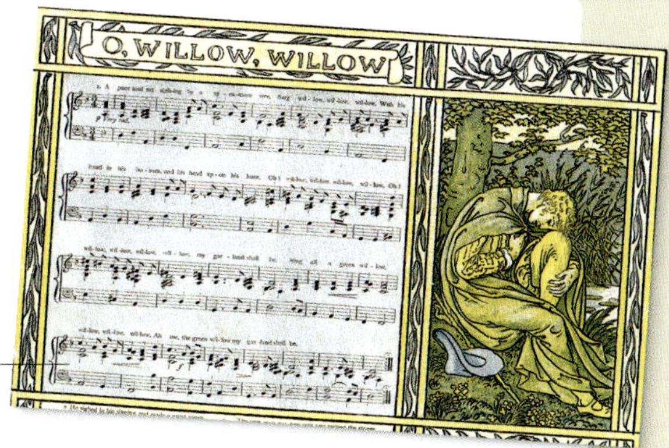

"O, the greene willow shall be my garland"

"O, WILLOW, WILLOW" SONGSHEET

> " ... the bark of an English tree which I have found... very efficacious in curing agues... "
>
> EDWARD STONE'S LETTER TO THE ROYAL SOCIETY, 1763

Following Stone's observations, salicin was isolated from white willow, and the active form, salicylic acid was later identified. A synthetic substitute for salicylic acid, acetylsalicylic acid, was then produced and given the commercial name aspirin.

◄ Willow bark
Dried willow bark is used as a herbal remedy for fevers and flu, and also to relieve back and muscular pain.

► Symbolic trees
Willows are highly valued trees around the world, and are often depicted in landscape art. In Japanese landscapes, such as this by Ryūryūkyo Shinsai (1764–1820), graceful willows are associated with warding off disaster and illness.

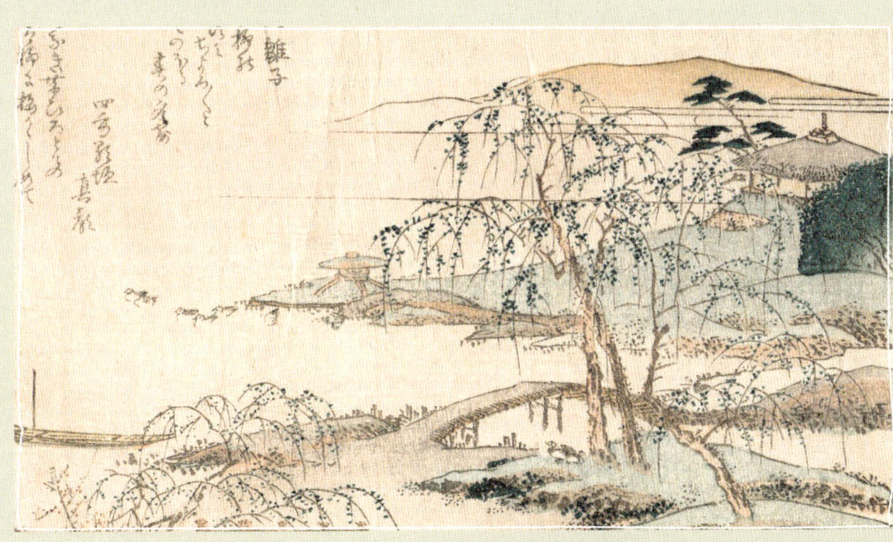

Similar herbs

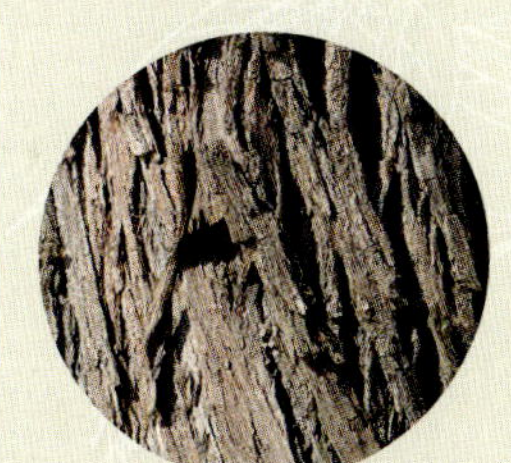

CRACK WILLOW
Salix × fragilis
This well-known willow shares medicinal properties with white willow. It is now thought to be a hybrid between that and *Salix euxina* from Turkey and the Caucasus.

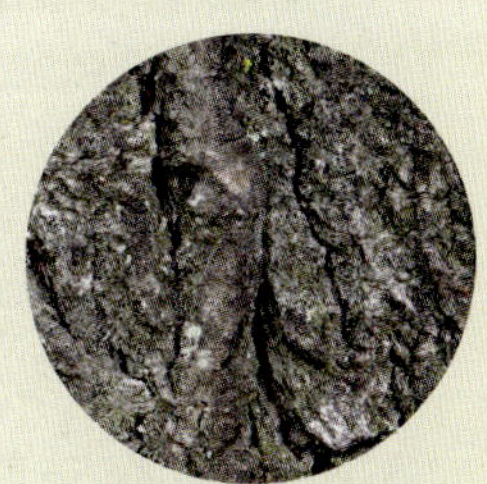

WEEPING WILLOW
Salix babylonica
Most of the spectacular weeping willows planted in parks and amenity areas are probably hybrids between this native from China and various other species of willows.

Eucalyptus

Eucalyptus globulus

Gum trees are the floral equivalent of kangaroos – both are widely recognized as symbols of Australia. They provide essential oils, which are widely used in medicines and cosmetics, as well as timber, and nectar for honey.

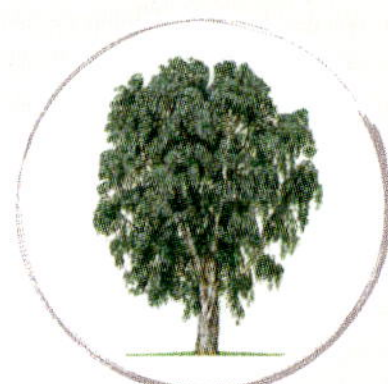

Uses Medicines, cosmetics, fragrances, food flavourings, disinfectants, insect-repellents, insecticides

Parts used Leaves, rarely bark

Active ingredients 1,8-cineole, p-cymene, pinene

Habitat Eucalypt-dominated evergreen forest in both uplands and lowlands

Nearly all the 750 or more eucalyptus species are endemic to Australia. Eucalyptus is now grown on every continent but Antarctica, due to its many useful properties, such as rapid growth, resistance to drought and bush fires, and long-burning firewood. Valued as an ornamental tree as well as a crop, eucalyptus has become a weed in some regions. Despite being an alien species, Eucalyptus provide an important winter shelter for the declining western population of monarch butterflies (*Danaus plexippus*) in coastal California.

Eucalyptus globulus, or southern blue gum, has dominated gum tree cultivation around the world. Native in southeastern Australia from New South Wales to Tasmania, where it is now the floral emblem. Its leaves are packed with volatile organic compounds (VOCs) that, when released, fill the air with the characteristic scent of eucalyptus oil. The main component of the oil is 1,8-cineole, also known as eucalyptol; it has fungicidal and insecticidal properties. VOCs released from damaged leaves may prompt adjacent eucalypts to produce toxic compounds as a defence against herbivore attack.

Essential oil

The oil of eucalyptus has many medicinal and culinary applications, although it is poisonous to humans in quantity; only tiny amounts are safe to take internally. For centuries, First Australians used eucalyptus medicinally to treat respiratory

➤ Mature leaves
The foliage gives the eucalyptus its distinctive appearance, but also battles drought. Each leaf surface intercepts less sunlight than if it were perpendicular to the sun's rays, so reducing leaf temperature and water loss.

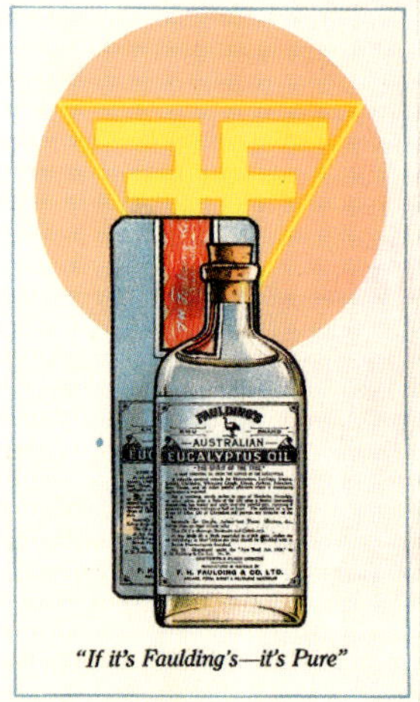

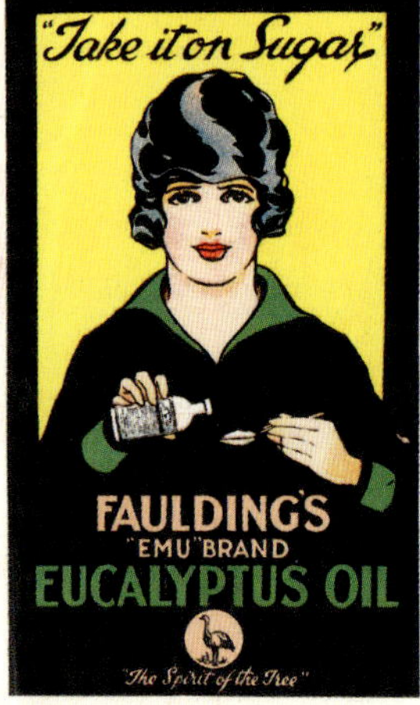

▲ Medicinal eucalyptus oil
In the 19th and early-20th centuries, eucalyptus oil became an important medicinal export for Australia. It was also used as a treatment and disinfectant during the 1918 Spanish flu pandemic.

Similar herbs

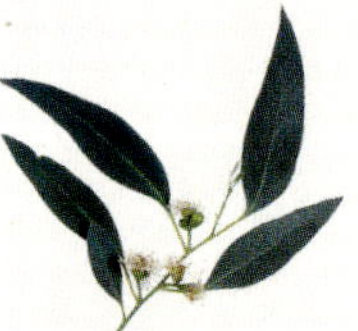

CIDER GUM
Eucalyptus gunnii
Named after a drink that was naturally fermented by First Australians after tapping the sweet sap, cider gum also yields an essential oil rich in 1,8-cineole.

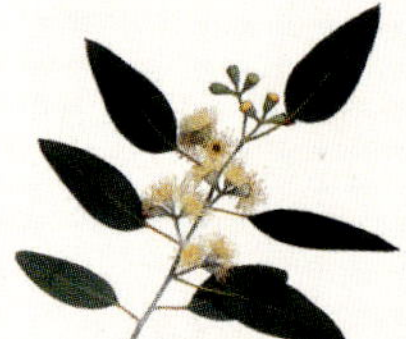

URN TREE
Eucalyptus urnigera
A popular ornamental, this eucalypt is named after its urn-shaped fruit capsules. Its oil has similar medicinal uses to that of southern blue gum.

Leaf stalk, or petiole, is long and flexible to allow the leaves to hang downwards
Leaf surfaces have few pores on both surfaces; they can close to reduce water loss

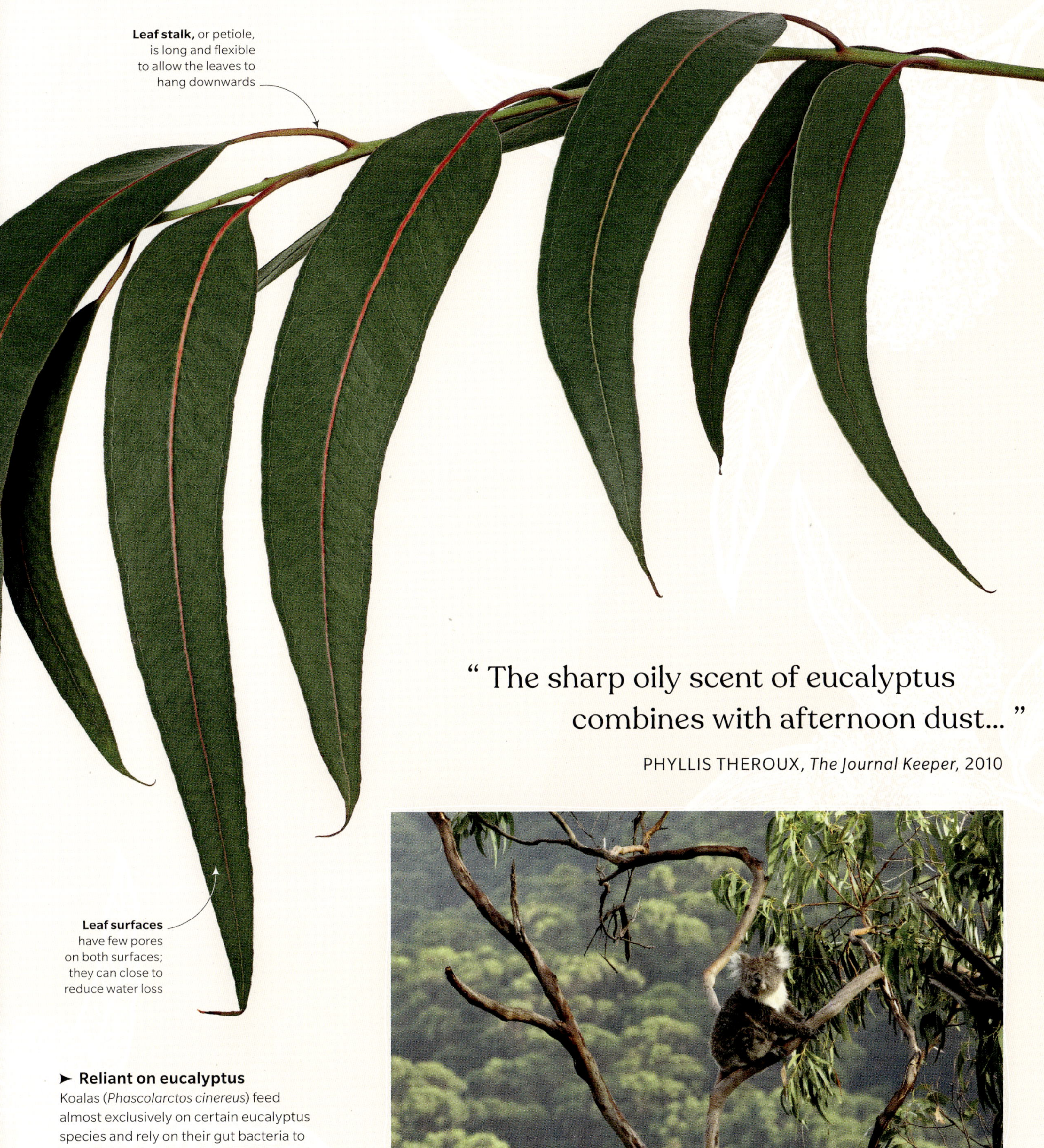

“ The sharp oily scent of eucalyptus combines with afternoon dust... ”

PHYLLIS THEROUX, *The Journal Keeper*, 2010

➤ **Reliant on eucalyptus**
Koalas (*Phascolarctos cinereus*) feed almost exclusively on certain eucalyptus species and rely on their gut bacteria to break down the toxins in the essential oils.

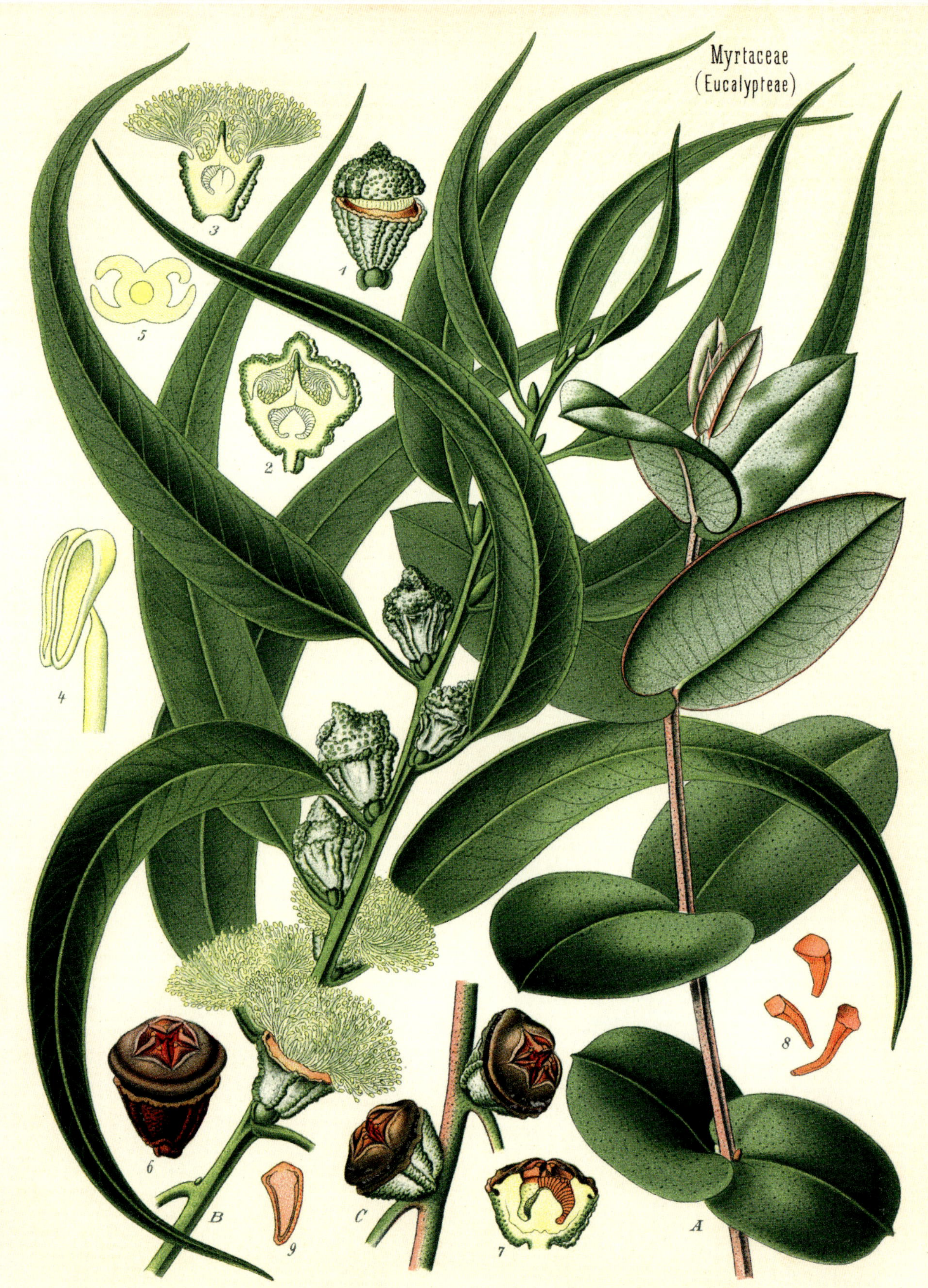
Myrtaceae
(Eucalypteae)
3
1
5
2
4
6
B
9
C
7
A
8
Eucalyptus Globulus Labillardière.
40

◄ Botanical study
In this illustration after *Köhler's Medicinal Plants* by Hermann Adolph Köhler (Vol. II, 1890), juvenile or immature leaves are pictured bottom right and the woody seed capsules, bottom left.

ailments, gastro-intestinal problems such as diarrhoea, aches and pains, and as an antiseptic for minor wounds. Poultices of blue gum leaves were applied to treat fevers and infections.

Europeans were quick to adopt this proven treatment. Eucalyptus oil is now produced by steam distillation: steam is passed over shredded leaves, causing the volatile oil to evaporate. The gas is then cooled to condense the oil, which is collected. The neat oil is added to boiling water for inhalation as an expectorant or mixed with a carrier oil to create a chest rub or aromatherapy massage oil. It is a key ingredient in several decongestants and can be dabbed on to the skin to treat insect bites and stings, boils, and wounds.

Today, China is the world's biggest producer of eucalyptus oil, which is utilized in a wide range of applications, from cosmetics, toothpaste, and insect repellents to cleaning products, and food flavourings. The oil is increasingly replacing more toxic insecticides to combat plant pests, and may have a future in high-energy, aviation biofuels. Eucalyptus oil's cooling, calming quality is much sought after by fragrance manufacturers. It can have quite pungent notes of camphor and citrus, depending on the gum tree species, and overwhelm other scents, but it is often used to mask undesired notes from other ingredients.

Bark and leaves

As a dominant plant in Australian ecosystems, gum trees provided many resources to First Australians. The bark of southern blue gum and other species peels off in strips, ridding the tree of external insect pests, lichens, and mosses, but also providing material for canoes. Blue gum trunks are made into didgeridoos, spears, and boomerangs. Many eucalyptus species have round juvenile leaves, while mature leaves are long and sickle-shaped. Gumleaf musicians play mature eucalypt leaves by vibrating them against the lips; the song in the past lured wild birds for capture.

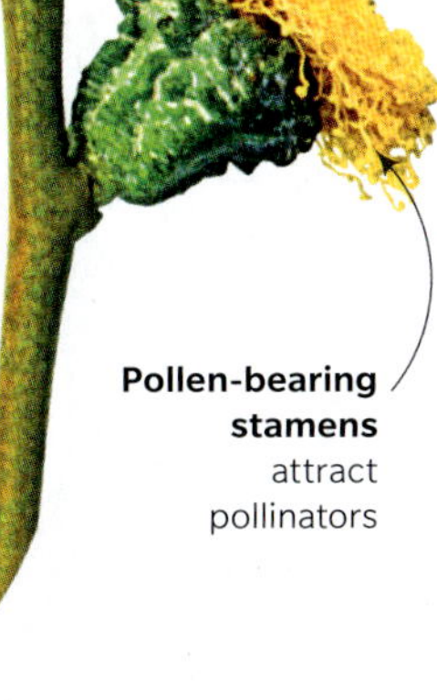

► Blue gum flowers
Eucalypt petals and sepals fuse to form a cap, or calyptra, which is shed when each flower opens to reveal the stamens (here, the leaves have been removed, for clarity).

Pollen-bearing stamens attract pollinators

Australia's tallest tree is a eucalyptus, a specimen of *Eucalyptus regnans* reaching over 100 m (328 ft)

BREATHING EASY

Eucalyptus oil evaporates readily, so is easily drawn into the lungs. Its decongestant and anti-inflammatory properties may be used to fight bacterial infections, reduce mucus and inflammation, as well as treat respiratory conditions, as with this hospital patient breathing in eucalyptus vapour in the 1930s.

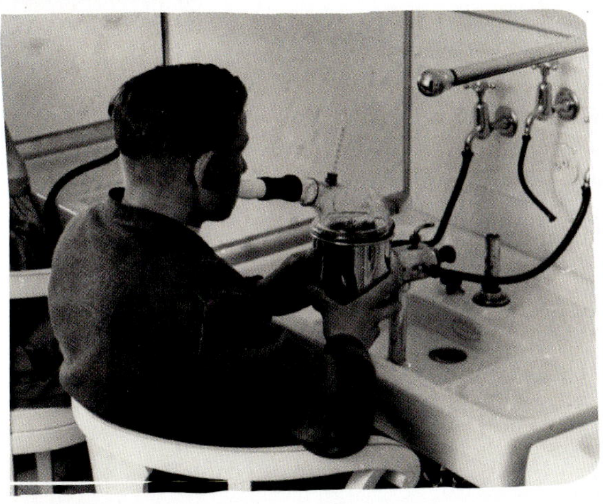

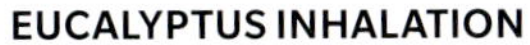

EUCALYPTUS INHALATION

Southern blue gum grows fast – up to 2.5 m (8 ft) a year, so its wood is **pulped** to **produce paper**

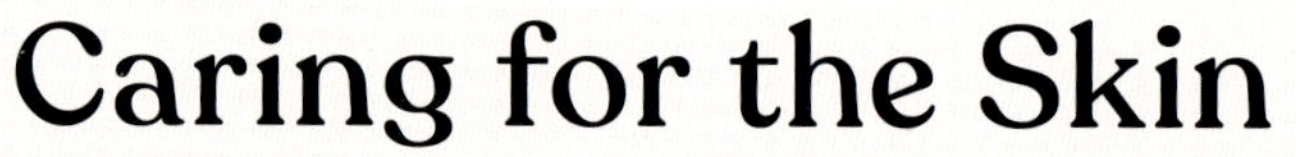

Caring for the Skin

Herbs have been used to soothe and beautify skin for thousands of years, through topical oils, balms, salves and poultices, or through antioxidant-rich teas, tinctures, and tonics. Many herbs are naturally antibacterial, antifungal, and anti-inflammatory, helping to heal irritation and wounds.

Pot marigold
Calendula officinalis
Extract of flowers; anti-inflammatory, antifungal, and antibacterial; plumps and softens skin; soothes eczema and nappy rash.

Witch hazel
Hamamelis virginiana
Extract of leaves, bark, or twigs; astringent, anti-inflammatory, and antioxidant to sooth irritation, removes oil, and tightens pores.

St John's wort
Hypericum perforatum
Flower tops; anti-inflammatory, antimicrobial, and astringent; used to heal wounds, sooth sunburn, and treat bruises and minor swellings.

Birch
Betula pendula
Extract of twigs and leaves; astringent, anti-inflammatory, and antibacterial; soothes sensitive and irritated skin and insect bites.

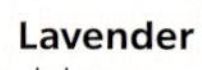

Lavender
Lavandula angustifolia
Essential oil from flowering tops; an anti-inflammatory, antimicrobial, and analgesic; helps heal minor burns, insect bites, and wounds.

Arnica
Arnica montana
Ointment made from flowers or rhizomes; anti-inflammatory; helps heal minor wounds, bruises, and insect bites.

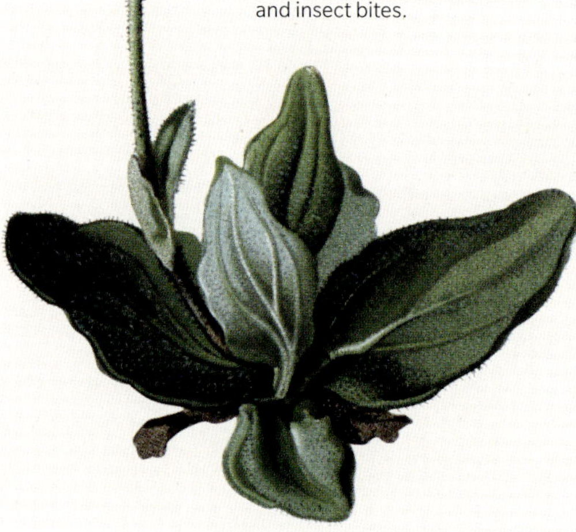

Oats
Avena sativa
Seed milk (colloidal oatmeal); emollient, anti-inflammatory, and antioxidant; moisturizes and maintains skin barrier, soothes dryness, and reduces itching and acne.

Evening primrose
Oenothera biennis
Seed oil; emollient and anti-inflammatory; hydrates, improves elasticity, and relieves itching and dryness.

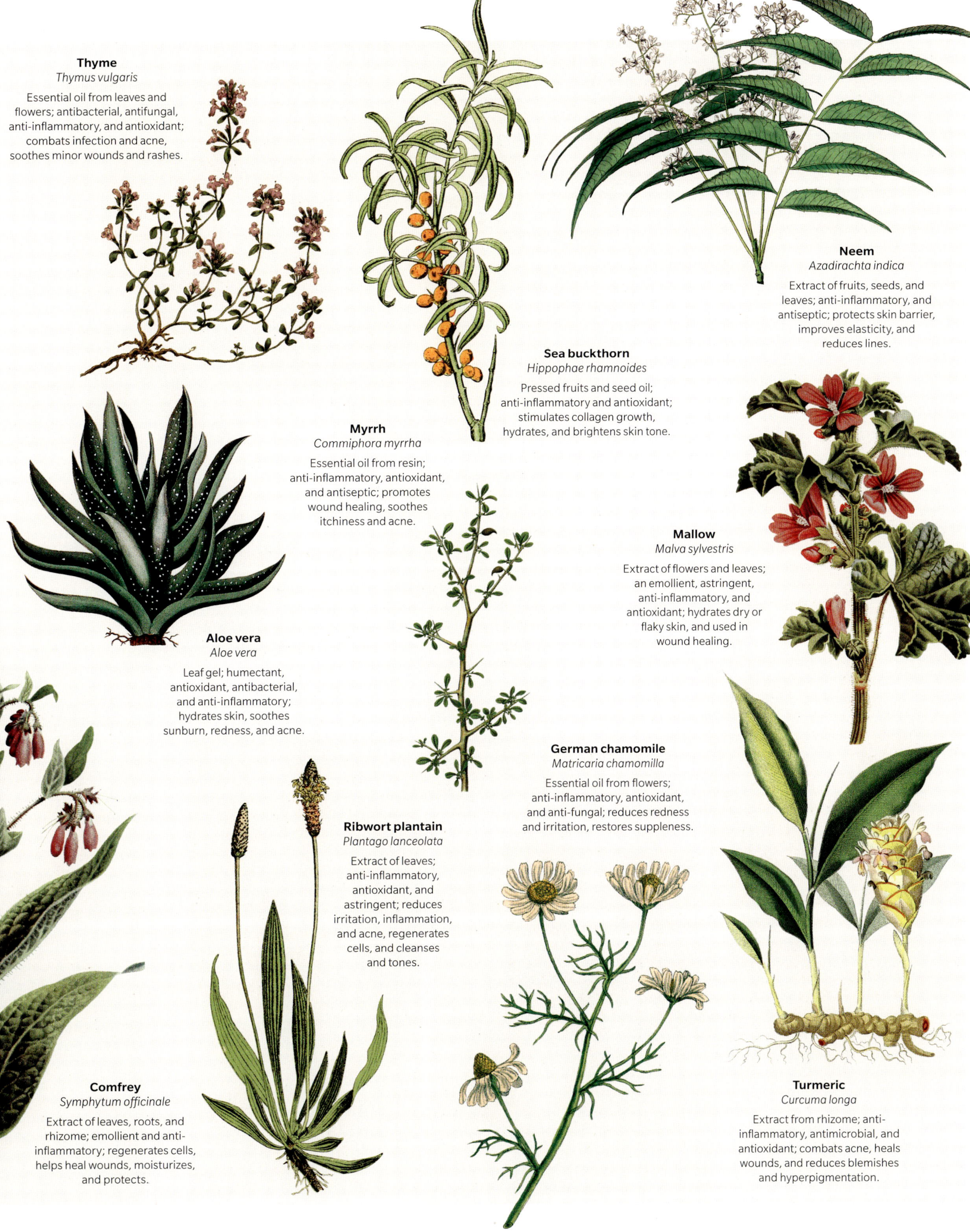

Thyme
Thymus vulgaris
Essential oil from leaves and flowers; antibacterial, antifungal, anti-inflammatory, and antioxidant; combats infection and acne, soothes minor wounds and rashes.

Neem
Azadirachta indica
Extract of fruits, seeds, and leaves; anti-inflammatory, and antiseptic; protects skin barrier, improves elasticity, and reduces lines.

Sea buckthorn
Hippophae rhamnoides
Pressed fruits and seed oil; anti-inflammatory and antioxidant; stimulates collagen growth, hydrates, and brightens skin tone.

Myrrh
Commiphora myrrha
Essential oil from resin; anti-inflammatory, antioxidant, and antiseptic; promotes wound healing, soothes itchiness and acne.

Mallow
Malva sylvestris
Extract of flowers and leaves; an emollient, astringent, anti-inflammatory, and antioxidant; hydrates dry or flaky skin, and used in wound healing.

Aloe vera
Aloe vera
Leaf gel; humectant, antioxidant, antibacterial, and anti-inflammatory; hydrates skin, soothes sunburn, redness, and acne.

German chamomile
Matricaria chamomilla
Essential oil from flowers; anti-inflammatory, antioxidant, and anti-fungal; reduces redness and irritation, restores suppleness.

Ribwort plantain
Plantago lanceolata
Extract of leaves; anti-inflammatory, antioxidant, and astringent; reduces irritation, inflammation, and acne, regenerates cells, and cleanses and tones.

Comfrey
Symphytum officinale
Extract of leaves, roots, and rhizome; emollient and anti-inflammatory; regenerates cells, helps heal wounds, moisturizes, and protects.

Turmeric
Curcuma longa
Extract from rhizome; anti-inflammatory, antimicrobial, and antioxidant; combats acne, heals wounds, and reduces blemishes and hyperpigmentation.

Uses Medicines, cooking, insect repellent, shade

Parts used Seeds, oil, leaves, flowers, bark

Active ingredients Limonoids, including azadirachtin, coumarins, glycerides

Habitat Well-drained, deep sandy soils, even in polluted urban areas

> " Considered a pharmacy in its own right in India, every part used medicinally. "
>
> ANDREW CHEVALLIER, *The Encyclopedia of Medicinal Plants*, 1996

Neem

Azadirachta indica

Related to mahogany, neem is a fast-growing tree that is native to Asia. The plant is used in cooking, in animal food, and as a poison, but is most valued for its numerous medicinal properties.

Powdered leaves are a bitter tonic for the prevention of infections

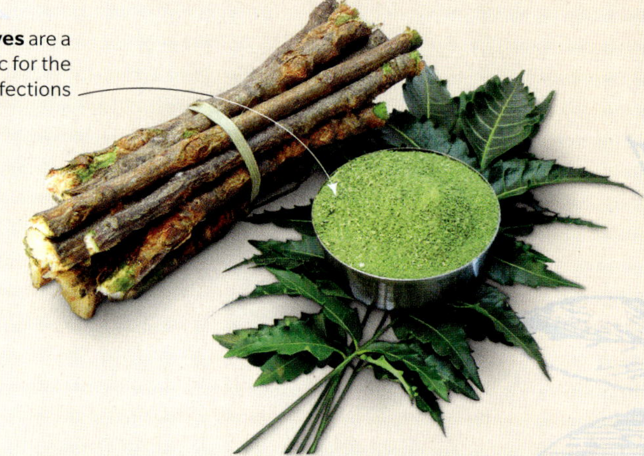

▲ **The neem pharmacy** All parts of the neem plant are valued in Ayurvedic medicine, from leaf juice to toothbrush twigs.

Neem grows wild in forests from Bangladesh to Vietnam, and is widely planted in India where it is used in medicine and as a shade tree in city streets. Because it can tolerate high temperatures, drought, and polluted groundwater, neem is also grown for shade in low rainfall areas of other tropical countries. In parts of the Middle East, sub-Saharan Africa, and tropical Australia, however, it has become a troublesome weed.

Since early times, neem has been a key plant in the traditional Ayurvedic medicine of India, where it is known as *nimba*, and Nepal. Infusions of its leaves are regarded as a powerful treatment against malaria, diabetes, intestinal worms, and skin diseases. An extract from its leaves is used to reduce plaque.

Insecticidal properties

In India, Europe, and elsewhere, neem seed oil is added to hair dressings to banish lice and mites. Dried leaves are left in cupboards to stop insects attacking clothes, in libraries to prevent insect damage to books, and in rice storage tins. Leaves and flowers are eaten in salads, usually mixed with other herbs to make them more palatable, and in a bitter Bengali vegetable dish called *shukto*.

Limited scientific studies suggest neem oil has anti-inflammatory, antibacterial, and anti-cancer properties. In common with other Ayurvedic medications, there is concern that Western drug companies are researching the benefits of neem and applying patents to restrict its commercial use, without giving recompense to the countries where it has been used for generations. Neem seeds contain up to 40 per cent oil, so offer potential in biodiesel production.

◄ **Traditional medicine** In traditional Ayurvedic medicine, local healers grind neem leaves and mix them with other herbs and minerals, according to the specific ailment to be treated.

Similar herbs

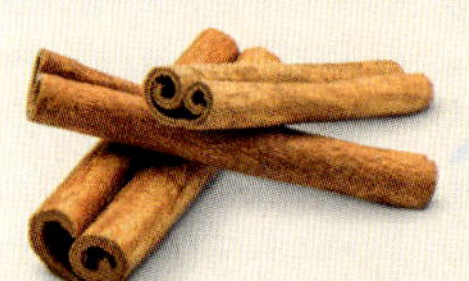

CINNAMON
Cinnamomum verum
This evergreen tree is native to Sri Lanka. Cinnamon is a widely traded spice, used to flavour curries and more. It is also a traditional remedy for digestive problems.

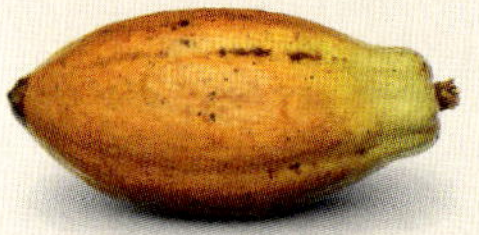

CACAO
Theobroma cacao
Chocolate is made from the ground roasted seeds of the cacao tree. The pulped seed is a stimulant to the nervous system, taken to treat angina and high blood pressure.

Leaf made up of asymmetric toothed leaflets
Dense cluster of small, white, fragrant flowers
Straight stems with bitter, astringent bark
Human-like round belly

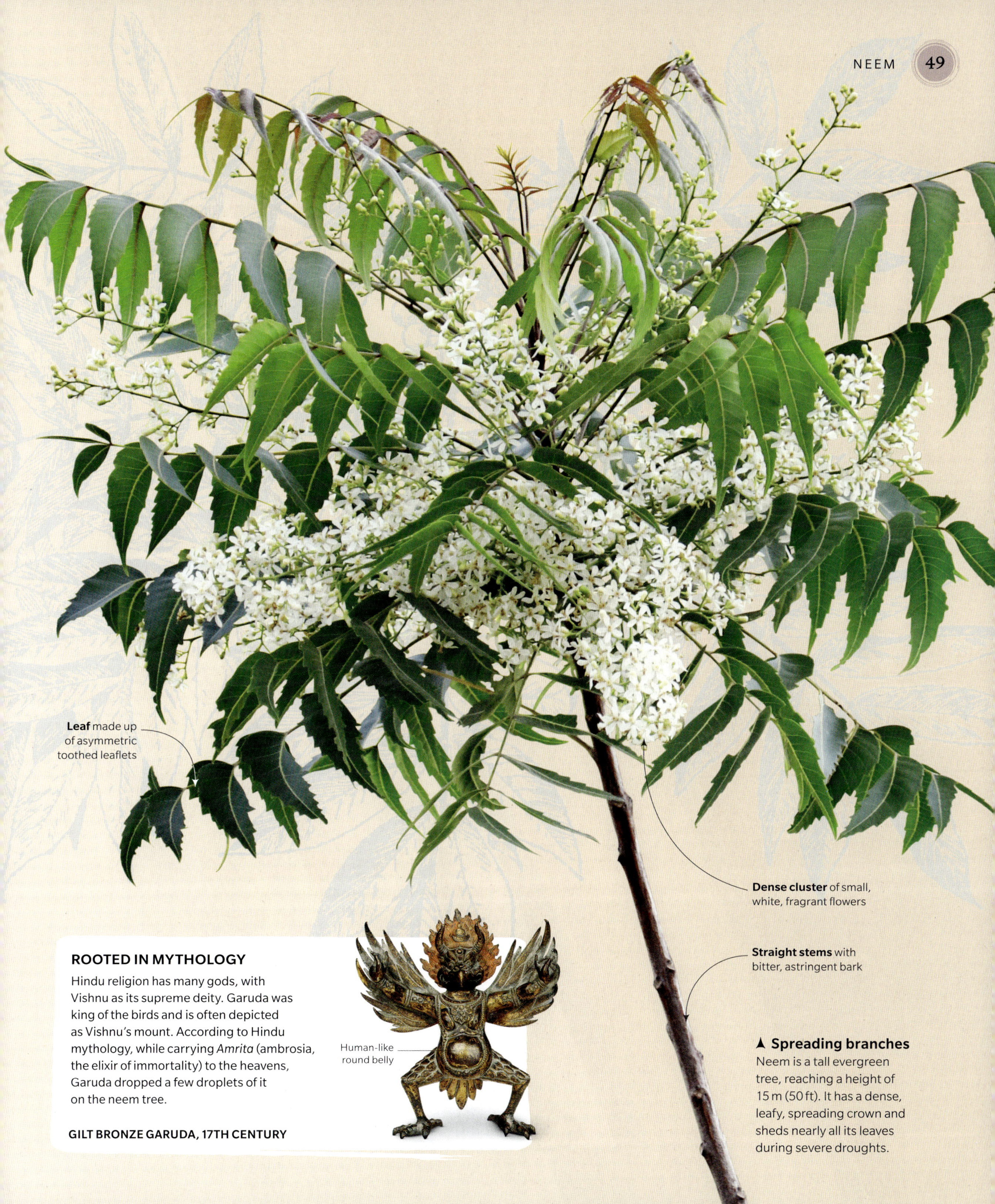

ROOTED IN MYTHOLOGY

Hindu religion has many gods, with Vishnu as its supreme deity. Garuda was king of the birds and is often depicted as Vishnu's mount. According to Hindu mythology, while carrying *Amrita* (ambrosia, the elixir of immortality) to the heavens, Garuda dropped a few droplets of it on the neem tree.

GILT BRONZE GARUDA, 17TH CENTURY

▲ Spreading branches
Neem is a tall evergreen tree, reaching a height of 15 m (50 ft). It has a dense, leafy, spreading crown and sheds nearly all its leaves during severe droughts.

Tea Tree

Melaleuca alternifolia

First Australians have utilized tea tree and its volatile compounds for centuries. However, what was once a local product is now being mass produced, and can be found in medicine cabinets around the world.

Uses Medicines for skin ailments; horticulture, honey-production

Parts used Leaves, wood

Active ingredients Terpinen-4-ol, terpinene, 1,8-cineole, terpinolene

Habitat Low-lying coastal swamps and rivers

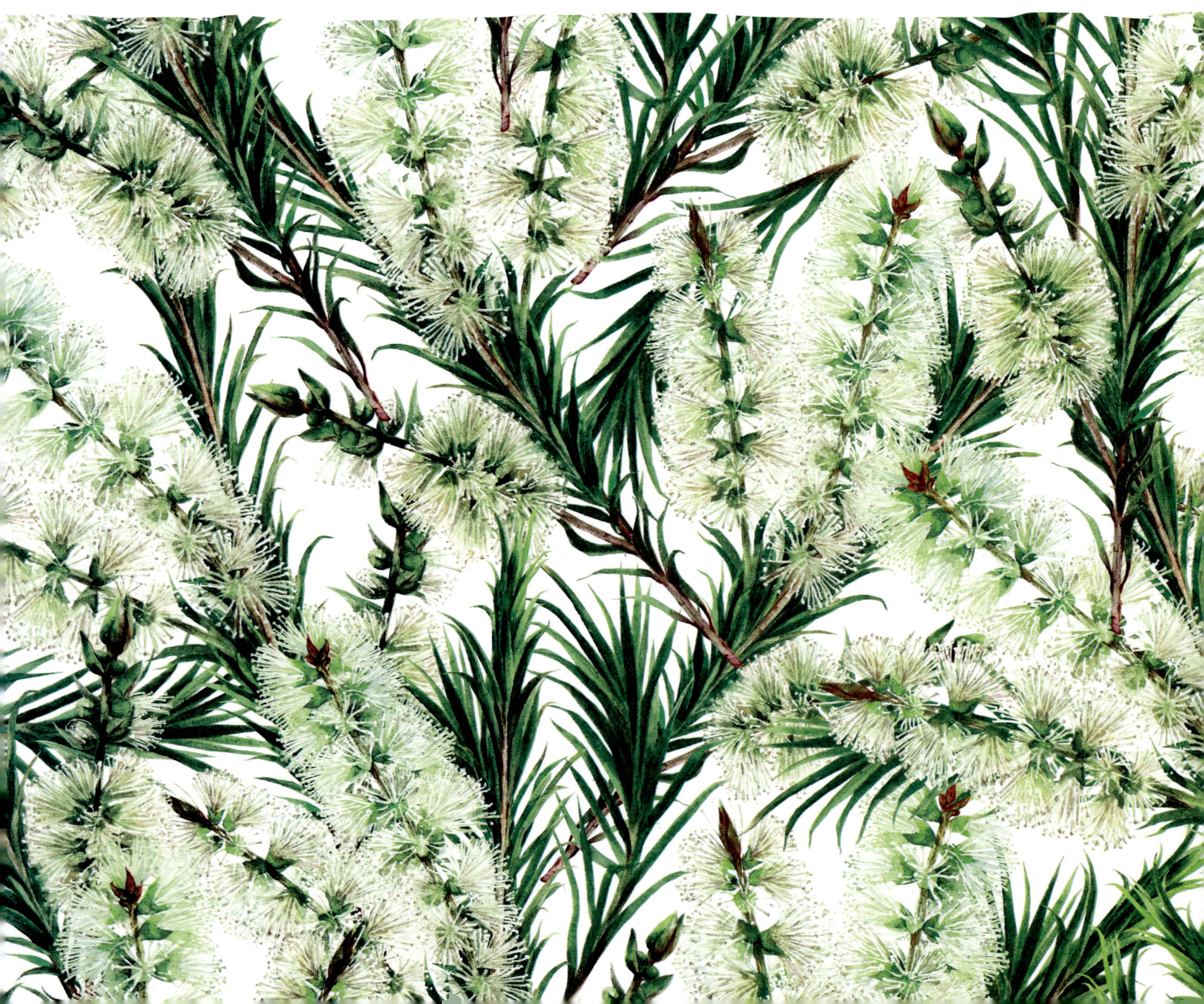

Tea tree, also known as narrow-leaved paperbark, is an evergreen shrub or small tree with a limited distribution in northeast New South Wales and southeast Queensland. Its common name may have been coined by British naval officer Captain James Cook, who prepared a tea from the leaves imitating the First Australians' use of the plant. Several other Australian *Melaleuca* species are also known as tea tree, as are species of *Leptospermum*, which also occur in New Zealand, where they are the source of manuka honey. But *M. alternifolia* remains the most commercially significant source of tea tree essential oil.

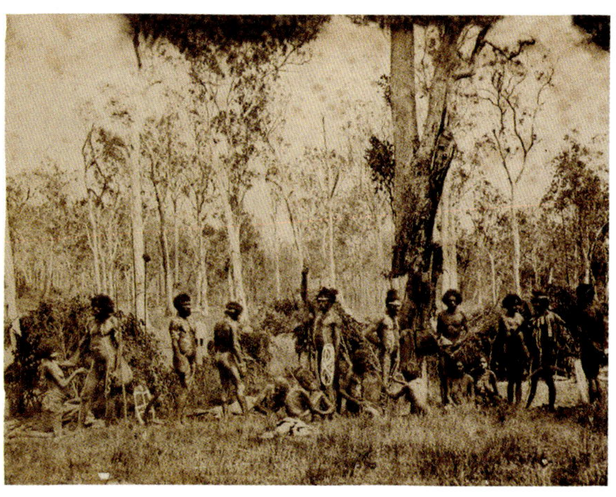

▲ Bandjalang people, c.19th century
As the original custodians of tea tree's native territory, the Bandjalang people have long utilized its medicinal properties.

Aromatic oils from Australia

Tea tree is a member of the same family as Eucalyptus (see pp.42–45) and both are known for their pungent essential oils, the benefits of which have been known to First Australians for centuries. The Bandjalang people treated coughs and colds by inhaling the vapour released from heated tea tree leaves and applied a poultice of crushed leaves to remedy skin conditions.

Scientific studies have demonstrated tea tree oil's antibacterial, antifungal, and antiseptic properties, and it is now produced commercially from *M. alternifolia* and other *Melaleuca* species. In addition to Australia, countries such as Egypt, Vietnam, and the US produce this oil. Species such as *M. cajuputi* are an important crop in several countries for their yield of the medicinal Cajuput oil. Other uses of tea tree oil include hair and skin care, as a cleansing agent for hands and surfaces, and as an insect repellent. It is also thought to be beneficial in the treatment of fungal skin conditions such as athlete's foot and nail fungus.

Tea tree wood is a locally important product as well. Durable in water, it is useful for making boats, flooring, and marine pilings – poles that bear structural weight. The wood is said to be termite-resistant, and tea tree wood chips are used as mulch to keep these insects away from homes. Several Melaleuca species are important garden plants, including bottlebrushes (previously in the genus *Callistemon*), while paperbark tea tree (*M. quinquenervia*) has become a significant invasive species in the Florida Everglades in the US.

Similar herbs

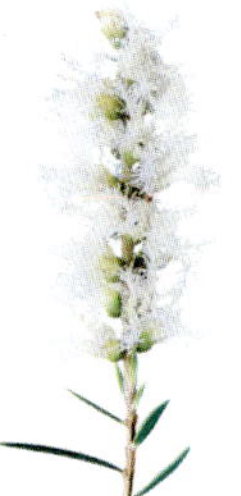

NARROW-LEAF PAPERBARK
Melaleuca linariifolia
Also known as snow-in-summer for its white blooms, this eastern Australia tea tree is a drought-tolerant alternative to *M. alternifolia*.

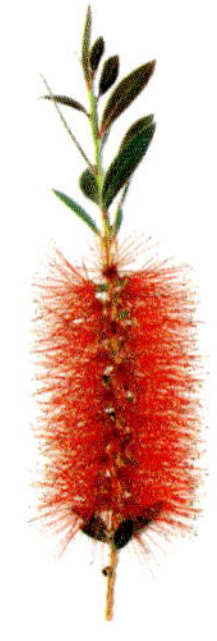

CRIMSON BOTTLEBRUSH
Melaleuca citrina
This eastern Australia ornamental has antifungal and antibacterial properties, and a modified form of leptospermone from its roots is used as a herbicide.

◄ White blossoms
The white flowers of tea tree derive their aesthetic appeal from the fluffy, white stamens, which carry the pollen. The petals are 2–3 mm (less than 1/10 in) long and difficult to see. The leaves of *M. alternifolia* are smaller in real life than depicted here.

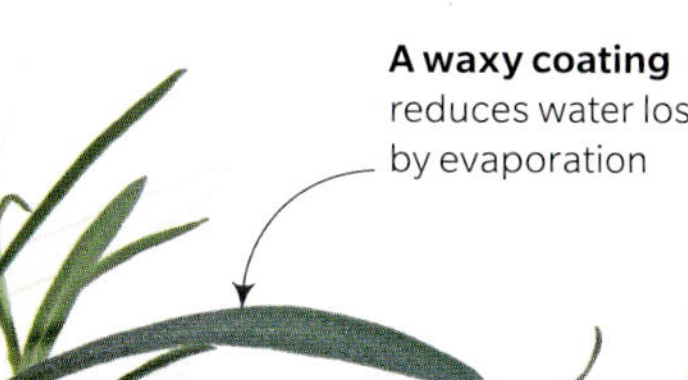

A waxy coating reduces water loss by evaporation

► Medicinal leaves
The leaves of tea tree and related species are rich in essential oil, produced from glands on both sides of the leaf, and extracted via steam distillation.

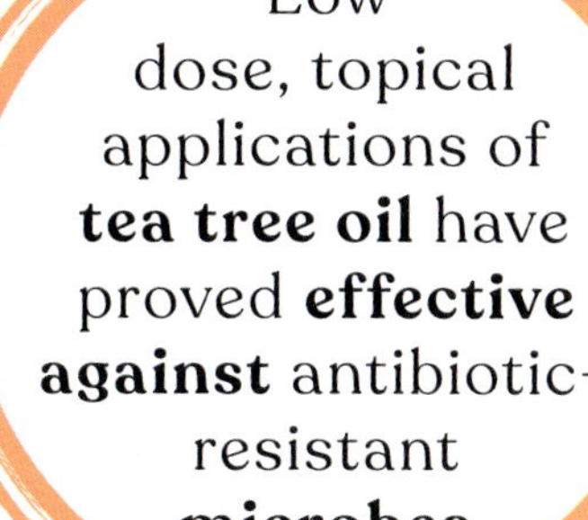

Low dose, topical applications of **tea tree oil** have proved **effective against** antibiotic-resistant **microbes**

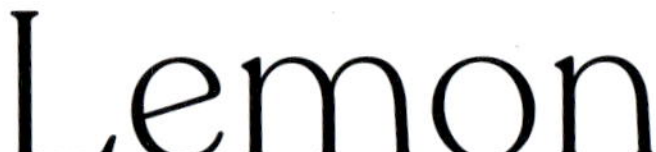

Uses Medicines for digestion; infusions, cooking; scents, cosmetics

Parts used Mainly fruits (including skins); leaves and flowers

Active ingredients Citric acid, ascorbic acid, hesperidin, D-limonene, diosmin

Habitat Not known in the wild; cultivated in tropical, subtropical, and Mediterranean regions

" It is probable that the lemon is the most valuable of all fruit for preserving health. "

MRS M. GRIEVE,
A Modern Herbal, Vol. II, 1931

Lemon

Citrus × limon

As it is a multipurpose plant, lemon has been a valued commodity for centuries. While the leaves and flowers have their uses, it is the fruits that are commercially significant.

Leaves release essential oils from surface glands

Lemons originated in Asia, from hybridization between citron (*Citrus medica*) and bitter or Seville orange (*C.* × *aurantium*). They first arrived in Europe during the time of the Roman Empire and travelled to the New World with Columbus. Now, lemons are cultivated around the globe.

The medicinal value of lemons is largely the result of two acids, citric and ascorbic (also known as vitamin C), considerable quantities of which can be found in the fruits. Lemon juice has more citric acid than almost any other citrus fruit, which accounts for the sour taste. Citric acid is a useful disinfectant, food additive (used as an emulsifier, flavouring, or preservative), and component of cosmetics. It was originally produced from lemons, but can now be synthesized artificially.

◄ **Citric-acid crystals**
Extracting citric acid, one of the active ingredients of lemon juice, involves a chemical purification process and crystallization.

Large crystals such as these are usually ground finer for use as a food additive

Sailors, scurvy, and ascorbic acid

Vitamin C is an antioxidant and helps collagen formation, tissue repair, and immune-system function in the body. Most animals produce their own vitamin C, but humans must ingest it as part of their diet. The disease scurvy results from insufficient vitamin C in the diet; symptoms include bleeding gums, lethargy, reopening of wounds, and aching joints. Scurvy is now uncommon, but was a leading cause of death for European sailors during the Age of Sail (late-15th to mid-19th centuries), when fresh fruit and vegetables were in short supply on long sea voyages. Once it was shown that sailors who were given lemon juice had very low incidences of scurvy, the UK's Royal Navy provided the juice regularly.

The lemon, especially the peel, is also a rich source of flavonoids, such as hesperidin, which act as antioxidants to fight the signs of ageing. They may aid vitamin-C absorption, help boost the immune system, and improve gastrointestinal function.

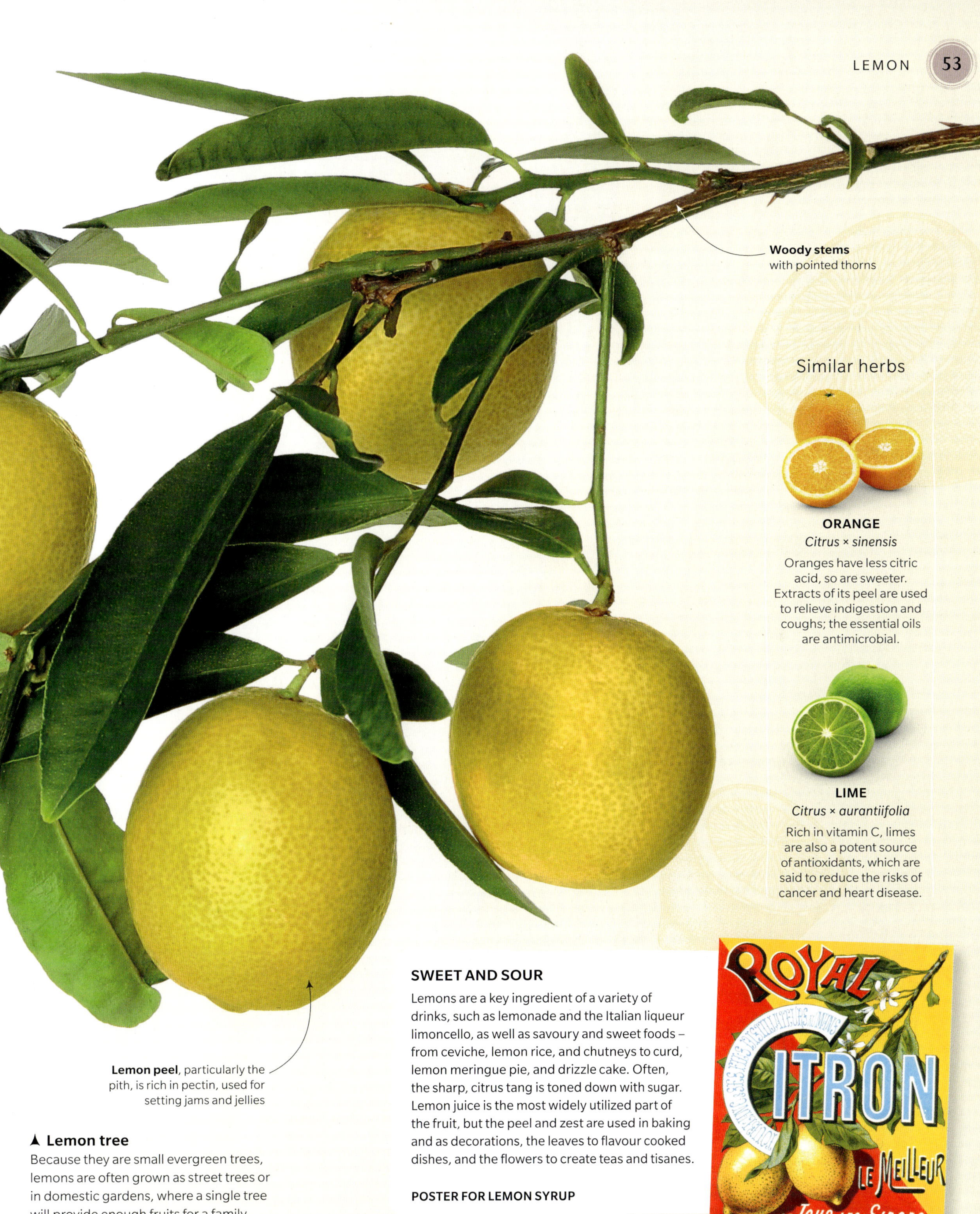

Woody stems with pointed thorns

Lemon peel, particularly the pith, is rich in pectin, used for setting jams and jellies

Similar herbs

ORANGE
Citrus × sinensis
Oranges have less citric acid, so are sweeter. Extracts of its peel are used to relieve indigestion and coughs; the essential oils are antimicrobial.

LIME
Citrus × aurantiifolia
Rich in vitamin C, limes are also a potent source of antioxidants, which are said to reduce the risks of cancer and heart disease.

▲ Lemon tree
Because they are small evergreen trees, lemons are often grown as street trees or in domestic gardens, where a single tree will provide enough fruits for a family.

SWEET AND SOUR

Lemons are a key ingredient of a variety of drinks, such as lemonade and the Italian liqueur limoncello, as well as savoury and sweet foods – from ceviche, lemon rice, and chutneys to curd, lemon meringue pie, and drizzle cake. Often, the sharp, citrus tang is toned down with sugar. Lemon juice is the most widely utilized part of the fruit, but the peel and zest are used in baking and as decorations, the leaves to flavour cooked dishes, and the flowers to create teas and tisanes.

POSTER FOR LEMON SYRUP

FEMALE FLOWERS
Young stems have green bark that later turns grey

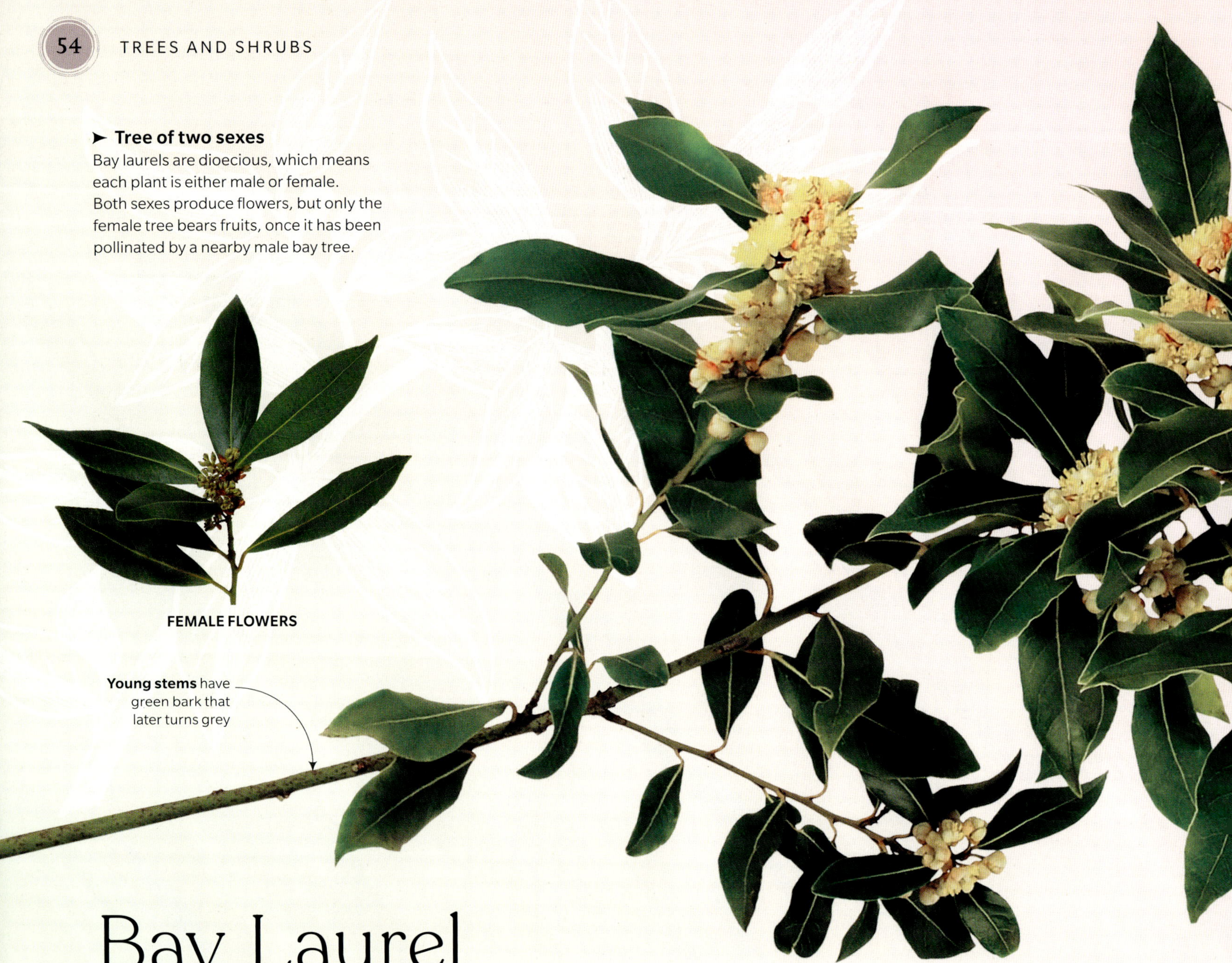

➤ Tree of two sexes
Bay laurels are dioecious, which means each plant is either male or female. Both sexes produce flowers, but only the female tree bears fruits, once it has been pollinated by a nearby male bay tree.

Bay Laurel

Laurus nobilis

Among the cultures of the ancient Mediterranean, bay laurel was an iconic tree symbolizing victory; its leaves provided the wreaths worn by Roman emperors and Greek gods. However, today it is best known as a culinary herb.

Bay leaves are widely used to flavour foods such as meat and fish dishes, soups, and pasta sauces. While bay leaves are often used dried, fresh leaves have a more pleasing scent, especially when they are torn or crushed. The flavour, a delicate mix of menthol, black pepper, and resinous pine, can be lost in strongly flavoured stews, and the herb is best used in milder dishes such as fish. A bay leaf is a primary ingredient in the *bouquet garni*, a classic European herb seasoning; the leaves are also popular in pickling spices and as garnishes for food and drinks. While technically edible, bay leaves are tough, fibrous,

In modern **Italy**, graduating **university students** still wear **wreaths** of **bay laurel leaves**

Male flowers are slightly larger than female ones and produce pollen
Evergreen leaves are leathery, aromatic, and often have wavy edges

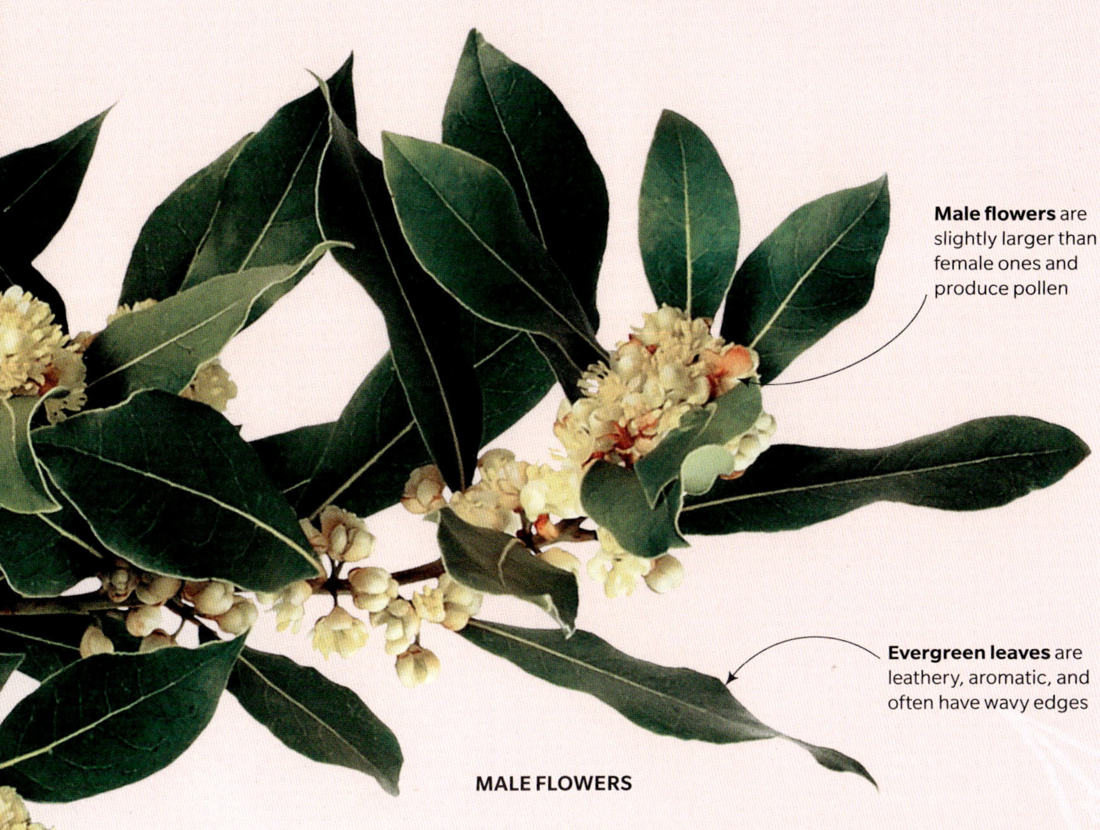

MALE FLOWERS

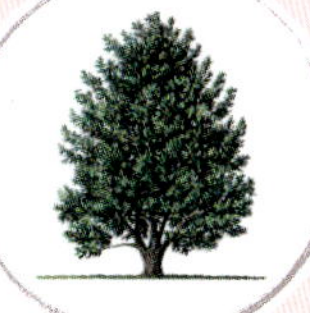

Uses Medicines for digestion and breathing; hygiene products; cooking; cosmetics

Parts used Leaves, fruits

Active ingredients 1,8-cineole, sabinene, pinene, linalool, terpinyl acetate, fatty acids

Habitat Subtropical and warm-temperate evergreen and mixed forest

and unpleasant to chew, so are usually removed prior to eating; the dried leaves may also be ground to a powder.

The laurel berry

The fruits are the source of laurel berry oil, produced from pressing the fresh berries and seeds. The oil is used to dilute more potently scented essential oils, especially in soaps and skin products. A soap from Aleppo in Syria, famed for its purity, traditionally contains laurel berry oil. The soap, also called laurel soap, is made from lye and olive oil, and the laurel berry oil is added just before the soap cools and hardens and is then stored for up to a year.

Medicinal uses

Essential oil derived from bay laurel leaves is extracted by steam distillation; it is typically diluted in a carrier oil for application to the skin or evaporated in a diffuser. In massage and aromatherapy, it is said to benefit those with respiratory conditions and aching joints and muscles. The oil may cause skin

Thwarted in love, Apollo swore always to wear a wreath of bay laurel leaves in tribute to Daphne

Daphne and Apollo

In the Ancient Greek myth, the god Apollo pursued the water nymph Daphne, who spurned his advances. She appealed to her father Peneus, who transformed her into a bay laurel tree to deter Apollo.

irritation, especially in high concentrations. Bay leaves in cooking may also help with digestion. Given its herbal uses, clipped bay trees are common components of formal herb gardens.

Laurels and bays

Bay laurel, also known as bay or sweet bay, is often confused with other plants that have "bay" or "laurel" in their names. *Magnolia virginiana* is called sweet bay in the US, while European *Prunus laurocerasus* is cherry laurel; both have leaves that resemble bay laurel leaves. When harvesting bay laurel, it is vital to select the correct tree. Cherry laurel leaves are rich in natural toxins, which are converted into toxic hydrogen cyanide if the leaves are chewed or crushed.

The lands around the Mediterranean have hot, dry summers, with most rain falling in winter. Bay laurel is among a handful of Mediterranean plants that persist from an earlier climatic period when rainfall was more frequent. During the Paleocene epoch, 65–56 million years ago, what is now the Mediterranean had a tropical climate with regular summer rain and a lush flora. The Eocene followed 55–34 million years ago and heralded a series of ice ages. The tropical flora receded and, today, all that remains are fragments in areas of high rainfall, such as the Canary Islands. Bay laurel is one of the few prehistoric species that adapted to the dryer climatic conditions and its presence in Mediterranean countries such as Greece, Italy, Morocco, and Turkey is a reminder of the rich forests of prehistory. The tree is now grown in temperate climates across Europe, Asia, and North America, and even in South Africa.

Similar herb

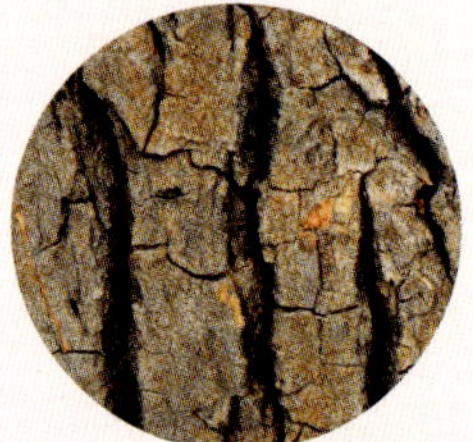

CAMPHOR TREE
Cinnamomum camphora
The bark and wood provides camphor, used in skin medications and as a decongestant, but also in pest deterrents and perfumery.

▼ Ancient Greek goddess Nike
As the goddess of victory in war and competition, Nike is often portrayed wearing a laurel wreath and bearing another symbol of victory, a palm leaf.

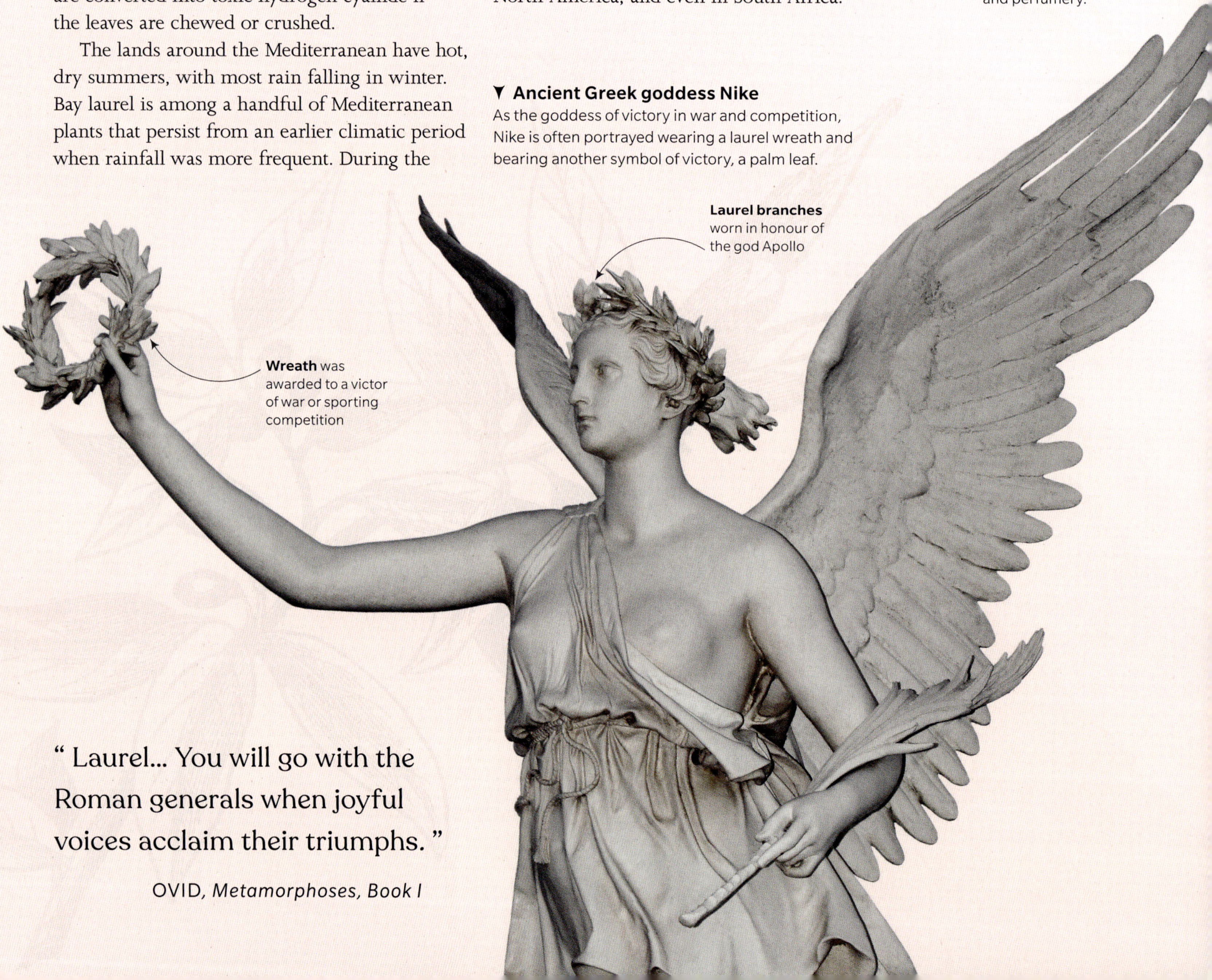

Laurel branches worn in honour of the god Apollo

Wreath was awarded to a victor of war or sporting competition

" Laurel... You will go with the Roman generals when joyful voices acclaim their triumphs. "

OVID, *Metamorphoses, Book I*

Uses Medicines, cooking, crafts, timber, shade tree

Parts used Primarily fleshy pulp from mature seedpods; also wood, leaves, flowers, seeds

Active ingredients Tartaric acid, malic acid, linalool, limonene

Habitat Semi-arid to moist tropical and subtropical woodland and savannas

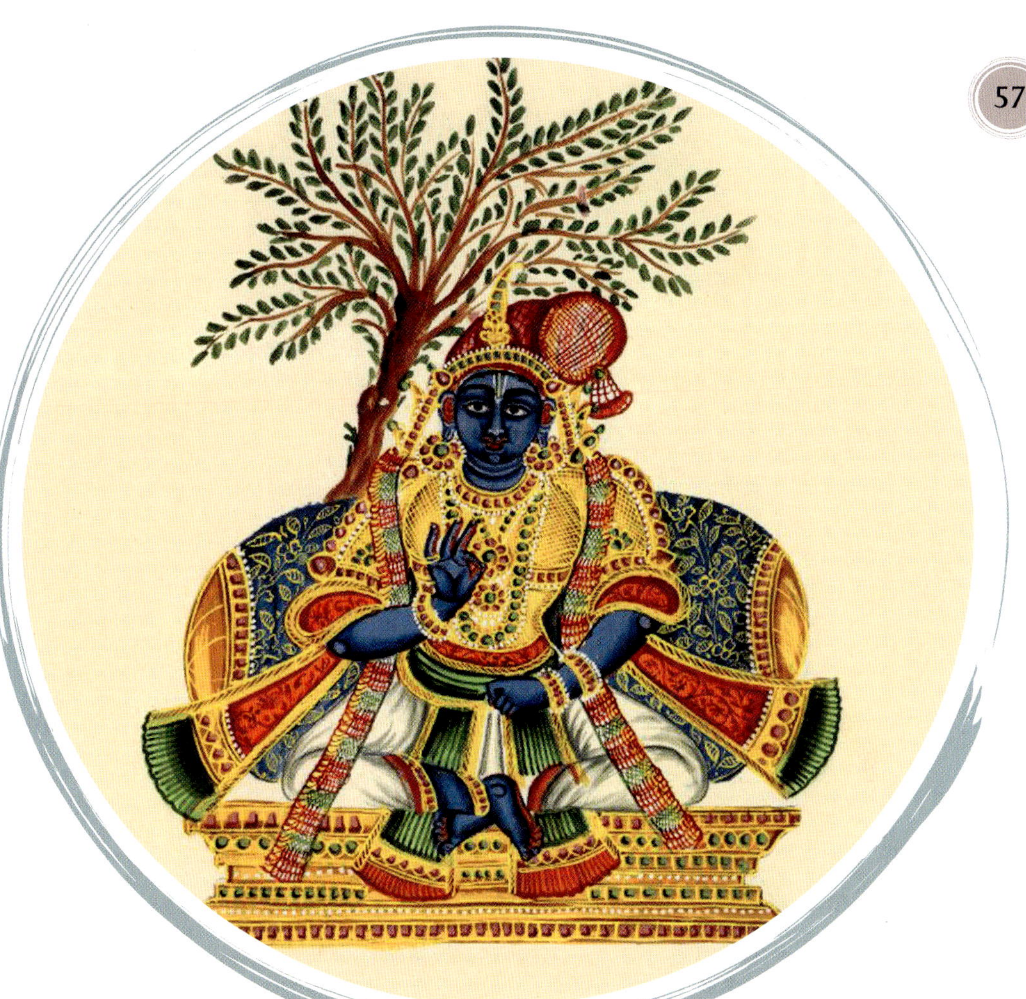

➤ **Saint Nammalvar**
According to religious texts, Hindu mystic Nammalvar spent his life from infancy under the protection of a tamarind tree. He did not speak for many years, until he answered a riddle posed by a scholar.

Tamarind

Tamarindus indica

The name tamarind derives from Arabic and means "Indian date". The tree has long been part of south-Asian culture, but scientists believe it originated in Africa or Madagascar and was then transported to Asia.

Today, tamarind is grown in tropical countries around the world; it is popular because almost every part of the tree has its uses. For the Mahafaly people of southwest Madagascar, tamarind trees are protected by a taboo, or *fady*, due to their enormous value.

Several parts of the tree are edible: tender young leaves flavour Indian dhals and Filipino *sinampalukang manok*, a chicken soup. Tamarind paste, the fleshy pulp around the flat seeds in mature seedpods, has a sour-sweet taste; it is used in Worcester sauce, Mexican candies, and Indian curries and chutney. *Tamarindo* is a popular flavour of *aguas frescas*, soft drinks in Latin America. Even the flowers are added to soups and relishes.

Seed extracts are used to improve digestion, treat dry eyes, and clean teeth; the seed oil is used as a biofuel. Tamarind fruit pulp has been used medicinally as a laxative and the leaves to control parasitic worms. The acidic pulp makes a good metal polish; the leaves and seedpod shells provide fodder; the dense heartwood is popular for making charcoal and for wood crafts. Tamarinds can reach more than 20 m (65 ft) and are valued ornamental shade trees.

➤ **Tamarind branch**
Tamarind trees have evergreen, compound leaves and red-veined, yellow flowers. Its large, fleshy seedpods reveal it to be a member of the bean family, Fabaceae.

" Tamarind rice is still a delicacy – and its preparation still an art form. "

BISHWANATH GHOSH, *Tamarind City*, 2012

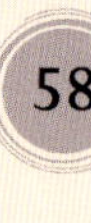

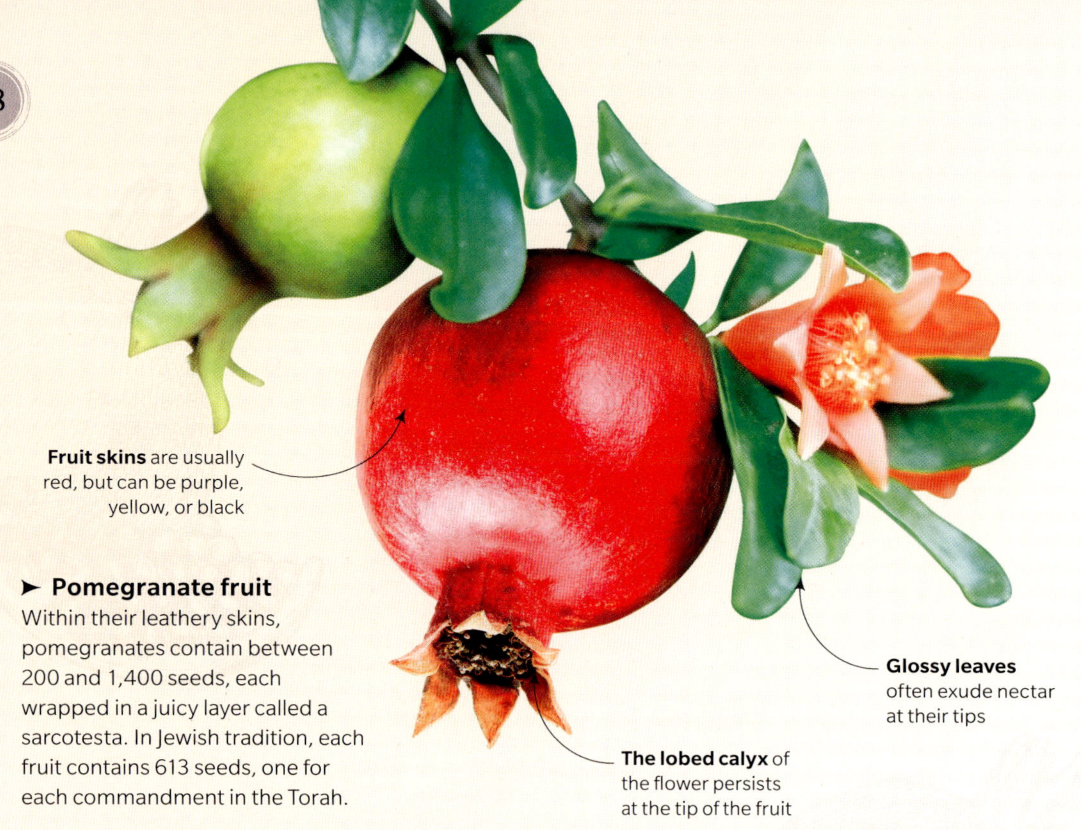

Fruit skins are usually red, but can be purple, yellow, or black

➤ **Pomegranate fruit**
Within their leathery skins, pomegranates contain between 200 and 1,400 seeds, each wrapped in a juicy layer called a sarcotesta. In Jewish tradition, each fruit contains 613 seeds, one for each commandment in the Torah.

The lobed calyx of the flower persists at the tip of the fruit

Glossy leaves often exude nectar at their tips

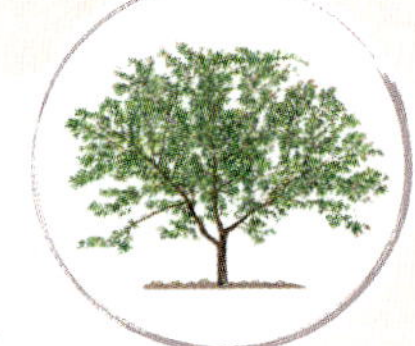

Uses Medicines for bleeding disorders, skin conditions, and dysentery; cooking; horticulture

Parts used Fruits, including juice, seeds, skins; leaves

Active ingredients Ellagic acid, punicic acid, punicalagin, polyphenols

Habitat Dry, limestone soils in scrub forest, in sun at mid- to low elevations

Pomegranate

Punica granatum

Native to central Asia, pomegranates have been cultivated for millennia and feature in traditions across the ancient world, including those of Judaism, Islam, and Christianity.

The early **French** name of ***pomme grenade***, derived from Latin, meant **"many-seeded apple"**

Notable for its bright red fruit, this small tree or shrub has long been used as a source of food and medicine. Remains excavated from Jericho prove that the plant was grown in the Middle East in the Bronze Age. Pomegranates feature in many cultures, especially in the Mediterranean and western Asia. The fruits are smashed in Greece at New Year to bring good luck, are eaten on the Jewish Rosh Hashanah as a sign of righteousness, and appear in paintings as a Christian symbol of resurrection. Black ink from the fruits was used for centuries to dye Oriental carpets. Pomegranate trees also make popular bonsai in Japan.

In Mexico, as an essential ingredient of the celebratory *chiles en nogada* (chillies with walnuts), the red, fleshy seeds represent the red in the Mexican flag. The juice is popular around the world and was the main ingredient of the cocktail syrup grenadine. The dried, fleshy seeds produce the spice *anardana*, used as a souring agent in India, Iran, and Pakistan, while many Middle Eastern dishes include pomegranate molasses. The leaves are infused to make a tea.

In Ayurvedic medicine, pomegranate is known as *dadima* and used to treat ulcers, haemorrhoids, intestinal parasites, dysentery, and diarrhoea. Experiments show that pomegranate extracts may slow or reduce the risk of some cancers and could tackle heart disease and osteoarthritis, but full clinical trials are lacking.

➤ **Iranian manuscript**
The pomegranate is valued in Iranian culture, cuisine, and medicine, symbolizing fertility and immortality. It features here in a 16th-century manuscript, *Javahir al Muusikat I Muhammadi.*

" ... of all trees, [pomegranate] is most salutiferous to mankind. "

PETER COLLINSON, botanist, in a letter, 18th century

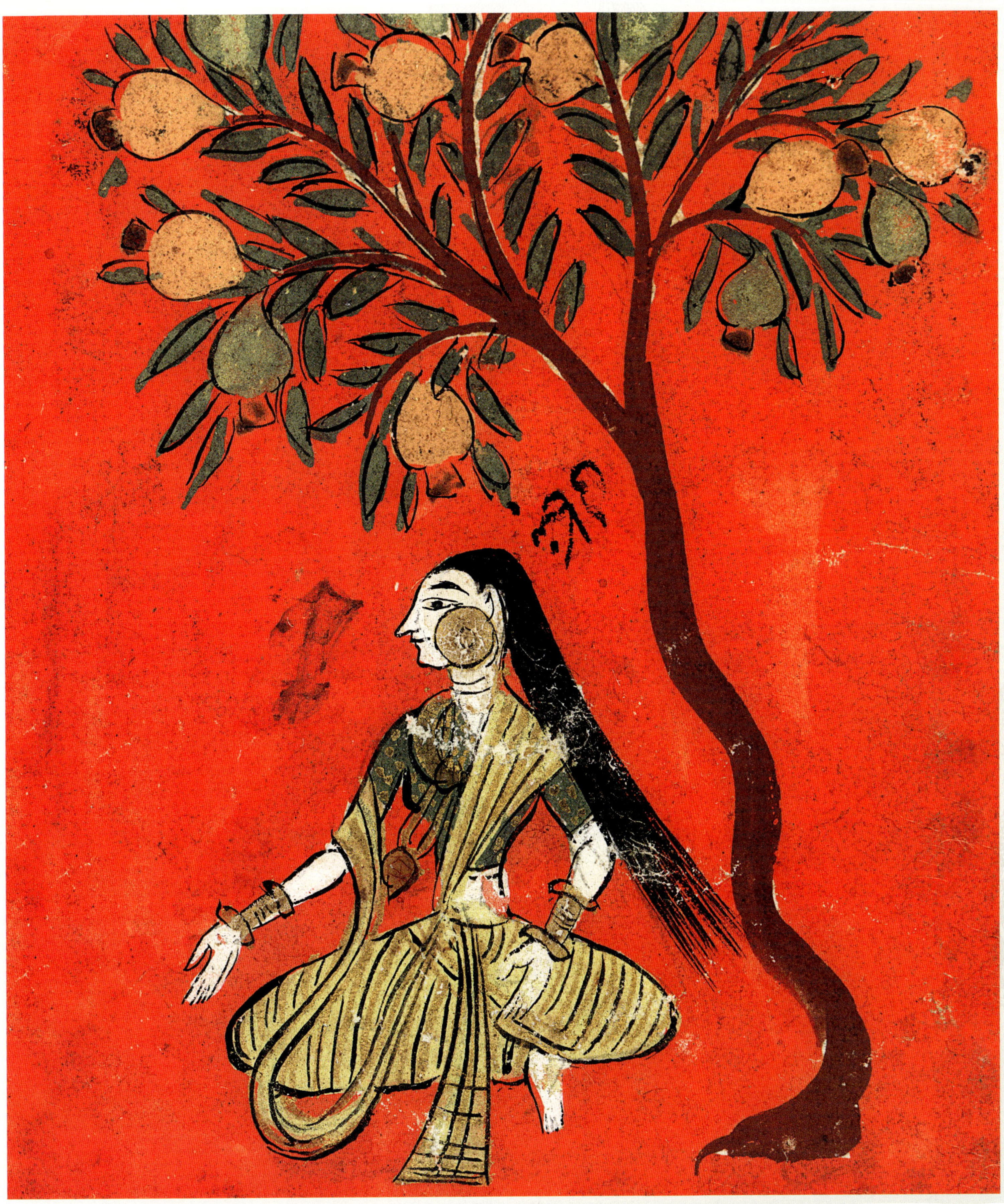

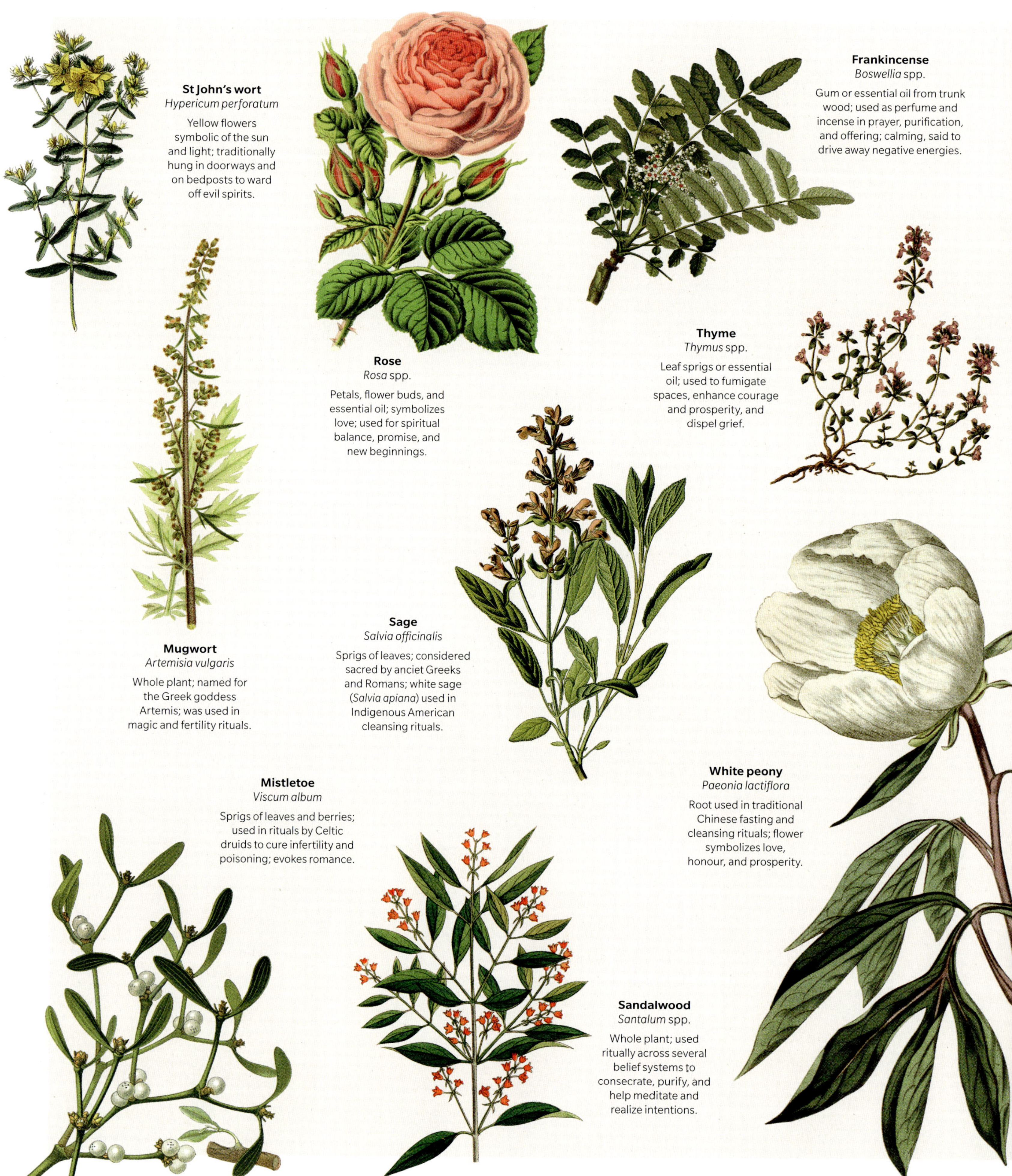

St John's wort
Hypericum perforatum

Yellow flowers symbolic of the sun and light; traditionally hung in doorways and on bedposts to ward off evil spirits.

Rose
Rosa spp.

Petals, flower buds, and essential oil; symbolizes love; used for spiritual balance, promise, and new beginnings.

Frankincense
Boswellia spp.

Gum or essential oil from trunk wood; used as perfume and incense in prayer, purification, and offering; calming, said to drive away negative energies.

Thyme
Thymus spp.

Leaf sprigs or essential oil; used to fumigate spaces, enhance courage and prosperity, and dispel grief.

Mugwort
Artemisia vulgaris

Whole plant; named for the Greek goddess Artemis; was used in magic and fertility rituals.

Sage
Salvia officinalis

Sprigs of leaves; considered sacred by anciet Greeks and Romans; white sage (*Salvia apiana*) used in Indigenous American cleansing rituals.

White peony
Paeonia lactiflora

Root used in traditional Chinese fasting and cleansing rituals; flower symbolizes love, honour, and prosperity.

Mistletoe
Viscum album

Sprigs of leaves and berries; used in rituals by Celtic druids to cure infertility and poisoning; evokes romance.

Sandalwood
Santalum spp.

Whole plant; used ritually across several belief systems to consecrate, purify, and help meditate and realize intentions.

Religion and Ritual

Some of the first uses of herbs were in religion and ritual, from associations with deities to use in cleansing or protection charms. Various parts of these herbs were consumed or used as incense, anointing oils, ceremonial offerings, and garlands.

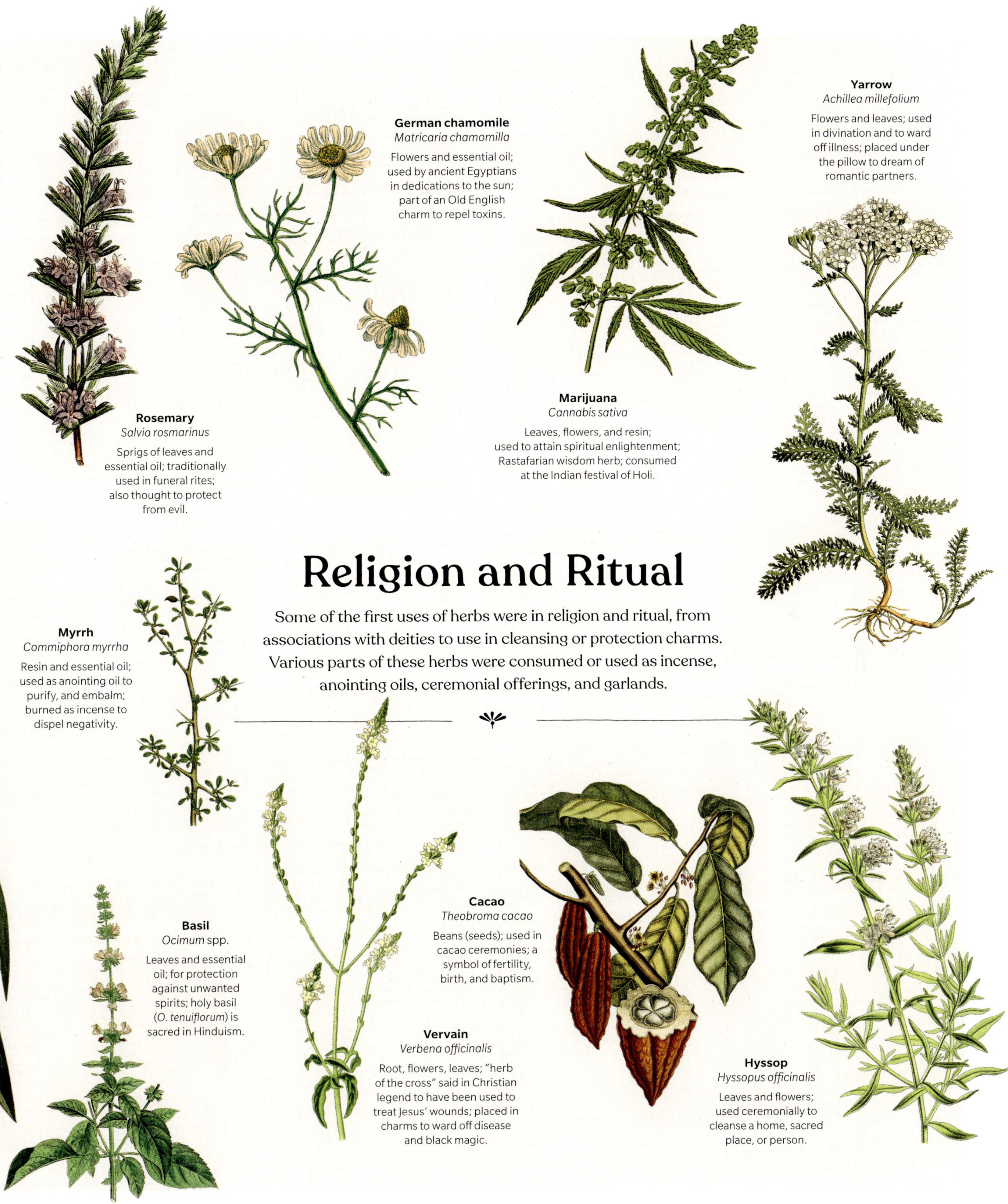

Rosemary
Salvia rosmarinus
Sprigs of leaves and essential oil; traditionally used in funeral rites; also thought to protect from evil.

German chamomile
Matricaria chamomilla
Flowers and essential oil; used by ancient Egyptians in dedications to the sun; part of an Old English charm to repel toxins.

Marijuana
Cannabis sativa
Leaves, flowers, and resin; used to attain spiritual enlightenment; Rastafarian wisdom herb; consumed at the Indian festival of Holi.

Yarrow
Achillea millefolium
Flowers and leaves; used in divination and to ward off illness; placed under the pillow to dream of romantic partners.

Myrrh
Commiphora myrrha
Resin and essential oil; used as anointing oil to purify, and embalm; burned as incense to dispel negativity.

Basil
Ocimum spp.
Leaves and essential oil; for protection against unwanted spirits; holy basil (*O. tenuiflorum*) is sacred in Hinduism.

Vervain
Verbena officinalis
Root, flowers, leaves; "herb of the cross" said in Christian legend to have been used to treat Jesus' wounds; placed in charms to ward off disease and black magic.

Cacao
Theobroma cacao
Beans (seeds); used in cacao ceremonies; a symbol of fertility, birth, and baptism.

Hyssop
Hyssopus officinalis
Leaves and flowers; used ceremonially to cleanse a home, sacred place, or person.

Uses Medicines, cosmetics, cooking

Parts used Flowers, fruit

Active ingredients Anthocyanins, flavonoids, phenolic acids, polyphenols, vitamin C

Habitat Woodland, hedgerows, scrub, wasteland

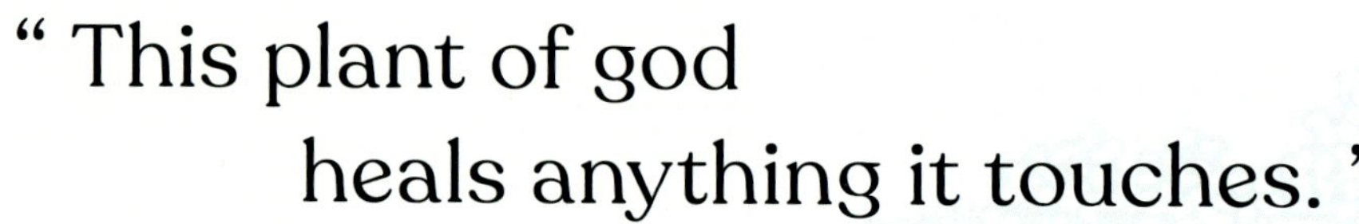

“ This plant of god heals anything it touches. ”

HIPPOCRATES,
Greek physician, 460–370 BCE

Elder

Sambucus nigra

An unremarkable plant for most of the year, this multipurpose hedgerow shrub comes into its own each summer with clusters of scented flowers and immune system-boosting berries.

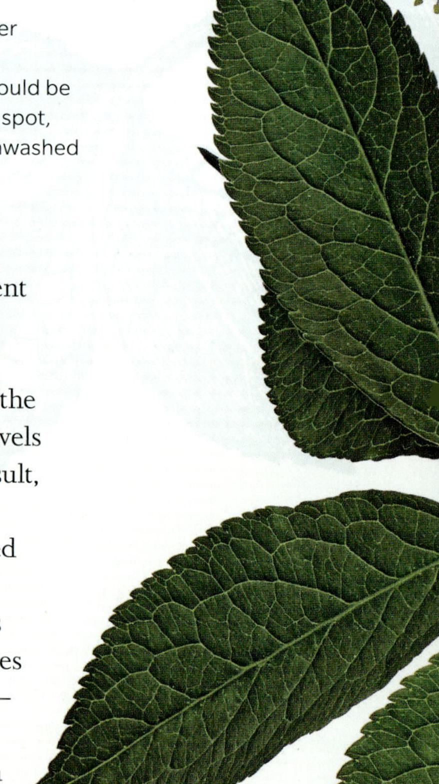

Leaves are toxic and ingesting them can induce vomiting. More serious symptoms are also possible

► Elder in flower
It takes around 20 elderflower heads to make about 4 litres (135 fl oz) of cordial. They should be picked from a pollution-free spot, free from insects, and left unwashed to preserve the fragrance.

Before the rise of modern medicine in the 19th century, certain plants were considered something of a rural medicine chest, with various parts harvested and prepared for a range of ailments, from coughs and colds to highly infectious or even fatal diseases. Elder was one such herb. In medieval times, its leaves, stems, roots, and bark were employed to purge fevers or expel phlegm – known as choler (angry bile).

The creamy-white, lacy flowers were used to perfume cordials and wines, and the subsequent clusters of deep red-purple berries were transformed into health-boosting robs (see below) and syrups, or jams and jellies. Today, the leaves and stems are known to contain high levels of toxic cyanide-producing glycosides. As a result, these parts are largely avoided and modern medicines concentrate on the benefits delivered by the blossoms and berries.

Scientific research has revealed elderberries to be antioxidant and antiviral. These properties are largely due to high levels of anthocyanins – plant pigments that give red, blue, or purple fruits their colouring. The berries are also rich

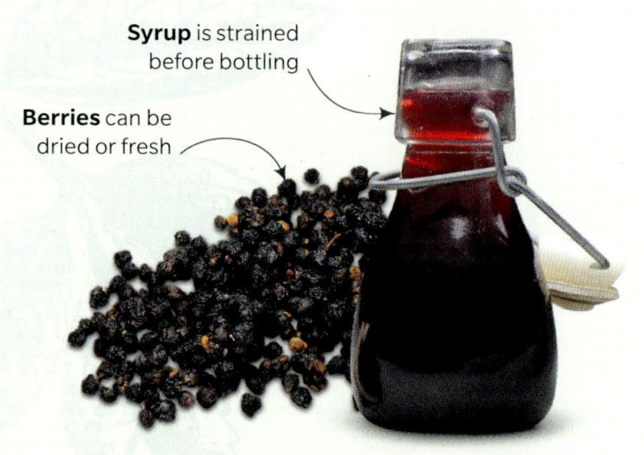

Syrup is strained before bottling

Berries can be dried or fresh

◄ Immunity booster
Elderberry rob (from the Arabic *robb,* meaning boiled down juice of a fruit or vegetable) and elder syrup (a sweetened rob) are used traditionally to relieve coughs and congestion.

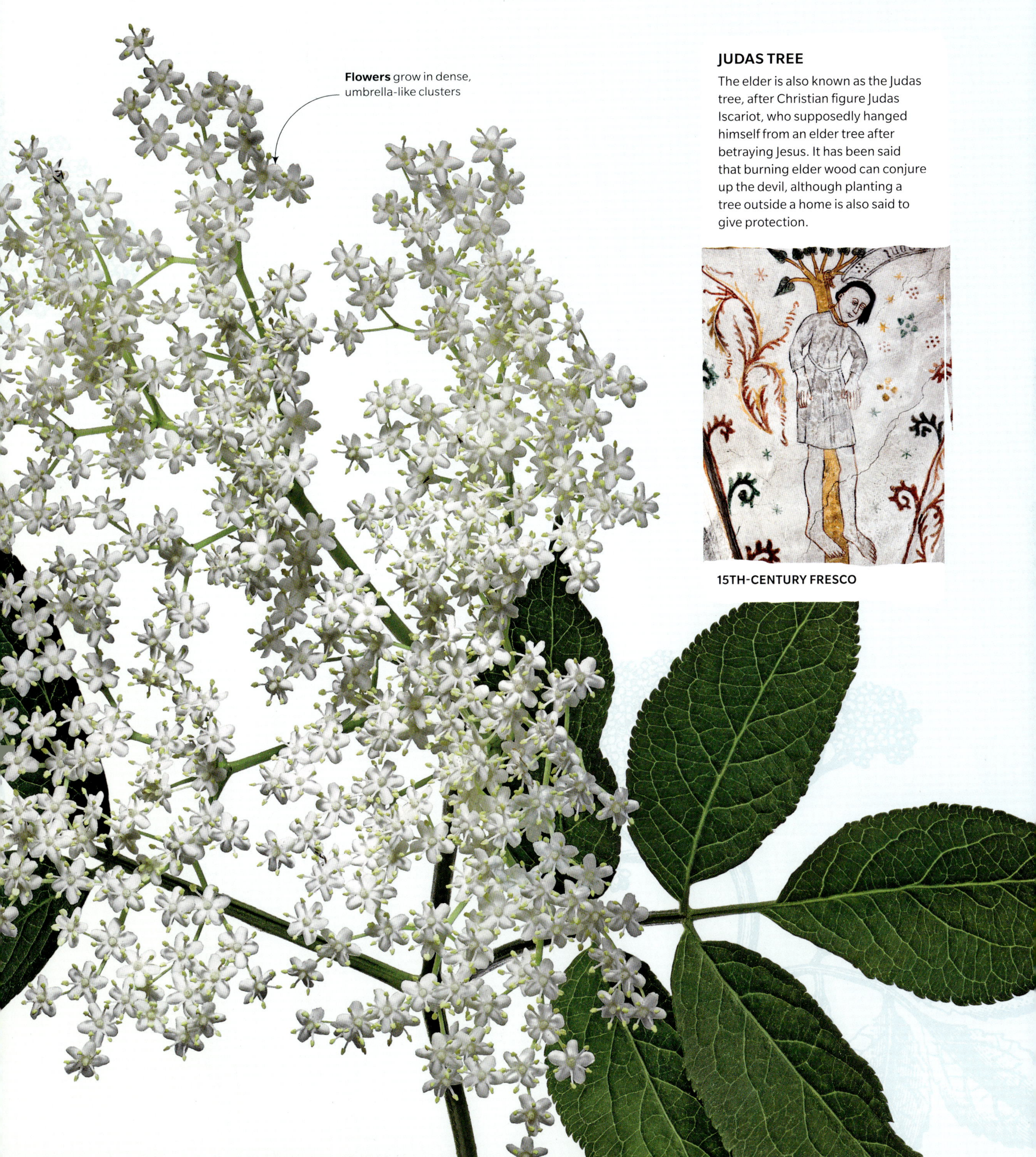

JUDAS TREE

The elder is also known as the Judas tree, after Christian figure Judas Iscariot, who supposedly hanged himself from an elder tree after betraying Jesus. It has been said that burning elder wood can conjure up the devil, although planting a tree outside a home is also said to give protection.

15TH-CENTURY FRESCO

➤ **Elder Tree Mother**
Made famous by Hans Christian Andersen's *Fairy Tales* (illustrated here in a 1935 edition), the Elder Tree Mother is said to protect the elder tree from harm.

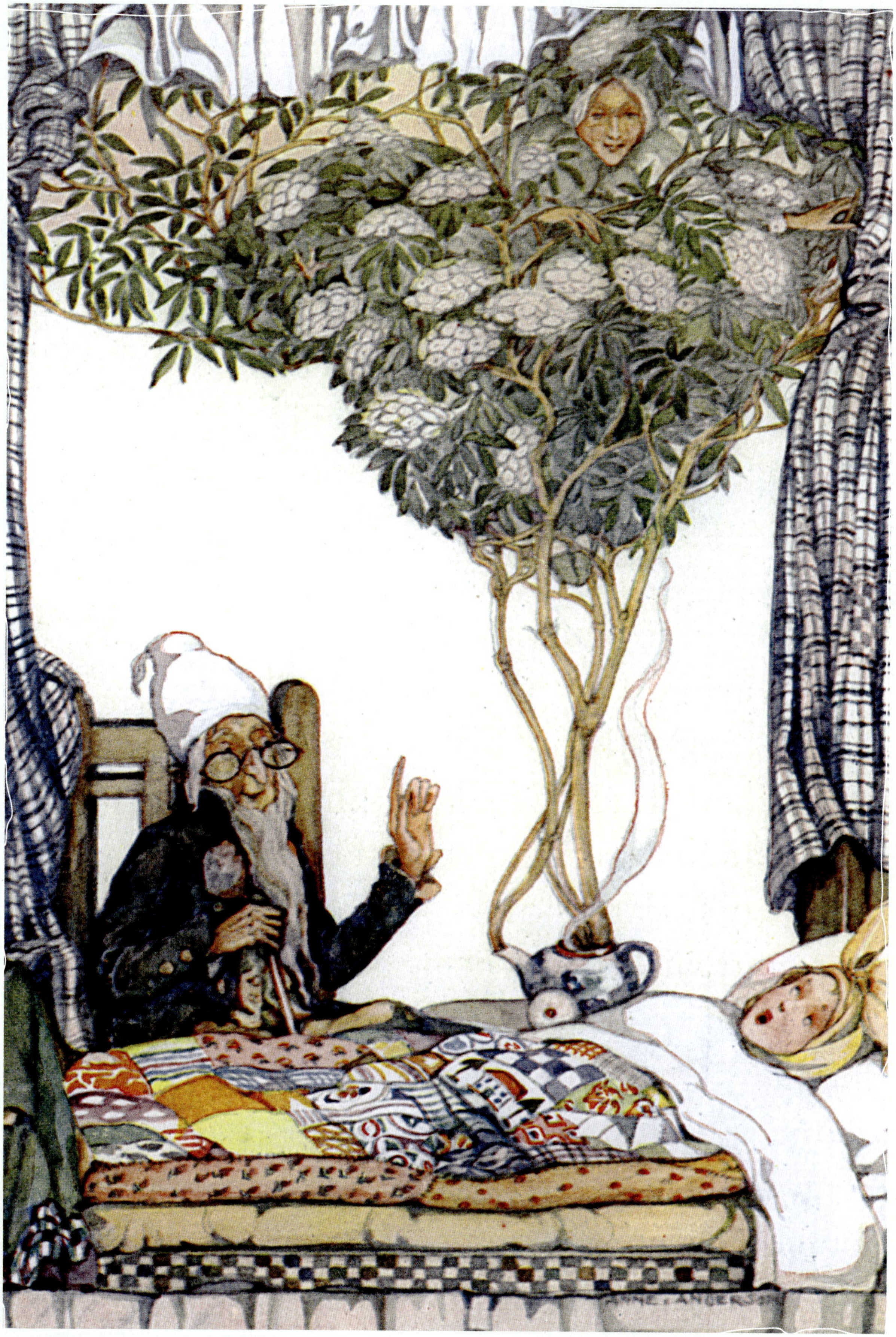

Similar herbs

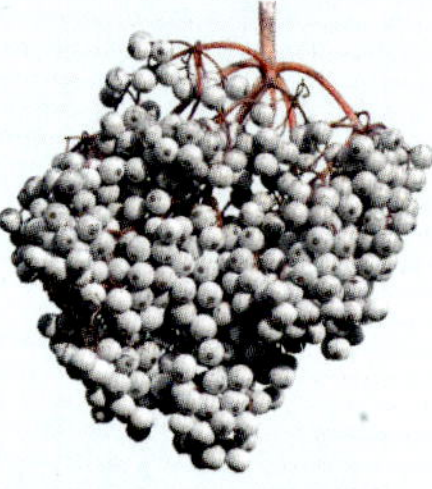

BLUE ELDERBERRY
Sambucus cerulea
Recognized by its powder-coated black-blue berries, this species is used by Indigenous American peoples for preparing traditional medicines.

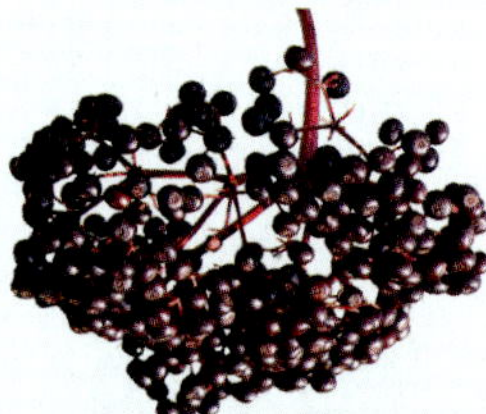

AMERICAN BLACK ELDERBERRY
Sambucus canadensis
Native to a large part of North America and down to Bolivia, it is used in the same way as *S. nigra*.

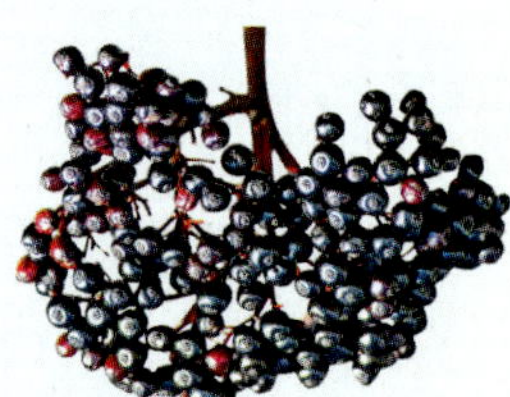

DWARF ELDER
Sambucus ebulus
From Europe to Turkmenistan, and north-west Africa, this herbaceous elder is seen as a more toxic species and is little used today.

> "... English summer is not here until the Elder is fully in flower, and ... ends when the berries are ripe."
>
> MRS M. GRIEVE, *A Modern Herbal*, 1931

in immune-boosting vitamin C and high in dietary fibre, the latter of which can help digestive health. As a result, elder is now not only foraged for personal or local use but also farmed as a commercial crop.

A cosmopolitan herb

Even with fewer plant parts used in modern times, *Sambucus nigra* is one of the world's most accessible and well-used herbs. It is native or naturalized across Western and Eastern Europe and parts of Eurasia, and is now also found in Northern Europe, North Africa, Western Asia, and parts of South America.

Known for thousands of years, the elder is shrouded in folklore and superstition. Its common name stems from the Anglo-Saxon word *aeld* meaning "fire", and harks back to the ancient practice of using the tree's hollowed-out stems to blow on flames. The generic name *Sambucus* can be traced back to Roman times: one theory links it to the sambuca, an ancient musical instrument of Asiatic origins, while *nigra* relates to the black tone of the berries.

Elderflower cordial also originated in Roman times, when a similar beverage was made from the highly perfumed early to mid-summer flowers. The drink became popular during the Victorian era in the UK as a sweetly fragrant concoction of elderflowers, sugar, and lemon, while a fermented, mildly alcoholic version, known as elderflower champagne, is also produced. In all cases, the potentially toxic stems must be removed first. In the kitchen, fresh berries should also be treated with caution and need to be cooked before eating to avoid stomach upsets.

In season from late summer to early autumn, berries can be dried in the sun, in a dehydrator, or in leftover heat from an oven. They can then be stored in an airtight jar for up to a year. Although the berries are ideal for preparing vitamin C-rich tea and tinctures, the most popular and historic way to enjoy their flavour and medicinal benefits is by combining the boiled-down juice with a sweetener, such as sugar or honey, to make a syrup. Flavour-enhancing ingredients such as ginger, cinnamon, and lemon peel can also be added.

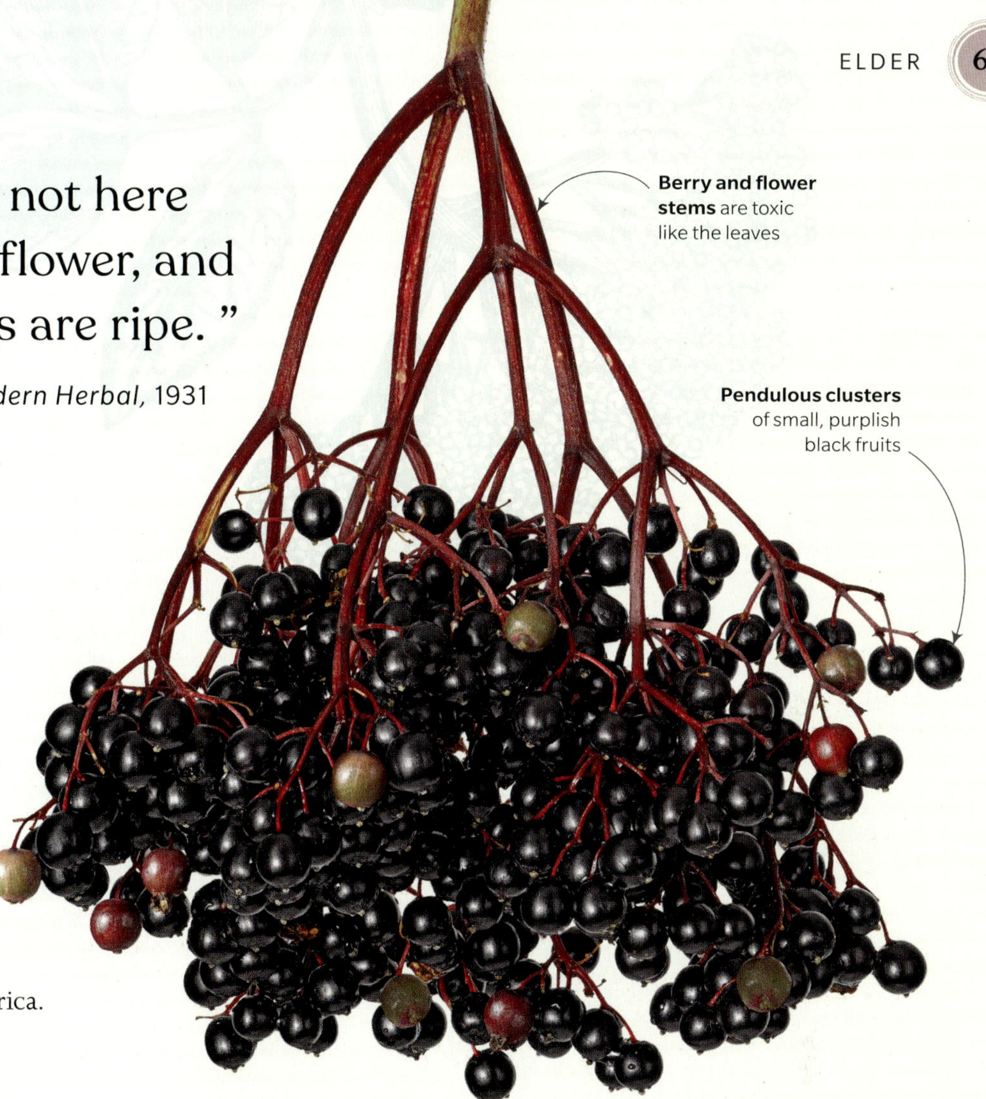

Berry and flower stems are toxic like the leaves

Pendulous clusters of small, purplish black fruits

▲ Natural dye
The richly coloured, almost black berries of *S. nigra* can be used to dye wool or silk lilac, blue, or purple. The Romans also used elderberries to dye their hair black.

Pastilles have a fruity taste and floral aroma

➤ Throat pastilles
Extracts of elderflower and lemon balm are combined with apple juice and natural glycerine to create a soothing (sugar-free) pastille to help combat a sore throat and hoarse voice.

Mistletoe

Viscum album

In winter, green balls of mistletoe can be seen blossoming in the bare branches of the plant's host tree. Historically, this was regarded as a sign of mistletoe's supernatural powers, inspiring herbalists, Celtic priests, and lovers.

Uses Medicines, cosmetics, herbal teas

Parts used Leaves, stems, berries

Active ingredients Lectins, viscotoxins, polysaccharides, oleanolic acid

Habitat Deciduous and evergreen trees

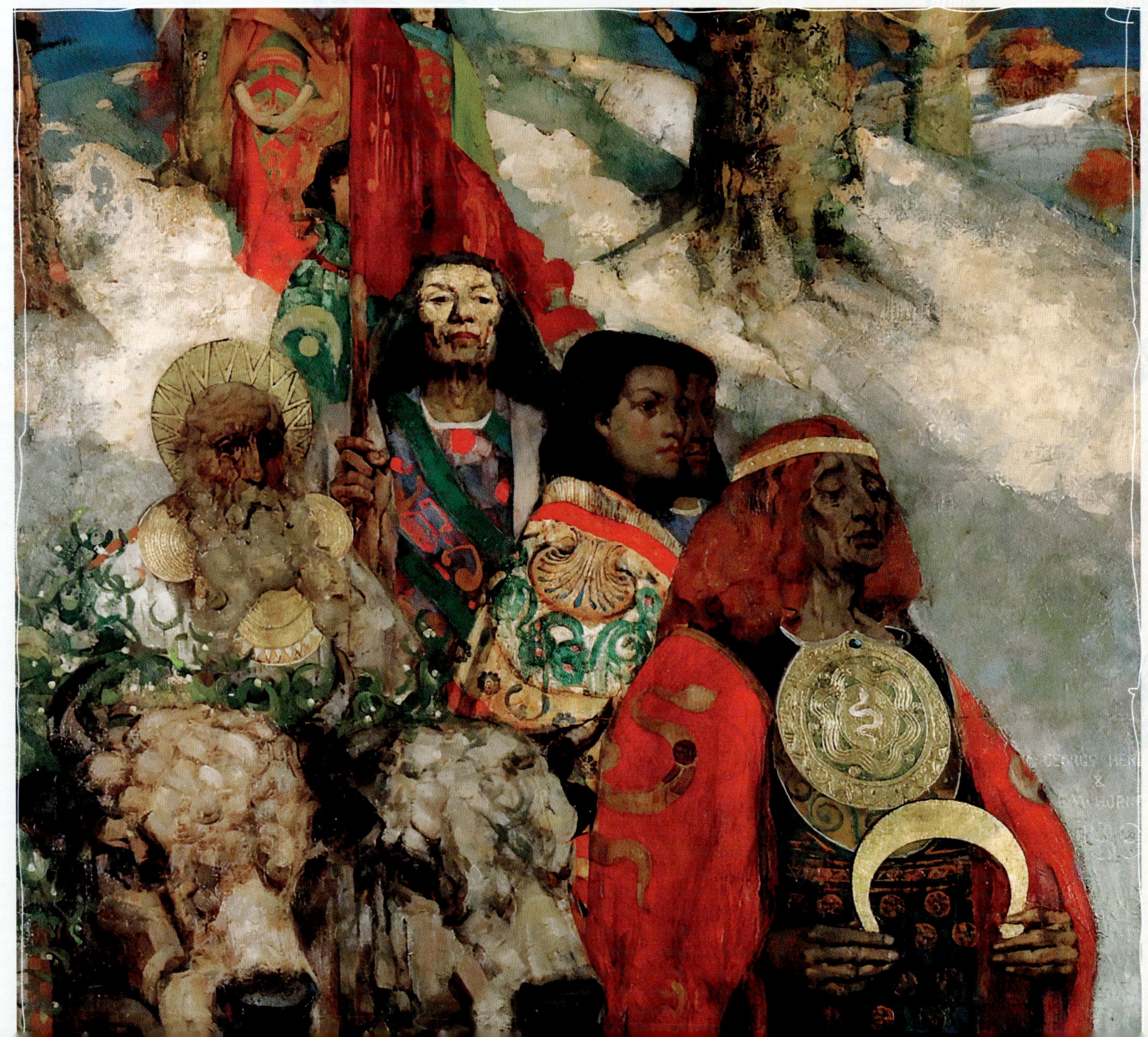

" Mistletoe traditions are amongst Northern Europe's last surviving remnants of plant magic. "

RICHARD MABEY, *Flora Britannica*, 1997

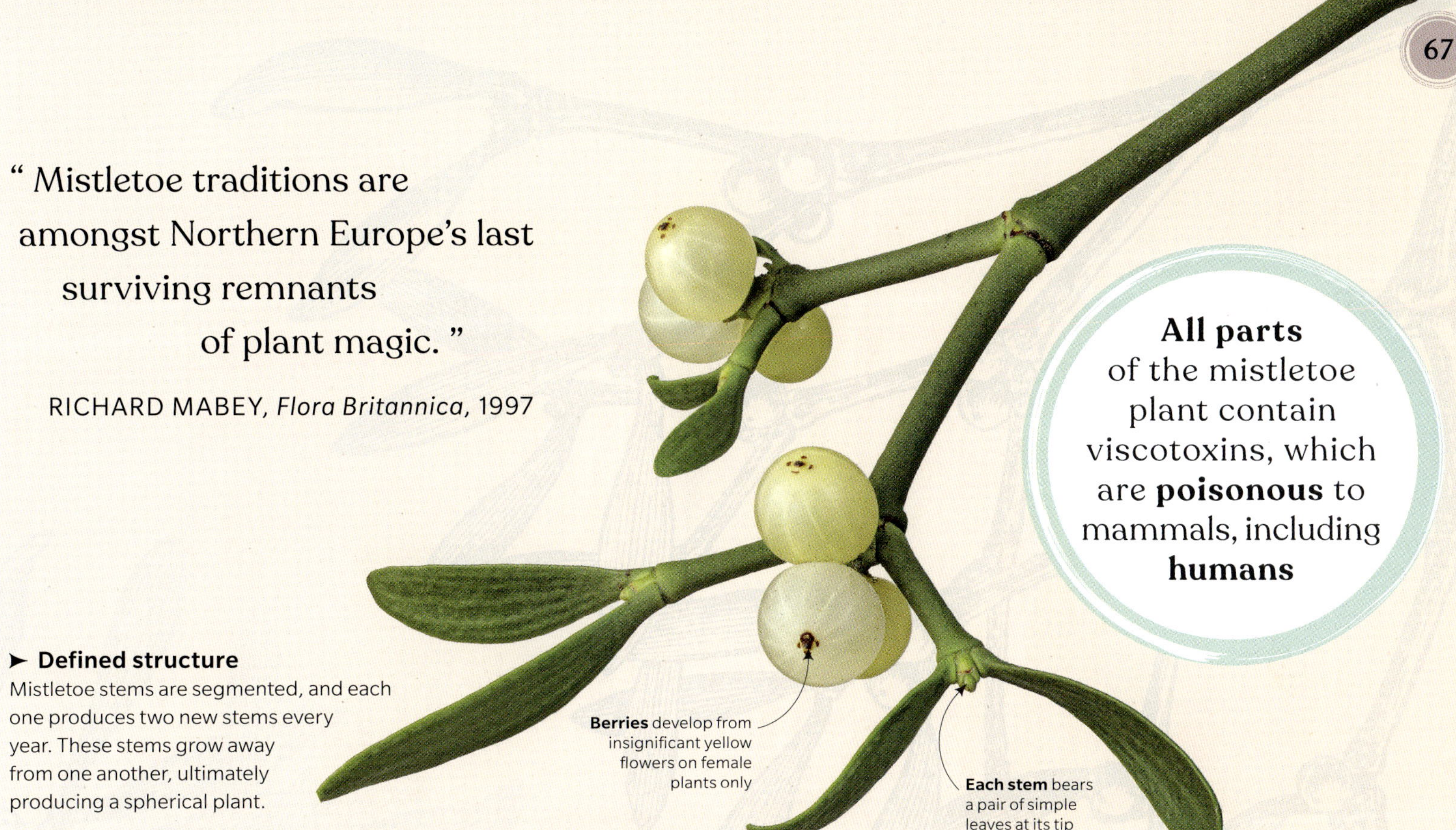

All parts of the mistletoe plant contain viscotoxins, which are **poisonous** to mammals, including **humans**

➤ **Defined structure**
Mistletoe stems are segmented, and each one produces two new stems every year. These stems grow away from one another, ultimately producing a spherical plant.

Evergreen plants have long inspired and enchanted people, who collected their boughs and brought them into their homes as a decorative reminder that life still exists during the cold heart of winter. Holly and ivy, for example, were revered in pre-Christian Europe, and when Christmas began to be celebrated more widely, these plants were incorporated into this Christian festival by attaching religious significance to their spiny leaves, red berries, and evergreen foliage. Among other evergreens, mistletoe was especially significant because its green leaves and stems sprout from the otherwise leafless branches of deciduous trees. However, early admirers were unaware that mistletoe is a hemiparasitic plant, one that gains sustenance from its host tree. Specifically, mistletoe can make some of its own carbohydrates via photosynthesis in its green leaves but relies on a host tree for water and soil minerals.

◄ **Bringing in the mistletoe**
In this 1890 painting by George Henry and Edward Atkinson Hornel, druids ceremoniously lead two bulls carrying mistletoe that has been cut from a sacred oak using a golden sickle.

In the past few years, biochemists have discovered that mistletoe is the only multicellular organism known to lack a protein complex vital for the release of energy within mitochondria (part of cell). Instead, mistletoe extracts from its host compounds that substitute for the missing complex – a wholly unique metabolic process. This may benefit the mistletoe because the plant avoids the "cost" of producing the protein complex, relying on its host in yet another way. Stealing from the host can reduce the vigour of that tree, and where there are multiple mistletoes on one host, this may cause whole branches to die. Usually, though, this only happens in conjunction with drought stress.

Sacred oak

Across its range in Europe, North Africa, and Asia, mistletoe is divided into several subspecies. Some grow on a variety of trees, while others are restricted to just one host species. In much of Northern Europe, mistletoe prefers apple, lime, or poplar trees, and oak is seldom chosen. The rare pairing of oak and mistletoe may partly explain the latter's significance in Celtic culture. Mistletoe was associated with the Celtic god of thunder, Taranis, and its white fruits were said to resemble his semen. According to Roman historian Pliny the Elder, writing in the 1st century CE, druids performed a religious ritual in which mistletoe was collected from a sacred oak and used to cure fertility issues. This may have led to the plant's association with kissing.

Birds and berries

Mistletoe cannot survive without a host, and the plant's berries allow it to spread from tree to tree. These berries contain viscin, a sticky cellulose-based substance that enables the seeds to adhere to bark. Hungry birds, such as the mistle thrush (*Turdus viscivorus*), act as couriers. After eating mistletoe berries, they excrete the seeds, which are left on the branches of other trees. The seed then germinates and its specialized root (haustorium) grows towards the host's stem, penetrating the bark to plug into water-conducting tissues within.

Birdlime is a viscous substance applied to tree branches to ensnare songbirds, which are then eaten or kept as pets. Sticky mistletoe berries are an ingredient of some birdlime mixes. The use of birdlime dates back to ancient Greece or earlier

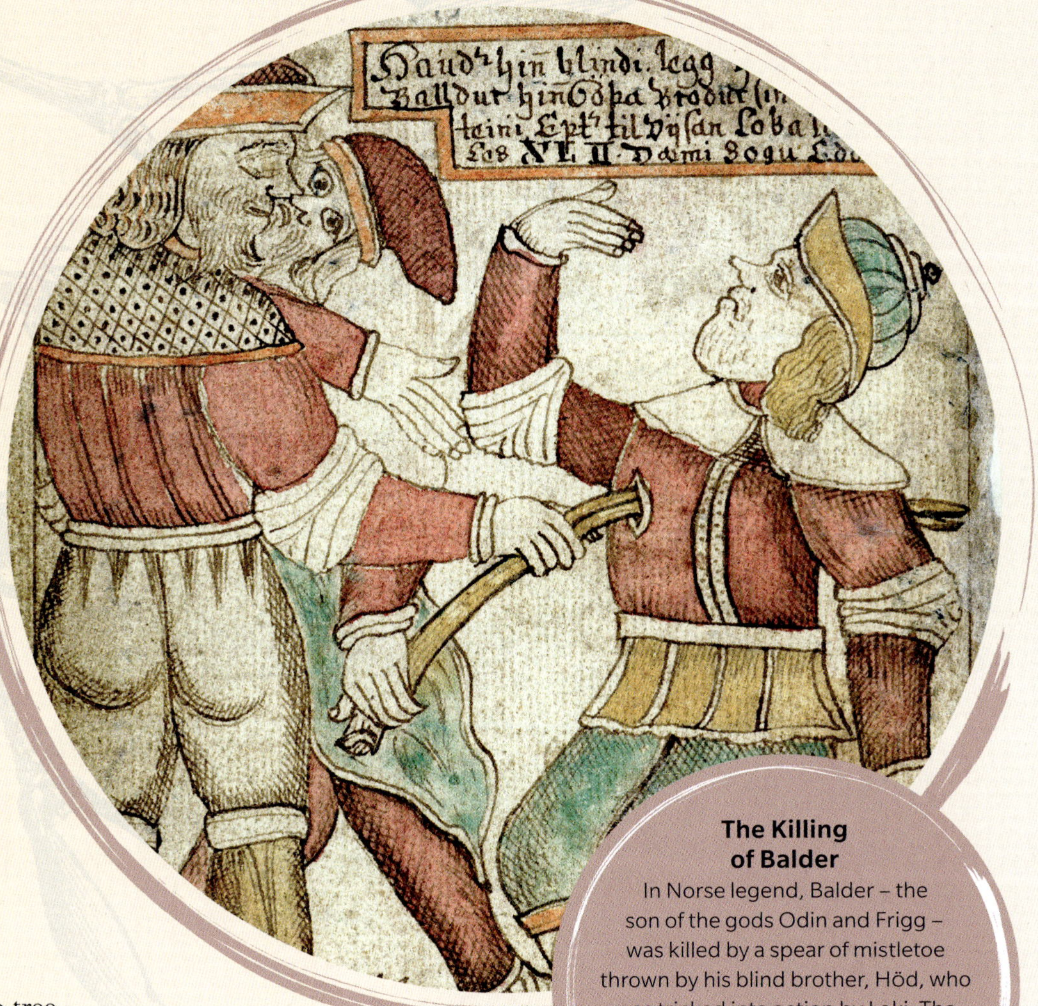

The Killing of Balder

In Norse legend, Balder – the son of the gods Odin and Frigg – was killed by a spear of mistletoe thrown by his blind brother, Höd, who was tricked into action by Loki. The myth is illustrated in the *Snorra Edda*, a textbook compiled by Snorri Sturluson in 13th-century Iceland.

> " Mistletoe should not be allowed to touch the ground; were it to... its healing virtue would be gone. "
>
> SIR JAMES GEORGE FRAZER, *The Golden Bough*, 1922

Similar herbs

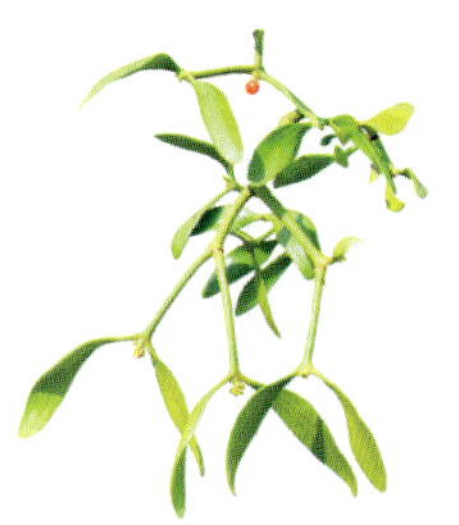

COLOURED MISTLETOE
Viscum coloratum
Native to East Asia, this plant is visually similar to common mistletoe. Extracts are used to treat ailments such as cancer and arthritis.

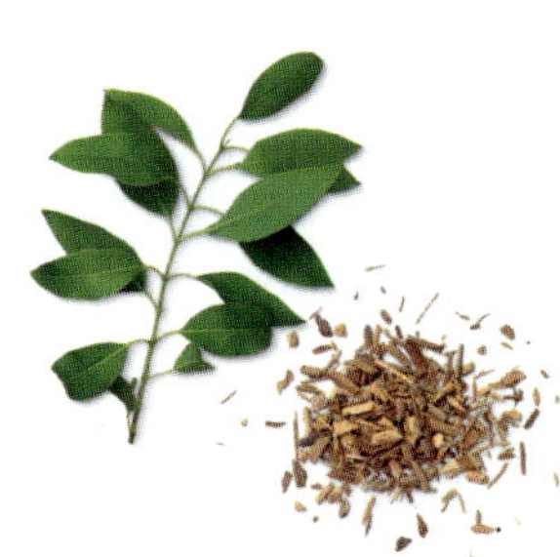

INDIAN SANDALWOOD
Santalum album
Oils from the wood of this Southeast Asian shrub, in the same plant family as mistletoe, are used as flavourings, in cosmetics, and for treating skin conditions.

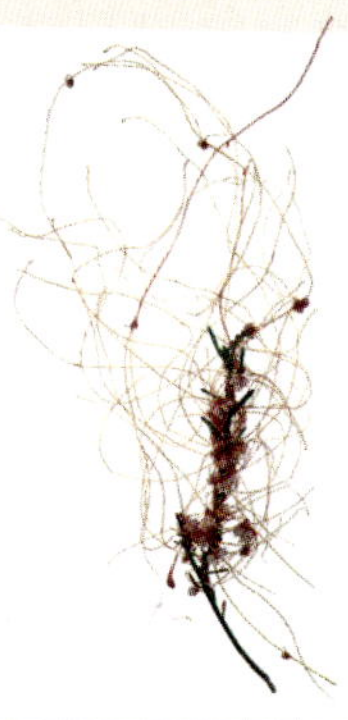

DODDER
Cuscuta spp.
These parasitic twining vines in the morning glory family are unable to photosynthesize. Medicinal uses include eczema and liver complaints.

and the practice inflicts a heavy toll on wild bird populations. Today, it is banned in many countries, including within the European Union.

Treating disease

Mistletoe has been attributed medicinal properties since the time of Greek physician Hippocrates, working in the 5th century BCE, and remedies for conditions such as hypertension, anxiety, and diabetes can include mistletoe extracts. The plant's use as a cancer treatment is controversial and originates with anthroposophic medicine, a discipline with spiritual and occult influences, developed in the 1920s in Austria. Practitioners saw a similarity between mistletoe gradually killing its host and cancer doing the same to the human body. Today, mistletoe extracts and preparations are widely used in cancer treatments in several countries, especially in Central Europe. Mistletoe therapy is said to stimulate the immune system, shrink tumours, and reduce side-effects of chemotherapy. While many scientific studies of mistletoe's cancer-fighting properties have been completed, few reach the standard required for widespread acceptance, and mistletoe cancer treatments should be treated with caution. Regardless, mistletoe is a common ingredient in cosmetics, herbal teas, and other complementary medicines.

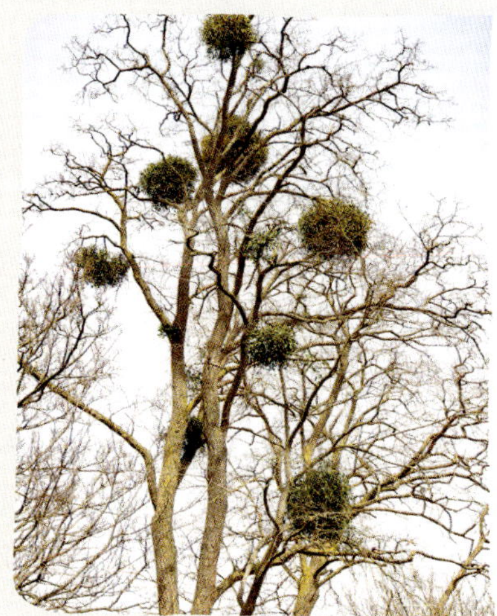

WINTER WONDERS

While mistletoe is present all year round, it becomes most noticeable during the winter months when host trees shed their foliage. This is also the time when the plant fruits, making its presence known to hungry birds. Like the majority of plants, mistletoe has leaves with pores that allow for gas exchange. In host tree leaves, these pores close during drought conditions to prevent water loss. Mistletoe, however, appears to lack this ability and continues to extract water from the host.

POPLAR TREE WITH BALLS OF MISTLETOE

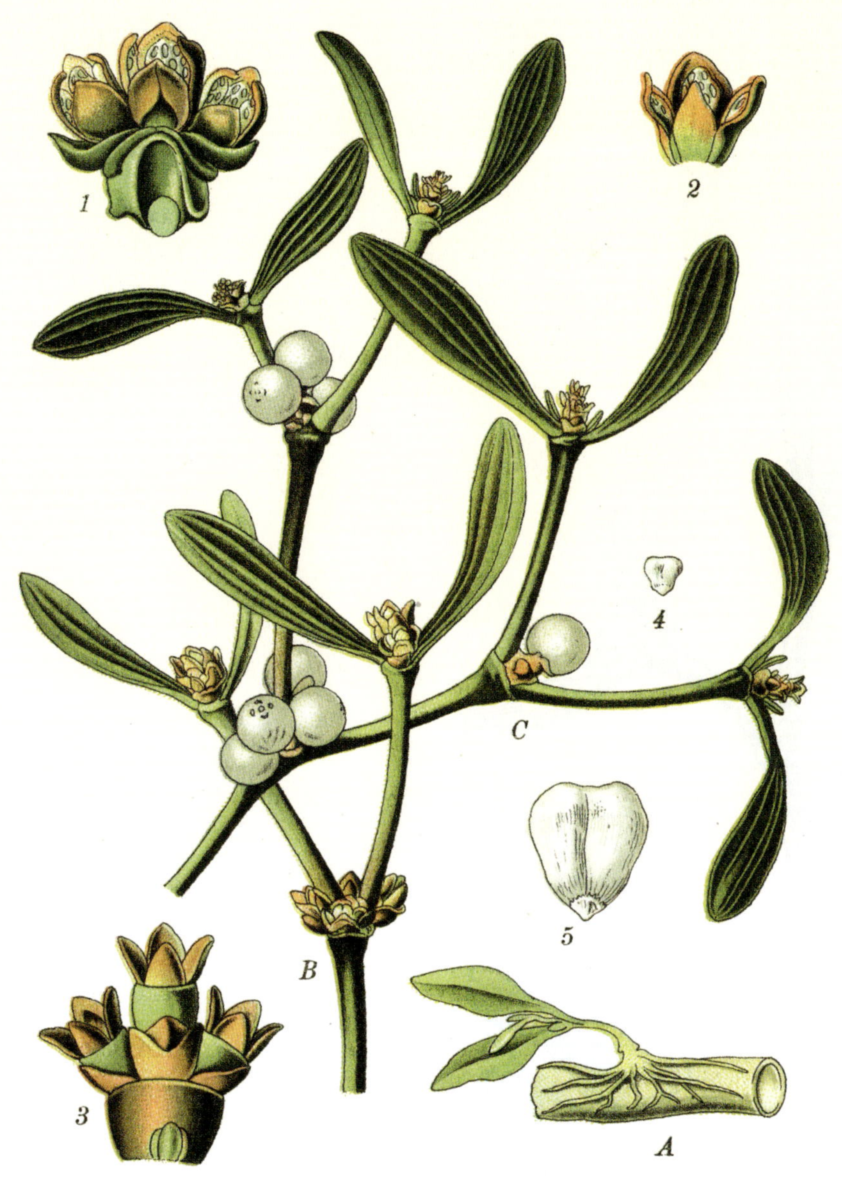

➤ European mistletoe

Mistletoe plants are dioecious: they have male (labelled 1 and 2 in this botanical illustration) and female (labelled 3) flowers on separate plants. Only female flowers produce berries, but males are required for pollination.

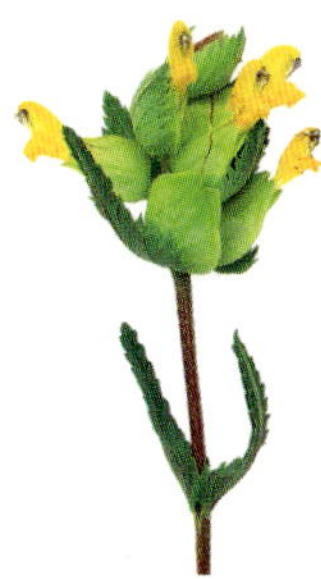

YELLOW RATTLE

Rhinanthus minor

A common component of European meadows, rattle parasitizes grasses, reducing their vigour and enabling wildflowers to compete. It has been used medicinally to treat eye conditions.

Uses Medicines for digestive and parturition problems, and altitude sickness; stimulant; ritual use

Parts used Leaves

Active ingredients Cocaine, cinnamoylcocaine, cuscohygrine, ecgonine, hygrine, hydroxytropacocaine, tropacocaine

Habitat Tropical, wet montane forest

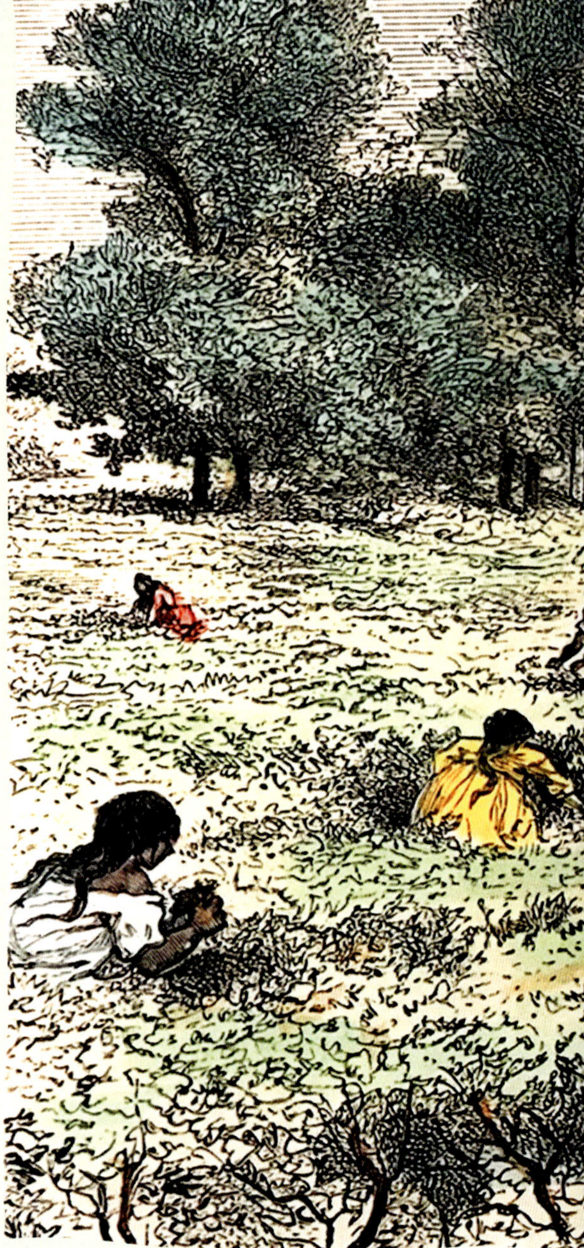

➤ Gathering coca
The manual harvest of coca leaves, pictured here in an illustration from 1863, is today carried out in a similar way and is still an important crop in many parts of the Andes.

Coca

Erythroxylum coca

Across its native Andes in South America, coca has a history that predates the Inca and remains an important cultural and medicinal herb in that region. It is also the source of a powerful narcotic, cocaine.

"Coca yes, cocaine no," was the slogan of Evo Morales, President of Bolivia from 2006 to 2019. As an Indigenous Aymara, he recognized coca's role in his country's heritage and protected the right to cultivate and sell native coca within Bolivia. He also encouraged economic rural development to reduce the total area of coca cultivation and stepped up seizures of cocaine paste and the destruction of illegal drug labs. The drug cocaine is a problem affecting many nations, but banning coca in Andean cultures is increasingly seen as futile.

Perhaps the most common traditional use of coca is to chew the leaves, forming a wad, or quid, in the cheek. An alkaline powder such as baking soda (bicarbonate of soda), quinoa ash, or quicklime, is often added to the quid to help

Sherlock Holmes, the fictional sleuth, often indulged in **cocaine**

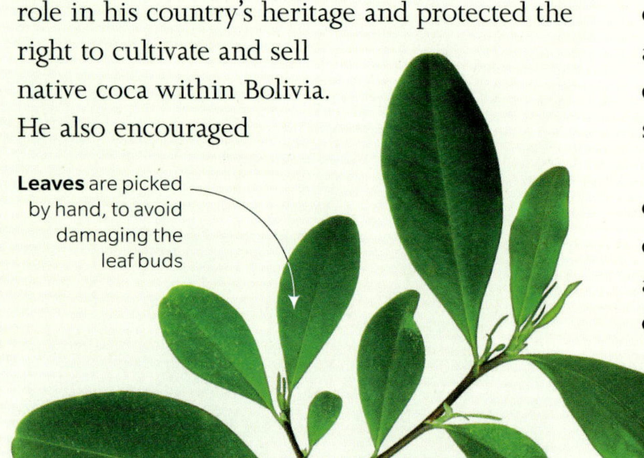

Leaves are picked by hand, to avoid damaging the leaf buds

◄ Evergreen foliage
Each leaf surface bears a pair of parallel lines composed of cells with thickened walls; they are more distinct on the underside. This shrub or small tree grows to around 5 m (16½ ft).

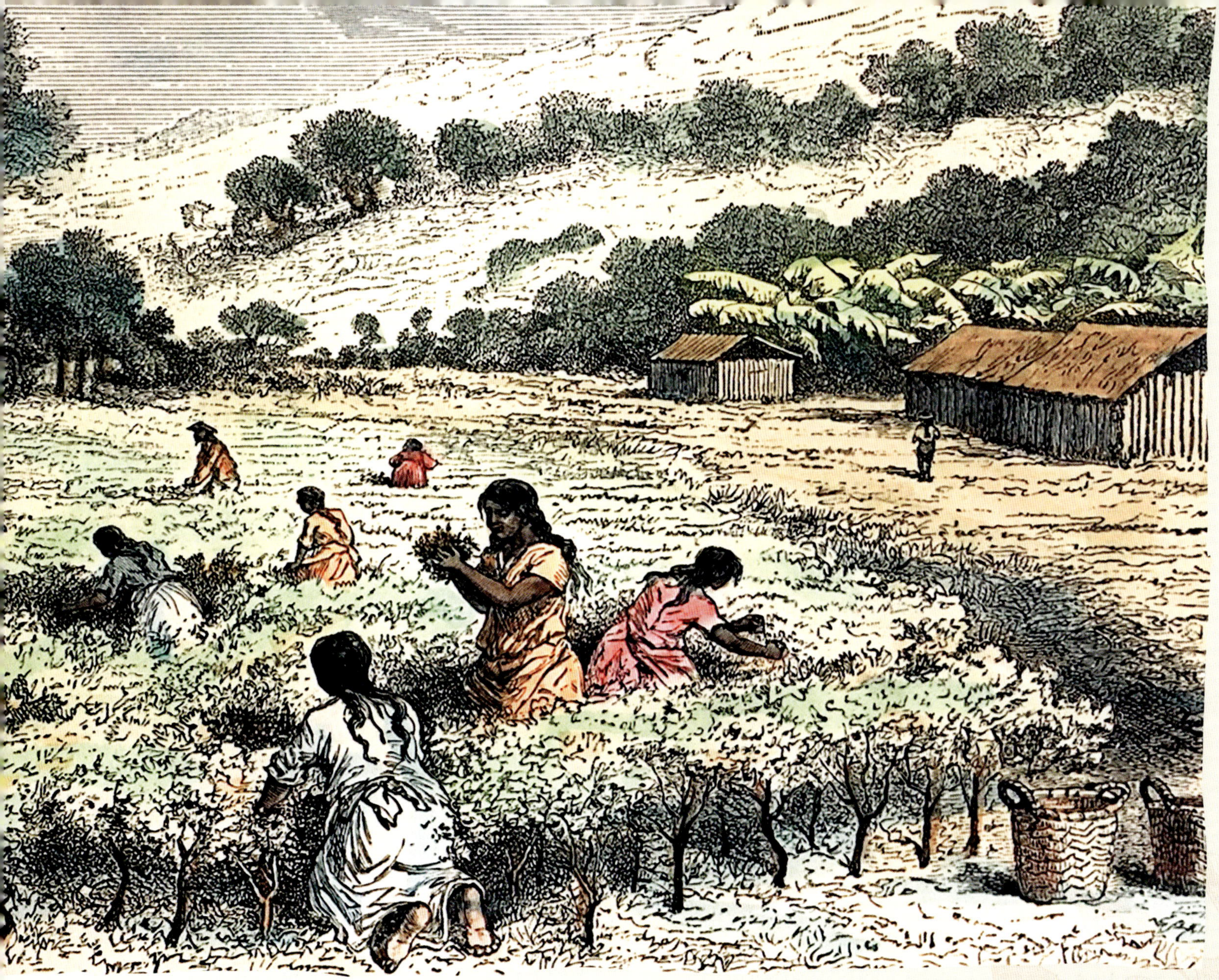

release the alkaloid ingredients, but has to be placed with care because the alkali is corrosive to skin. A coca quid provides mild stimulation and reduces fatigue, hunger, thirst, and pain, such as childbirth pains. Chewing coca alleviates the symptoms of altitude sickness, so is important in Indigenous communities at high elevations in the Andes. This herb has many other medicinal uses, including as an analgesic and anaesthetic, to stop bleeding, and treat depression. Awareness of its addictive qualities has meant that coca and its derivatives are rarely used outside South America.

The history of coca

The history of coca use is long: leaves recovered from archaeological sites in Peru date to 3,000 years ago – before the time of the Inca, one of several Andean cultures to adopt coca. The plant

" North American interest in coca and cocaine grew after 1860, explosively after 1884. "

PAUL GOOTENBERG, *Andean Cocaine*, 2009

A HEALTH TONIC

First formulated in Atlanta in 1886, Coca-Cola was marketed in the US as a temperance drink during the prohibition era. It was initially sold at soda fountains in drug stores and ascribed many medicinal properties. Its two key ingredients were cocaine from coca leaves and caffeine from kola nuts – the seeds of two West African trees, *Cola nitida* and *C. acuminata*. Modern Coca-Cola still utilizes coca-leaf extracts, but it no longer contains any cocaine.

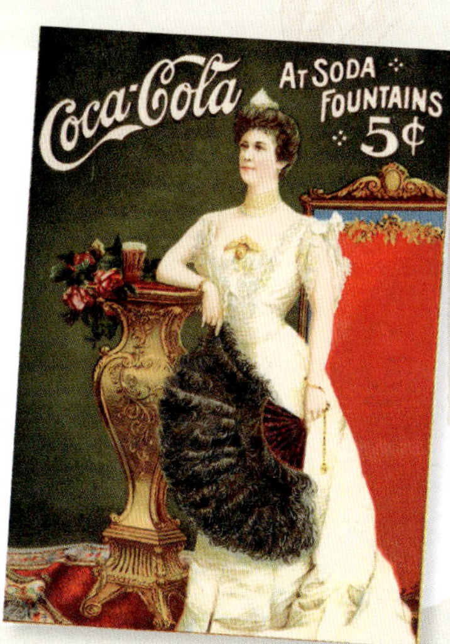

COCA-COLA VINTAGE POSTER

➤ Coca pouch
For centuries, Andean men have carried special, often ornate bags, or *chuspas*, designed to hold coca leaves for medicinal and ritual purposes, as shown in this 17th-century woodcut.

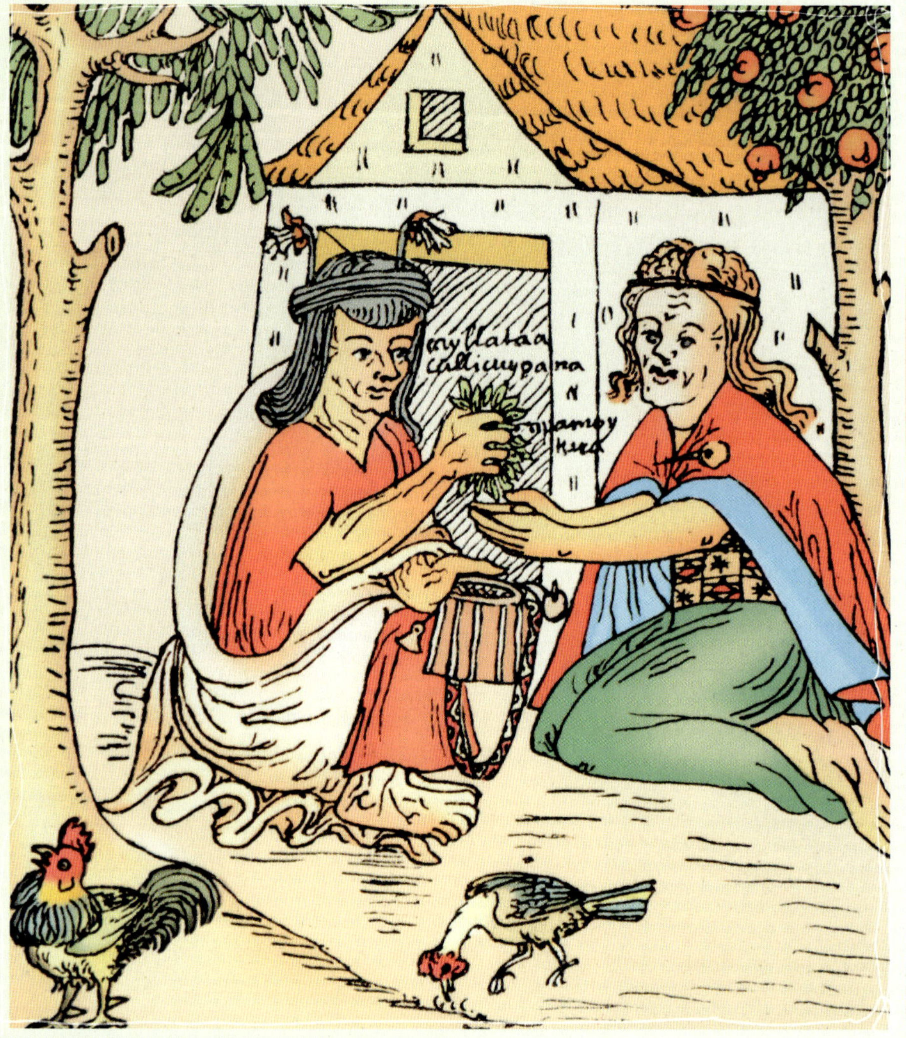

Similar herbs

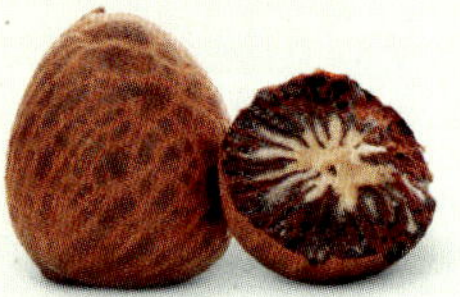

BETEL NUT
Areca catechu
The nut, or seed, of this palm grown in South and Southeast Asia is chewed with leaves of betel (*Piper betle*) for its stimulating effects. Regular use carries the risk of oral cancers and dental maladies.

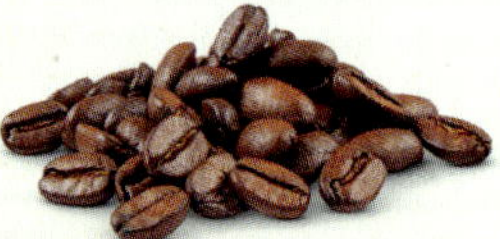

ROBUSTA COFFEE
Coffea canephora
Native to tropical West and Central Africa, this coffee species produces almost half of the world's coffee beans. Coffee is a popular drink because it is rich in caffeine, which is a stimulant. Caffeine is also used in some painkillers.

brought about significant developments in Incan culture. The Inca believed the plant was of divine origin, so reserved its use to royalty, priests, and other people vital to society. Coca enabled men conscripted into military service or labour each year to increase their productivity. Messengers got coca rations to boost their stamina while travelling across rugged and vertiginous terrain and keeping communications open between distant parts of the empire. Inca priests burned coca to divine the future, and coca leaves were chewed by children prior to their ritual sacrifice.

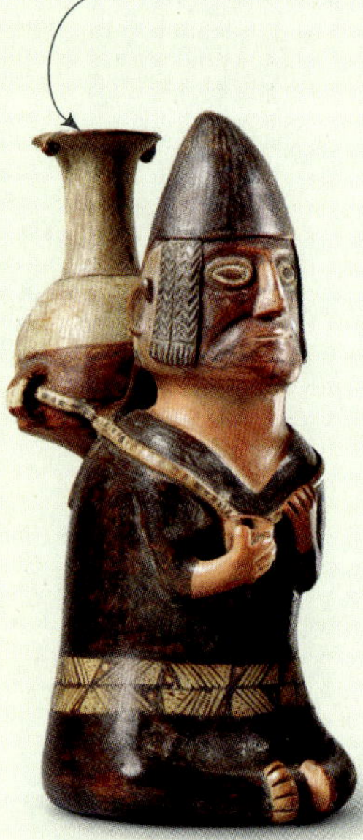

Large urpu made to hold *chicha*, a ritual drink made from fermented corn

◄ Incan ceramic figurine
This figure from 15th- or 16th-century Peru is shown holding a small container for carrying coca leaves. He also carries a large *urpu* – a ceramic vessel made around Cusco, the former Inca capital.

Cocaine was first extracted from coca around 1860, and soon became viewed as a wonder drug. It was an ingredient in medical and food products, for example as a painkiller and local anaesthetic, to control bleeding (as a vasoconstrictor) or help morphine users escape addiction, and in wine and lozenges. The US pharmaceutical company Merck produced 83,343 kg (83 tonnes) of cocaine in 1885. "Forced March" tablets, containing cocaine and caffeine, were popular with World War I soldiers because they increased endurance and combatted cold and hunger. Antarctic explorers Ernest Shackleton and Robert Scott had the tablets in their medical kits, as well as cocaine eye drops to relieve snow blindness. However, the harmful effects of habitual cocaine use soon became obvious, and by 1914 the US government legislated to restrict cocaine's use.

Indian Snakeroot

Rauvolfia serpentina

Possessing a cocktail of powerful alkaloids, this shrub from South and Southeastern Asia has proven potency in treating high blood pressure and may help scientists to create other significant medicines.

Indian snakeroot is important in Ayurvedic medicine, where it is known as *sarpagandha*; it is valued as a traditional treatment for gastro-intestinal and mental disorders, insomnia, and snakebites. The popularity of the herb has led to a decline in its wild populations and an increase in the marketing of counterfeit roots, but new cultivation methods and DNA barcoding of the roots are addressing these problems.

Creating modern medicines

Reserpine, which is derived from Indian snakeroot, has been established as an effective drug for treating high blood pressure, or hypertension. That alkaloid has also been used to treat psychosis, but may have a depressive side effect; in horses, it acts as a tranquilizer. Naturally occurring plant alkaloids such as reserpine are hugely important compounds in medicine, but it is not always easy to synthesize them. Scientists studying Indian snakeroot may have found the key to manufacturing alkaloids. The plant contains up to 150 alkaloids and studies have identified an enzyme that is key to their production. This discovery may allow more of these drugs to be created safely in laboratories without harvesting from plants in the wild. It also offers the opportunity to create new drugs based on those that are already known in snakeroot.

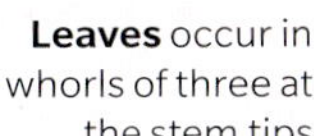

Leaves occur in whorls of three at the stem tips

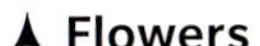

Flowers
The flower is pollinated by long-tongued butterflies that can reach the nectar, although some bees pierce the floral tube to steal it.

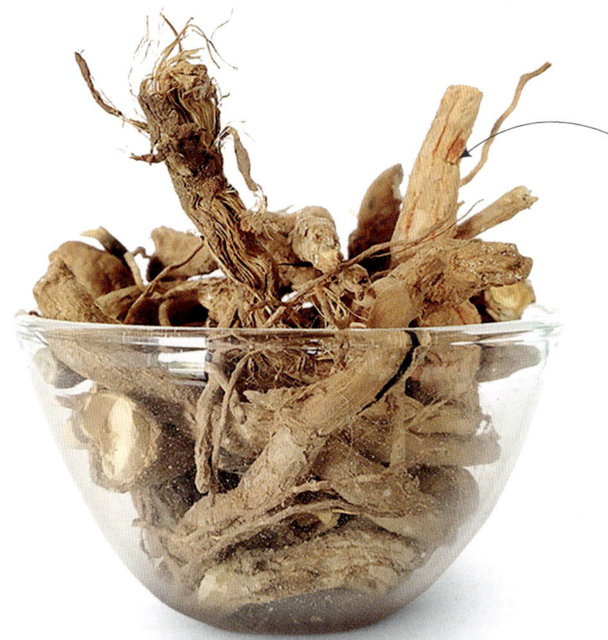

Roots contain key alkaloid

The plant roots
Indian snakeroot is typically harvested around 18 months after planting. The stems are cut down and the roots lifted and dried ready for processing and drug extraction.

Uses Medicines for high blood pressure, and for circulatory and mental health issues

Parts used Roots

Active ingredients Alkaloids including ajmalicine, ajmaline, deserpidine, rescinnamine, reserpine, serpentine

Habitat In the shade of evergreen and deciduous forests, in tropical and subtropical regions

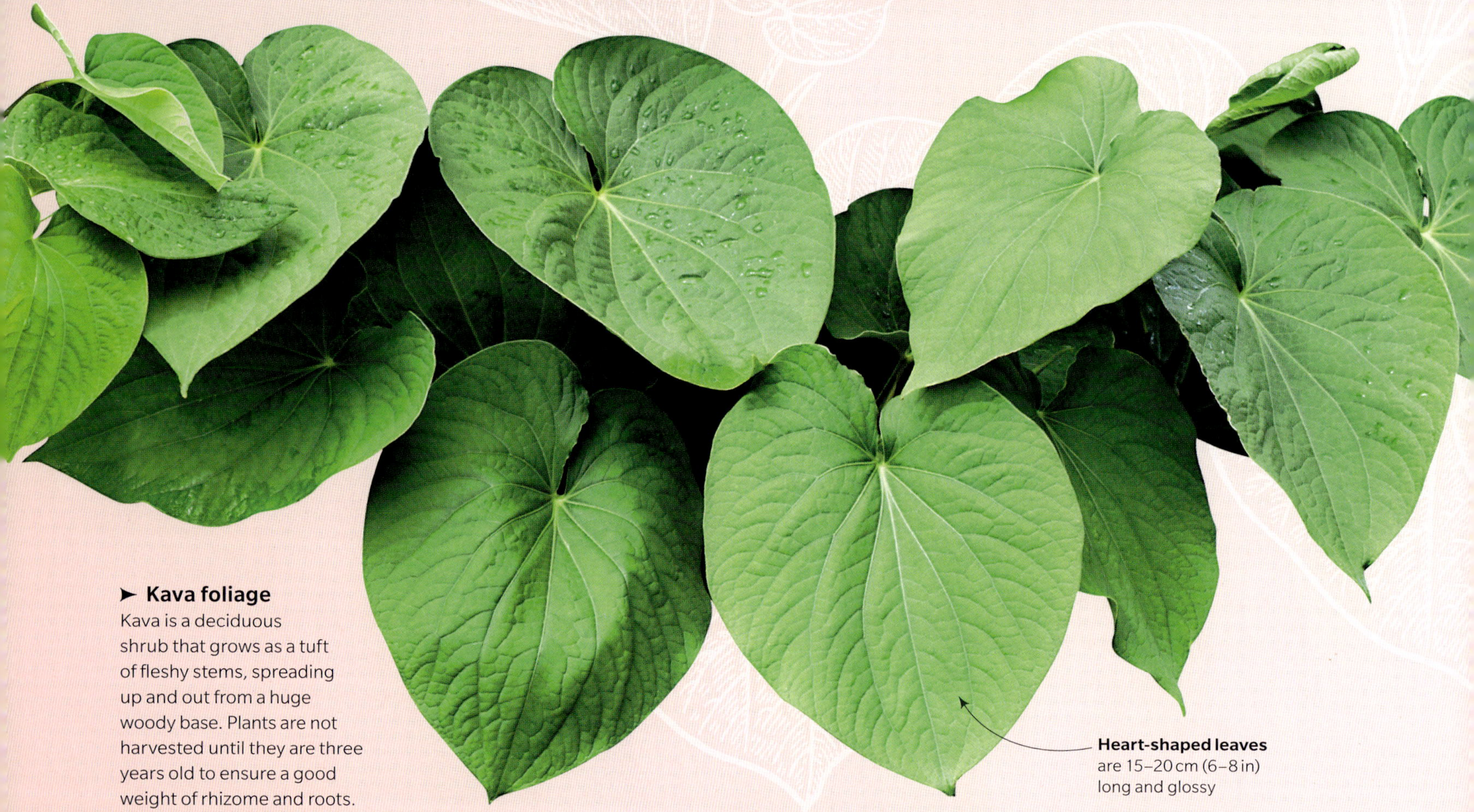

➤ Kava foliage
Kava is a deciduous shrub that grows as a tuft of fleshy stems, spreading up and out from a huge woody base. Plants are not harvested until they are three years old to ensure a good weight of rhizome and roots.

Heart-shaped leaves are 15–20 cm (6–8 in) long and glossy

Kava

Piper methysticum

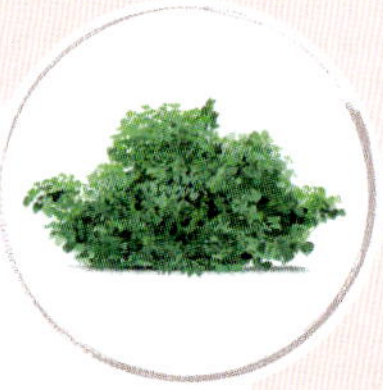

Uses Intoxicant, stimulant, sedative

Parts used Rhizome, roots

Active ingredients Kawain and other kava lactones

Habitat Equatorial and wet subtropical forest habitats in rich soils

People in the Pacific Islands have been consuming a potion from ground kava roots for hundreds of years as a ceremonial beverage and social drink, renowned for its mood-altering and stress-relieving properties.

Evidence suggests that kava, also called kava kava, originated on the islands of Vanuatu and perhaps Santa Cruz in the Pacific but was introduced for use socially and in religious and civic ceremonies to many other islands around Oceania, where it is known by many names, including *sakau* and *yaqona*. It was one of the plants carried by ancient Polynesian voyagers who colonized Hawai'i, where it is known as *'awa*, meaning "bitter", referring to its taste.

Traditionally, the rhizome or root was chewed and the macerated mass was spat into a bowl and diluted with coconut milk for consumption. Today, the rhizome or root is more typically ground or pounded into a coarse powder, then infused in water. The drink was imbibed as a sacrament before religious rituals, when it was said to enable participants to communicate with their gods, and in many other ceremonial occasions, as well as at social

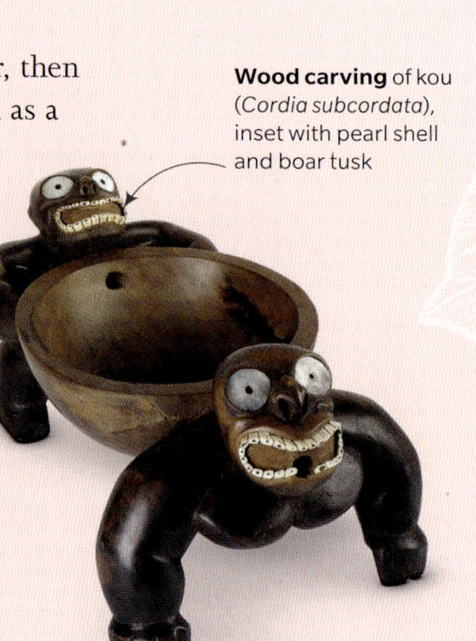

Wood carving of kou (*Cordia subcordata*), inset with pearl shell and boar tusk

➤ Ritual drinking bowl
This 18th-century bowl from Kaua'i Island in Hawai'i was probably used for ritual kava drinking. Kava was traditionally gulped rather than sipped, and liquid left in the bowl was poured onto the earth in thanks.

gatherings. Kava is a calming and stimulating intoxicant and, if taken in large quantity, may produce a euphoric state, which could explain why it is also considered to be an aphrodisiac.

Intoxicating pepper

In the 1770s, Captain James Cook was the first European to report encountering kava. Botanists on his ship gave it the name *Piper methysticum* meaning "intoxicating pepper".

Kava is grown as a cash crop in Vanuatu, Fiji, and some parts of the US, to be bottled and sold. The plant is also grown by tissue culture in Fiji for export. Kawain from the plant has been shown to act as a sedative, help to relieve anxiety and reduce pain. Kava sale is banned in some countries because of reports that it can cause serious liver damage, although this may result particularly from overindulgence, especially when kava is mixed with alcohol or other drugs.

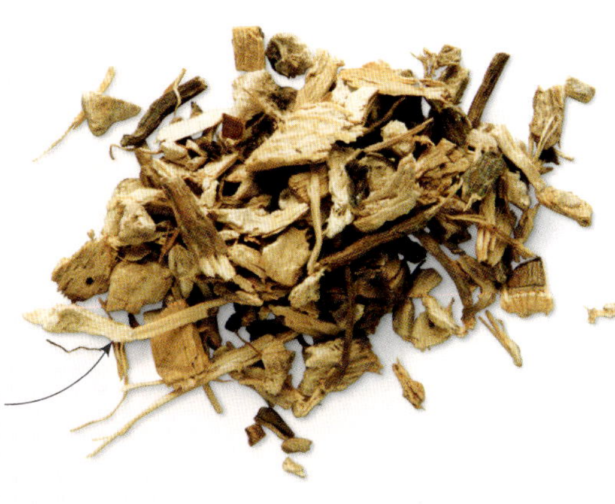

➤ Pulverized kava rhizome and roots
The roots and rhizome have a hot, bitter taste and a numbing effect on the mouth. Taking kava is said to calm anxiety and promote mental awareness.

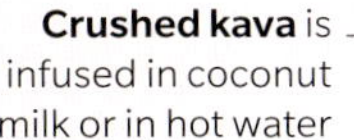

Crushed kava is infused in coconut milk or in hot water

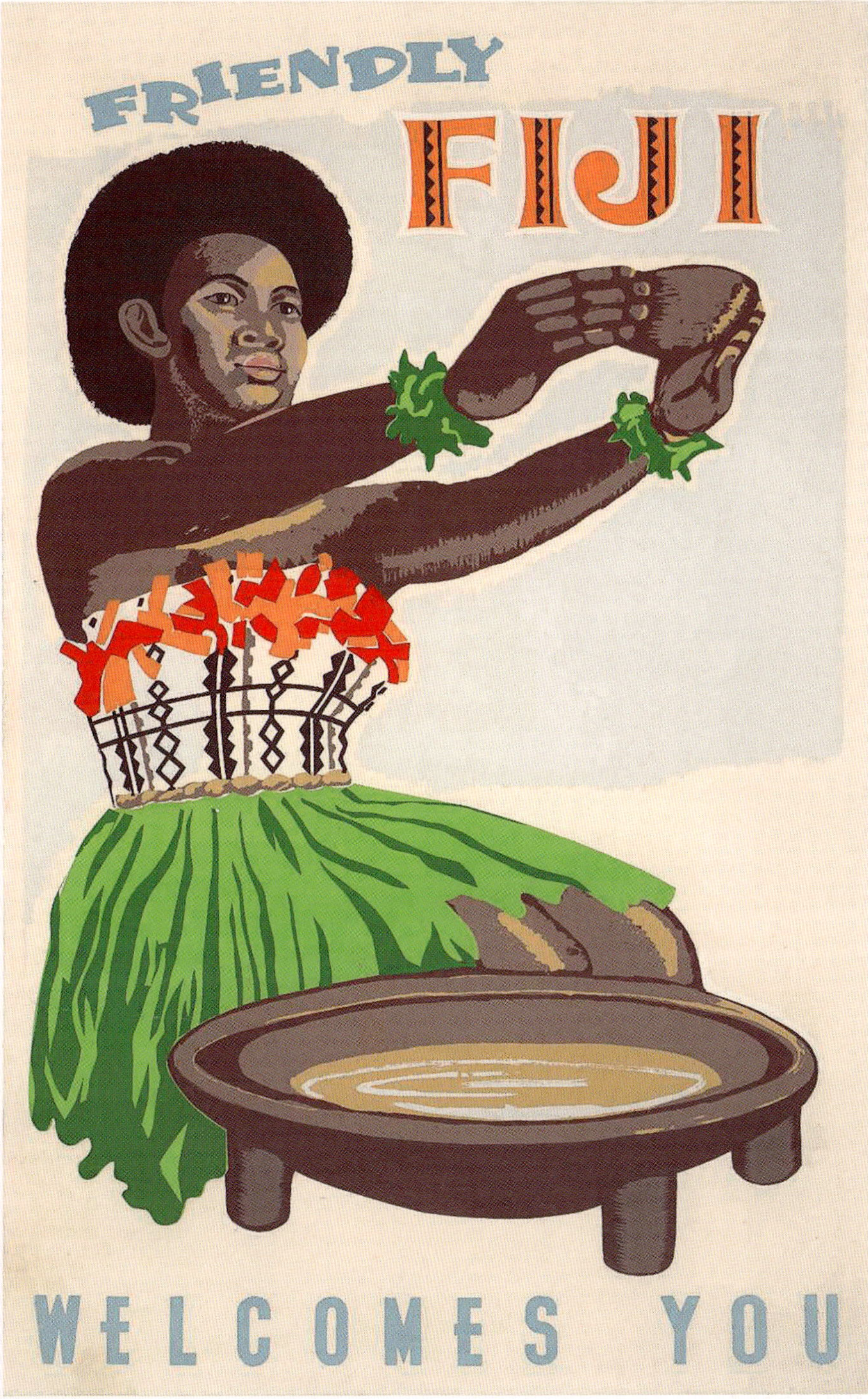

➤ Welcome drink
In Fiji, kava heralded the installation of a new chief. It is still drunk in ceremonies to honour distinguished visitors, and may be included in social occasions such as marriages and funerals.

> " [Kava induces] a state of somnolent torpor accompanied by incoherent dreams. "
>
> J.K. ARONSON, *Meyler's Side Effects of Drugs*, 16th edition, 2015

Similar herb

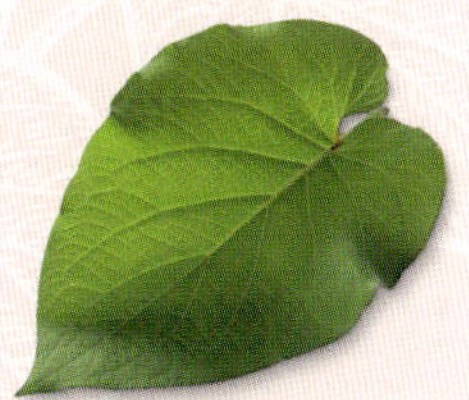

HOJA SANTA
Piper auritum
Native from Mexico to Ecuador, *hoja santa*, or "sacred leaf", is an invasive weed, but its leaves are popularly used in cooking, for example as a spice or as wraps in fish and meat cookery.

Goji Berry

Lycium barbarum

Native to China, the sprawling, suckering shrub *Lycium barbarum*, also known as Chinese box thorn, matrimony vine, or wolfberry, produces the commonly used goji berry fruits.

Uses Medicines, food, flavouring in food and drink

Parts used Ripe berries, sometimes leaves and root bark

Active ingredients Zeaxanthin, beta-carotene, phenolic compounds such as caffeic acid, chlorogenic acid, and rutin, polysaccharides

Habitat Dry forest margins and coastal areas; semi-arid habitats

The name goji berry derives from the Chinese *gou qi zi* and the plant has long been cultivated in China, Korea, and Japan, and is now grown widely across the world. Traditional Chinese medicine has esteemed goji berries for their remarkable properties for at least two thousand years. Unripe, green berries may contain toxins, so only red, ripe berries are gathered. They are dried to preserve them, consumed raw as a dietary supplement, or added to herbal teas and soups that are sometimes taken as tonics.

Goji berries are packed with polysaccharides and antioxidants such as vitamin C, phenolic compounds, and carotenoid pigments, which include zeaxanthin and beta-carotene (a pre-cursor for vitamin A). Carotenoid pigments give the berries their red colour and could contribute to eye health. In traditional Chinese medicine, goji berries are used to tone the liver and kidney channels, and moisten the lung channel. They are used for coughs, dizziness, tinnitus and blurred vision, infertility and impotence.

➤ Goji berry stem
This branch is *Lycium barbarum*; the leaf width and flower size vary only slightly from other species of *Lycium*. Sometimes the stems have thorns.

Goji-berry tonic was used for blood and liver deficiencies

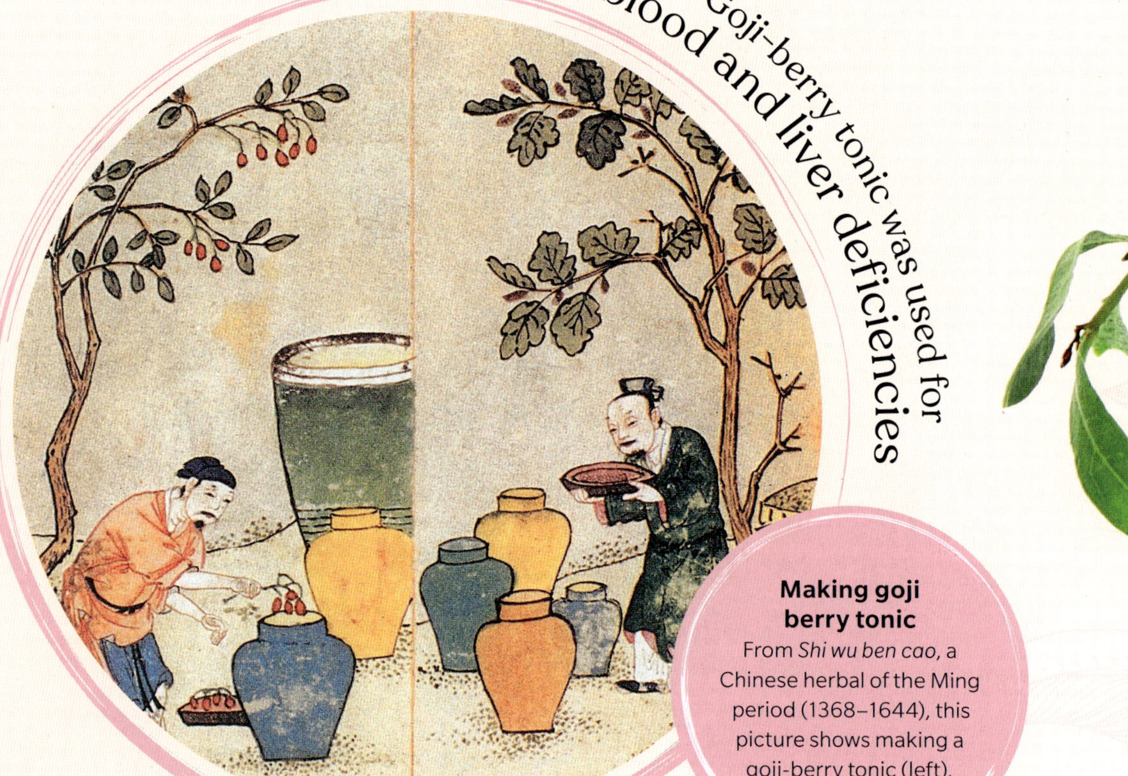

Making goji berry tonic
From *Shi wu ben cao*, a Chinese herbal of the Ming period (1368–1644), this picture shows making a goji-berry tonic (left).

Leaves are sometimes steamed or boiled before being consumed as a spinach-like vegetable

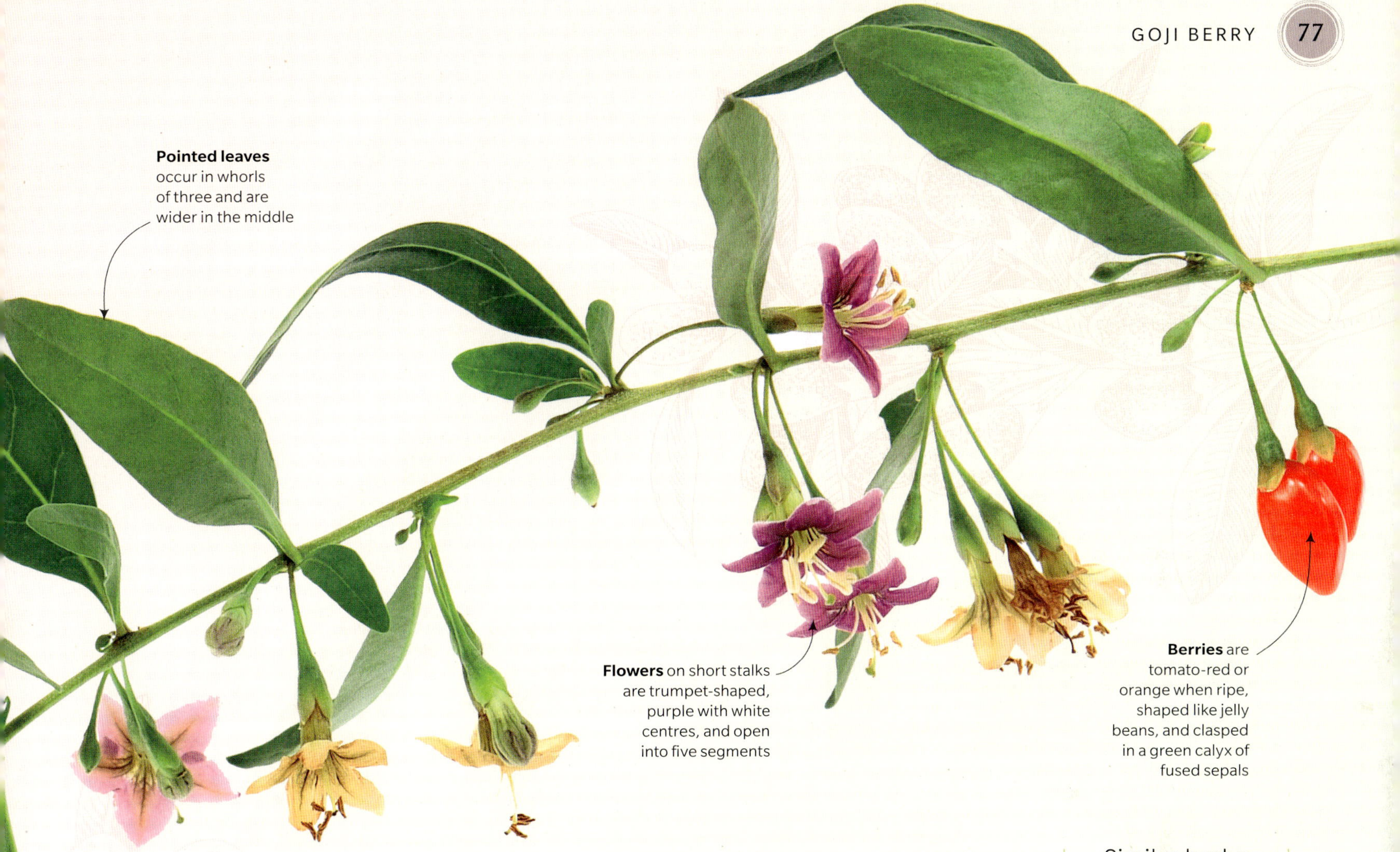

Pointed leaves occur in whorls of three and are wider in the middle

Flowers on short stalks are trumpet-shaped, purple with white centres, and open into five segments

Berries are tomato-red or orange when ripe, shaped like jelly beans, and clasped in a green calyx of fused sepals

" He who travels far from home should not eat goji berries. "

ANCIENT CHINESE PROVERB

One study found that elderly people who drank goji-berry juice daily for 90 days boosted their antioxidants by the end of the trial. There is also some evidence that the berries help eye conditions such as glaucoma.

The root bark, or *di gu pi*, of *L. barbarum* and its relative *L. chinense* are used to clear heat and cool the blood. It is used for fevers and night sweats, coughs, and nosebleeds.

In the West, although goji has been grown as a garden plant for several centuries, its berries were reputed to be poisonous because the plant is in the same family (Solanaceae) as deadly nightshade and henbane. Only in recent decades has goji berry been hailed in the West as a "superfruit". Its health benefits remain unproven, but goji berry is now established in Western alternative medicine.

Rehydrated berries are used in cakes, jellies, and bread or to flavour congee (rice porridge); the juice is used for smoothies and tonic wines.

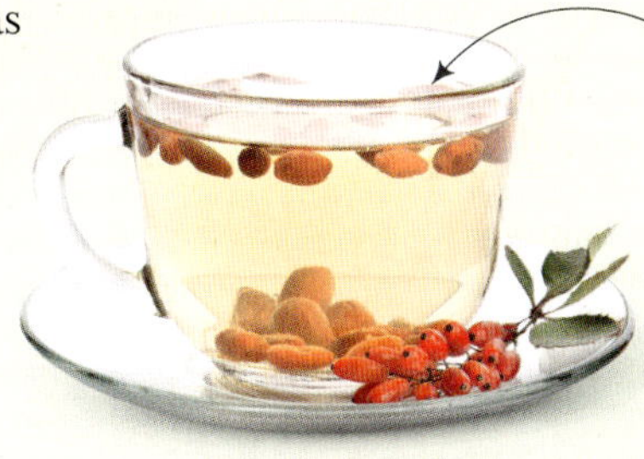

Ripe berries impart a natural sweetness

◄ **Goji berry tea**
The dried berries are chewy, with a sour-sweet taste. Dried berries, when steeped in boiling water, produce a traditional Chinese herbal tea.

Similar herbs

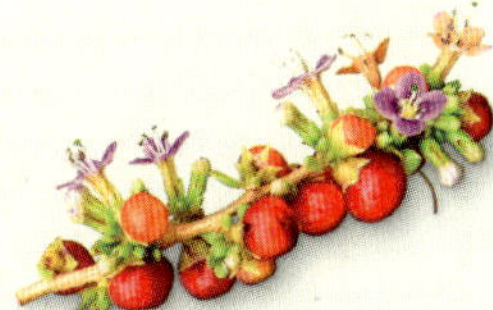

FRÉMONT'S DESERT THORN
Lycium fremontii
This species occurs naturally in desert scrub in the south-west of North America and in spring produces masses of sweet berries rich in vitamin C.

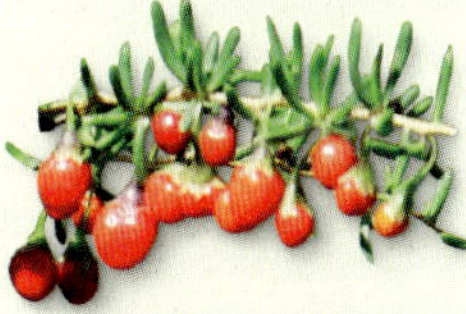

CHRISTMAS BERRY
Lycium carolinianum
Native to southern North America and Cuba, often on the coast, this shrub's berries ripen in December and can taste like sweet, slightly salty tomatoes.

Smooth Sumac

Rhus glabra

Indigenous Americans found numerous uses for the chemicals that evolved in the foliage and roots of this widespread North American shrub to deter grazing animals.

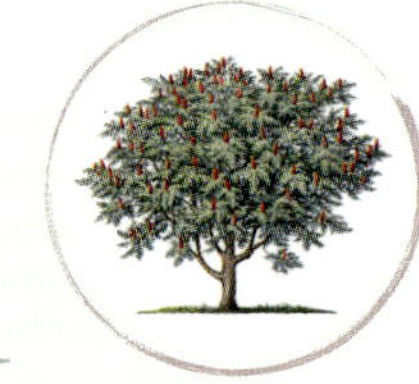

Uses Medicines for respiratory and stomach issues, cooking, leather tanning, dyes

Parts used Root, bark, fruits

Active ingredients Phytols, gallic acid, tannin

Habitat Woodland edges, prairies, fields, wasteland

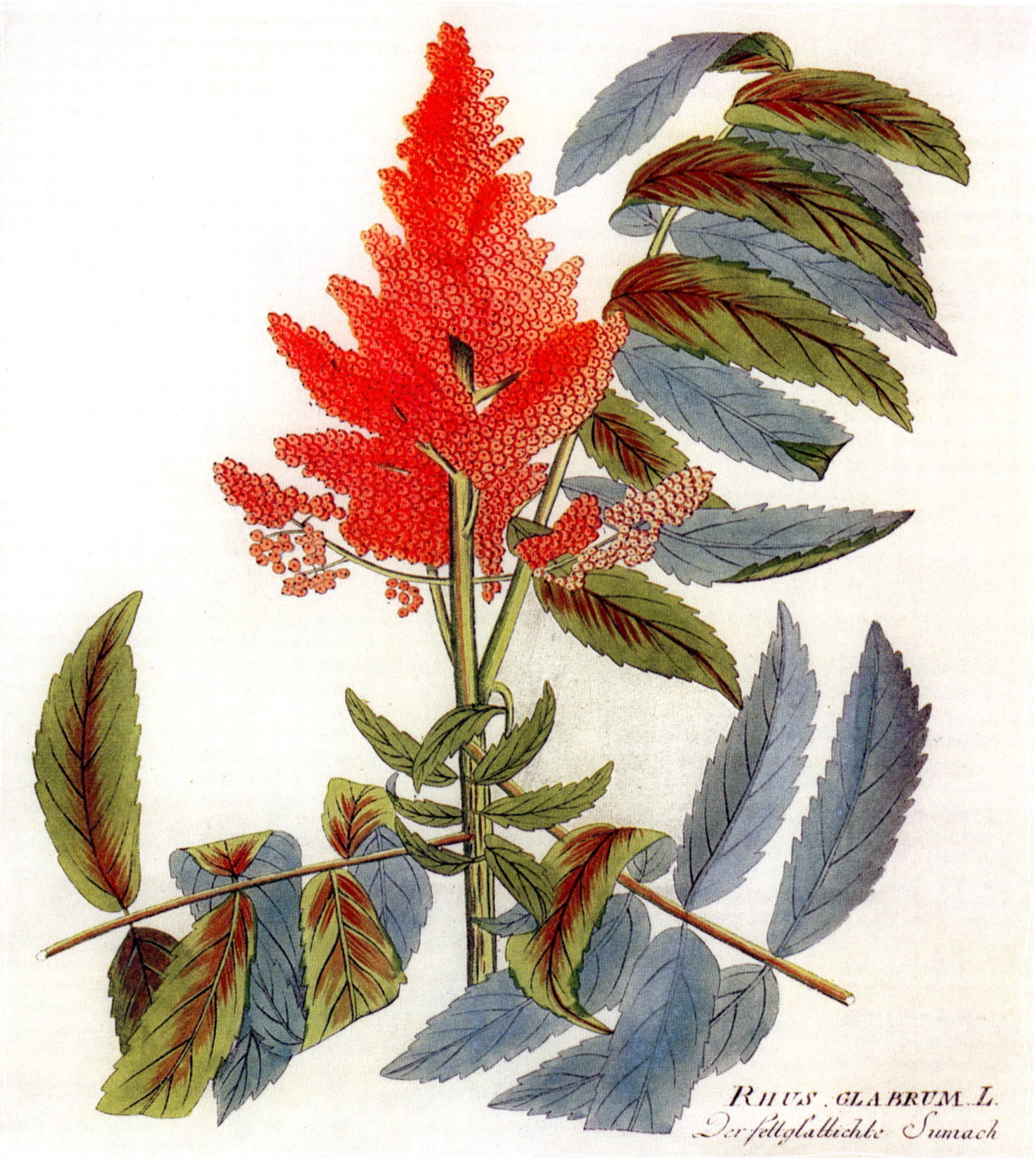

◄ **Bright berries**
This 19th-century botanical engraving depicts the long leaves, smooth stems, and distinctive red berries typical of this species.

Similar herbs

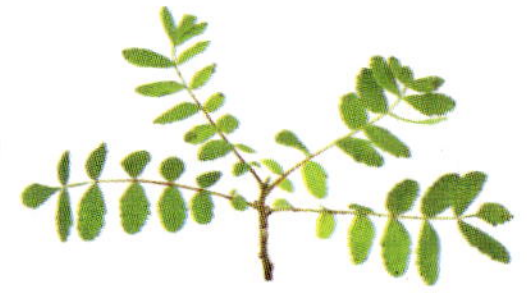

SICILIAN SUMAC
Rhus coriaria
Traditionally used in leather tanning, this eastern Mediterranean species is also known as tanner's sumac. *Coriarius* is Latin for "tanner".

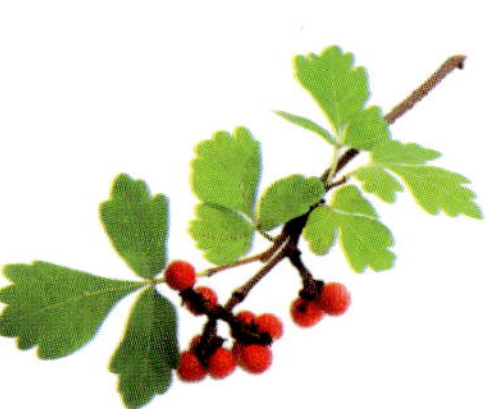

FRAGRANT SUMAC
Rhus aromatica
The aromatic leaves of this North American species have only three leaflets. They turn orange to red or purple in autumn, and produce hairy red berries.

Smooth sumac is a leggy shrub found from southern Canada across the US to northern Mexico. It spreads by root suckers to form dense thickets, and in autumn its foliage turns vividly red. Female plants produce clustered spikes of fleshy scarlet fruits, which are an important food for many birds, small mammals, and deer. Few creatures graze its leaves, however, because they are full of distasteful chemicals.

Indigenous uses

Indigenous Americans put these chemicals to various uses. Tea prepared from different parts of the plant was thought to be effective against a range of illnesses including diarrhoea, asthma, and tuberculosis. Boiled roots were used for their antiseptic properties, and a rinse made from boiled berries was applied to stop bleeding after childbirth. The leaves, roots, and crushed twigs also made yellow or brown dyes.

Picked in autumn, the berries can be eaten by humans, but they are very tart. A refreshing alternative to lemonade, sometimes called "sumac-ade", can be made by crushing the fruits and soaking them in cold water. They should never be boiled, however, as this releases acrid tannins. Extracted from a related species, the spice known as sumac is also a familiar sight in kitchens. It consists of a bright red powder made from the dried ground berries of Sicilian sumac (*Rhus coriaria*), which imparts a tangy flavour to savoury and sweet dishes.

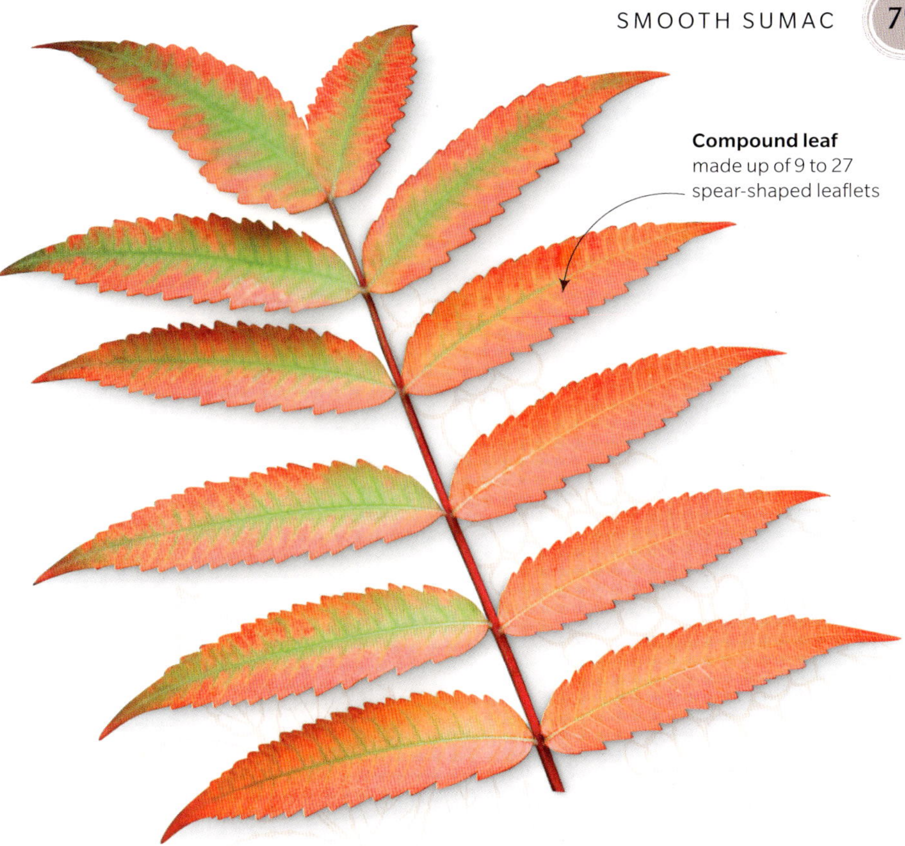

Compound leaf made up of 9 to 27 spear-shaped leaflets

▲ **Jagged leaves** Smooth sumac's large leaves can be identified by their jagged edges. Their colour varies from deep green to red.

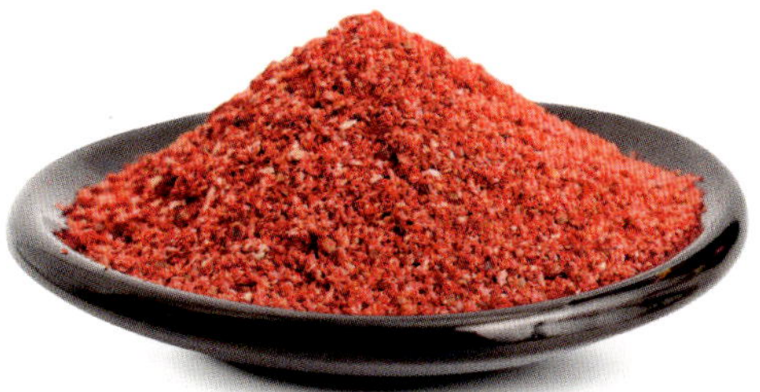

► **Aromatic sumac spice** Popular in the Middle East, this spice has a citrus flavour and is used in dry rubs and blends, such as *za'atar*.

> " This deep red spice is... the 'red thread' that connects every dish. "
>
> ANAS ATASSI, *Sumac: Recipes and Stories from Syria*, 2021

TANNIN AND TANNING

The leaves and bark of various species of sumac contain up to 25 per cent (by weight) of tannins. These are used in the leather industry. Prepared skins are soaked in tannic acid, which makes the leather flexible and lightens its colour. The finest Moroccan leather, used for gloves, shoes, and bookbinding, is goat skin tanned with sumac.

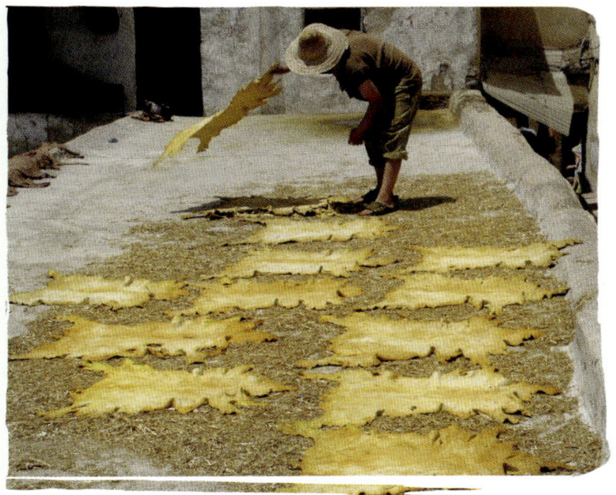

TANNER LAYING OUT HIDES

Sumac is closely related to **poison ivy** (*Toxicodendron* spp.), whose sap can cause **painful blistering** in humans

Perfumes and Scents

Many powerful herbs are highly recognizable by scent. Their aromatic leaves, stems, flowers, and distinctive essential oils have been harvested and harnessed for centuries for use in aromatherapy, perfumes, cosmetics, bath and body products, and home fragrance.

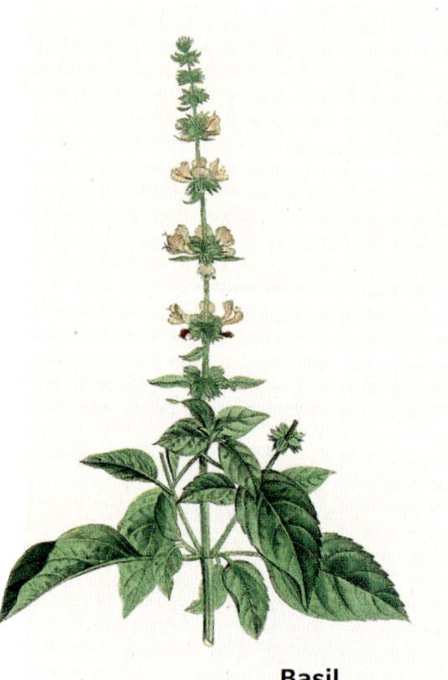

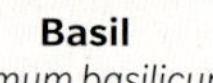

Basil
Ocimum basilicum

Essential oil from leaves; used in aromatherapy, cosmetics, and perfume; sweet, herbaceous, balsamic aroma energizes and uplifts.

Rose geranium
Pelargonium graveolens

Essential oil from leaves; rose aroma but with herbaceous, lemony notes; soothes anxiety and promotes relaxation.

Bergamot
Citrus × bergamia

Essential oil from rind; energizes and calms; delivers citrus, lightly floral, slightly bitter notes.

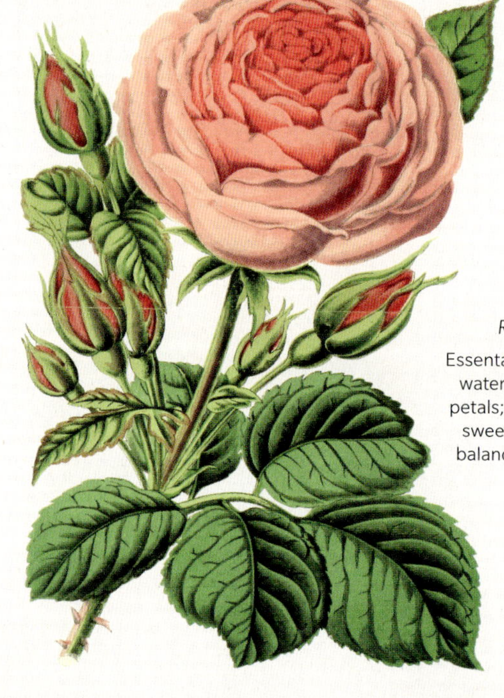

Rose
Rosa spp.

Essentail oil and flower water distilled from petals; typically floral, sweet, and musky; balances and calms.

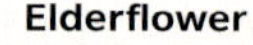

Elderflower
Sambucus nigra

Midsummer flowers; floral-herbal, honey-sweet, musky aroma; used to enhance beverages, bakes, and perfumes.

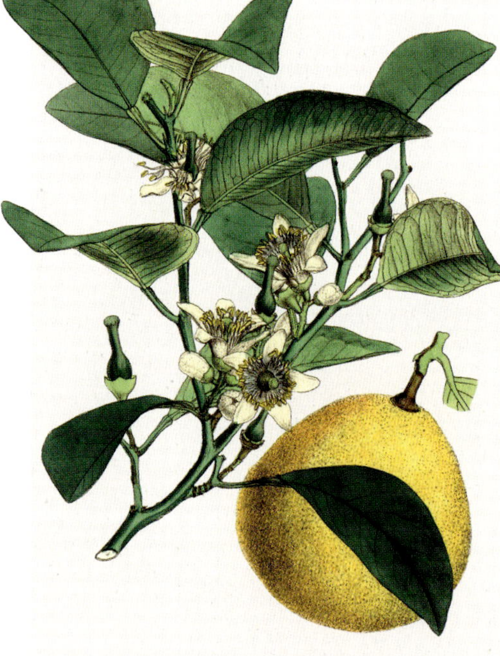

Eucalyptus
Eucalyptus globulus

Essential oil from leaves; opens sinuses and clears head; delivers a camphor, citrus note to perfumes.

Marjoram
Origanum majorana

Essential oil from leaves and flowers; a sweet, floral, warm scent; relieves stress and soothes nerves.

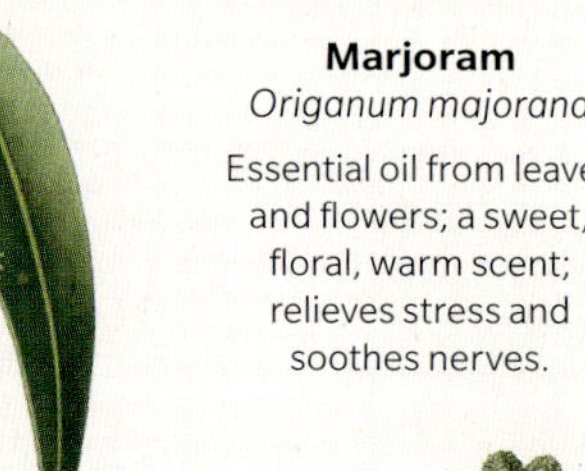

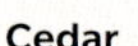

Cedar
Cedrus spp.

Essential oil from wood chips and shavings; smells warm and woody; used in perfumes and as a decongestant; repels moths.

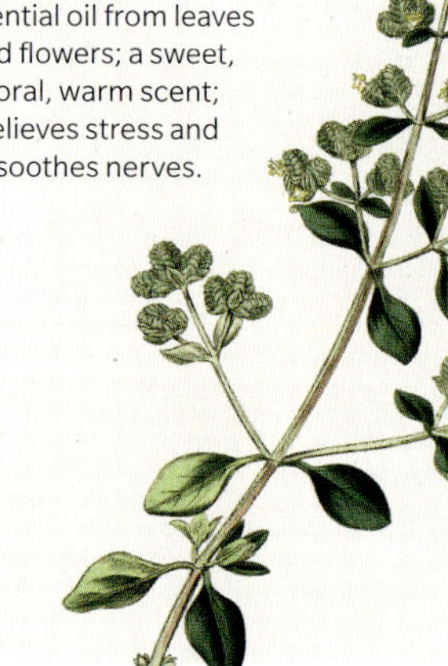

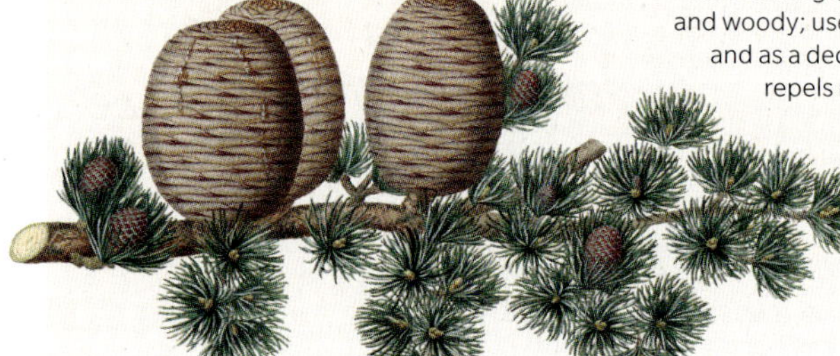

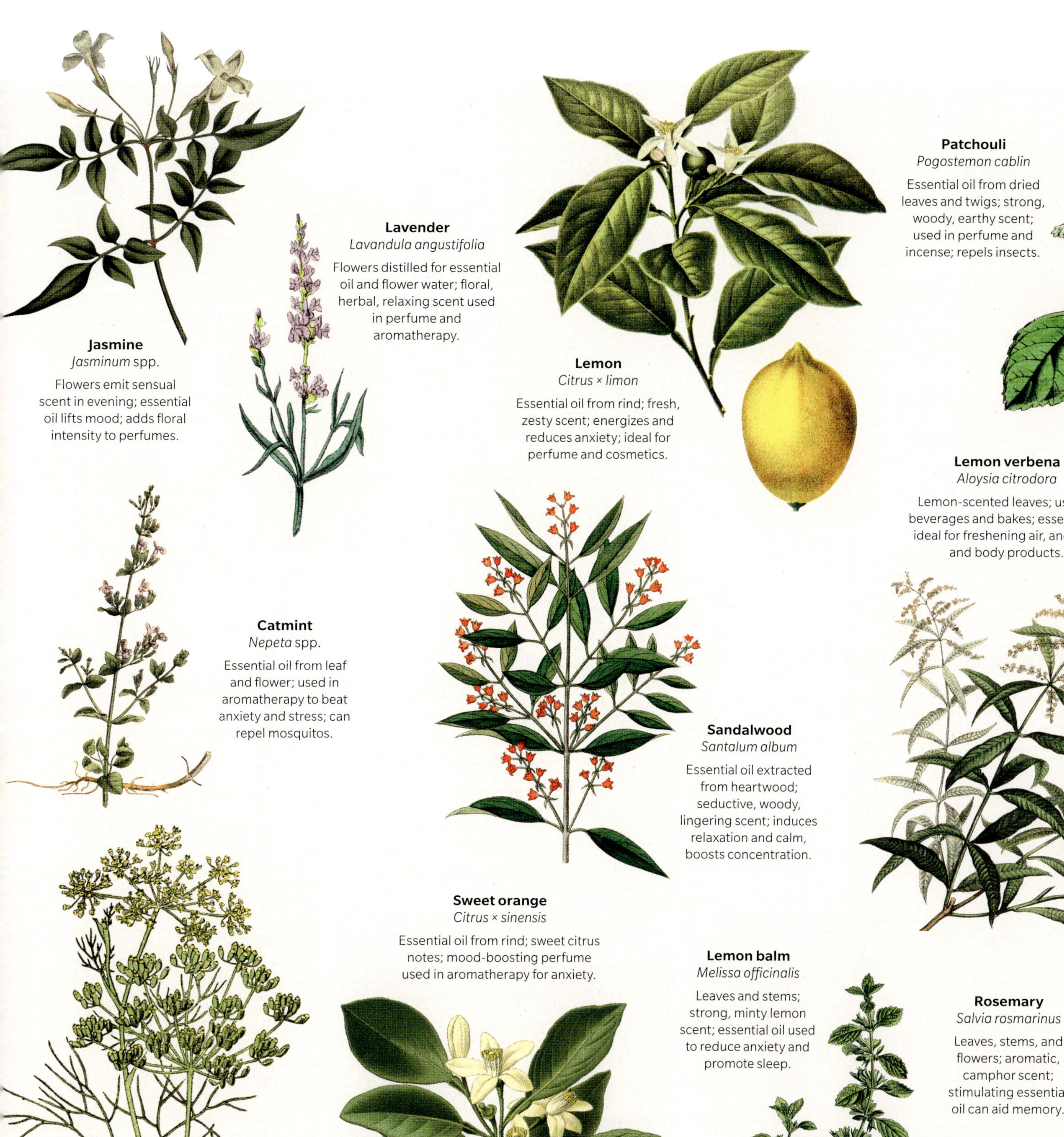

Jasmine
Jasminum spp.
Flowers emit sensual scent in evening; essential oil lifts mood; adds floral intensity to perfumes.

Lavender
Lavandula angustifolia
Flowers distilled for essential oil and flower water; floral, herbal, relaxing scent used in perfume and aromatherapy.

Lemon
Citrus × limon
Essential oil from rind; fresh, zesty scent; energizes and reduces anxiety; ideal for perfume and cosmetics.

Patchouli
Pogostemon cablin
Essential oil from dried leaves and twigs; strong, woody, earthy scent; used in perfume and incense; repels insects.

Lemon verbena
Aloysia citrodora
Lemon-scented leaves; used in beverages and bakes; essential oil ideal for freshening air, and bath and body products.

Catmint
Nepeta spp.
Essential oil from leaf and flower; used in aromatherapy to beat anxiety and stress; can repel mosquitos.

Sandalwood
Santalum album
Essential oil extracted from heartwood; seductive, woody, lingering scent; induces relaxation and calm, boosts concentration.

Sweet orange
Citrus × sinensis
Essential oil from rind; sweet citrus notes; mood-boosting perfume used in aromatherapy for anxiety.

Lemon balm
Melissa officinalis
Leaves and stems; strong, minty lemon scent; essential oil used to reduce anxiety and promote sleep.

Rosemary
Salvia rosmarinus
Leaves, stems, and flowers; aromatic, camphor scent; stimulating essential oil can aid memory.

Fennel
Foeniculum vulgare
Leaves and flowers; an anise, liquorice scent; spicy, peppery essential oil ideal for home fragrance and bath products.

Indian Frankincense

Boswellia serrata

From very ancient times, various varieties of frankincense were prized in civilizations such as ancient Egypt and Greece, in the Ayurvedic tradition, and in Christianity. Indian frankincense was well known for its medicinal properties, and remains in widespread use today.

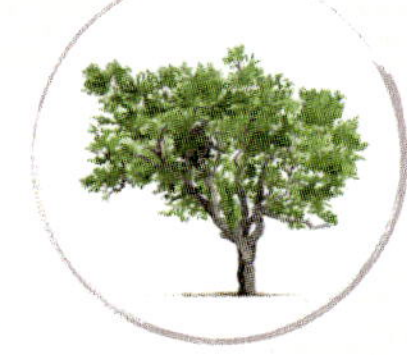

Uses Medicines, incense, fumigants, mummification preparations, cosmetics, and perfumes

Parts used Gum resin and oils

Active ingredients Terpenoid acids including boswellic acids; terpenes; polysaccharides

Habitat Dry tropical forests, but widely grown as an avenue tree in India

Frankincense comes from small trees of the genus *Boswellia*, found in hot, arid zones including central Africa and the Indian subcontinent. The trees have clusters of composite leaves along their tangled branches and produce gum-resin from their trunks and branches. This is extracted three times a year by scrubbing or making cuts in the bark. The aromatic, milky gum-resin, or olibanum, that oozes out and dries is collected in lumps – this is the herb known as frankincense.

Frankincense scent is said to induce a sense of calm and spirituality, enjoyed by gods and people alike, especially if inhaled as incense and an altar offering. Greek historian Herodotus recorded the trade of frankincence in the 5th century BCE. Since the Middle Ages, many Christian churches have burned frankincense. The thousands of tonnes of this highly valued substance traded today are still mainly used in religious ceremonies.

Frankincense is also a key ingredient in the perfume industry and for scenting items such as luxury candles. It is a natural deodorizer and makes a room smell clean and healthy.

Colour ranges from white to amber yellow

▲ **Dried gum-resin**
When burned, the semi-translucent frankincense releases a smoke with a rich and sweet, woody or spicy balsamic fragrance.

Fragrant vapour released by small pieces of gum-resin

➤ **Indian incense burner**
This burner holds pieces of dried coconut husk, and sometimes a few hot coals to light the husks. Frankincense is scattered on the top to produce scented smoke.

> " Frankincense... though fashioned of dreams, is raiment and food for your soul. "
>
> KAHLIL GIBRAN, *The Prophet*, 1923

Similar herbs

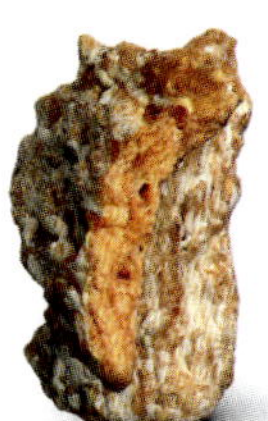

MAYDI RESIN
Boswellia frereana
The resin of the yagcar tree (native to Somalia) is used medicinally and as incense in the Coptic Orthodox Church in Egypt.

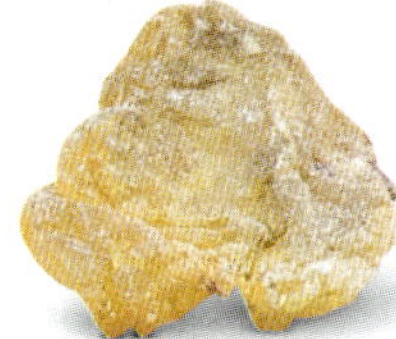

SUDANESE FRANKINCENSE
Boswellia papyrifera
The fragrance of this gum-resin from central Africa smells of spices and fresh lemon or pine. It has a translucent, yellow colour.

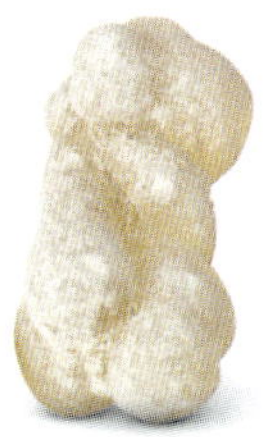

FRANKINCENSE
Boswellia sacra
Usually known as simply "frankincense", the most expensive resins come as white lumps from a small tree growing in Oman, Yemen, and Somalia.

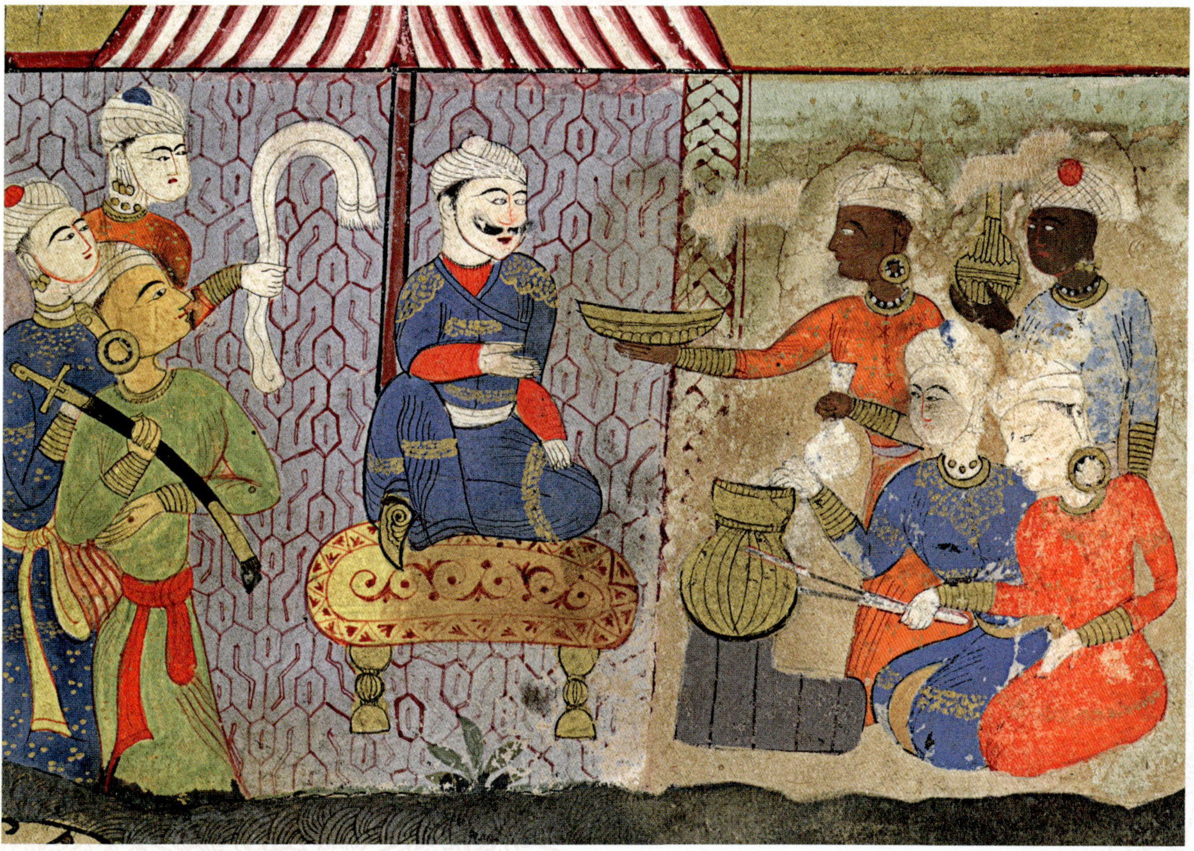

◄ Delights for a sultan
Frankincense here features as a treat fit for a sultan in a late-15th-century Indian manuscript, entitled the *Ni'matnāma-i Nasir al-Din Shah*. It details recipes for many culinary delicacies, remedies, and aphrodisiacs, to be prepared for Sultan Ghiyath Shahi and, later, his son Nasir Shah.

In ancient Egypt, it was used to clean and fumigate body cavities in preparation of the body for mummification, and in embalming. The female pharaoh Hatshepsut in 15th century BCE also added charred frankincense to kohl.

Medicinal applications

Frankincense has long featured in traditional medicine – *B. serrata* in Ayurvedic medicine and *B. sacra* in Middle Eastern and Western practices. Breathing its incense helped to calm patients and its uses ranged from healing wounds to alleviating pain. Indian frankincense's Ayurvedic uses include salving wounds and sores, balancing female hormones, and as an anti-inflammatory.

Today, oil obtained by steam distillation of the gum-resin is used medicinally, in cough drops and throat lozenges, and in aromatherapy to relieve anxiety. Clinical studies have indicated it is effective in treating rheumatoid and osteoarthritis, asthma, inflammatory bowel, and other afflictions. Its antibacterial properties make frankincense a useful ingredient of mouthwash. Extract of Indian frankincense is also sold in tablet or capsule form.

The highly valuable trade in varieties of frankincense still depends primarily on the wild population of slow-growing trees. Some trees are being heavily tapped, with the result that they produce fewer fruits and seeds and are prone to beetle attack. The current rate of harvest is believed to be unsustainable in the long term, especially as it is combined with other pressures such as habitat destruction and climate change.

SYMBOL OF DIVINITY

Frankincense occurs in the Hebrew and Christian Bibles as a prized and holy spice. It was the second of three gifts to the infant Jesus, given to him by the Magi (depicted here in the 1375 CE *Catalan Atlas* by Jewish illustrator Abraham Cresques). The "Book of Exodus" says God gave Moses an incense recipe: a mixture of frankincense, other gum-resins, scented spices, salt, and mollusc shells.

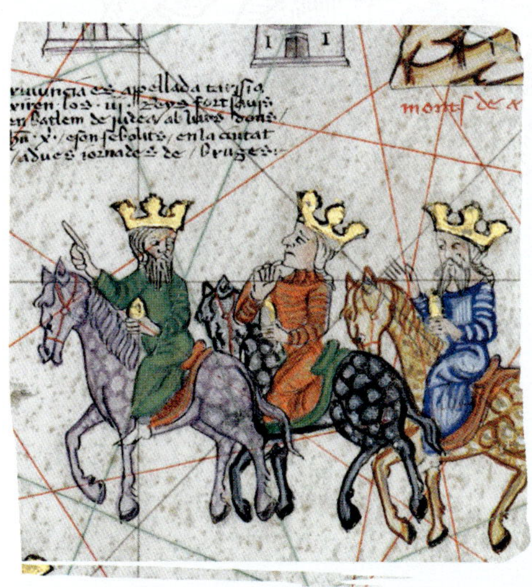

THE THREE MAGI, OR WISE MEN

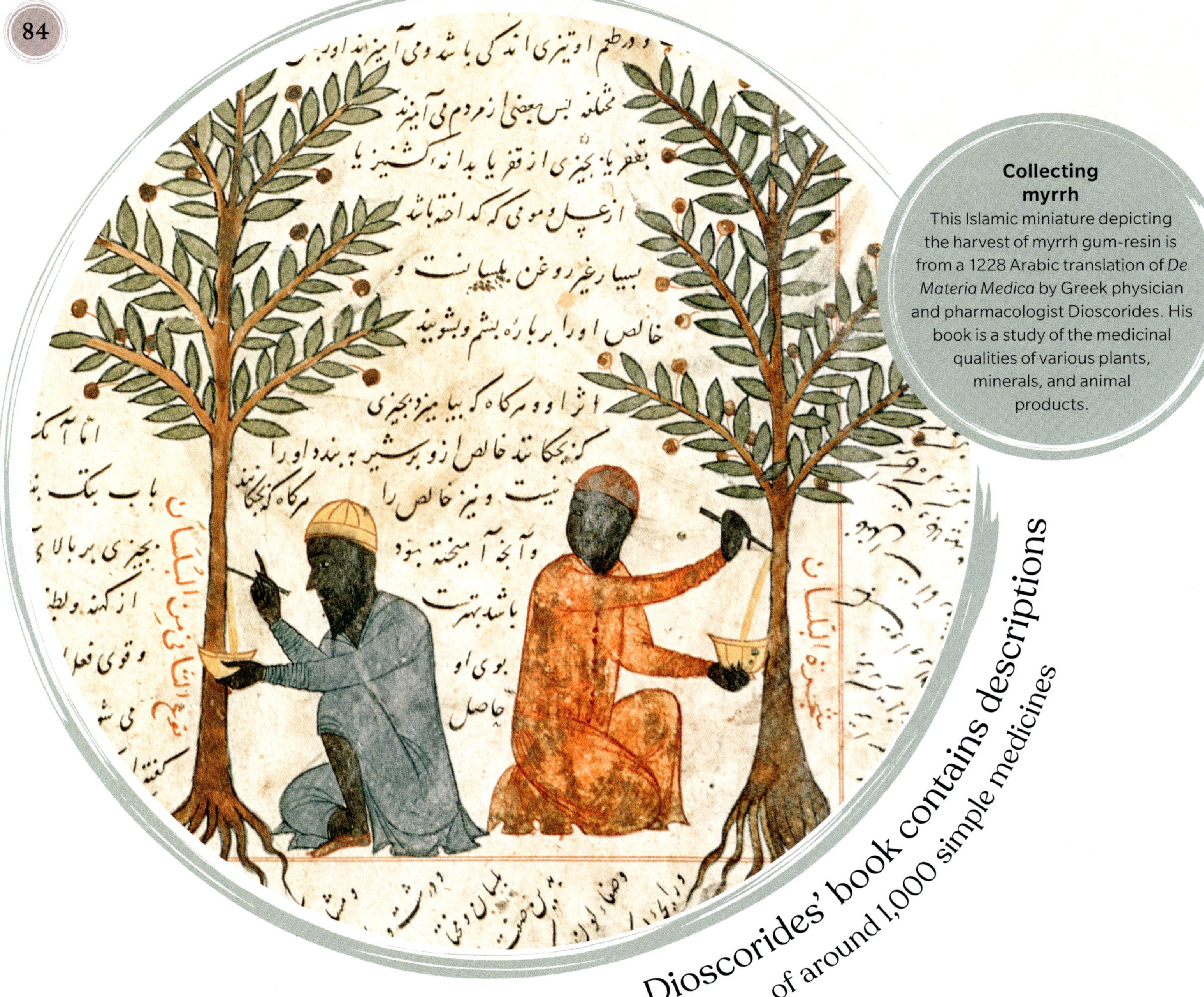

Collecting myrrh
This Islamic miniature depicting the harvest of myrrh gum-resin is from a 1228 Arabic translation of *De Materia Medica* by Greek physician and pharmacologist Dioscorides. His book is a study of the medicinal qualities of various plants, minerals, and animal products.

Dioscorides' book contains descriptions of around 1,000 simple medicines

Myrrh

Commiphora myrrha

Uses Medicines for pain, wound healing, and general health; perfume and incense, cosmetics

Parts used Dried resin, oil

Active ingredients Curzerene, limonene, and other terpenoid oils

Habitat Dry, rocky hillsides on limestone in tropical zones

Myrrh is the name for several small, thorny trees, as well as for the aromatic gum-resin that leaks from wounds in their bark. From ancient times, the resin has been prized as a perfume, incense, and medicine.

All *Commiphora* trees and shrubs exude a gum-resin, but the most valuable species is *C. myrrha*, named after the perfumed substance long known as myrrh. In turn, that word is derived from an Aramaic root, *murr*, meaning "bitter", referring to its taste. This species of myrrh is native to the Middle East and the Horn of Africa: it has knotty, fissured bark and the desert wind batters some of the wild trees into almost leafless, twisted shapes. The gum-resin from *C. myrrha* is called herabol

> " Myrrh and incense are accounted among the most ancient of the sweet-smelling spices. "
>
> EDMUND S. PURCELL, *The Antiquary, Volume 11*, 1885

myrrh; it is reddish-brown, darkens with age, and sometimes has white streaks. Another type of myrrh available is bisabol myrrh, from *C. kataf*: also called sweet myrrh, it is usually clear or opaque yellow with a glossy or waxy sheen and comes in smaller, pea-sized lumps. All myrrhs are members of the Burseraceae family, which also includes frankincense (see pp.82–83).

Myrrh is harvested, or tapped, by wounding the tree with a blade. The tree responds by bleeding a waxy resin, a natural, wound-healing glue. It dries quickly and can be scraped off. *C. myrrha* is now scarce in some places, due to drought and pressures on the land from agriculture and grazing.

The Incense Road

Myrrh, as well as frankincense, was a valuable commodity, traded between the Mediterranean, North Africa, and eastwards to the Persian Gulf, India, and beyond. The route, the Incense Road, flourished between the 7th century BCE and the 3rd century CE, after which economic decline ended much of the trade. The Bible mentions myrrh loaded for trading on to camels along with spices and balm. Myrrh traded to the Levant, and by sea to southern Europe, was vital to the economy of ancient Yemen. After the 6th century CE the trade partly resumed, with myrrh exported as far away as Spain.

Pliny the Elder in his *Natural History* (around 77 CE) described many kinds of myrrh gum-resin. Myrrh from wild trees, he said, was superior to that of cultivated plants and commanded a higher price. Some dry, dirty lumps of myrrh were more powerfully scented than more sightly ones. Pliny noted that experts could assess myrrh's quality and price from its scent and "unctuousness".

To Christians, myrrh is famed as one of the three gifts brought to the baby Jesus by the three kings, or Magi. In Biblical times, myrrh was used as an anointing oil in religious rituals, and to embalm the dead, so was a symbol of death and suffering. The gift of myrrh prefigured Jesus Christ's suffering. Mark's Gospel (15:23) describes how when Christ was on the cross, "they gave him to drink wine mingled with myrrh". The Gospel of Saint John relates how Nicodemus anointed Jesus's body with myrrh according to Jewish custom.

Incense and perfume

When combined with mugwort and thyme, myrrh served as a fumigant in the ancient Middle East. The gum-resin was also burnt over hot coals to produce a scented incense with a meditative influence suited to prayer. In some Christian churches, the incense burner is swung on a

▲ Myrrh resin
The tree's resin seeps from fissures in its bark, and is collected and dried. It can be dissolved in water or alcohol to form a hydrosol (suspension in water) or tincture.

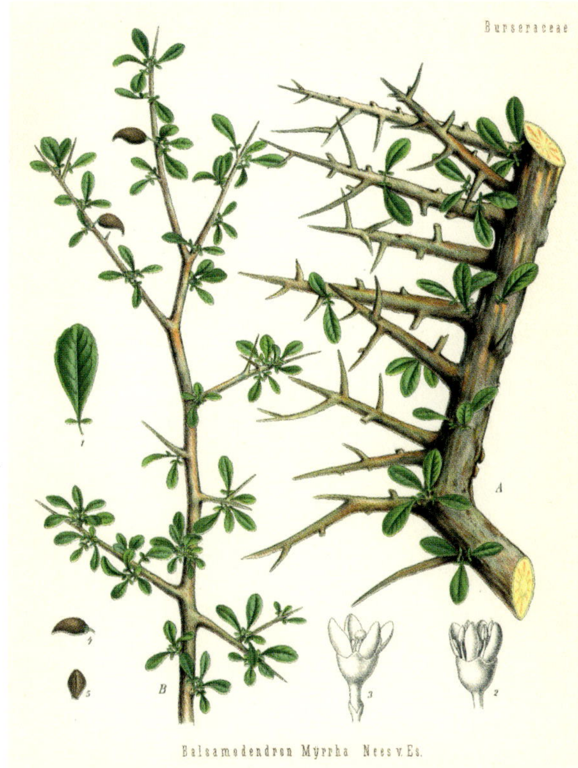

◄ Spiny, shrubby trees
The myrrh tree (*C. myrrha*) and its near relatives have quite variable characteristics. *C. myrrha*'s flowers are white, but some myrrhs have greenish yellow or pale red blooms.

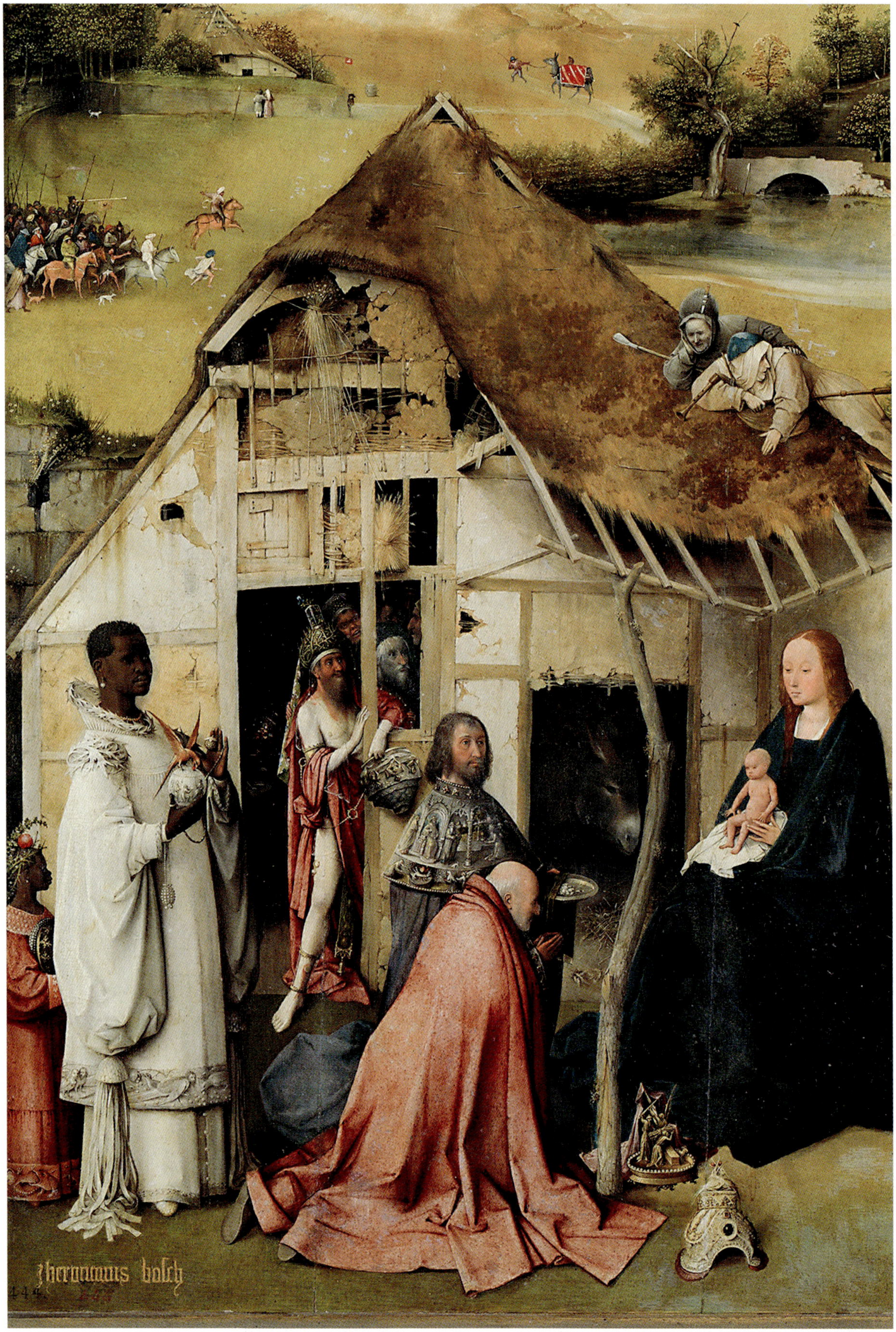

Similar herbs

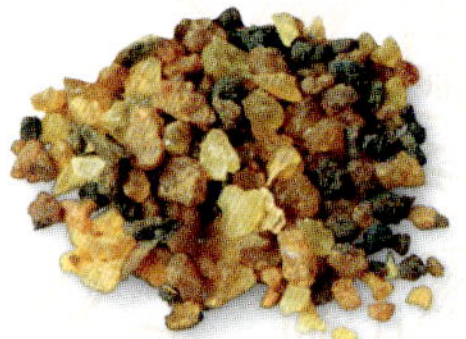

ABYSSINIAN MYRRH RESIN
Commiphora kua
Dried resin from this small tree was used in traditional medicine in Arabia. A liquid in which a small quantity of resin had been dissolved was painted over the affected part of the body.

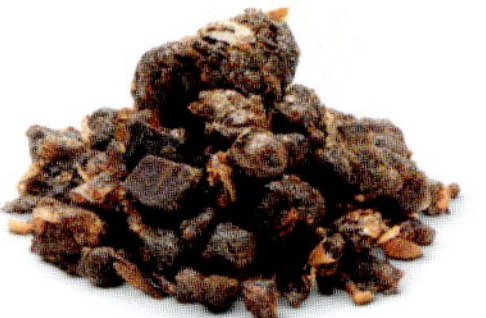

GUGGUL RESIN
Commiphora wightii
This resin, from Oman, Yemen, India, Pakistan, and Bangladesh, occurs in traditional medicine, including Ayurvedic. It is used to treat acne and arthritis.

◄ **Myrrh and the Magi**
In the Christian Bible story, the gift of myrrh from the wise men (Magi) to the newborn Jesus has been interpreted as a symbol of humanity and mortality. Here the scene is depicted by Dutch painter Hieronymus Bosch in a work from c.1495–1500.

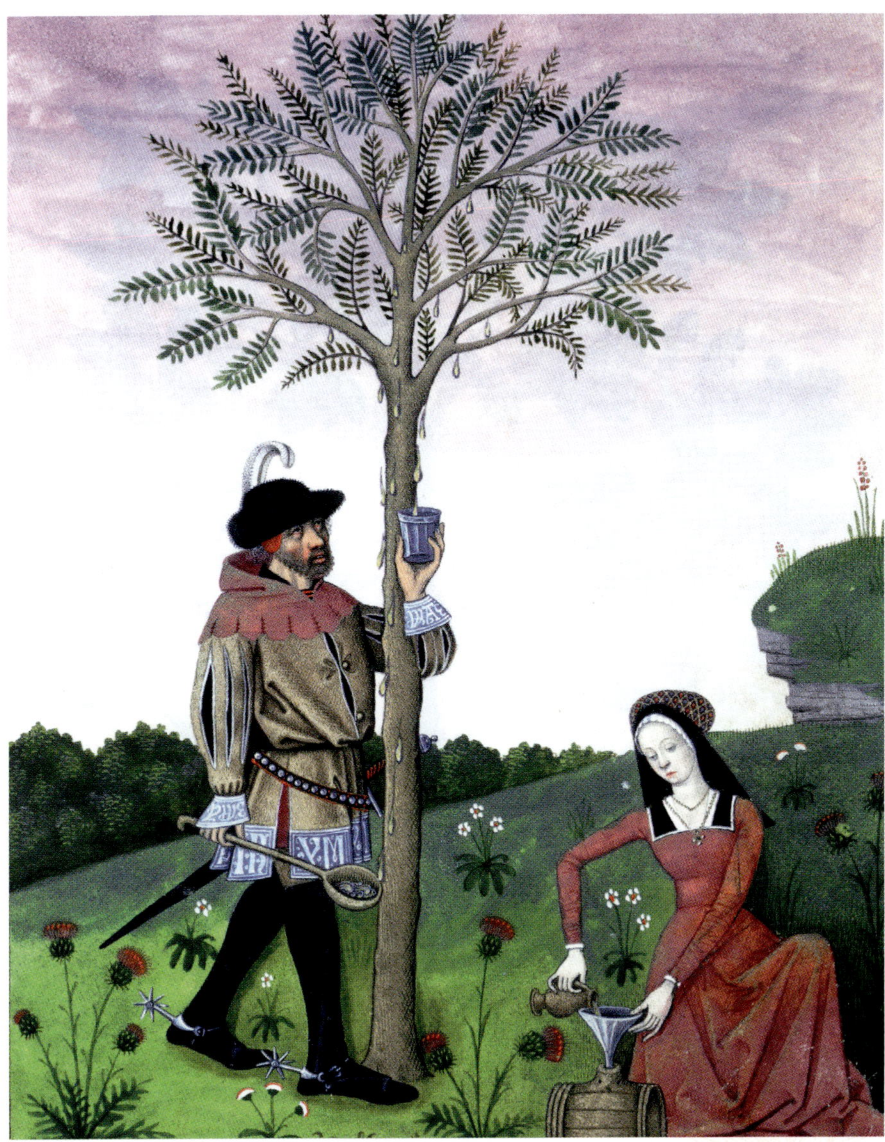

➤ **Medieval herbalism**
This depiction of collecting myrrh from Arabian balsam (*C. gileadensis*) is from a 15th-century edition of *The Book of Simple Medicines*, a 12th-century compendium of herbs and their medical applications by Matthaeus Platearius.

chain or suspended from the ceiling. To this day, myrrh is a key perfume ingredient and is often combined with frankincense in incense sticks.

Medicinal applications

Myrrh in traditional Chinese medicine is said to have "blood-moving" powers, as when purging stagnant blood from the uterus. Mixed with spices and alcohol, oil of myrrh was taken internally or rubbed on the skin as balm. It was judged most powerful if mixed with frankincense: while myrrh moved the blood, frankincense moved the *qi*, or life force. Together they offered a remedy for arthritis.

By contracting tissue, myrrh could strengthen hair roots to reduce hair loss. It is reputed to heal wounds by the same astringent action, restricting bleeding and increasing white-blood-cell function. Myrrh's astringency is also used to improve the health of gums, muscles, and internal organs.

Steam distillation of the gum-resin creates the warm, earthy, bittersweet scent of myrrh oil, used in aromatherapy to ease congestion and as a mild sedative. In the toothpaste industry, it is used as a flavouring and antibacterial agent. A dilute preparation rubbed into the skin is said to aid wound healing and prevent fungal infections; rubbed into joints, it may relieve pain. As with many natural drugs, scientific proof lags behind belief, but myrrh oil is known to be rich in antioxidants and anti-inflammatory compounds.

" The mirrhe sweete-bleeding in the bitter wound. "

EDMUND SPENSER, *The Faerie Queene*, 1590

WHAT IS AN ASTRINGENT?

Astringents are substances that cause contraction or shrinking in organic tissue and restrict secretion of fluids. Certain herbs have astringent properties and are used in herbal treatments, applied topically or internally. They are said to reduce skin inflammation and irritation, and create a barrier against infection. Herbs with astringent qualities include myrrh (see above), neem (pp.48–49), nettle (pp.200–203), prickly pear (pp.124–25), and rosemary (pp.92–93).

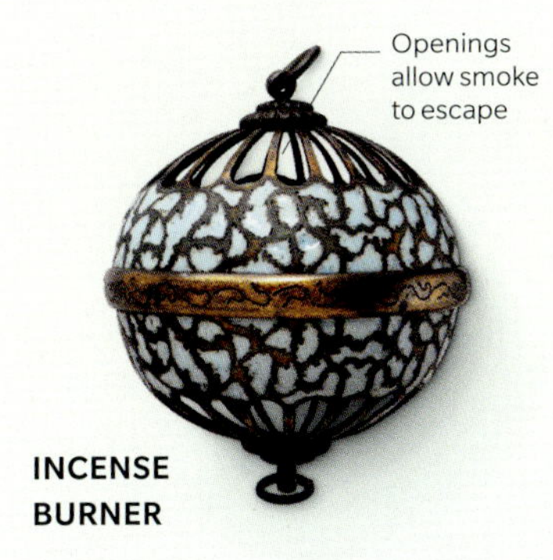

INCENSE BURNER

BURNING INCENSE

Myrrh has been burned in incense burners in many cultures for hundreds of years. Burning charcoal or coals heat the myrrh and the fragrant smoke escapes through openings in the vessel. Incense burners vary from simple earthware bowls or fire pots to elaborate enamelled and gilded devices (left). Middle Eastern or Chinese burners in stone, pottery, or metal often take the forms of various beasts.

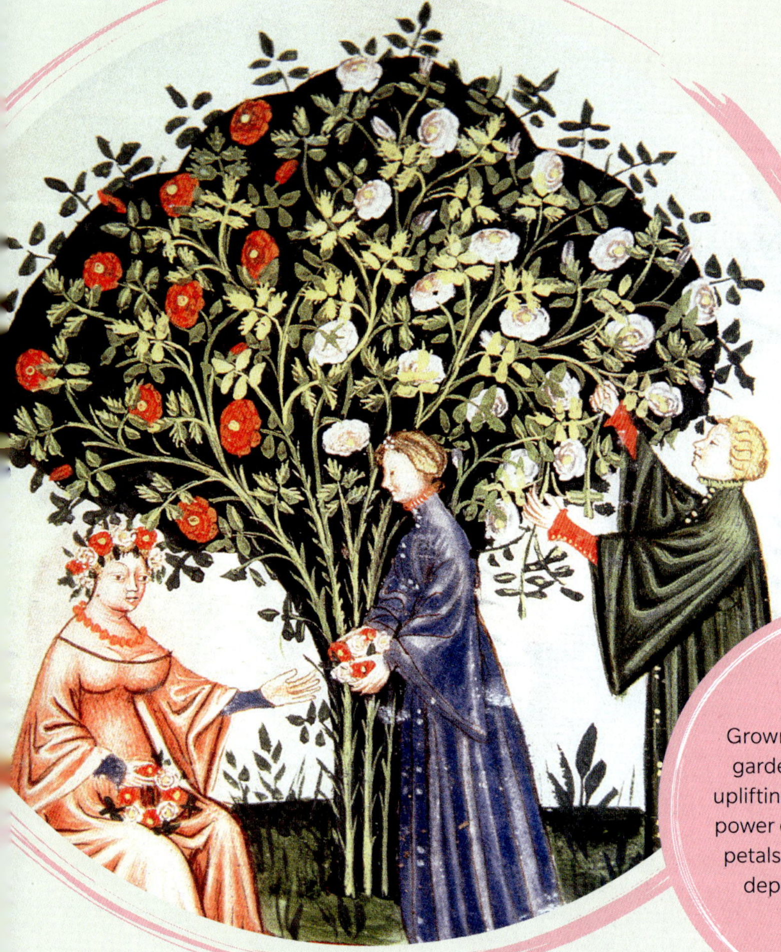

Rose gathering

Grown in medieval monastic gardens across Europe, the uplifting and anti-inflammatory power of essential oil from rose petals was harnessed to treat depression, sore throats, indigestion, and skin rashes.

➤ **French rose**

The Apothecary's rose is a variety of French rose (*Rosa gallica*) so named for its popularity in France, although it is thought to have originated in Persia.

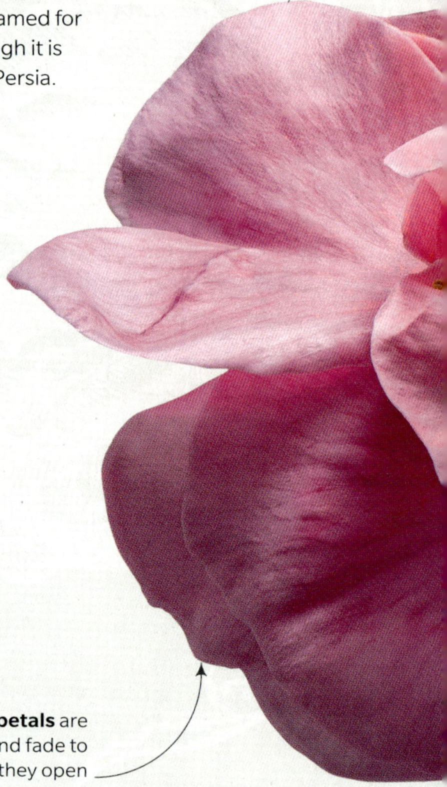

Light crimson petals are highly fragrant and fade to paler pink as they open

Apothecary's Rose

Rosa gallica var. *officinalis*

Although named for its widespread use by 19th-century French apothecaries, the medicinal, cosmetic, and culinary benefits of this ancient, cultivated, deeply fragrant shrub rose have been documented for hundreds of years around the world.

Of the thousands of wild and cultivated roses found worldwide, *Rosa gallica* var. *officinalis* is perhaps the most well known as a herb. Thought to have originated in ancient Persia, it was brought to western Europe during the 13th century by returning Crusaders, where it was grown in the gardens of medieval monasteries for use in various rituals, and in herbal and cosmetic preparations. When apothecaries began to emerge in Europe in the 15th century, the rose's medicinal benefits became known to a much wider audience. Grown in pots outside 19th-century French apothecaries, and later adopted as the emblem

The rose has compound leaves that divide into leaflets. They are discarded seasonally (deciduous) and appear as new foliage in spring

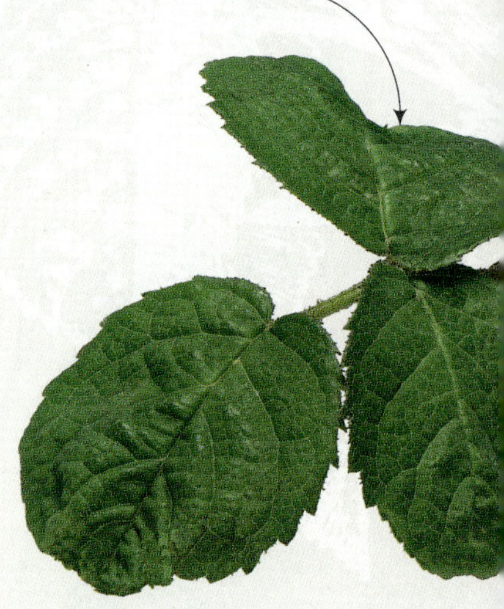

Prominent yellow stamens in semi-double flowers – cup-shaped flowers with two or more rows of petals – give bees easy access to pollen and nectar

Stems can be bristly but have few true thorns

" The dry conserve called the sugar of roses is a very good cordial against faintings, swooning, weakness and trembling of the heart. "

NICHOLAS CULPEPER, *Complete Herbal*, 1653

Uses Medicines for skin conditions, cooking sweet dishes, perfume

Parts used Petals, hips, leaves

Active ingredients Citronellol, geraniol, nerol, eugenol, linalool; vitamins C, B, E, K

Habitat Prefers full sun and moist, humus-rich conditions, but will grow in poor, dry soil with some shade

of a burgeoning pharmaceutical profession, *Rosa gallica* var. *officinalis* gained the name "Apothecary's rose".

This crimson-petalled, deeply scented shrub rose is still grown in herb gardens today, although its modern-day uses are more fragrant than those outlined in such early herbals as Pliny the Elder's *Natural History* (79 CE), *The Canon of Medicine* (1025) by Ibn Sina (also known as Avicenna), John Gerard's *Herball, or, Generall Historie of Plantes* (1597), or Nicholas Culpeper's *Complete Herbal* (1653). These herbal guides include rose-based panaceas for dysentery, scurvy, indigestion, heart palpitations, anxiety, constipation, fainting, insomnia, and melancholy. In the modern era, more palatable uses were found with recipes for crystallized roses and rose-petal sandwiches, and directions for making dry and moist potpourri, featured in Mrs M. Grieve's book *A Modern Herbal* (1931). She directs readers on the preparation of roses for the distillation of essential oil and scented water, and therapeutic, cosmetic, or culinary uses. She advises that in dry weather, in the morning, only the flower-buds that are just about to open and fragrant, should be "plucked from the calyx so that they remain united in small conical masses, leaving the stamens behind", kept in a fresh state for "confection", but "dried carefully and quickly on trays in a good current of warm air".

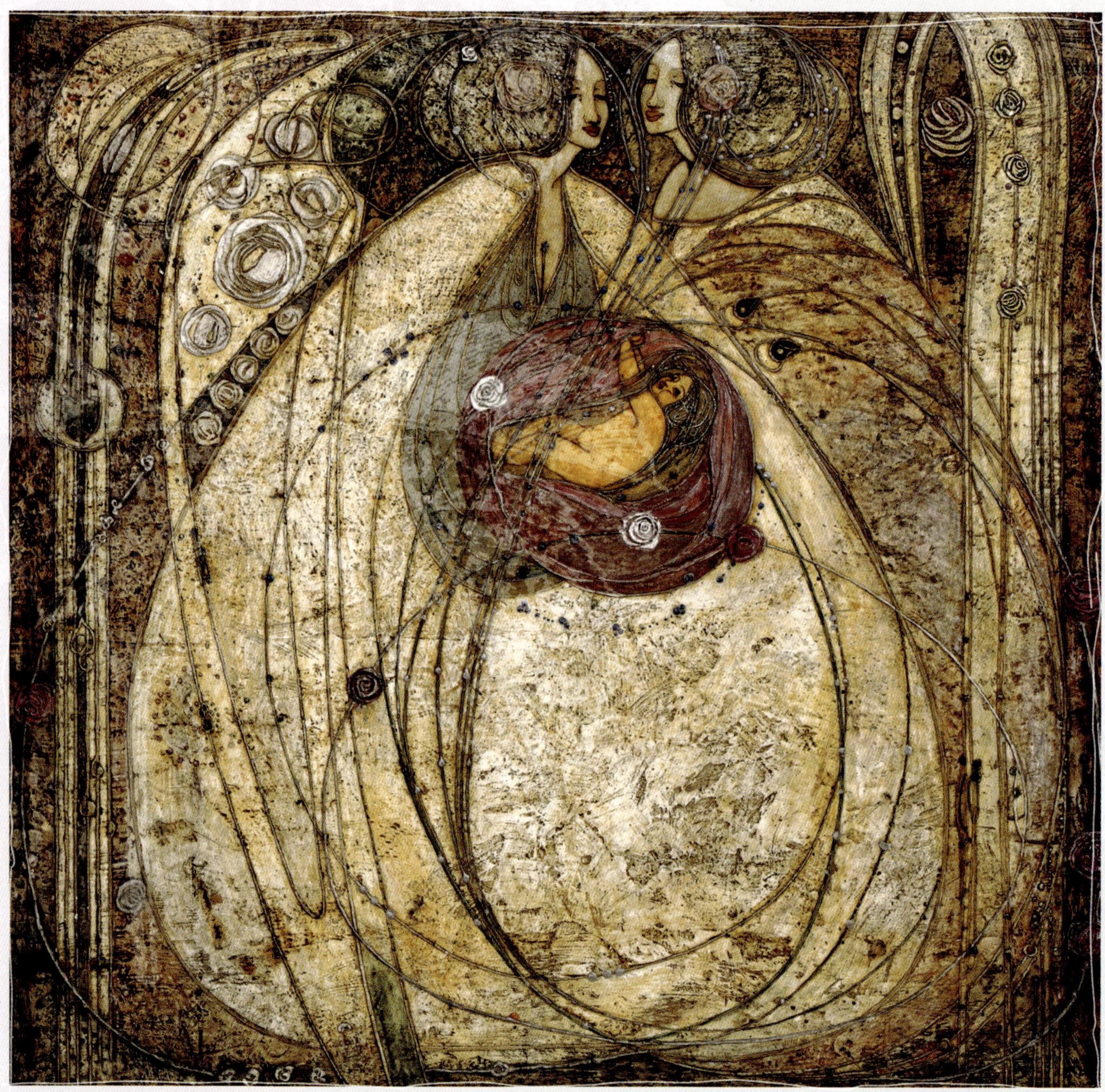

◄ Heart of the rose
Roses commonly symbolize love, romance, sensuality, beauty, and religion in art. *Rosa gallica*, particularly, was revered during the Renaissance era where it appeared in notable works by botanical illustrator Pierre-Joseph Redouté. Art Nouveau motifs, such as Margaret MacDonald Mackintosh's *The Heart of the Rose* (1902), left, often used roses to symbolize maternal and sensual love.

The elongated or globular orange-red hips of roses such as *Rosa gallica* have also historically been used to make vitamin C-rich syrup and tea, or to produce oils for use on the skin, while leaves can be infused into a restorative tea.

An illustrious past

Rosa gallica is a direct ancestor of Apothecary's rose and has been used to heal and beautify since antiquity; other wild roses have also been used for this including beach or Japanese rose (*Rosa rugosa*), China rose (*Rosa chinensis*), dog rose (*Rosa canina*), and briar rose (*Rosa rubiginosa*). Native to an area encompassing central and southern Europe and spanning the Caucasus and the Middle East, many societies used *Rosa gallica*. The ancient Egyptians, Persians, Greeks, and Romans cultivated the fragrant and naturally antibacterial, astringent, and tonic buds and petals to make perfumed oils, waters, wines, and cordials. Petals were scattered on the floor to mask unpleasant smells and used lavishly in ceremonies and celebrations. Such ancient practices, alongside the teachings of Ayurveda, which considers rose to be balancing, and traditional Chinese medicine, for which uses include for diarrhoea, dysentery, and menstrual regulation, found their way across continents and oceans through exploration, conquest, and writings.

DISTILLING ROSES

Many ancient civilizations made rose water by soaking petals. The first distilled version is credited to Persian physician Ibn Sina (980–1037 CE), leading to the production of "rose otto" essential oil some five centuries later. Miniatures from the Bundi school of art (17–19th centuries) depict women sprinkling rose water.

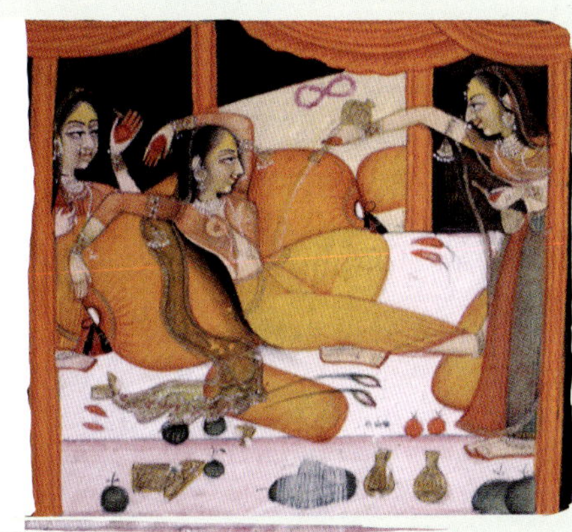

INDIAN MINIATURE SHOWING ROSE WATER

The Romans spread *Rosa gallica* across their empire, using it to adorn villas and make medicine. The red rose (the word "pink" was not widely used until the 17th century) has since been used widely in art, culture, and religion as a symbol of love, passion, romance, sensuality, healing, spirituality, and the divine. In 15th century Britain, the Church of England adopted the "rose without thorns" to represent the purity of the Virgin Mary, and two rival branches of the house of Plantagenet fighting for the English throne assumed red and white roses as emblems of power. The red rose, thought to be *Rosa gallica* var. *officinalis*, and the white rose, thought to be *Rosa alba*, were later combined into the emblem of the Tudor Rose as the two houses unified.

> " It is necessary to distil about 10,000 lb of roses to obtain 1 lb of oil. "
>
> MRS M. GRIEVE, *A Modern Herbal*, 1931

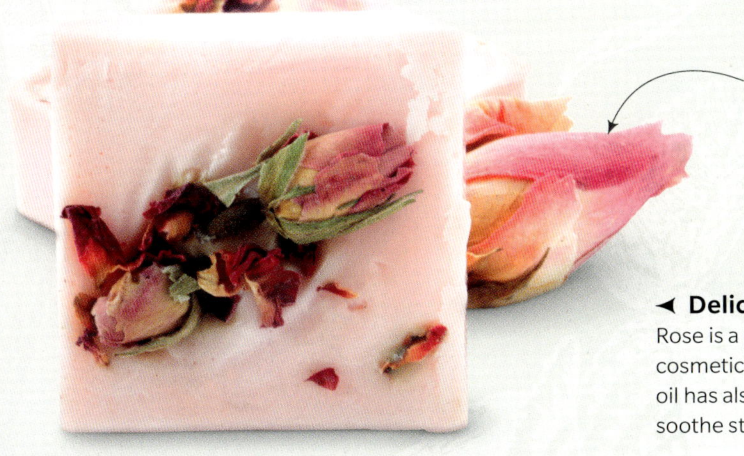

Rose buds and petals are often added to decorate soaps

◄ Delicate scent
Rose is a popular scent used to fragrance cosmetics. Soap made with rose essential oil has also long been thought to help soothe stressed skin.

Similar herbs

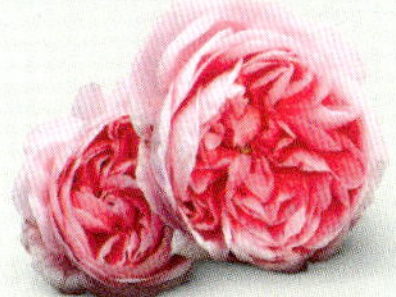

PROVENCE ROSE
Rosa × centifolia
Also known as the cabbage rose, this highly perfumed, multi-petalled hybrid is widely cultivated in Grasse, France, to produce rose oil.

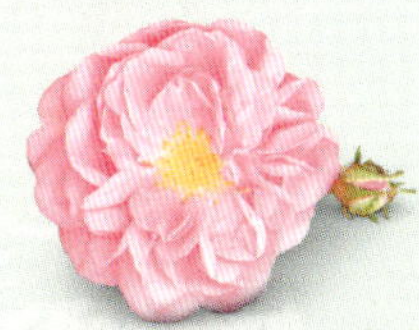

DAMASK ROSE
Rosa × damascena
Originating from the Syrian city of Damascus, this ancient, cultivated red rose hybrid is revered for its medicinal, edible, and highly scented qualities.

CHEROKEE ROSE
Rosa laevigata
Native to parts of East Asia, this rambling white rose has been used in Chinese traditional medicine and is the state flower of Georgia, US.

Uses Medicines for joint and stomach health; cooking; cosmetics

Parts used Leaves, stems, flowers

Active ingredients Rosmarinic acid, caffeic acid, carnosic acid, rosmanol, carnosol, pinene, camphor, limonene, borneol

Habitat Dry, sunny mountainous or hilly slopes near coast; in sandy, well-drained soil

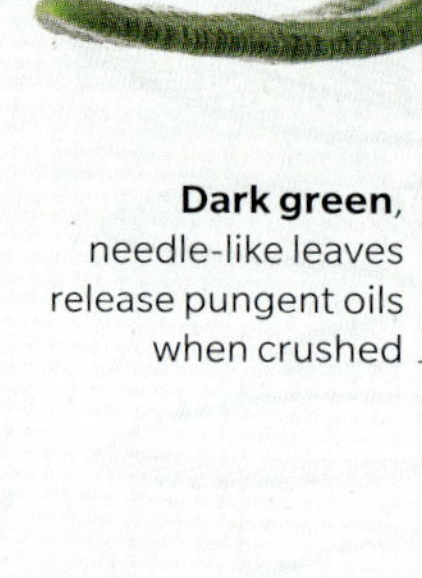

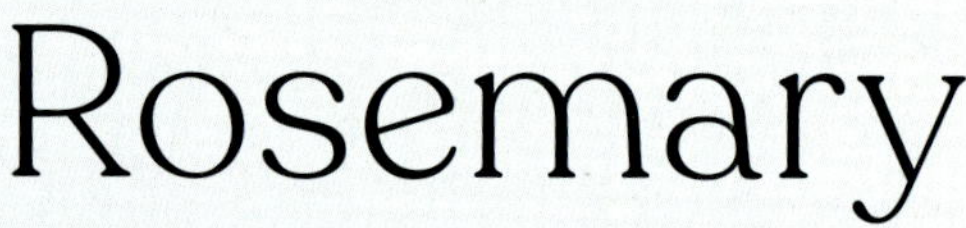

Rosemary

Salvia rosmarinus

Steeped in symbolism, this blue-flowered evergreen is a culinary herb with medicinal properties. Its pungent taste imparts a punch of flavour, while its fragrance has aromatherapeutic applications.

Native to the Mediterranean, including parts of Europe, the Middle East, and North Africa, rosemary takes its name from the Latin words *ros* and *marinus*, meaning "dew of the sea" – referring to its perceived ability to thrive in dry, coastal areas by drawing water from moisture in the air. Rosemary is an upright, woody shrub, although cultivars such as 'Prostratus' have a low-growing habit that can drape over the walls.

Multipurpose herb

This member of the Lamiaceae, or mint, family is an aromatic herb widely used in cooking – lending an earthy-floral, lemon-pine taste to roasts, breads, and sauces. Also known for its medicinal and cosmetic properties, rosemary is used in bath oils and ointments to warm the joints. It can also be used as a stimulating hair tonic, a soothing tea, and an air purifier. Such benefits largely stem from the constituent rosmarinic acid, which has anti-oxidant, anti-inflammatory, and antifungal properties.

Although ancient civilizations were yet to discover the science behind their herbs, they did gravitate towards such useful plants. Rosemary was seen as a token of love and virility. The Greek goddess Aphrodite was said to have rosemary draped around her neck as she rose from the sea, and Roman brides carried a sprig in their bouquets or in crown garlands, signifying the groom's prowess. It was also believed to boost memory and became symbolic of rememberance (see panel).

◄ Flavouring agent
A rosemary sprig can be used to coat the surface of breads with oil to add flavour. Its stems and leaves are included in fresh herb mixes, or *Herbes de Provence*, to infuse flavour in stocks and sauces.

Similar herbs

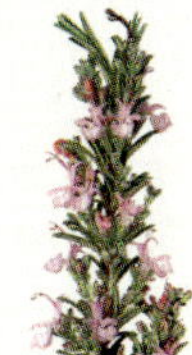

PINK ROSEMARY
Salvia rosmarinus 'Rosea'

This hardy cultivar bears small pink flowers and grows to a height of about 0.8 m (2 3/5 ft). Its short, bright green leaves are highly aromatic.

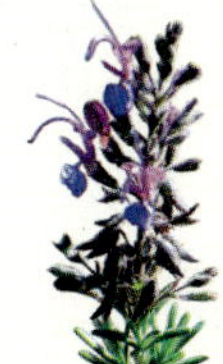

JORDAN'S ROSEMARY
Salvia jordanii

Native to southern Spain and North Africa, this medicinal rosemary has a two-lipped flower with a violet top and a lavender bottom lip.

" Where rosemary flourished, the woman ruled. "

ANON, cited in *A Modern Herbal*, Mrs M. Grieve, 1931

A HERB FOR REMEMBRANCE

William Shakespeare's play *Hamlet* (1603) makes reference to rosemary's traditional symbolic associations: "There's rosemary, that's for remembrance. Pray you, love, remember", proclaims the ill-fated young noblewoman Ophelia to her brother Laertes, foreshadowing her tragic death. British painter John Everett Millais depicted Ophelia drowning, surrounded by symbolic wild herbs and flowers.

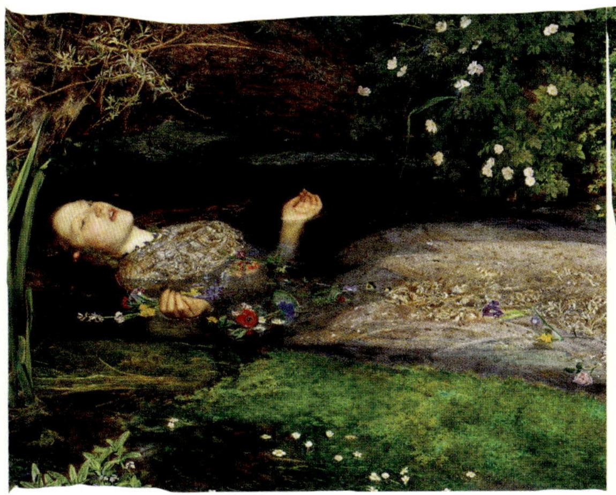

OPHELIA **(1851–52), PAINTING BY J. E. MILLAIS**

▲ Aromatic leaves
This versatile herb grows as a small to medium shrub, providing herbal supplies and ornamental interest through the year. Its nectar-rich flowers are also edible.

Woody stems make for fragrant cocktail stirrers

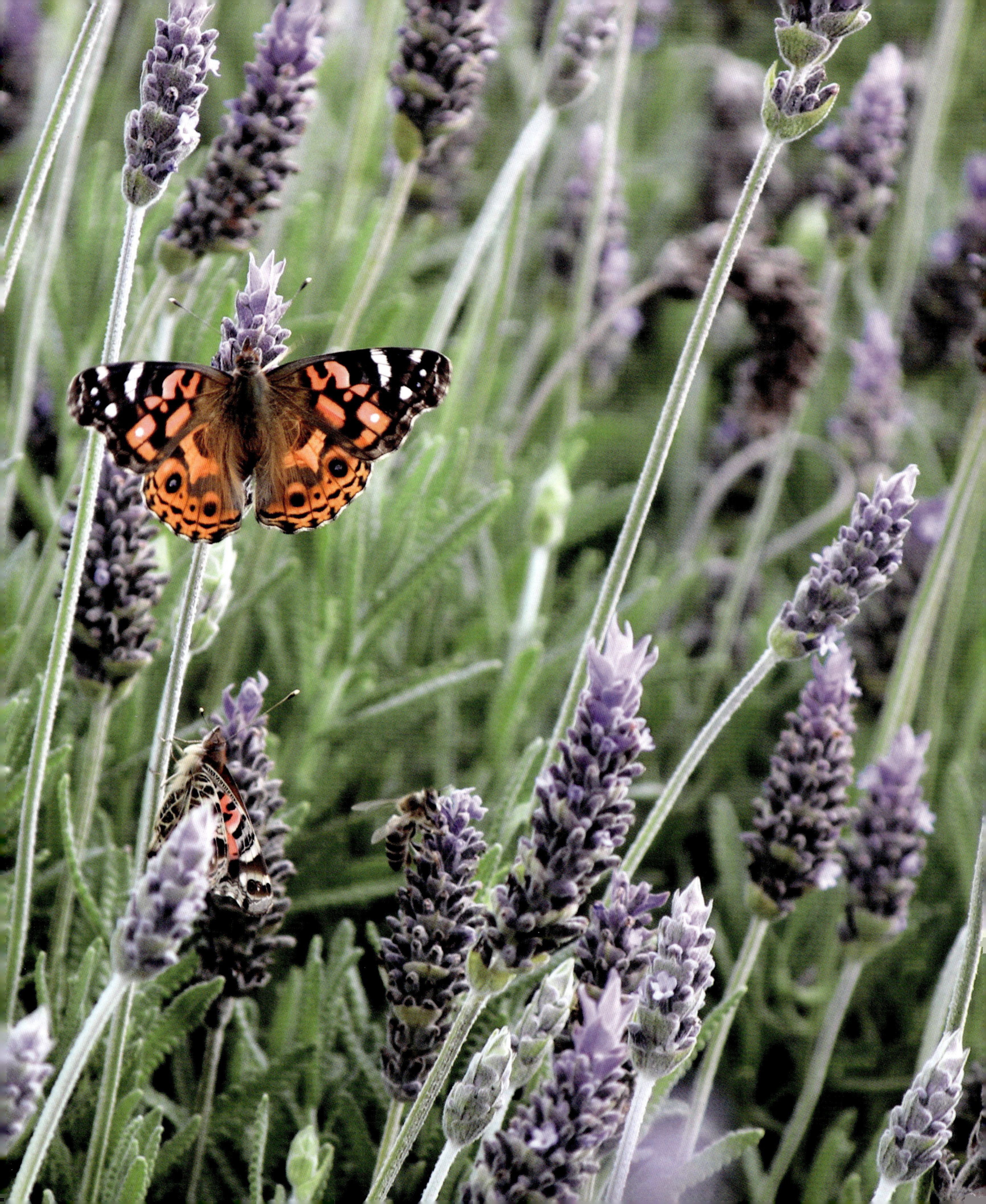

Uses Medicines, insect repellent, cosmetic, aromatherapy, perfumes, and cooking

Parts used Flowers, leaves

Active ingredients Linalool, linalyl acetate, geraniol, 1,8-cineole

Habitat Flourishes on sunny, mountainous slopes and in free-draining, sandy, or chalky soil

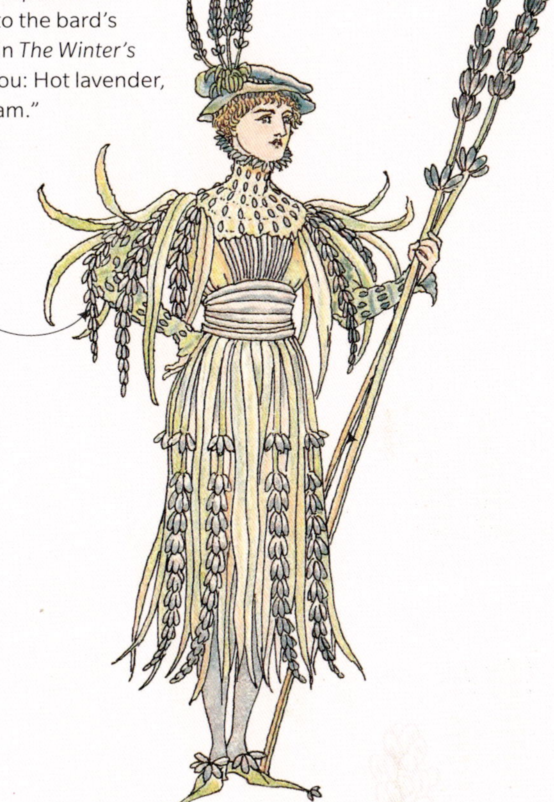

➤ Shakespearean flower
Lavender is one of the numerous herbs depicted in British illustrator Walter Crane's *Flowers from Shakespeare's Garden* (1906). It alludes to the bard's words spoken by Perdita in *The Winter's Tale*: "Here's flowers for you: Hot lavender, mints, savory and marjoram."

Aromatic herbs such as lavender were classified as "hot" in Elizabethan times for their restorative properties

Lavender

Lavandula angustifolia

Calming, cleansing, and sweetly scented, lavender has been used for thousands of years and remains popular today. True, common, or English, lavender is one of the most widely cultivated herbs.

Although often referred to as English lavender, *L. angustifolia* is native to the Mediterranean regions of France, Italy, and Spain. It has also been known as *L. officinalis* – from the Latin *officīna* meaning "storeroom for medicines" – owing to its medicinal properties. However, its previously published and current accepted name *L. angustifolia* refers to its narrow leaves, setting it apart from other known medicinal species, such as the wider-leaved spike lavender (*L. latifolia*) and the tuft-flowered French lavender (*L. stoechas*).

True lavender is one of around 40 species of the genus *Lavandula*, and there are also numerous cultivar and hybrid forms. They include the naturally occurring *L.* × *intermedia*, the white-flowered *L.* × *intermedia* 'Alba', the compact *L. angustifolia* 'Hidcote', and the slow-growing culinary favourite, *L. angustifolia* 'Munstead'. Various forms of lavender are grown across the world – for commercial use, for use at

➤ Pollinators' favourite
In full bloom, flowers, like those of this fringed lavender (*L. dentata*) attract a host of potential pollinators, including bumblebees, honey bees, and butterflies.

A PURIFYING OINTMENT

In the Gospel of John, 12:3, it is said that Mary Magdalene anointed Jesus with a perfumed oil days before his Crucifixion – to purify, heal, and make fragrant – in preparation for his impending death and burial. Here, Jesus anoints the feet of the Apostles with such an oil at the Last Supper (John 13:1–15). Different sources identify this oil as either lavender or spikenard, a member of the valerian family.

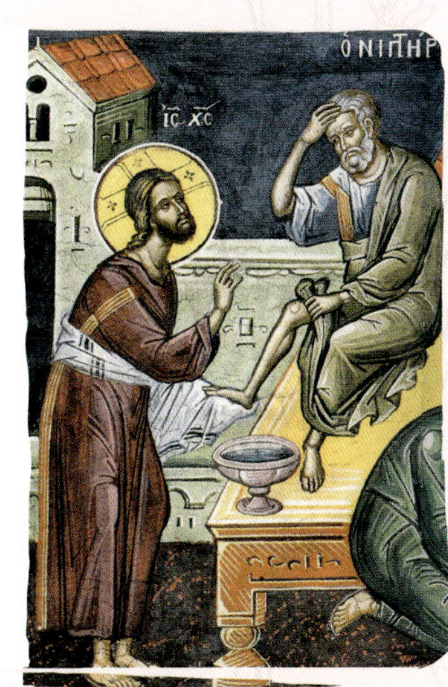

CHRIST ANOINTS AN APOSTLE

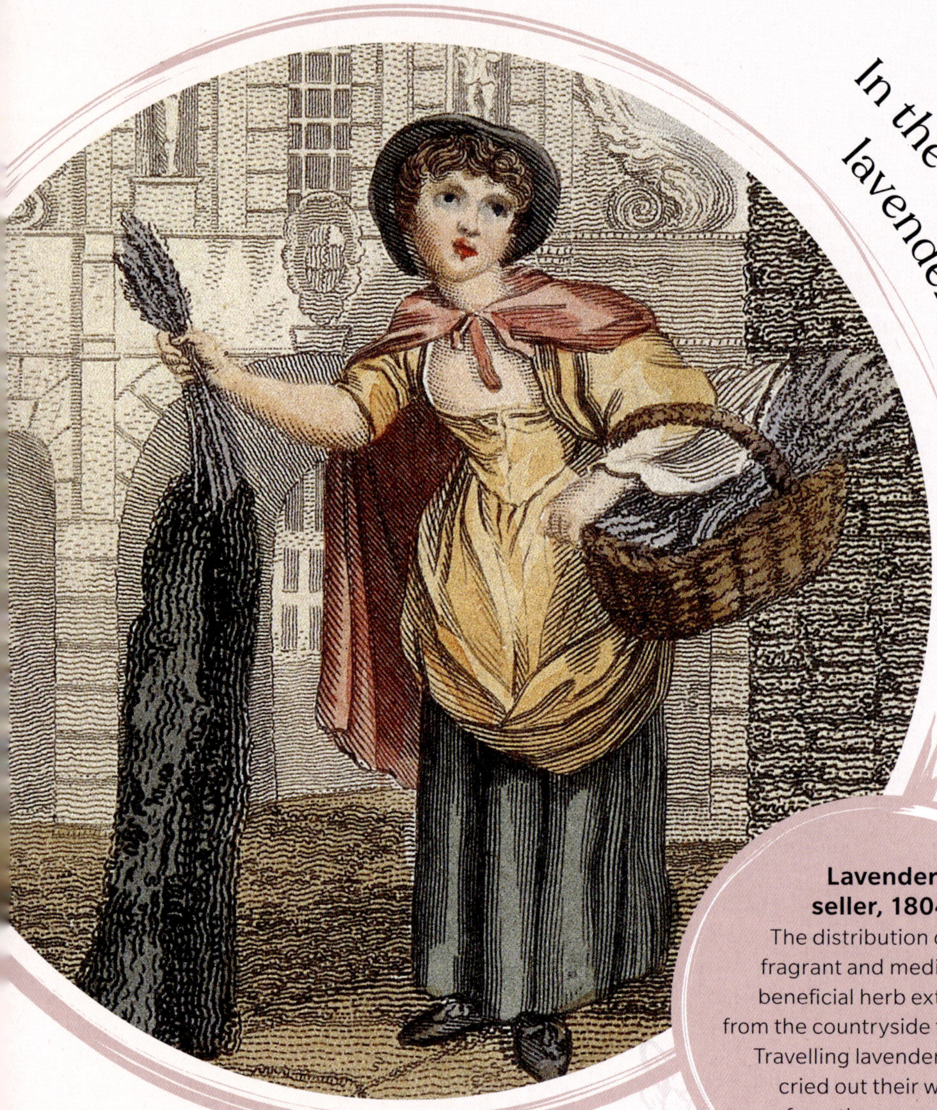

In the Victorian language of flowers, lavender signified devotion

Lavender seller, 1804
The distribution of this fragrant and medicinally beneficial herb extended from the countryside to the city. Travelling lavender sellers cried out their wares from the corners of busy streets.

home, and as a garden ornamental. The use of this multipurpose herb has been documented over thousands of years.

Spreading the word

In his *Canon of Medicine* (1025 CE), Persian polymath Ibn Sina, also known as Avicenna, describes lavender as a treatment for "melancholia". There are accounts indicating lavender was part of the mixture used by Italian polymath Leonardo da Vinci to preserve the cadavers he studied. In ancient Greece, lavender was referred to as *nardus* – after the Syrian city of Narada, where it was traditionally sold.

Although its use as a medicinal and culinary herb had already been established and passed down over hundreds of years in other civilizations, it was the Romans who were responsible for spreading lavender further afield by introducing it across their empire, which encompassed North Africa, western Asia, the Mediterranean region (from Greece to Portugal), and Britain. Known for their appreciation of perfumes, Romans utilized lavender's aromatic essential oil to scent hair, clothes, linen, floors, and walls. They also used lavender to scent, cleanse, and disinfect the water in private and communal bathhouses, harnessing its antibacterial and antiviral properties (see p.98). In fact, lavender gets its name from this usage – the Latin *lavare* meaning "to wash". Lavender water, prepared by steeping the dried or fresh herb in water, was also used on Roman battlefields and in hospitals to help prevent infection in wounds. Books such as Greek physician Dioscorides' *De Materia Medica*

Pale to deep purple flowers form dense spikes
Flowers are tubular and fragrant

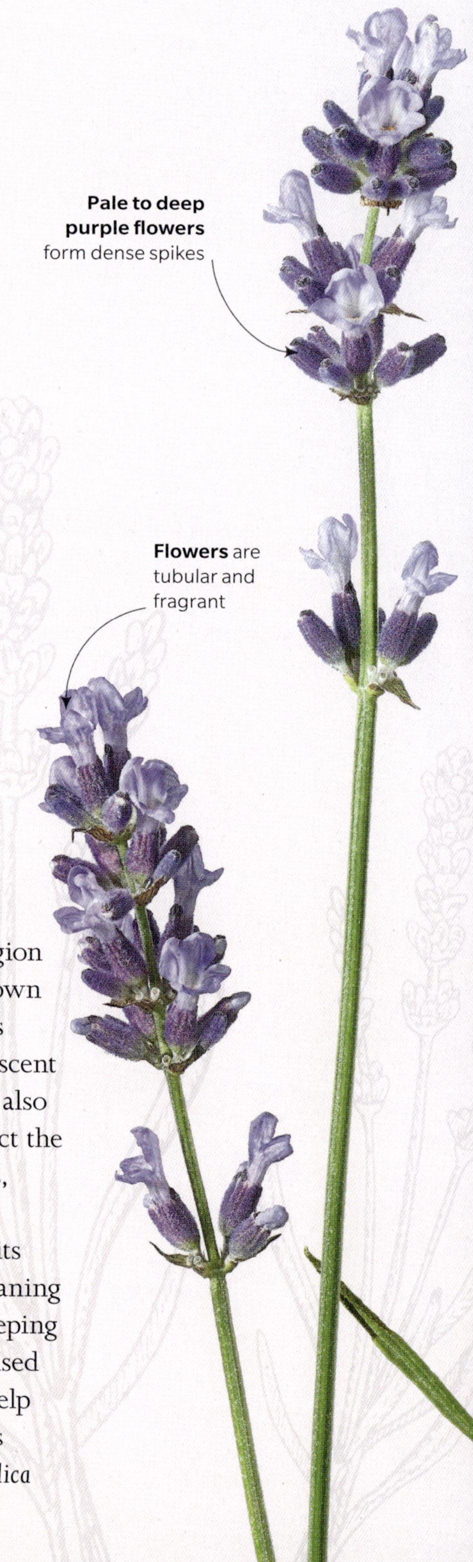

▼ Distinctive flowers
This easy-to-grow, compact woody shrub extends to about 1 m (3 ft) high, producing long unbranched stalks of flowers in mid to late summer.

Flower buds are often harvested as they retain their colour and scent well. The oil from immature flowers may have a "green" note

Narrow, grey-green leaves are highly aromatic

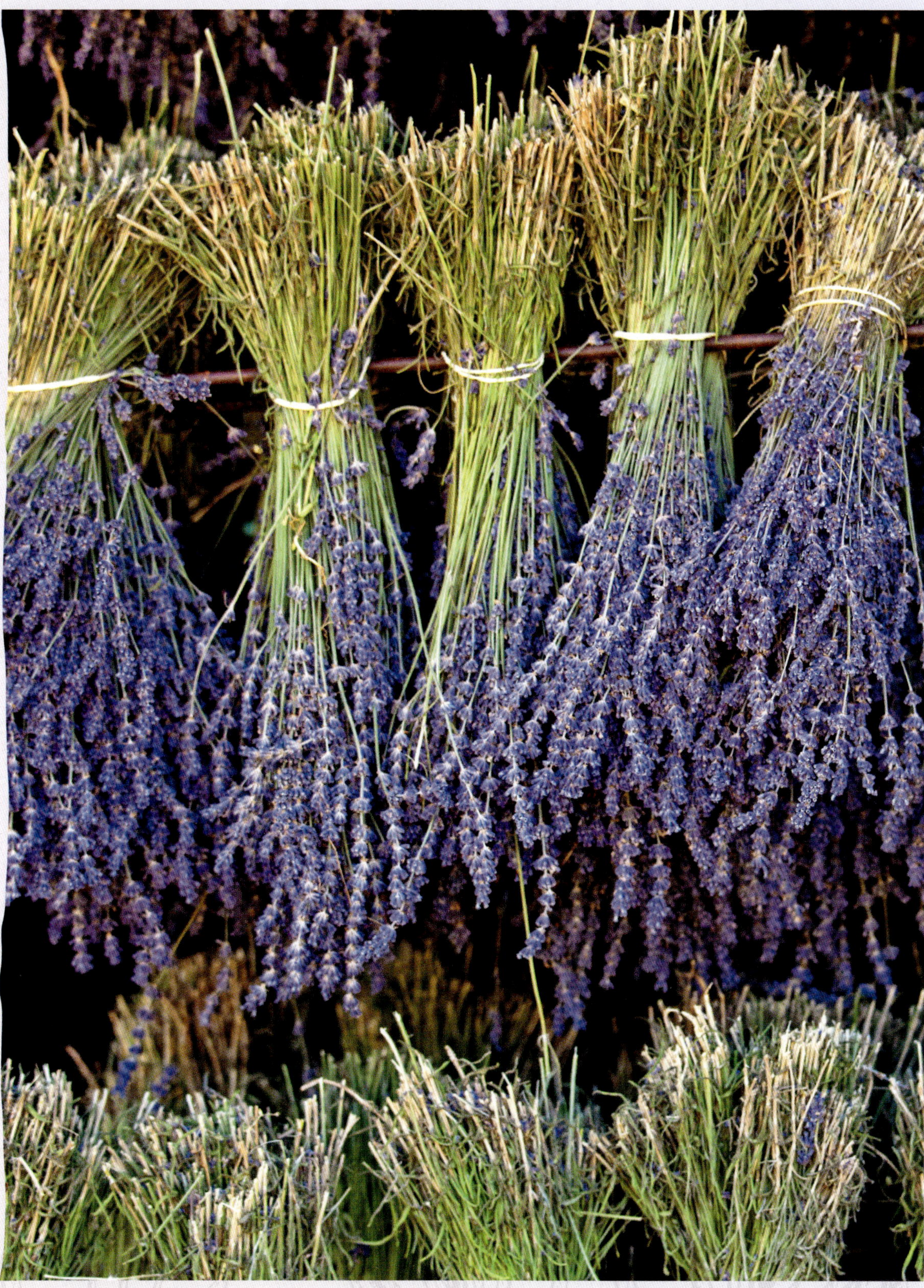

▲ Lavender bundles
Once harvested, bundles of lavender are hung upside down to maintain their shape, and stored away from direct sunlight to preserve their fragrance and colour.

Similar herbs

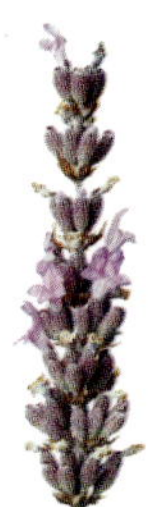

LAVANDIN
Lavandula × intermedia
This hybrid of true lavender (*L. angustifolia*) and the broad-leaved spike lavender (*L. latifolia*) exudes a more intense smell.

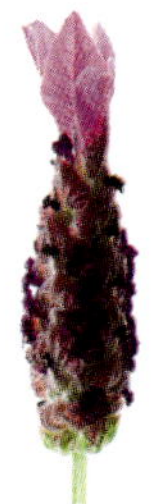

FRENCH LAVENDER
Lavandula stoechas
Easily recognized by its narrow grey leaves and deep purple barrel-shaped flower spires and bright purple tufted bracts, it is mainly used for its oil.

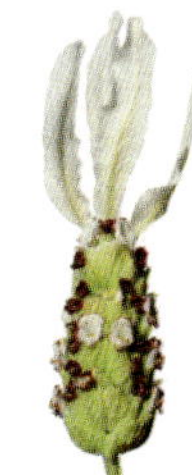

GREEN LAVENDER
Lavandula viridis
Native to southern Portugal and southwest Spain, this greenish white lavender has a high concentration of essential oils.

> " Being an inhabitant almost in every garden, it is so well known, that it needs no description. "
>
> NICHOLAS CULPEPER, *Complete Herbal*, 1653

(77 BCE) are thought to be the origin of lavender's use as a treatment for indigestion, headaches, sore throats, and skin conditions. Its reputation as a "cure-all" was echoed by the first printed herbals – manuscripts detailing herbal use – by British herbalists John Gerard, Nicholas Culpeper, John Parkinson, Elizabeth Blackwell, and Mrs M. Grieve.

A global phenomenon

By the Middle Ages, lavender was commonly used across Europe, the Middle East, North Africa, and Asia. During the Renaissance, it was used for protection against infections from cholera and the plague. It was used to treat early medical gloves and was a crucial component of the Four Thieves Oil – an essential oil concoction that is said to have prevented thieves from becoming infected while robbing the sick and dying during the plague.

Lavender was also popular with various monarchs, including Charles VI (1368–1422) of France, who used a pillow of lavender to help him sleep. Queen Elizabeth I of England (1553–1603) had daily bouquets and vases of the fresh flower placed throughout her castle, and had it strewn on the floors to ward off foul smells and the plague. She reportedly even drank lavender tea in an effort to treat her migraines. Queen Victoria (1819–1901) created a heightened awareness of lavender, both as a flavouring in food and as a scent. It is said that she preferred lavender jelly in place of mint with her roast mutton. She used lavender as a deodorant and perfume. The floors

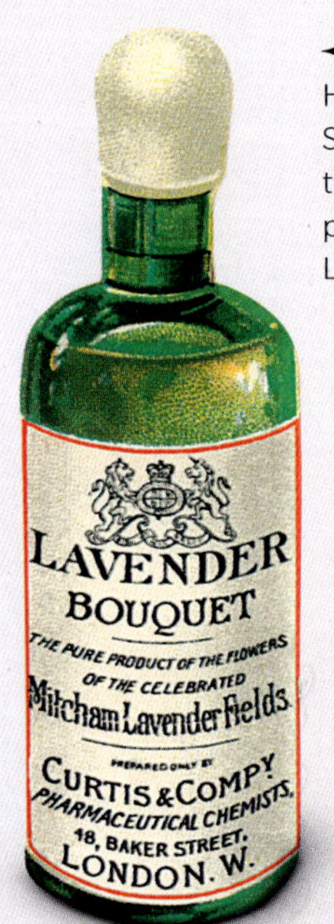

◄ **Pretty perfume**
Historically, the fields in Mitcham near Surrey, England, became synonymous with the production of quality lavender used in perfumes such as Crown's Mitcham Lavender Bouquet.

HOW DO ANTIBACTERIAL HERBS WORK?

Lavender, as with rosemary (pp.92–93) and thyme (pp.100–103), has antibacterial properties. The key ingredients in lavender essential oil, such as linalool and linalyl acetate, inhibit the growth of certain bacteria and pathogens by destroying their membranes. This includes harmful food-borne bacteria like *Escherichia coli* (*e-coli*), which can cause severe stomach cramps and vomiting, and the skin-infecting *Staphylococcus aureus*.

and furniture in the royal residence were washed in lavender, and linens spritzed with it. A Purveyor of Lavender Essence to Her Majesty the Queen was appointed to keep Victoria well stocked with lavender water and essential oils. Flower sellers on street corners procured basketfuls of budding lavender flower stems from farms and sold them as nosegay bouquets.

With the colonization of the Americas, Pacific regions, and parts of Asia and Africa, knowledge of the herb spread. As the demand for lavender increased, production needed to keep up. Lavender farms were established across Provence in France, around London, and then further afield, from which stems could be cut and oil and water distilled.

The birth of aromatherapy

In 1910, French chemical engineer René-Maurice Gattefossé successfully treated the gangrene developing in burns he sustained during a laboratory explosion, by smearing lavender essential oil on the wounds.

This confirmed his hypothesis that lavender had antiseptic and healing properties. He conducted further experiments – detailed in his 1937 book entitled *Aromatherapy* – which documented lavender's therapeutic benefits and its importance across the ages.

Today, lavender is widely used in soothing and healing bath and skincare products; as a relaxing, stress-relieving aromatherapy treatment; and to make perfumes and home fragrances. In the kitchen, it can lend a rich aroma and flavour to cooked and baked goods, and its restorative qualities are useful in treating small burns, insomnia, and menstrual problems.

◄ Lavender oil glands
This micrograph of a lavender calyx shows its oil-producing glands (in blue). While humans harness this essential oil for its aroma, flavour, and medicinal properties, insects such as mosquitoes are repelled by it.

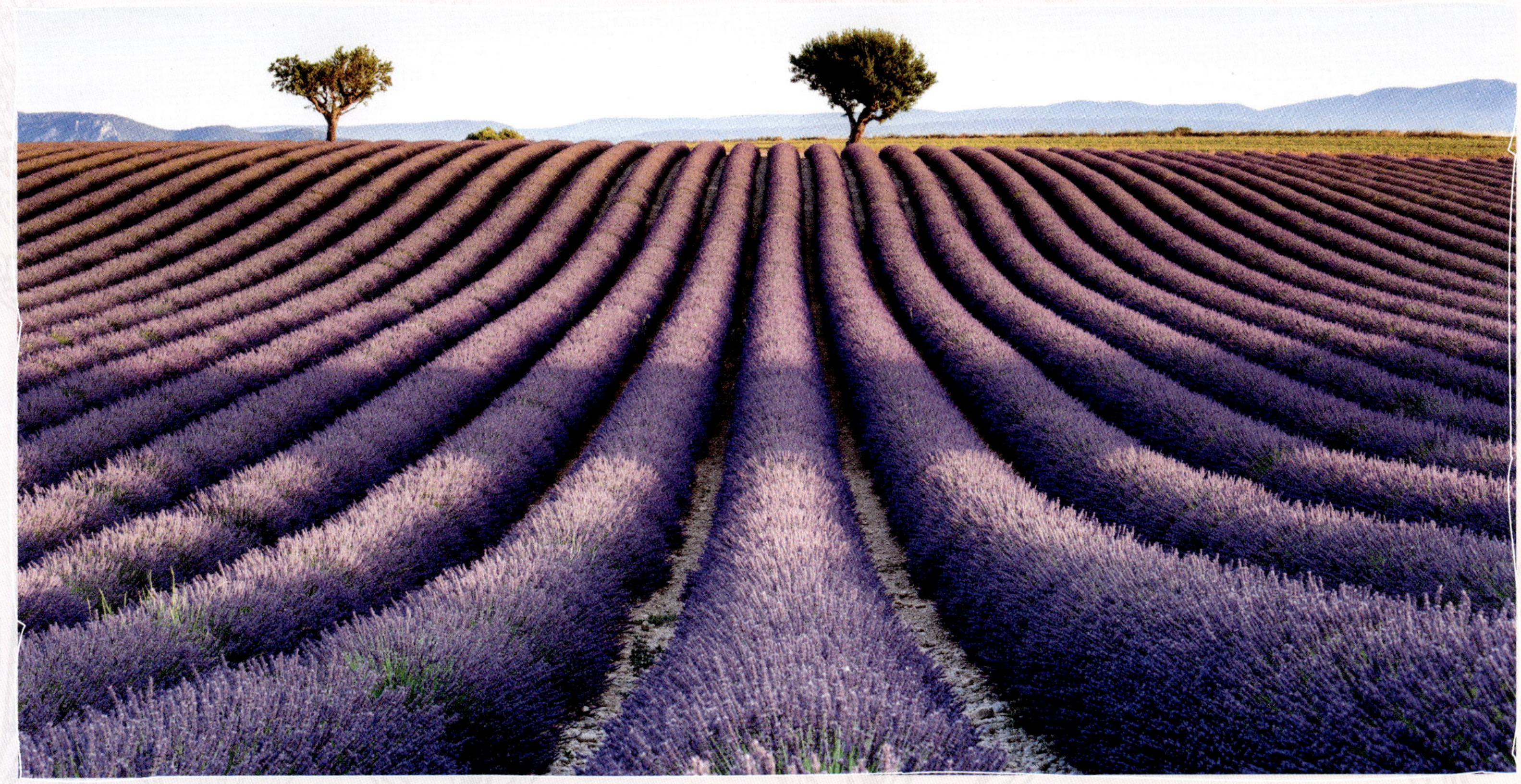

▼ Fields of violet
In 1747, with the establishment of the first perfume factories in the French town of Grasse, fragrant herbs such as lavender, initially harvested in the wild, were soon being farmed across the region of Provence.

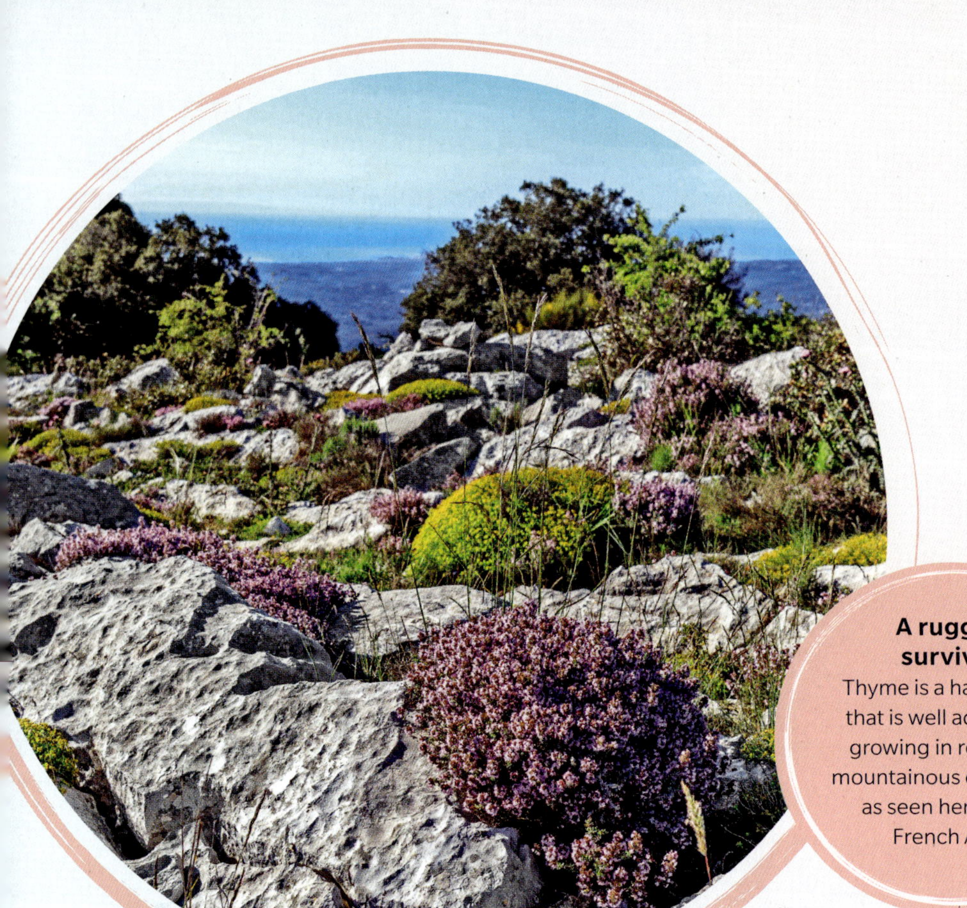

A rugged survivor
Thyme is a hardy plant that is well adapted to growing in rocky and mountainous conditions, as seen here in the French Alps.

Thyme is traditionally associated with vigour and bravery

Uses Medicines for respiration and digestion, flavouring savoury dishes, herbal teas, essential oils

Parts used Leaves, flowers

Active ingredients Thymol, carvacrol

Habitat Warm climates, rocky soil

Flowers are attractive to bees, butterflies, and other pollinators

Common Thyme

Thymus vulgaris

Thyme is one of the oldest and most commonly used herbs. Deliciously fragrant fresh or dried, it is an important food flavouring throughout the Mediterranean region and its oil has medicinal value.

The thyme most often found in shops and garden centres is the Mediterranean species common or garden thyme (*Thymus vulgaris*). Cultivated and sold fresh or dried, this is the thyme that is typically used in cooking – although many other wild and cultivated thyme species are equally aromatic, especially in dried form.

People first noticed the sweet aroma of thyme in prehistoric times, rising from beneath their feet as they walked. They swiftly identified the source as a small mat-like plant with clusters of lilac flowers. Indigenous not only to the Mediterranean area but also to North Africa, common thyme is a perennial herb that has

Grey-green leaves grow in pairs along the stems
Flower heads bloom in early summer

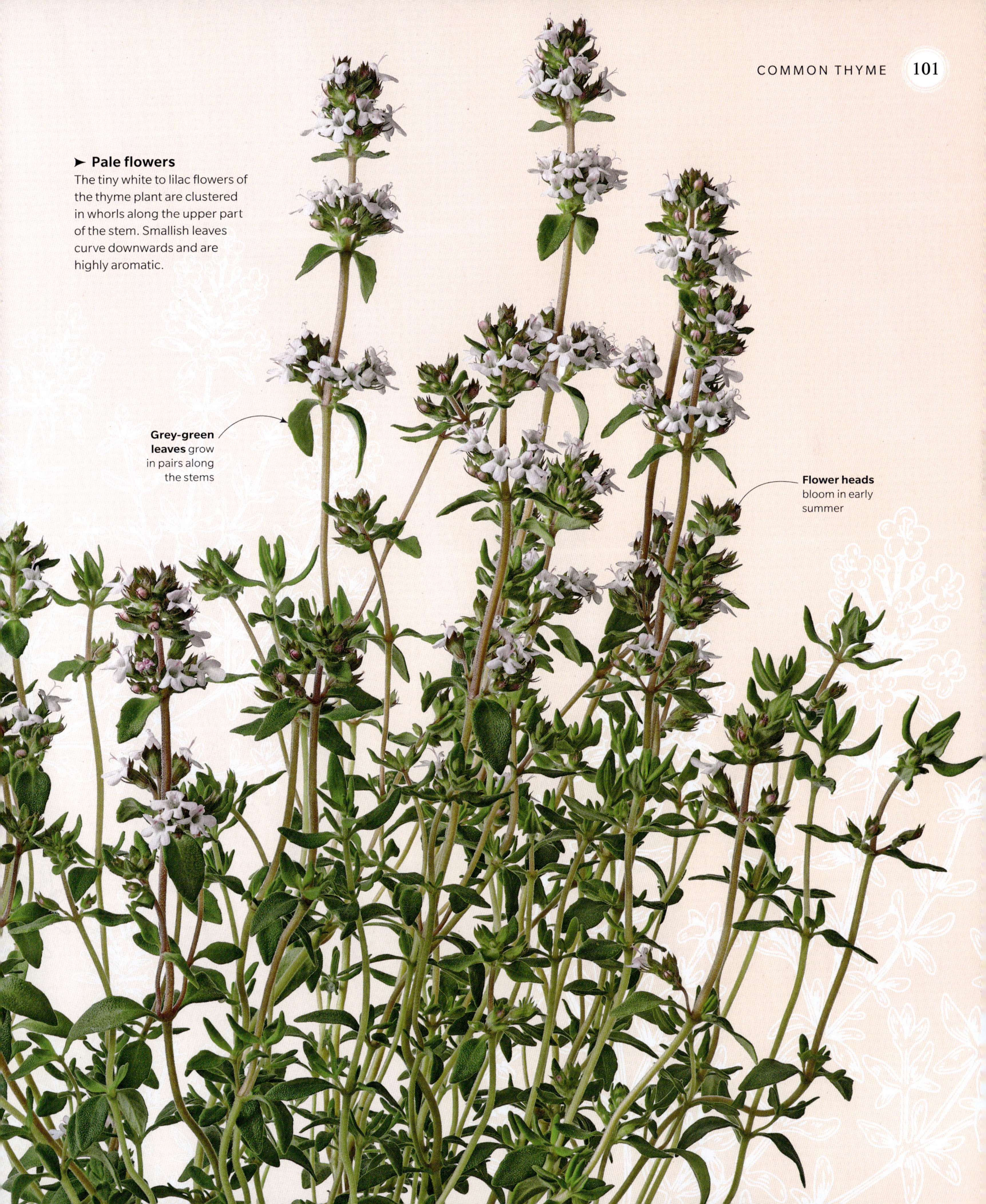

➤ Pale flowers
The tiny white to lilac flowers of the thyme plant are clustered in whorls along the upper part of the stem. Smallish leaves curve downwards and are highly aromatic.

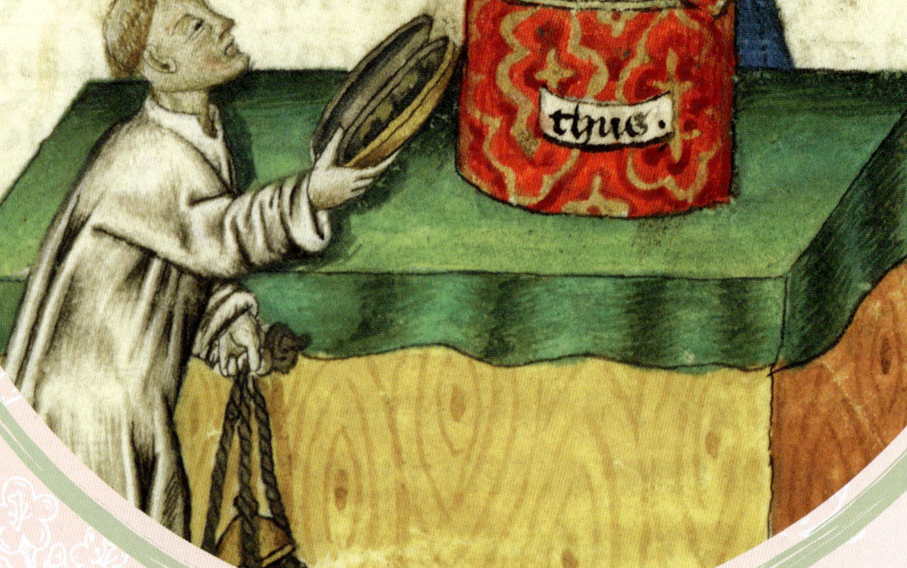

Dioscorides and thyme
The ancient Greek physician Dioscorides, seen here in the 15th-century Latin manuscript *Tractatus de Herbis*, described two kinds of thyme. One was *serpyllum*, a creeping form used medicinally. The other was a small shrub called *thumos*, used as a flavouring.

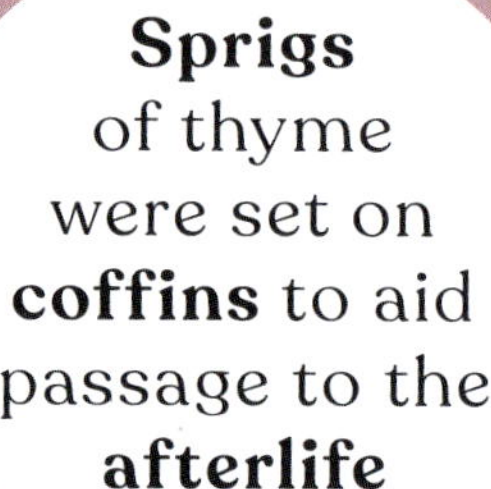

been widely grown since ancient times and carries a number of cultural associations. The Egyptians used thyme as an embalming herb, whereas the Greeks added it as a scent to their baths and burnt it as incense in their temples. It was assumed that the gods themselves would enjoy the fragrance as much as humankind. The cultivation of thyme spread throughout Europe during Roman times, when it was used as an air purifier and to flavour alcoholic drinks and cheeses.

Roman writer Pliny the Elder, working in the 1st century CE, recommended the burning of thyme in the home to deter poisonous creatures, and by the Middle Ages, knights in Europe were being given a sprig of thyme by their ladies as a symbol of strength and courage. Later, the herb reportedly became associated with the French Republican movement, with a tuft of thyme being sent to members with the call to meetings. In Scotland, thyme was considered a tonic that could help to prevent bad dreams, and it was either made into a tea or a sprig or two of fresh thyme was placed under the pillow at night.

HERBAL ANTISEPTIC

The phenol thymol, derived from the leaves of thyme plants, is well known for its antiseptic qualities. It was first isolated in the 1700s and later became the key ingredient in Thymol Dore, a popular eau de toilette used for personal and home hygiene (right). Thymol is also used in the modern antiseptic and antiviral product Thymox.

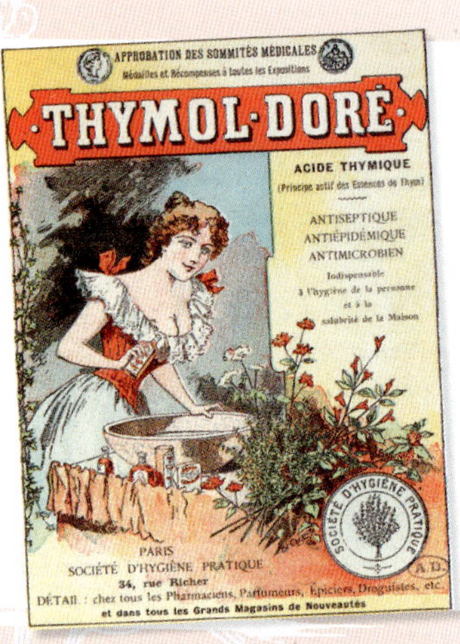

THYMOL DORE ADVERTISEMENT, 1908

Similar herbs

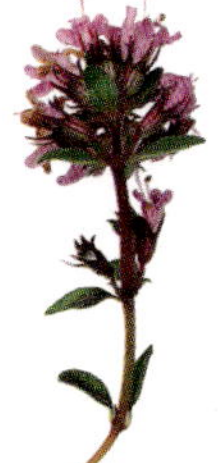

WILD THYME
Thymus polytrichus
Widespread throughout the UK and mainland Europe, this mat-forming plant has creeping, four-angled stems. Its clusters of flowers appear throughout the summer.

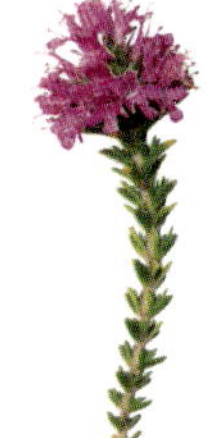

CONEHEAD THYME
Thymbra capitata
A Mediterranean plant, this compact species has longer leaves than some thymes and a distinctively cone-shaped cluster of purple flowers.

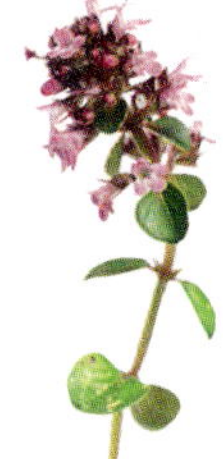

LARGE THYME
Thymus pulegioides
Native to Europe, this is a larger, looser plant than wild thyme. Its purple flowers grow in long clusters and it is found most commonly on chalky ground.

> "I know a bank where the wild thyme blows... There sleeps Titania sometime of the night, Lull'd in these flowers with dances and delight."
>
> WILLIAM SHAKESPEARE, *A Midsummer Night's Dream*, Act 2, Scene 1, 1600

Essential oils

Thyme belongs to the Lamiaceae family and, like many of its members, such as mint (pp.180–85), basil (pp.256–61), oregano (pp.126–28), and sage (pp.132–35), it contains volatile oils with antibacterial properties. These oils also make the plant taste bitter. Despite this, thyme tea is still taken as a herbal medicine, especially in the Scottish Highlands, where it is used as a stomach-settler. A stronger infusion in vinegar is good for respiratory complaints, although some say it must be prepared outdoors because bringing freshly gathered thyme into the house is unlucky.

The sources of thyme's delicious scent are its volatile monoterpene phenols, especially thymol, otherwise known as oil of thyme. This has long been used as an ingredient of cough medicine. In times past, thyme was strewn in drawers to scent linen and handkerchiefs before being overtaken for this purpose by lavender. Today, thyme is used in the cosmetic industry as an ingredient of scented soap, oils, pot pourri, diffusers, and lotions, as well as some perfumes. However, large quantities of fresh or dried thyme are needed to produce just a few grams of thyme oil. Fortunately, the scent is strong enough that most products require only a small amount of the oil.

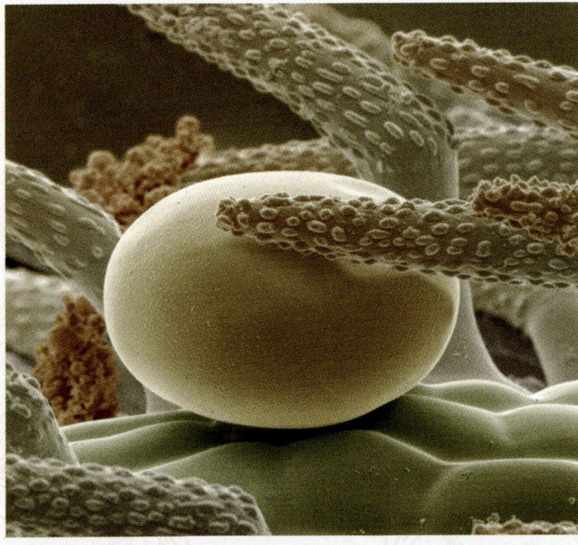

◄ **Thyme leaf oil gland**
Thyme's oils are contained in tiny spherical glands, known as trichomes, embedded in the leaf surface. They rupture when touched, releasing their fragrance.

Cooking with thyme

The most important modern use of thyme is in cooking. It lends a sparkle to stews and soups, to fish, pasta, and, particularly, potato dishes. It pairs well with tomatoes and beans, and is a principle ingredient of *bouquet garni* and *Herbes de Provence*. Dried thyme is also an ingredient of the Middle Eastern spice mixture called *za'atar*. Lemon thyme (*T.* × *citriodorus*) brings a citrus element, while Corsican thyme (*T. herba-barona*) has a distinct flavour of caraway seed. There are also varieties of thyme that smell of coconut, orange, or even rose petals.

CHAPTER 3

Perennial Flowering Herbs

Perennial plants live for several years, usually flowering every year. They are non-woody and in temperate regions may die back to roots in autumn, growing back in spring.

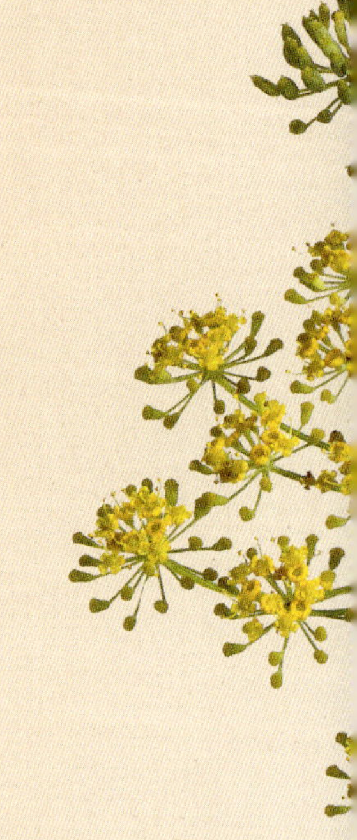

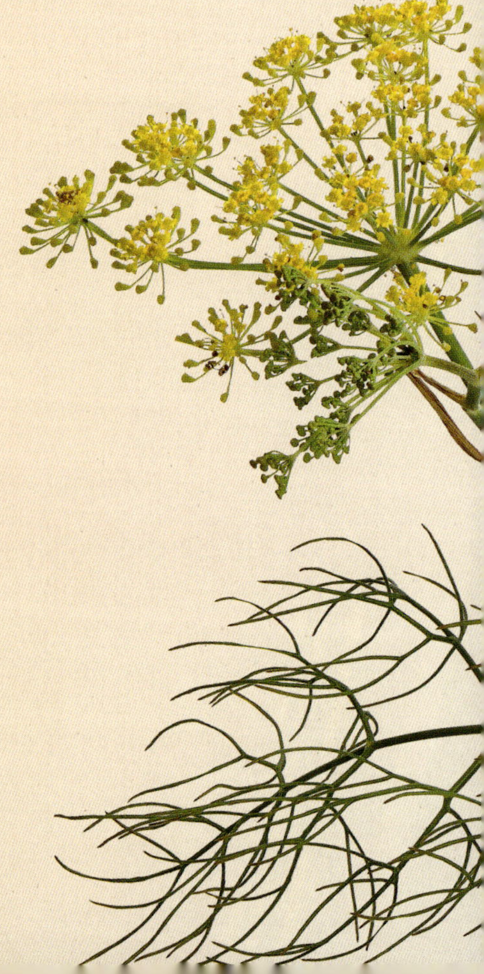

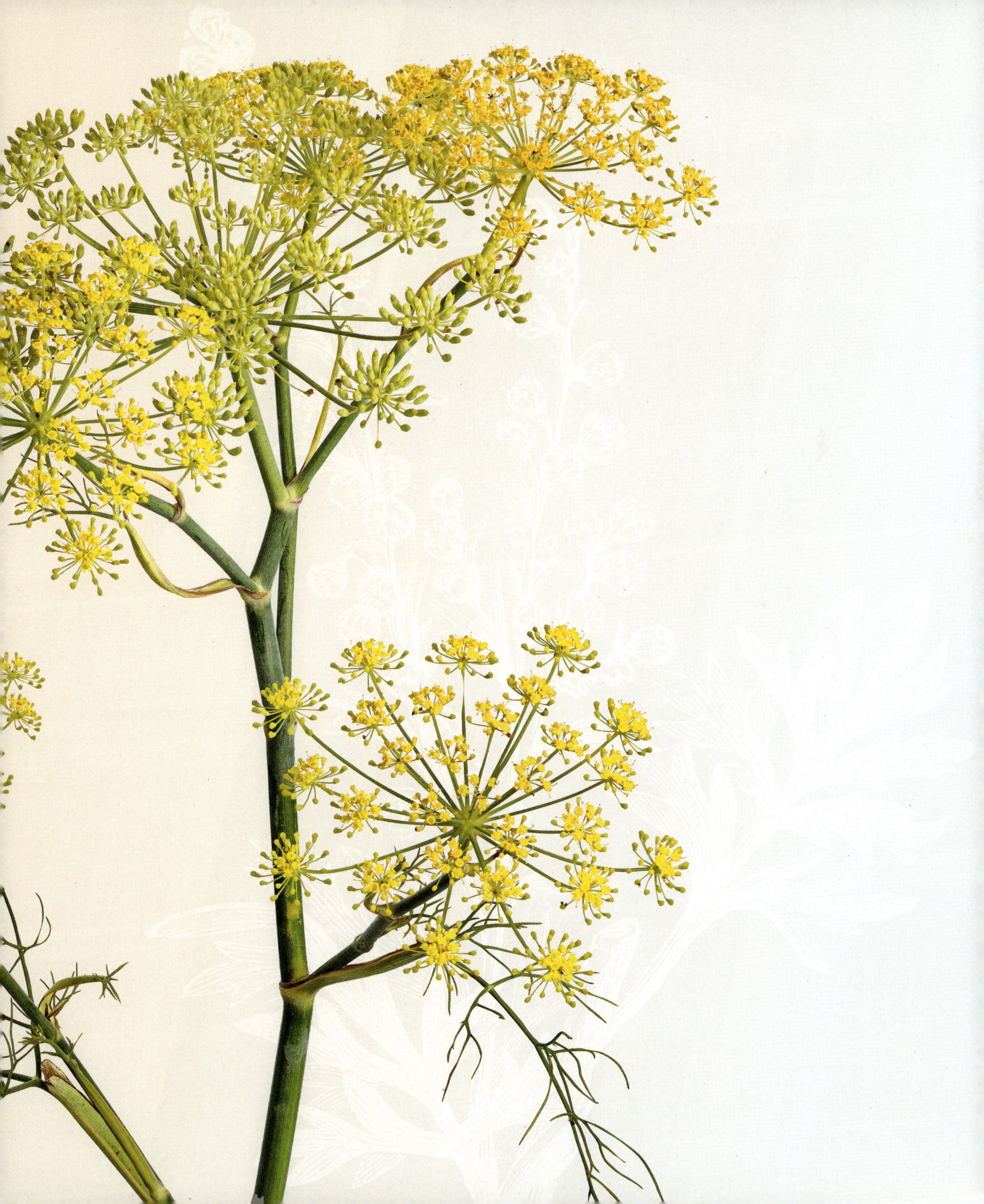

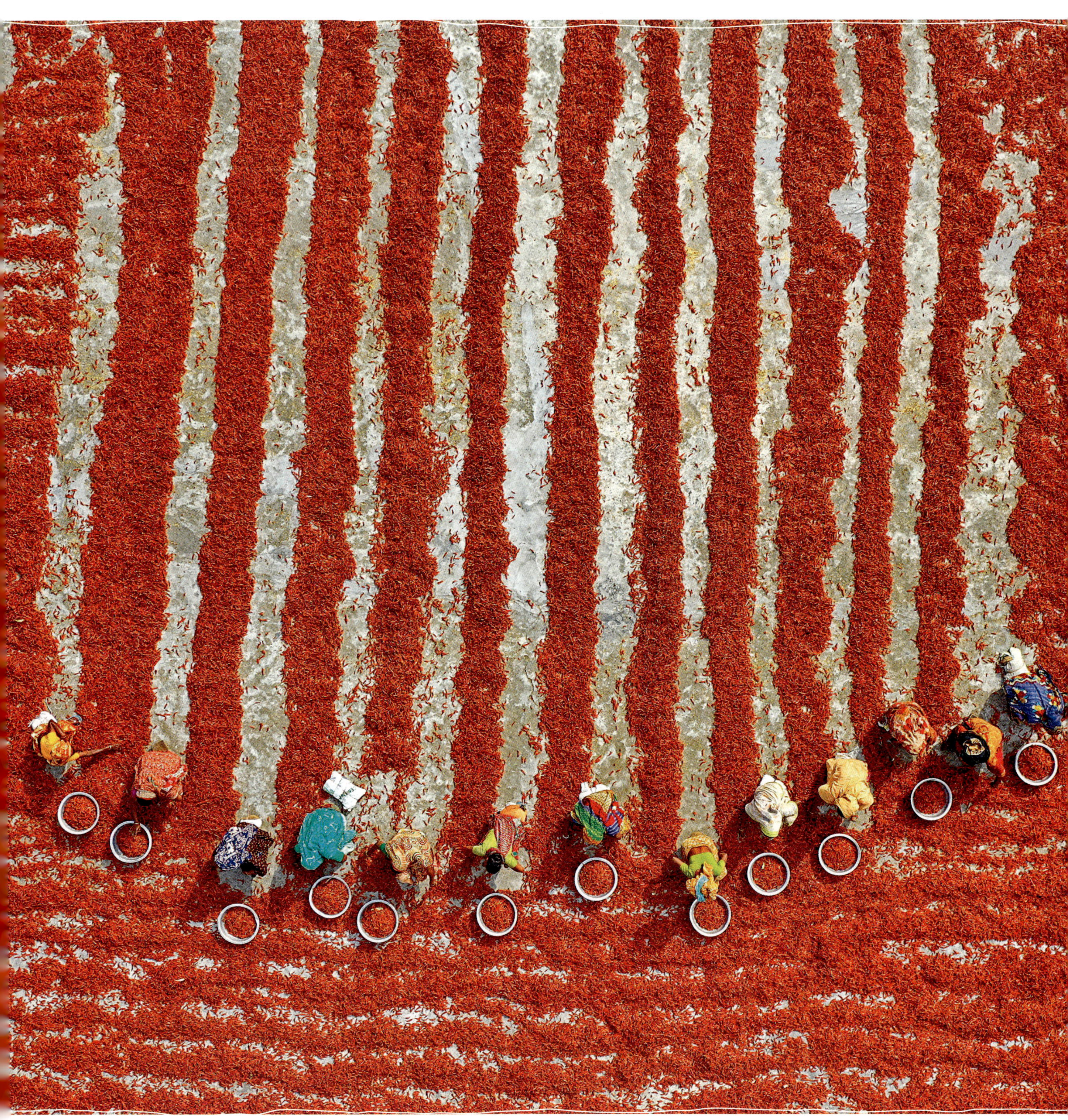

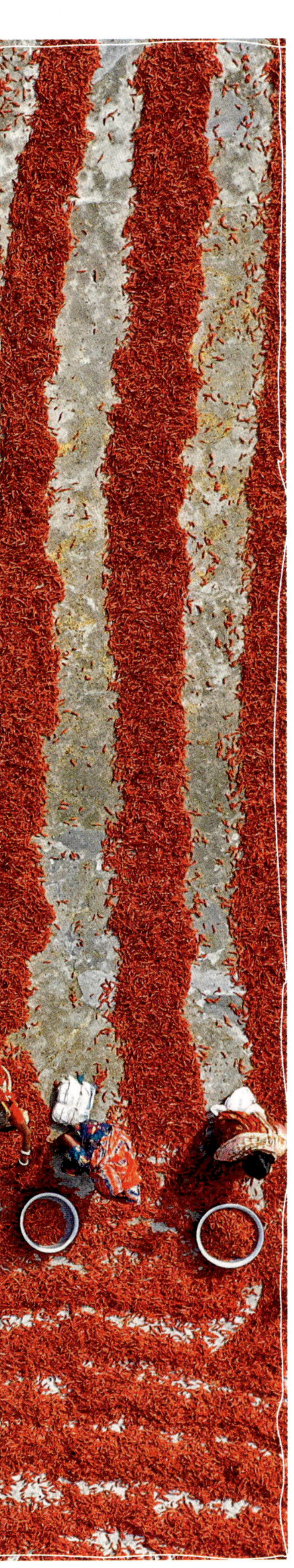

◄ Vibrant harvest
Freshly harvested chillies are dried in the sun for preservation. These women in Bangladesh clean, sort, and turn the chillies, removing any spoiled fruits.

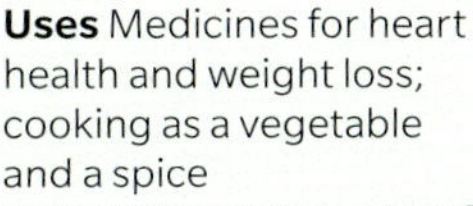

Uses Medicines for heart health and weight loss; cooking as a vegetable and a spice

Parts used Fresh and dried fruits including seeds

Active ingredients Capsaicin, capsiate, capsanthin, capsorubin

Habitat Well-drained soils in tropical and sub-tropical areas

Chilli

Capsicum annuum

From pepperoni to pepper spray, chillies have a wide range of uses. Their fiery flavour has influenced many cuisines around the world, and inspired eating competitions and plant breeders seeking to break the record for the world's hottest chilli.

Members of the Solanaceae family, which also includes tomatoes and potatoes, chillies form the genus *Capsicum* with around 40 different species. Several species produce edible fruits, but most peppers in cultivation derive from five domesticated species, the most important of which is *Capsicum annuum*, producer of bell peppers, jalapeños, and cayenne peppers. *C. chinense* brings habaneros and scotch bonnets, while *C. frutescens* is the parent of piri-piri and tabasco peppers. The final two species are *C. baccatum* (aji-amarillo, lemon drop) and *C. pubescens* (rocoto, manzano). Chilli breeders use these five species to develop new strains and the world record for hottest chilli is regularly topped.

Chillies derive their heat from the chemical compound capsaicin, which is formed in blisters on some parts of the inner fruit walls. With the exception of humans, mammals dislike the heat of capsaicin and avoid eating chillies, but birds are unaffected and provide a seed-dispersal service for the plants. As chilli powder inhibits mammals but not birds, it can be used to keep squirrels off bird feeders. The reason why chillies produce a mammal deterrent is unknown, but may be because some mammals chew fruits, potentially destroying the seeds, while birds swallow fruits whole or in small pieces, preserving the seeds. Given the presence of this chemical deterrent, it

◄ Heat source
The pungent chemical capsaicin is concentrated in the inner segment walls and pale placental tissues holding the seeds. Removing these tissues greatly reduces the heat of the chilli on eating.

Seeds of chilli peppers do not contain hot capsaicin

Similar herbs

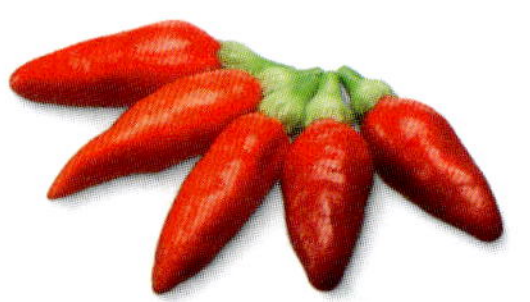

TABASCO PEPPER
Capsicum frutescens

Native to Central and South America, tabasco produces clusters of small, upward-pointing, cone-shaped peppers. They are popular in Ethiopia and southern India.

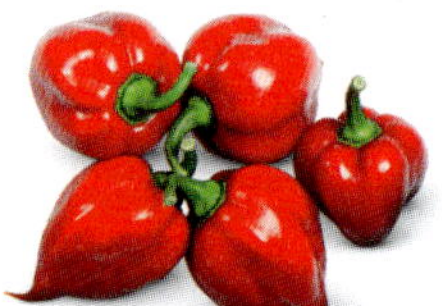

HABANERO CHILLI
Capsicum chinense

Originating in the Americas, this pepper has fruits that vary extensively in shape, colour, and piquancy. Some are non-spicy, while others are extremely hot.

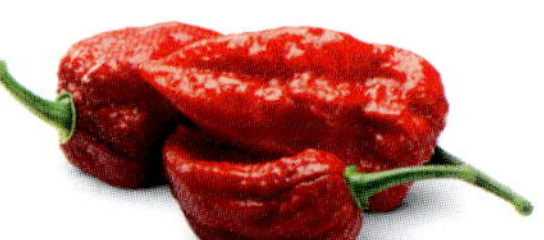

GHOST PEPPER
Capsicum chinense × Capsicum frutescens

Once considered the world's hottest chilli, this hybrid is popular in India where it is known as *bhut jolokia*. It has red, yellow, or purple fruits.

HOW DO RUBEFACIENT HERBS WORK?

Rubefacients redden the skin and are commonly used to relieve chronic pain by acting as counterirritants. They stimulate dilation in blood vessels, releasing a flow of blood and causing the skin to redden. This soothing warmth is said to counteract pain in adjacent areas of the body. Some studies have demonstrated their efficacy, and capsaicin in chilli is used in herbal medicine as a rubefacient.

may seem strange that so many humans regularly consume fiery chillies, and this behaviour has proved enlightening to psychologists who study human decision making and pleasure-pain responses.

Measuring heat

The heat of an individual chilli is measured on the Scoville scale using Scoville heat units (SHUs), named after the American pharmacist Wilbur Scoville (1865–1942) who created both the scale and a method of determining capsaicinoid levels. His test has been superseded, but the scale remains and today's hottest chillies rate above 2 million SHUs. Not all peppers are hot – bell peppers, also known as sweet peppers or capsicums, rate zero on Scoville's scale.

Chilli peppers were given part of their common name as they taste similar to spicy black pepper (*Piper nigrum*), an unrelated plant native to tropical Asia. Sichuan peppers (various *Zanthoxylum* species) also produce a similar hot, spicy effect, but are unrelated to chilli and, like black pepper, do not contain capsaicin. The word chilli (*chile* in Spanish) is thought to derive from the Aztec Nahuatl word for the plant and is not connected to the South American nation of Chile.

Ancient cuisine

Peppers are known to have been used for at least 6,000 years and they are best known as a foodstuff. They can be eaten raw, both when green and when ripe, and also dried, pickled, or made into jams and jellies. Dried chillies are often ground into flakes or a fine powder, known variously as chilli powder, paprika, cayenne, or pimento, depending on which chilli variety is used. Some chilli powders also include other ingredients such as salt, garlic, or cumin.

Chillies are core components of many cuisines, from Mexico to Spain to Thailand and beyond. Sweet peppers are used as vegetables, but it is the hot varieties that are most sought after. Significant dishes include *chiles rellenos* and *mole* sauce in Mexico, chicken *paprikash* in Hungary, pasta *arrabiata* in Italy, jerk meat from Jamaica, and Korean *kimchi*. In the US, pepperoni, which is flavoured with paprika, is the nation's favourite pizza topping. The spicy stew *chilli con carne* is also popular in many states.

Hot sauces flavoured with chillies are also available in a bewildering variety and encourage

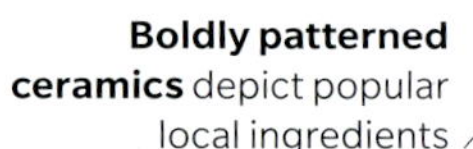

Boldly patterned ceramics depict popular local ingredients

➤ Pepper motifs
Made in Peru between 180 BCE and 500 CE by the Nazca people, this ceramic bowl is painted with stylized chillies and reflects the long history of chilli use.

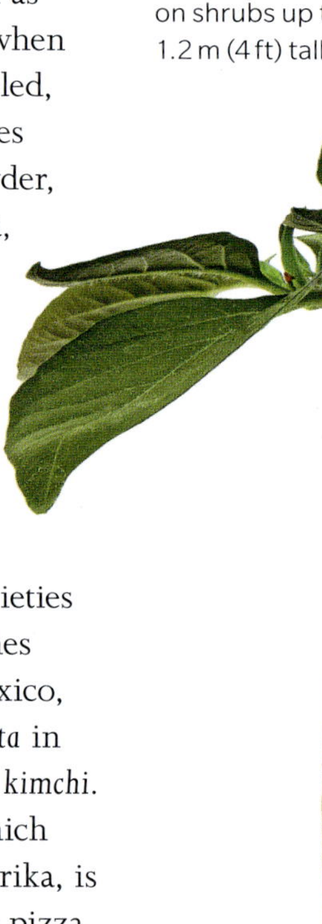

➤ Medium hot fruit
Cayenne is a form of *Capsicum annuum* grown for its long, red, moderately spicy fruits, which are dried and ground to make cayenne pepper. The fruits grow on shrubs up to 1.2 m (4 ft) tall.

> " They have hot peppers in Louisiana. Little red devils with fire in their skin and hell in their seeds. "
>
> JAMES STREET, *The Grains of Paradise*, 1955

Branches are weak and benefit from support canes, especially when bearing heavy fruits
Leaves are glossy and hairless on this evergreen shrub
Cayenne peppers change colour, starting out green then ripening to red

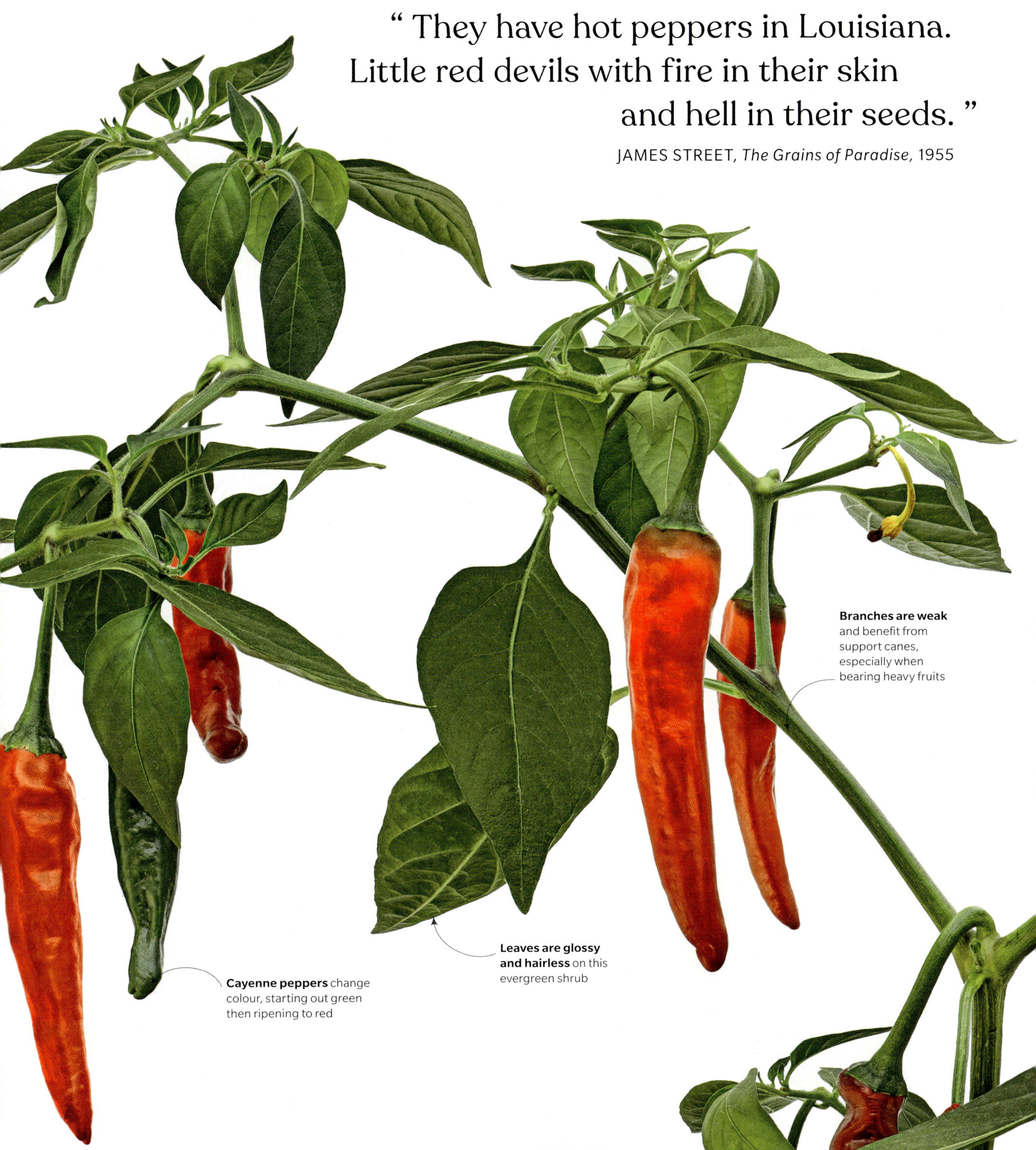

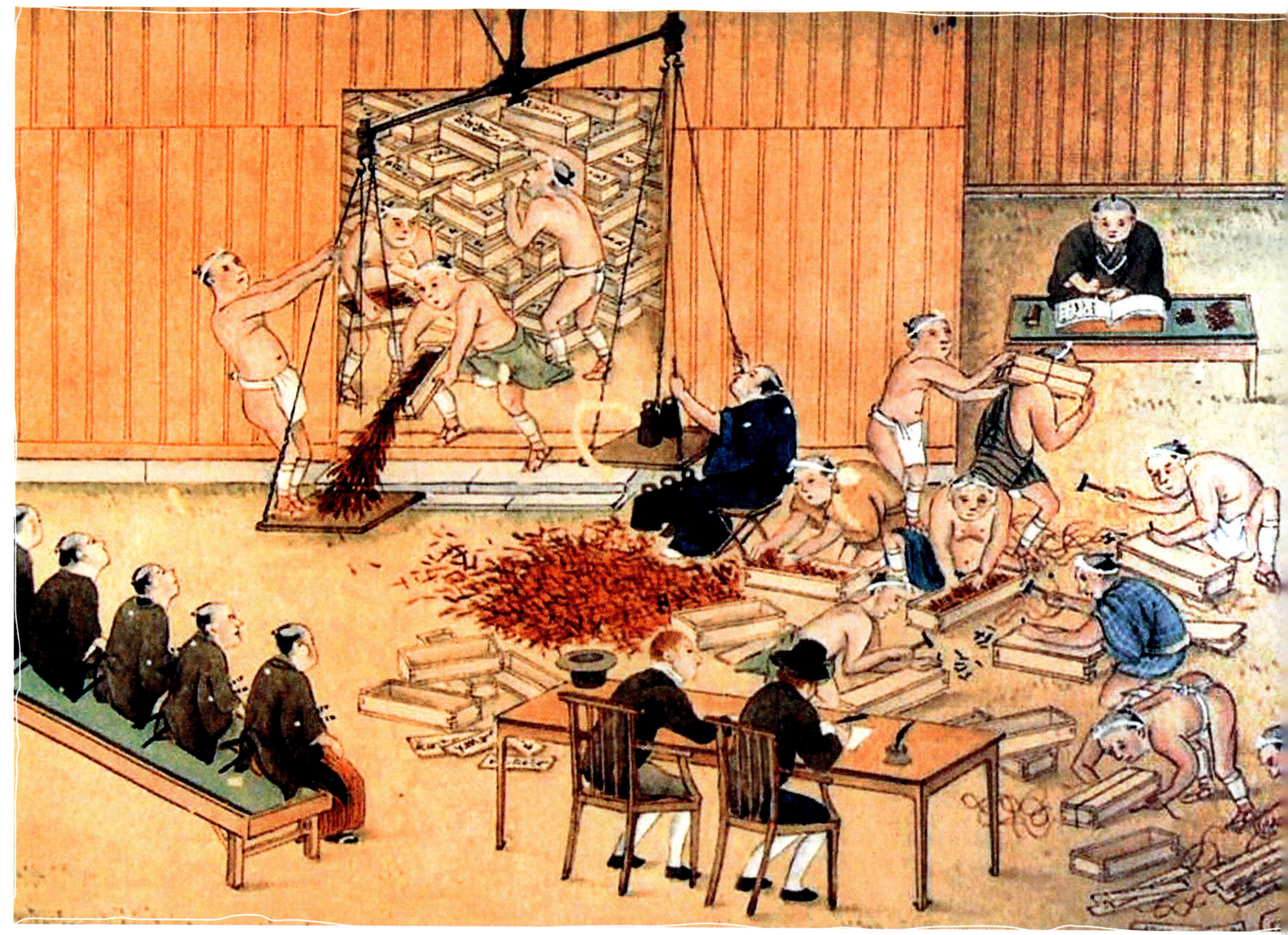

Unlike most chillies, this cultivar has silvery hairs all over its stems and leaves

Cultivated pepper flowers are usually white but can be purple or green

➤ Colourful plant
Chilli flowers will generally self-fertilize, although bees and other insects can transfer pollen. The cultivar Black Cobra (right), produces fruits that change from green, through red, to black.

the consumption of ever hotter foods, which is also apparent in the growing appetite for chilli eating competitions. One chilli combination now having a renaissance hearkens back to the Aztec and Mayan civilizations, where roasted cacao beans were used to make chocolate beverages flavoured with local spices, including vanilla and chilli. Chilli-flavoured chocolate bars are now widely available, while cocoa is increasingly used in chilli sauces to enhance flavour complexity.

From cancer to crowd control

Chillies also have a long history of medicinal use and contain significant quantities of vitamin C – more than in citrus fruits. Chilli may reduce the

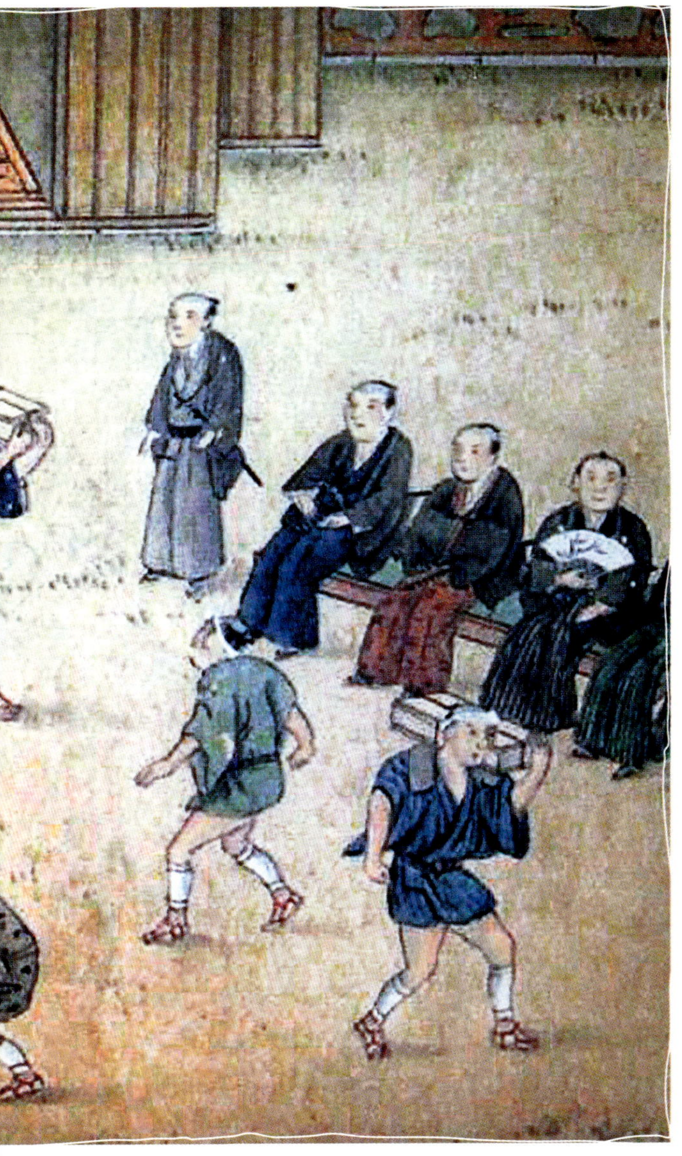

▲ Processing for trade
In this picture from Nagasaki, Japan (c.1700), Dutch factors (with hats) and Japanese officials observe the weighing, sorting, and packaging of chilli peppers prior to their export to Europe.

CHILLI IN SPAIN

When Christopher Columbus reached the Americas, he was looking for trade routes to Asia and supplies of black pepper (*Piper nigrum*) that could be sourced there. He failed to find Asia, but he did find chilli peppers, which had been in cultivation in Central and South America for centuries. He took them back to Spain after his second voyage and they rapidly became a notable part of Spanish cuisine, featuring in popular foods such as chorizo and many soups and stews.

SPAIN

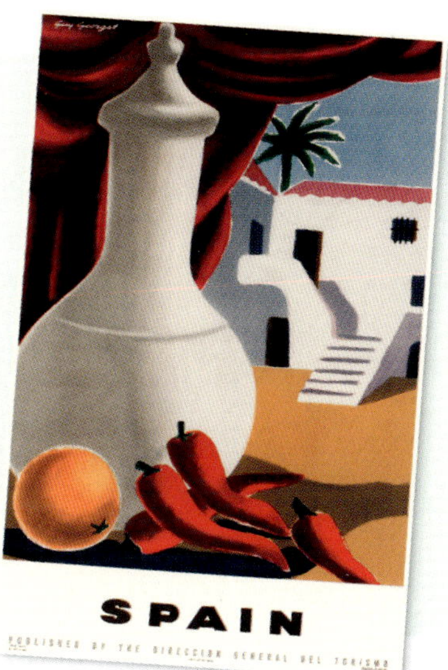

SPANISH TRAVEL POSTER, 1951

The world's hottest chilli is the Carolina Reaper, at 2.2 million Scoville heat units

Sliced chillies are dried in an oven or dehydrator before being crushed

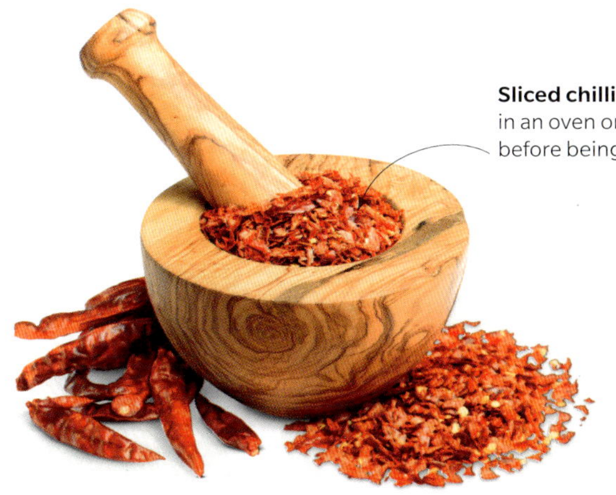

◄ Flavoursome flakes
Dried chillies can be ground into flakes used in cooking or as a condiment. Their relative hotness depends on the variety of chilli.

risk of prostate and lung cancers; however, high doses could increase the risk of gastric cancer and exacerbate irritable bowel syndrome. People with chilli-rich diets may be less likely to die of heart disease, possibly due to capsaicin reducing inflammation, and although it may cause heartburn, chilli can protect from gastric ulcers.

Chilli has also long been thought to contribute to weight loss. The capsaicin in chilli has been shown to stimulate the metabolism, increasing metabolic rate by up to eight per cent, although this marginal increase is only temporary. Chilli can act also as an appetite suppressant and may help the body's regulation of insulin, when both factors are combined with the impact on the metabolism, it may cause some weight loss.

Pepper spray, also known as mace, is widely used for self-defence and by police agencies for crowd control. Banned in some countries and states, the spray contains capsaicin and an emulsifier, suspended in water. Capsaicin will dissolve in fats (lipophilic), and so milk is sometimes recommended to wash the faces of those affected by pepper spray; milk is also the treatment of choice for those who have eaten too much hot chilli.

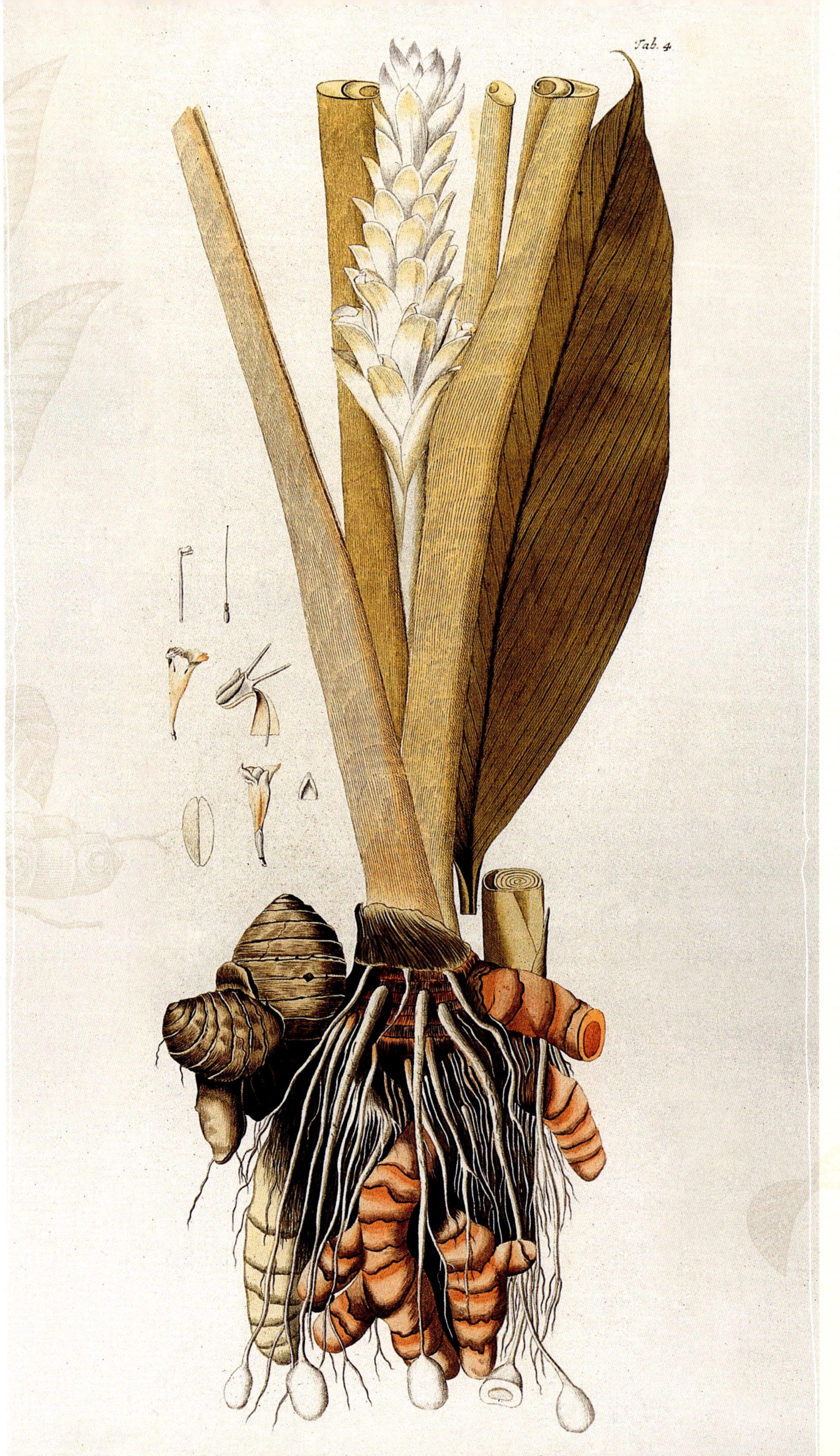

◄ **Useful rhizome**
Turmeric is a herbaceous perennial grown from a thickened underground stem called a rhizome. The spice derives from the rhizomes, which are harvested and processed, though some are replanted for future cropping.

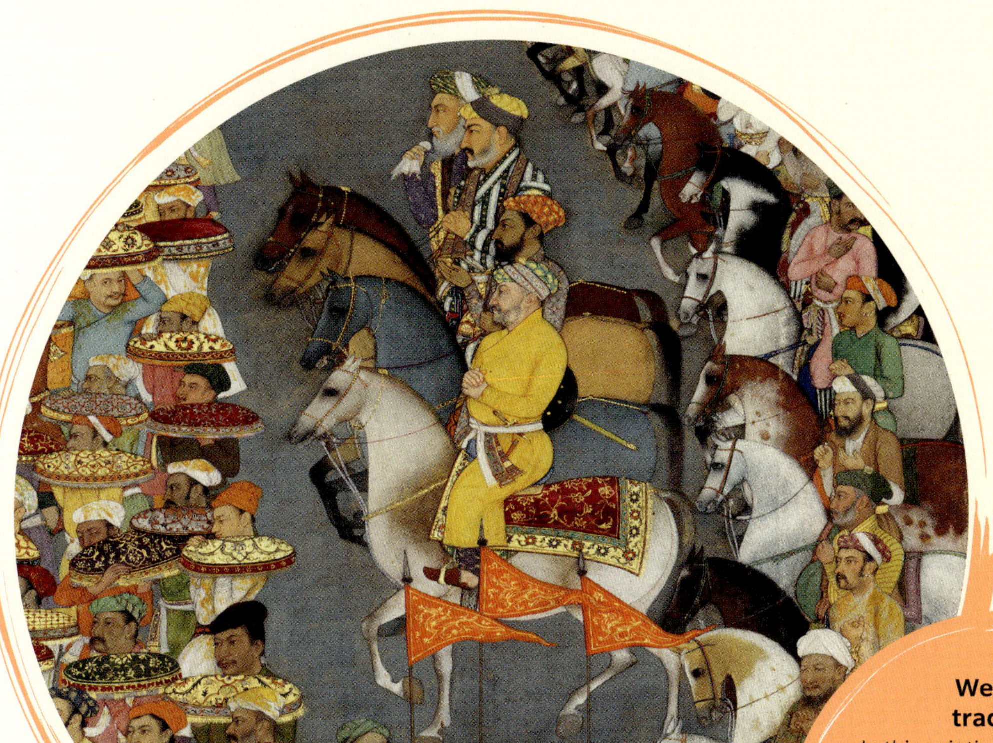

Wedding traditions
In this painting of the marriage of Prince Dara Shikoh in 17th century India, an array of rich wedding gifts are presented. Turmeric is seen on the some of the figures' clothes from the pre-wedding *haldi* where a mixture of turmeric, oil, and water is placed on the bride and groom.

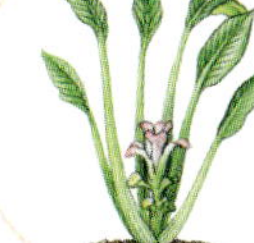

Uses Medicines for arthritis and gastrointestinal problems, cooking, colourant

Parts used Rhizomes, leaves

Active ingredients Curcumin, volatile oils including zingiberene and turmerene

Habitat Tropical deciduous and evergreen forest

Turmeric

Curcuma longa

Now commonly used around the world, this spice has its origins in South Asia, where it is an essential ingredient in curries, dyes, and a variety of cultural events from feast days to marriages.

With its warm, earthy, peppery flavour and fragrance of ginger and citrus, turmeric has long been a key element of South Asian cooking. Together with ginger, coriander, fenugreek, and cumin, it is a core component of curry powder, though the exact content of these mixes varies. Archaeological excavations in the Indus Valley dating between 2600–2200 BCE found turmeric residues inside preserved cooking pots, revealing the long history of use of this pungent spice. However, the precise origins of the plant and its wild distribution remain mysterious.

Curcuma longa seems to have originated in southern India. The country is home to more than 40 species of *Curcuma*, several of which are used to manufacture turmeric, and the precise identification of these species is challenging. Today, *Curcuma longa* is cultivated in tropical countries around the world. In the North Pacific

Grinder is used to process dried rhizome into a powder

▲ **Turmeric powder**
Rhizomes of turmeric are harvested from the soil, cleaned, boiled, and dried. Dried whole turmeric can be stored and then powdered when required.

island chain of Micronesia, turmeric is thought to have been brought to the islands by the first human settlers to be used medicinally and to colour the skin. The people that populated the Pacific islands took only those plants and animals considered essential when making long oceanic journeys; as turmeric is not a critical foodstuff, it may have had significant health uses or cultural importance to justify its presence on such journeys.

Long-distance trading of turmeric may also have early origins. Analysis of plaque on human teeth from archaeological sites in Israel, dating to around 1630–1550 BCE, shows evidence of turmeric consumption indicating trade between South Asia and the Levant much earlier than previously thought.

Colour and flavour

Turmeric's twin traits of flavour and colour have long been important in Asian and Middle Eastern cuisines. In Iran, it is often paired with meat or vegetables in *khoresh*, or stew, though it is used with caution as it can impart a bitter flavour. Thai yellow curries take their colour from fresh turmeric, while in Sumatra, turmeric leaves bring flavour to curries from the city of Padang. In Goa, India, turmeric leaves are stuffed with rice, palm sugar, and coconut and cooked to make *patoleo*, which is served during the Catholic Feast of the Assumption. *Patoleo* is also presented to icons of the Hindu goddess Parvati, who craved sweet dishes during her pregnancy. Turmeric powder flavours the Lebanese semolina cake *sfouf* and also Indian golden milk, a popular health drink and common home remedy for childhood ailments.

Beyond its traditional uses, turmeric and its derivative curcumin, also known as the food additive E100 within Europe, are commonly used to colour processed foods. These can

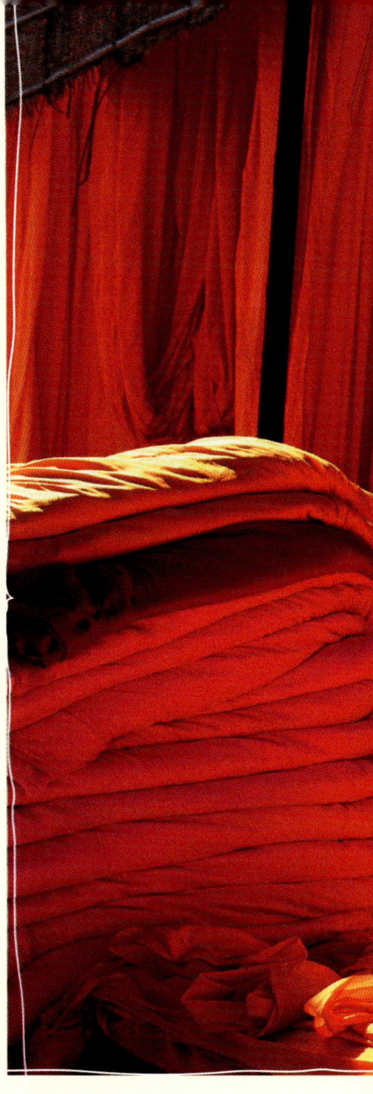

➤ Vivid dye
Turmeric has long been used as a dye, especially in India, and notably to colour the robes of some Buddhist monks. However, it is an impermanent pigment that fades quickly with age and washing.

Turmeric is a **pH indicator** – **yellow** in **acid and neutral pHs**, but turns **red when it becomes alkaline**

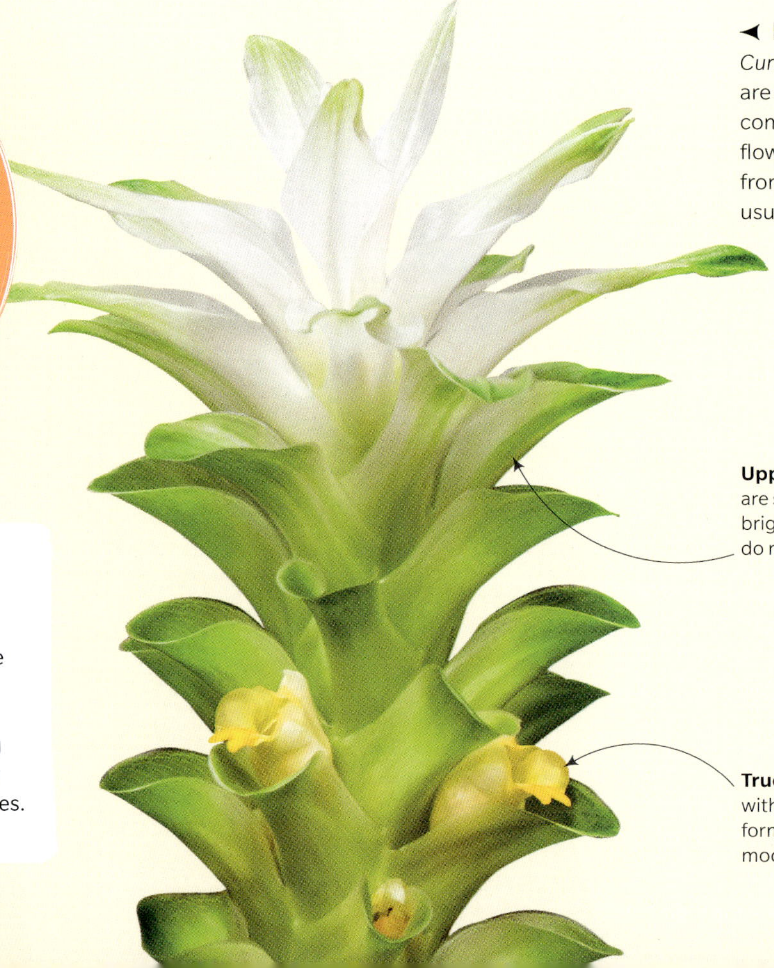

◄ Bracts and flowers
Curcuma flower heads are tall and elegant spikes comprising small, individual flowers barely emerging from within bracts that are usually green and white.

Uppermost bracts are sometimes brightly coloured but do not contain flowers

True flowers are tubular with a with a lip (labellum) formed from fused, modified stamens

HOW DO ANTIOXIDANTS WORK?

Free radicals are highly reactive molecules as they contain an unpaired electron. They are produced naturally in the body but are also the result of some diseases and of exposure to x-rays, smoking, and other external sources. Antioxidants react with the oxygen-containing free radicals before they can cause damage by reacting with DNA or other important molecules.

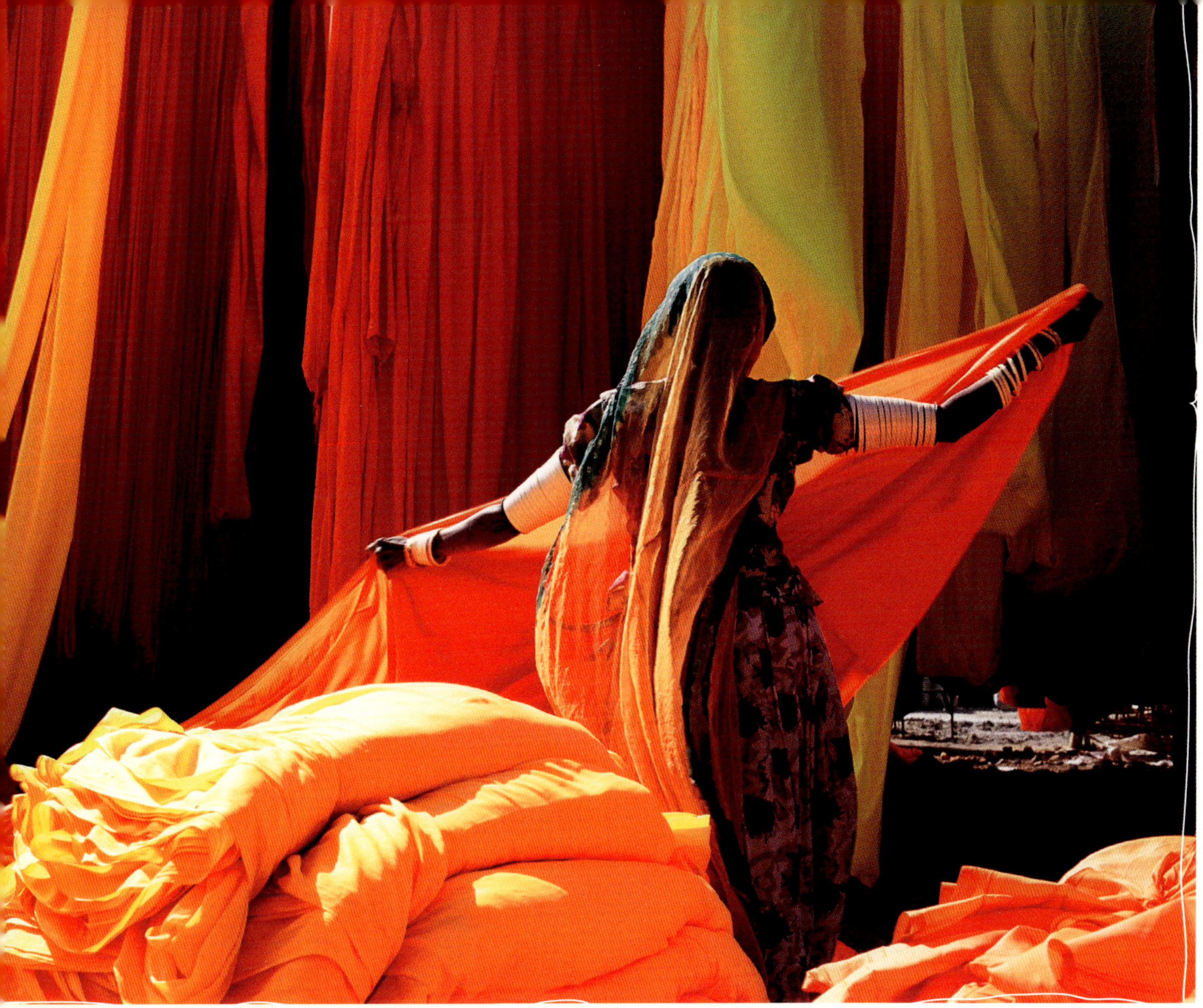

include cheese, margarine, butter, yellow cake, and mustard. It is also sometimes used as an inexpensive alternative to the golden spice saffron, though the two taste very different.

Curcuma in medicine and culture

Turmeric has a long history of use in Ayurveda for respiratory and skin conditions and also for sprains and swelling, and in Chinese traditional medicine to treat abdominal pain. Turmeric is an antioxidant and it has become a popular herbal remedy around the world. Although few scientific studies support the many claims made about this spice, it is used to treat several conditions including arthritis, inflammation, psoriasis, and gastrointestinal and respiratory conditions. Turmeric is also used as an antiseptic and, in Pakistan and Afghanistan, turmeric is traditionally added to bandages to cleanse wounds and stimulate healing. As a rich source of antioxidants, turmeric is an increasingly popular component of sunscreens and cosmetic preparations for cleansing and brightening.

Beyond food and medicine, turmeric has earned a place within the cultural practices of several countries. In Bangladesh and neighbouring India, within Bengali families, it has a crucial role in the wedding tradition *gaye holud*. Brightly coloured turmeric paste is applied to the face and body of a bride by invited family and guests in a ceremony observed by Bengalis of all religions. A similar ceremony is held in other parts of India where it is known as *haldi*.

The Hindu god Shiva, in his manifestation Khandoba, is venerated in north-western India where statues of him bear a turmeric bowl in one of his four hands. At the temple in Jejuri, worshippers scatter powdered turmeric in the air and over one another in praise of him.

Similar herbs

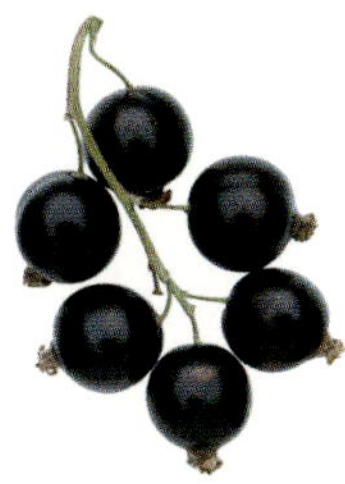

BLACKCURRANT
Ribes nigrum
A native of northern Europe and Asia, the fruits are rich in antioxidant vitamin C and are used to make cordials, jams, and desserts.

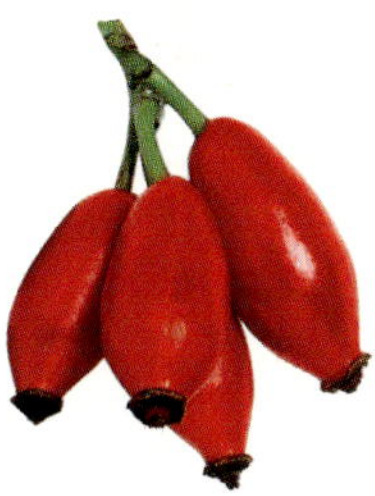

DOG ROSE
Rosa canina
A thorny shrub from Europe, western Asia, and North Africa, the hips are a source of potent antioxidants, and are often made into a syrup.

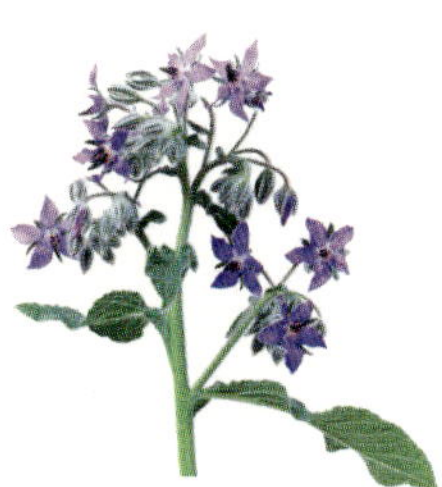

BORAGE
Borago officinalis
An annual from Africa and Mediterranean Europe, its seed oil is used for eczema and psoriasis. Its leaves can be used as a vegetable and flowers, as garnish.

> “Turmeric the auspicious spice, placed on the heads of newborns for luck.”
>
> CHITRA BANERJEE DIVAKARUNI, *The Mistress of Spices*, 1997

Flavouring Dishes

Herbs and spices are particularly valued for their taste. Used even in tiny quantities, they can introduce bold, complex flavours to plain dishes and are an indispensable part of cuisines around the world. This is a small selection of popular culinary herbs.

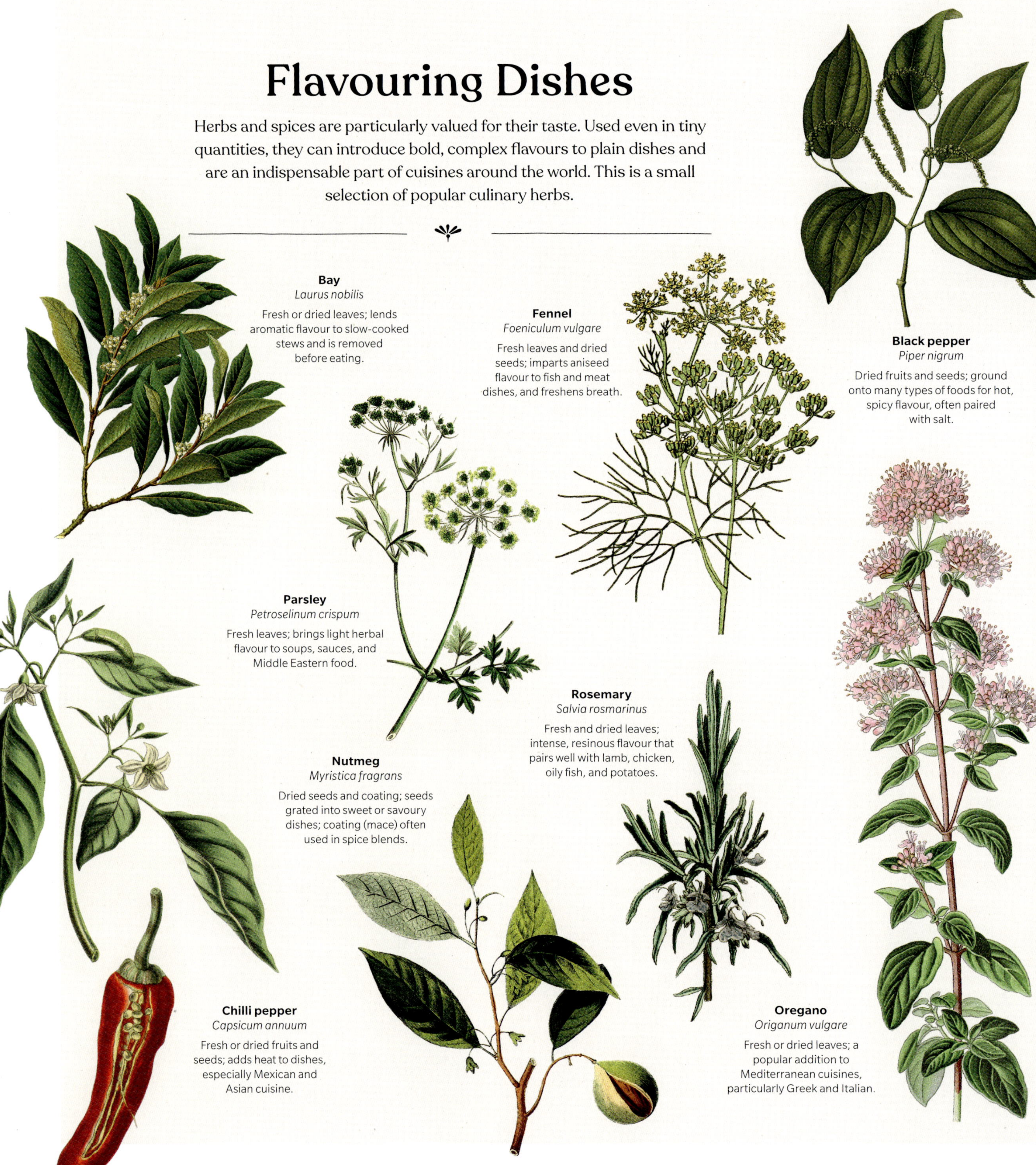

Bay
Laurus nobilis
Fresh or dried leaves; lends aromatic flavour to slow-cooked stews and is removed before eating.

Fennel
Foeniculum vulgare
Fresh leaves and dried seeds; imparts aniseed flavour to fish and meat dishes, and freshens breath.

Black pepper
Piper nigrum
Dried fruits and seeds; ground onto many types of foods for hot, spicy flavour, often paired with salt.

Parsley
Petroselinum crispum
Fresh leaves; brings light herbal flavour to soups, sauces, and Middle Eastern food.

Rosemary
Salvia rosmarinus
Fresh and dried leaves; intense, resinous flavour that pairs well with lamb, chicken, oily fish, and potatoes.

Nutmeg
Myristica fragrans
Dried seeds and coating; seeds grated into sweet or savoury dishes; coating (mace) often used in spice blends.

Chilli pepper
Capsicum annuum
Fresh or dried fruits and seeds; adds heat to dishes, especially Mexican and Asian cuisine.

Oregano
Origanum vulgare
Fresh or dried leaves; a popular addition to Mediterranean cuisines, particularly Greek and Italian.

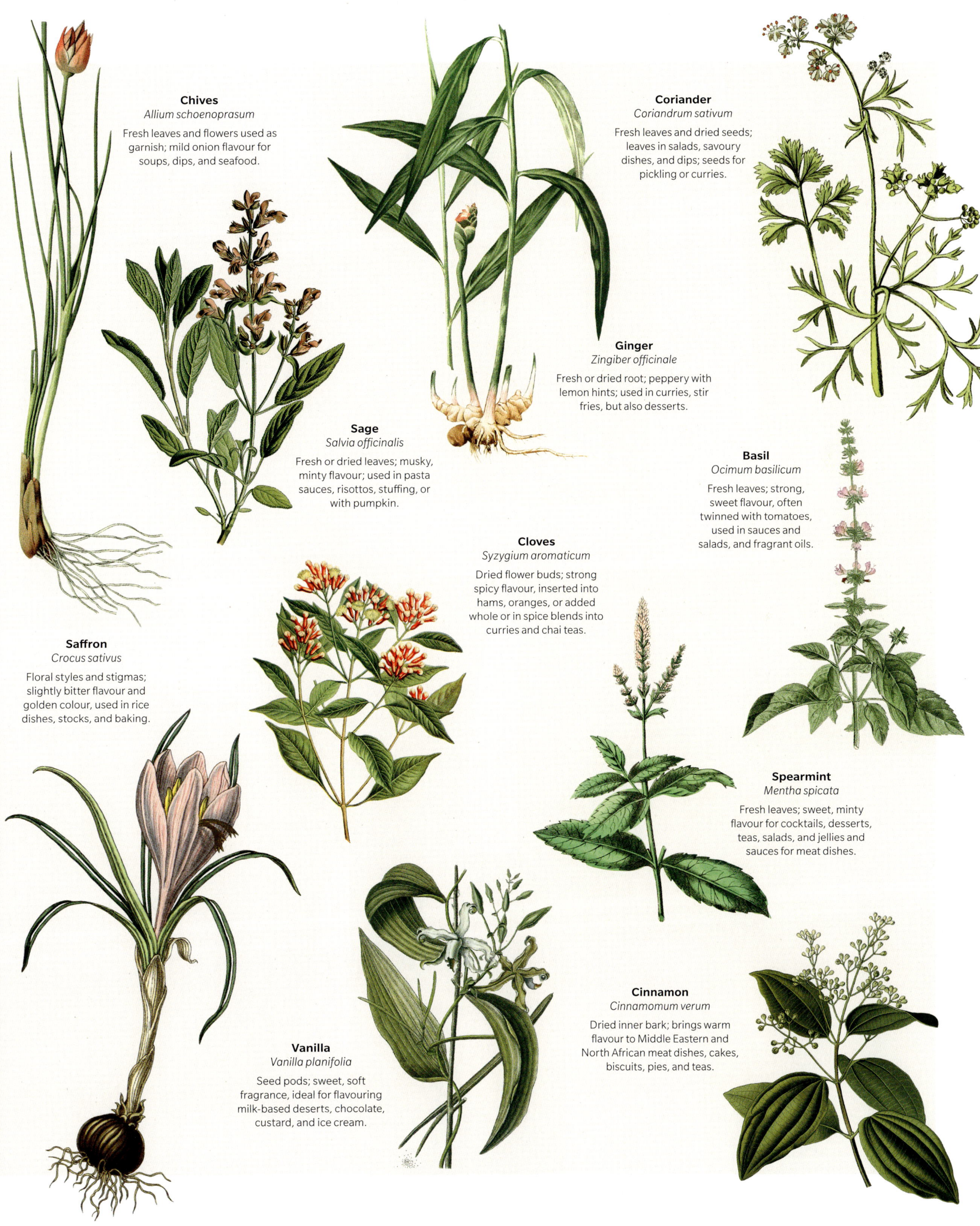
Chives
Allium schoenoprasum
Fresh leaves and flowers used as garnish; mild onion flavour for soups, dips, and seafood.
Coriander
Coriandrum sativum
Fresh leaves and dried seeds; leaves in salads, savoury dishes, and dips; seeds for pickling or curries.
Ginger
Zingiber officinale
Fresh or dried root; peppery with lemon hints; used in curries, stir fries, but also desserts.
Sage
Salvia officinalis
Fresh or dried leaves; musky, minty flavour; used in pasta sauces, risottos, stuffing, or with pumpkin.
Basil
Ocimum basilicum
Fresh leaves; strong, sweet flavour, often twinned with tomatoes, used in sauces and salads, and fragrant oils.
Cloves
Syzygium aromaticum
Dried flower buds; strong spicy flavour, inserted into hams, oranges, or added whole or in spice blends into curries and chai teas.
Saffron
Crocus sativus
Floral styles and stigmas; slightly bitter flavour and golden colour, used in rice dishes, stocks, and baking.
Spearmint
Mentha spicata
Fresh leaves; sweet, minty flavour for cocktails, desserts, teas, salads, and jellies and sauces for meat dishes.
Cinnamon
Cinnamomum verum
Dried inner bark; brings warm flavour to Middle Eastern and North African meat dishes, cakes, biscuits, pies, and teas.
Vanilla
Vanilla planifolia
Seed pods; sweet, soft fragrance, ideal for flavouring milk-based deserts, chocolate, custard, and ice cream.

Garlic

Allium sativum

In continuous use throughout much of recorded history, this pungent bulb plays an essential role in kitchens worldwide and is thought to inhibit both viruses and vampires.

Uses Medicines; cooking as a flavouring and a vegetable

Parts used Bulbs, scapes

Active ingredients Allicin, alliin, ajoene, diallyl sulphide, diallyl disulphide, diallyl trisulfide

Habitat Arid steppe and grasslands

Garlic has been utilized as a herb for much of human history. It was found among the treasures of Tutankhamun's tomb, dating to 1325 BCE, and it is thought that garlic was regularly consumed by labourers and enslaved people in ancient Egypt to maintain their strength. Garlic has also been found in Middle Eastern archaeological sites dating from as early as 3000 BCE and features in one of the world's oldest-known recipes: a Babylonian recipe for lamb stew.

The precise geographical origins of garlic, and the wild species it derived from, remain mysterious, although central or southwestern Asia are likely locations for the bulb to originate from. Today, semi-wild garlic is found growing in several countries including Egypt, India, and Turkey. However, the name "wild garlic" is also applied to several other garlic-scented *Allium* species that are distinct from culinary *A. sativum*, such as *A. ursinum*, also known as ramsons.

The pungent taste of garlic has assured its place in the culinary traditions of many nations, and it is the segmented bulb that is of most importance, though the flowering stalks, or scapes, are also of use. While whole bulbs are sometimes roasted, as with Korean black garlic, more often individual cloves are added whole, sliced, or crushed to impart flavour to various dishes. A crucial component of many dishes, it adds flavour to soups, stir frys, marinades, sauces, and meat dishes. In the absence of fresh bulbs, garlic powder, garlic salt, and garlic oil are also widely used and the cuisines of eastern and southern Asia, the Middle East, North Africa,

▼ Garlic bulb
Plants produce bulbs as storage organs, allowing them to preserve food and nutrients that later fuel the production of flowers and seeds. In garlic, the bulb is segmented into units called cloves, which are separated by papery tunics.

Neck above the bulb may be soft or hard depending on the variety

" Without garlic, I simply would not care to live. "

LOUIS DIAT, chef at the Ritz-Carlton Hotel, New York, US, from 1910–51

China is the biggest producer of garlic, harvesting 80 per cent of the world's supply

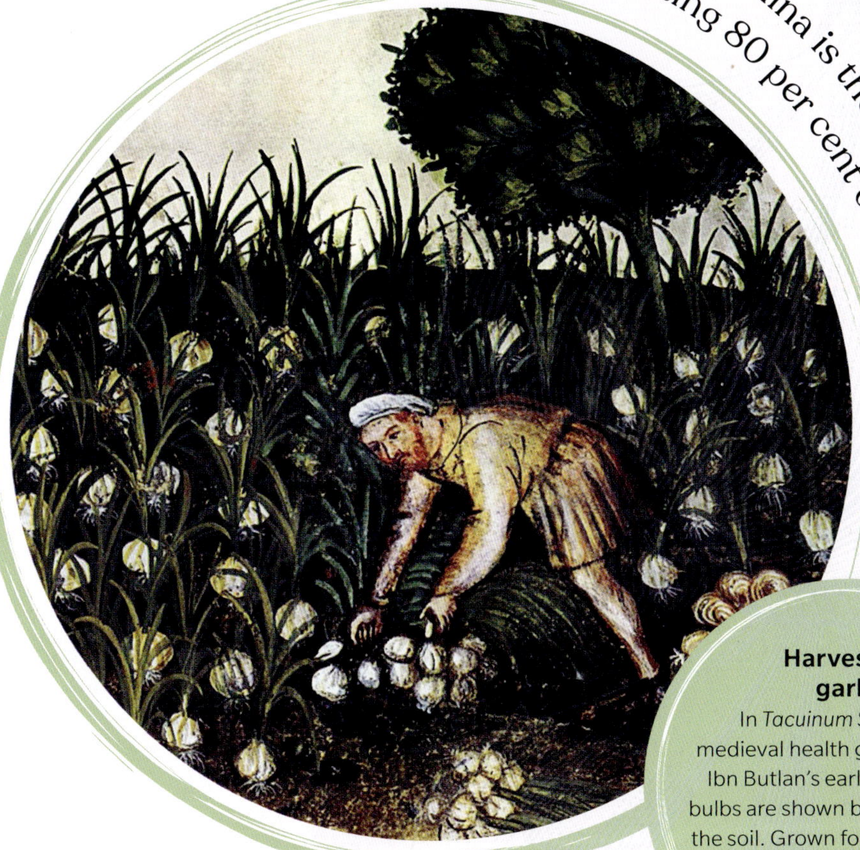

Harvesting garlic

In *Tacuinum Sanitatis*, a medieval health guide based on Ibn Butlan's earlier text, garlic bulbs are shown being lifted from the soil. Grown for both food and medicine, it was popular throughout Europe.

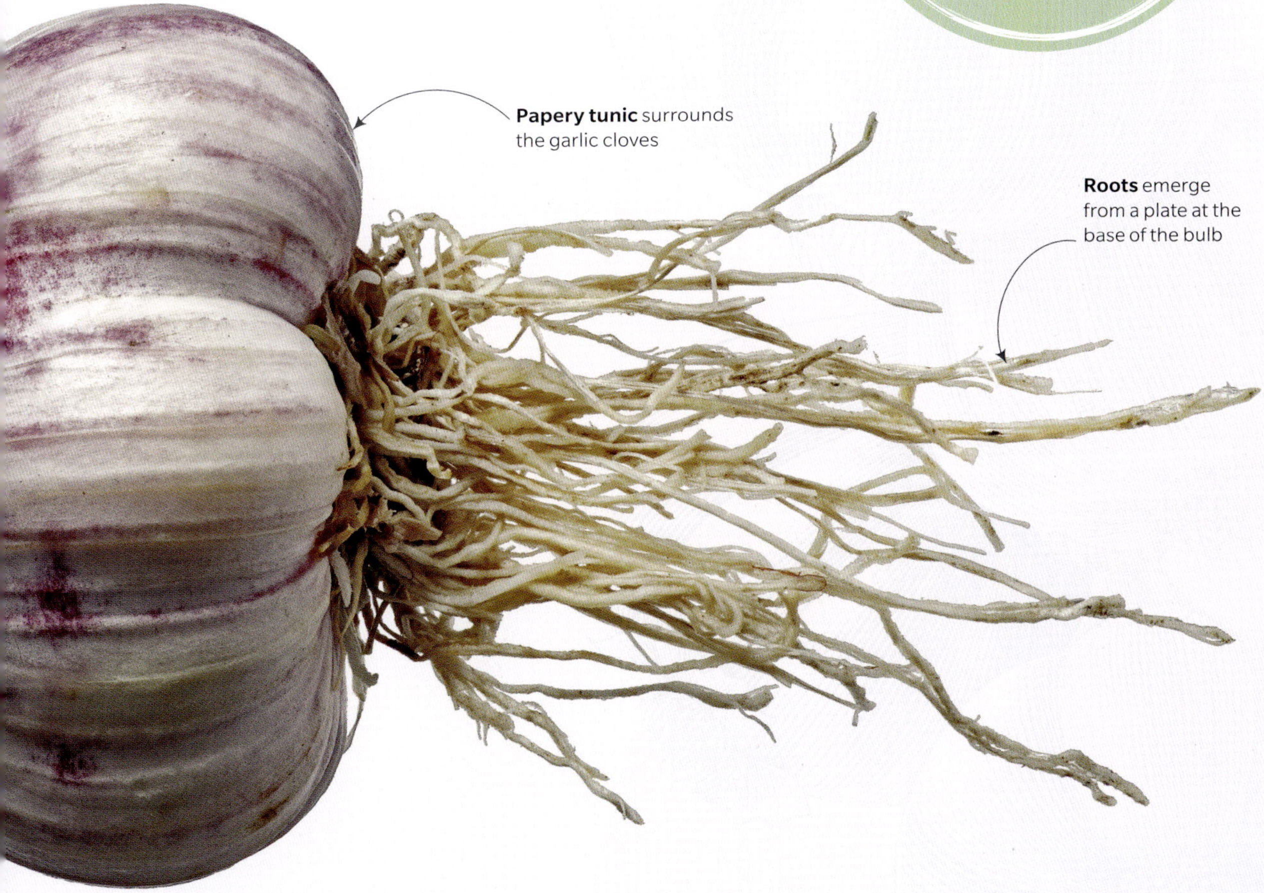

Papery tunic surrounds the garlic cloves

Roots emerge from a plate at the base of the bulb

Similar herbs

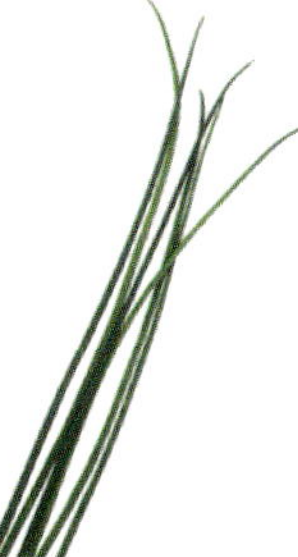

CHIVES

Allium schoenoprasum

Grown primarily for their edible leaves and flowers, which have a mild onion taste and are often used as garnish, chives form small but seldom-eaten bulbs.

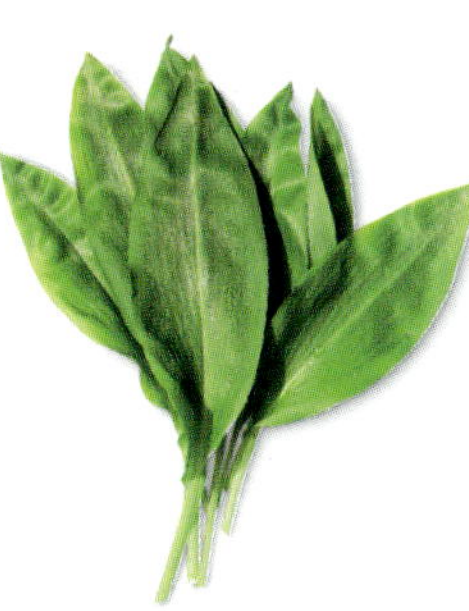

RAMSONS

Allium ursinum

Also known as wild garlic, this European native has edible leaves and flowers with a mild garlic taste. It produces a notable garlic fragrance when crushed.

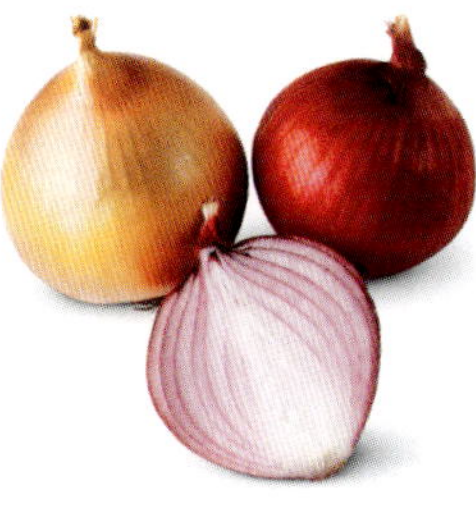

ONION

Allium cepa

Exclusively known from cultivation, the wild origins of commercial onions are uncertain; they may be red, yellow or white-skinned and are sometimes harvested when immature.

Mediterranean Europe, and Latin America all rely on garlic's distinctive bouquet. Especially significant garlic-based foods include Lebanese *toum*, a garlic sauce; Philippine *adobo*, a marinade for meat or seafood; and aioli, a simple Mediterranean sauce that is made from garlic and olive oil.

The chemistry of "garlic breath"

The strong scent of garlic is a product of several sulphur-bearing compounds found in the bulb, and these are also the unfortunate cause of "garlic breath". Allicin, the compound formed when garlic is crushed, breaks down in the stomach to produce allyl methyl sulphide, a potent scent that can last for several hours or even days. It produces distinctive halitosis and is also excreted through the skin and in urine. Mouthwash seldom relieves garlic breath, as allyl methyl sulphide is distributed in the blood stream, allowing it to be expelled via the lungs. However, consuming foods such as milk, parsley, and peppermint can alleviate the symptoms. Garlic produces these chemical products to deter herbivores from eating the bulbs, and there is some evidence that this defence mechanism is effective. Garlic solution is commonly used as a home-made insecticide, and garlic plants are said to dissuade insect pests from other crops in companion planting systems. However, eating garlic is unlikely to deter mosquitoes, as often claimed.

Cultivated garlic comes in two main forms: hard-neck and soft-neck. Both refer to the stem above the bulb, formed from numerous overlapping leaves. In hard-neck varieties, a hard flower stem forms in the centre of the bulb with a single ring of cloves surrounding it. Hard-necks produce edible scapes. Soft-necks do not flower and produce many cloves that are not in a ring arrangement. Hard-necks grow better in cooler climates but do not store well, while soft-necks prefer warm growing conditions and keep for longer. Another popular *Allium*, elephant garlic (or giant-headed garlic), is outwardly similar to normal garlic, though with bigger bulbs. It has a milder flavour and is technically a form of wild leek (*Allium ampeloprasum*).

Colds, cancers, and cardiovascular disease

Garlic has long been used medicinally. Ancient writers including Pliny the Elder in Rome, Ibn Sina (or Avicenna) in Persia, and Huangdi (the Yellow Emperor) in China all spoke of its usage as a stimulant and treatment for a wide range of ailments.

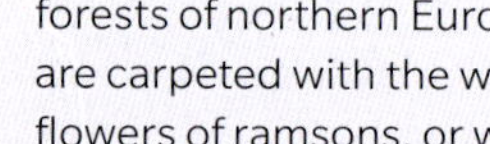

▲ Garlic explosion
In spring the deciduous forests of northern Europe are carpeted with the white flowers of ramsons, or wild garlic (*Allium ursinum*).

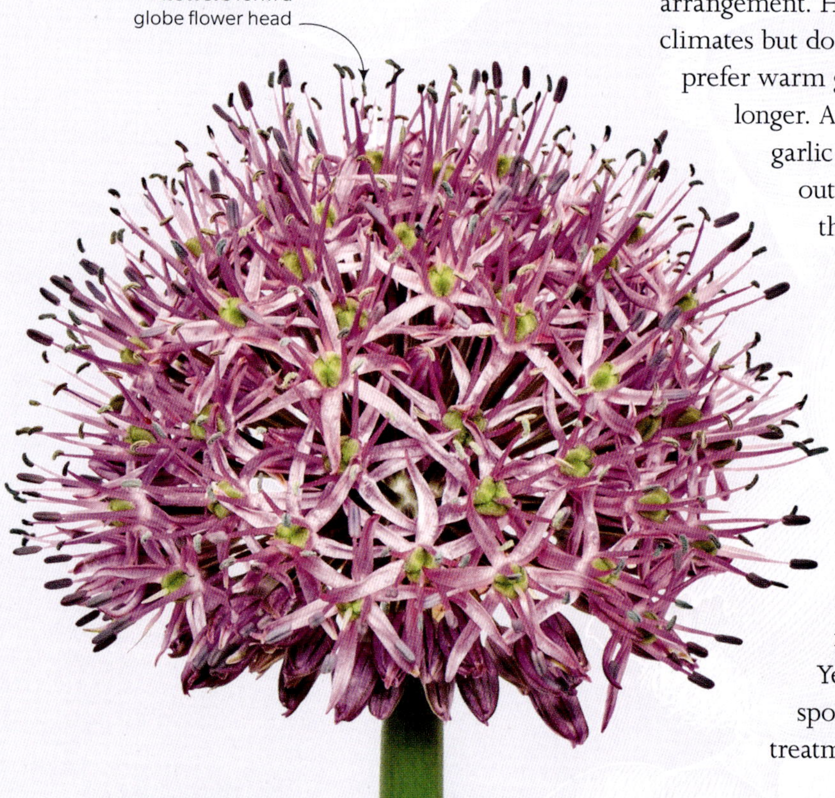

Tiny, star-shaped flowers form a globe flower head

Long single stalk can grow to around 1 m (3 ft) tall

◄ Ornamental flowers
The flowers of edible garlic and onion have limited horticultural appeal, but by hybridizing several wild species, numerous ornamental forms have been developed. Also grown from bulbs, these plants are not consumed.

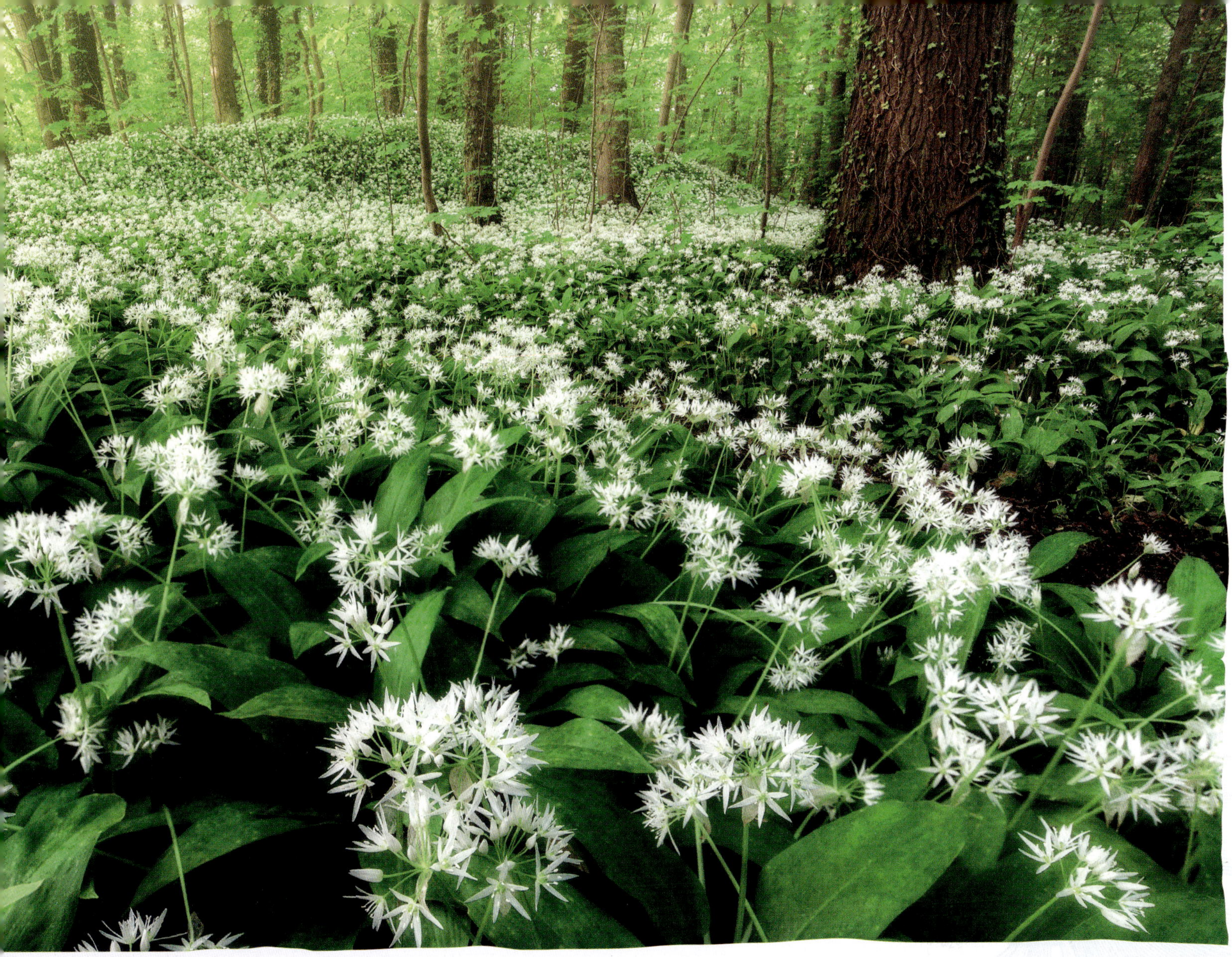

However, in modern medicine the evidence for garlic's effectiveness in treating disease is scant. Despite this it remains a popular component of traditional herbal medicine.

Some studies indicate that components of garlic have antiviral properties that can combat colds, influenza, and even herpes. It may also reduce the growth of cancerous tumours and prevent the development of cardiovascular disease by helping to reduce blood pressure, cholesterol levels, and inhibiting thrombosis. However, garlic can have negative side effects; its prevention of thrombosis is due to a reduction in the clumping of blood platelets, and this effect may increase the risk of bleeding in patients taking blood thinners. Occasional allergies to garlic have also been recorded, as has skin irritation after the application of garlic-based acne preparations.

> " Eat no onions nor garlic, for we are to utter sweet breath. "

BOTTOM in William Shakespeare's
A Midsummer Night's Dream, 1595 or 1596

POPULAR FICTION

The use of this common kitchen vegetable to ward off terrors may seem far-fetched. Bram Stoker's *Dracula* popularized garlic as a vampire deterrent, but across much of Europe, garlic was said to provide protection from several different horrors in traditional folklore, including werewolves and evil spirits. Although the idea of garlic's supernatural powers is widely known and is regularly depicted in popular culture, its origins are uncertain.

MAGAZINE COVER, 1936

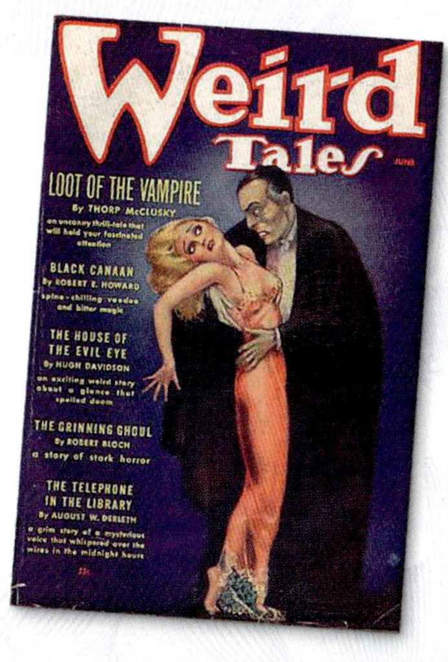

Saffron

Crocus sativus

Famously said to have been used by Cleopatra in a beautifying bath and by the Romans to enhance love, this spice has been cultivated since antiquity and is still used to add earthy flavour to food and drinks, as a natural dye, and to boost health.

Uses Medicines; cooking; cosmetics; natural dyes

Parts used Styles and stigmas, petals

Active ingredients Carotenoids, apocarotenoids, including crocin, crocetin, picrocrocin, and safranal

Habitat Mediterranean climates with hot, dry summers; fields and lightly shaded woodlands on free-draining soil

Best known for adding a golden colour and warm, comforting flavour to dishes such as Iranian jewelled rice, Cornish saffron buns, Spanish paella, and Indian *kahwa* tea, saffron is also used as a skin-enhancing and immune-boosting tonic. Studies have shown it can also be used in the treatment of depression.

A legendary spice

Saffron was possibly used as a yellow pigment in cave art dating back some 50,000 years, and as a natural dye for expensive clothes. Buddha is said to have been wrapped in a saffron-dyed cloak after his death. In *A Curious Herbal* (1737–39), Elizabeth Blackwell said it was "esteemed a great Cordial, Strengthening ye Heart & vital Spirits, resisting Putrefaction, & useful in all Kinds of malignant & contagious Distempers, Fevers, Small Pox, & Measles".

Saffron probably originates from Greece and is naturalized in parts of Europe, Asia, and North Africa. It is associated with the colour yellow – its name derived from the ancient Arabic *zahafaran*. However, the spice is collected from the orange-red styles and stigmas, which are harvested as "threads". Each thread is picked and processed by hand to preserve its carotenoid-rich properties, making it a costly spice. A little goes a long way: just a few strands impart its warming tones to a savoury or sweet dish, drink, or herbal remedy.

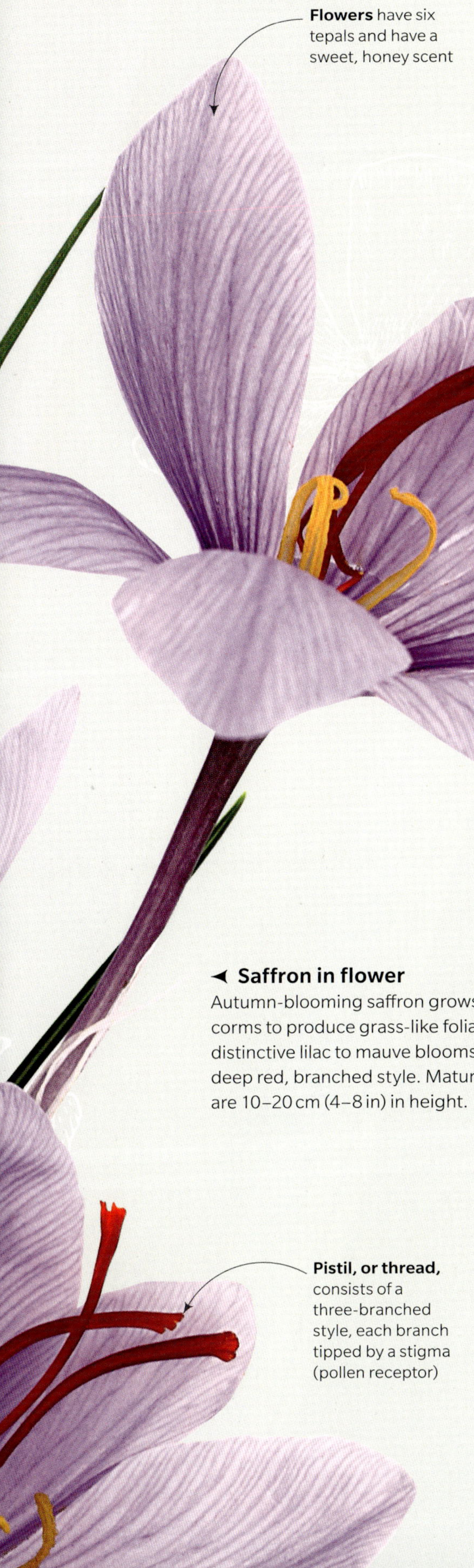

Flowers have six tepals and have a sweet, honey scent

Edible petals are crystallized or brewed into a flavonoid-rich tea

Pistil, or thread, consists of a three-branched style, each branch tipped by a stigma (pollen receptor)

➤ Cure by crocus
By the 15th century, saffron was well known as a useful herb for ailments such as liver disease, as illustrated by this herbal *De Herbis*, based on the writings of Ancient Greek physician and botanist Dioscorides.

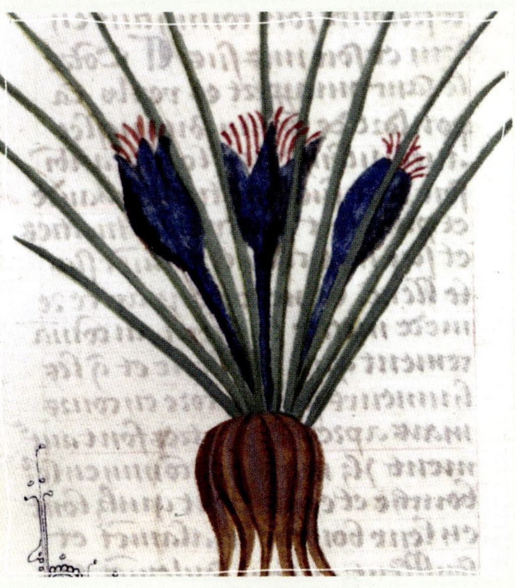

Saffron is the world's **most costly spice** by weight; about **72,000 flowers** make **450 g (1 lb)**

◄ Saffron in flower
Autumn-blooming saffron grows from corms to produce grass-like foliage and distinctive lilac to mauve blooms with a deep red, branched style. Mature plants are 10–20 cm (4–8 in) in height.

" It is with good successe given to procure bodily lust. "

JOHN GERARD, *The Herball, or Generall Historie of Plantes*, 1597

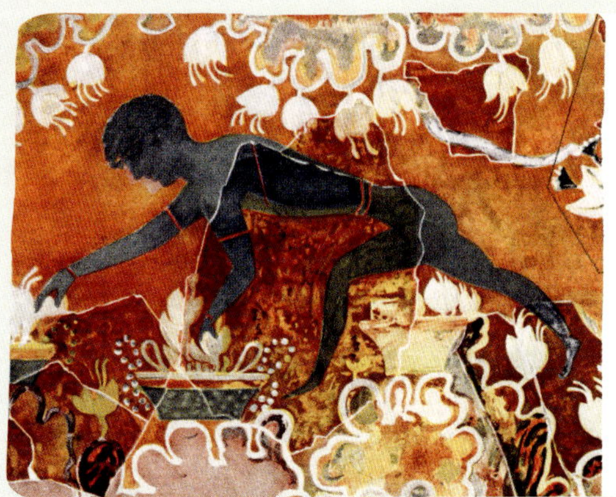

ANCIENT HARVEST

Saffron has been cultivated for more than 3,000 years, as is evidenced by this reproduction of an ancient fresco known as the "Saffron Gatherer", which was found at the Palace of Minos at Knossos, Crete, and dates back to at least 1650 BCE.

FRESCO, PALACE OF MINOS

Uses Medicines; food; animal feed; controlling soil erosion; producing cochineal

Parts used Fruits, stems

Active ingredients Quercetin, isorhamnetin, gallic acid, protocatechuic acid, p-coumaric acid, vitamin C

Habitat Seasonally dry tropical forest, desert

➤ Sweet fruits
The fruits of prickly pear are the source of the botanical name *ficus-indica*, meaning "fig of the Indies", in this case the West Indies. They can be eaten raw, usually peeled to remove any spines, or made into jams, jellies, and juice.

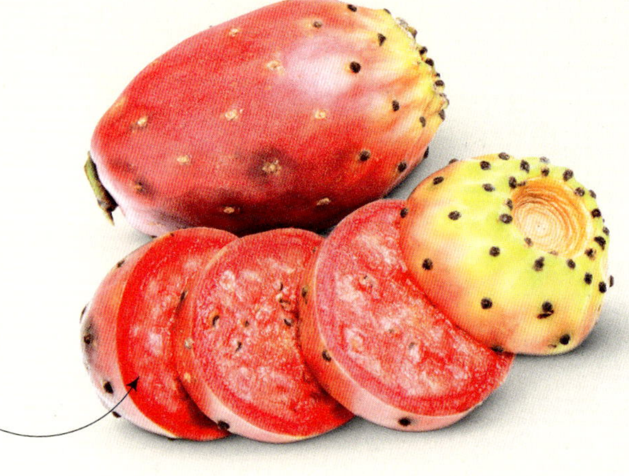

Reddish flesh has a sweet taste, similar to watermelon

Prickly Pear

Opuntia ficus-indica

An important food source for people and animals living in arid areas, prickly pear may also provide treatments for type 2 diabetes, high cholesterol, and even hangovers.

Originating in Mexico, prickly pear now grows wild in more than 40 nations, from Australia through Algeria to the US. This is testament to its ability to survive in some of the world's harshest habitats. In arid areas, the plant efficiently converts limited amounts of water into usable biomass, providing food for people, livestock, and wild animals. However, prickly pear has also become an invasive weed that threatens biodiversity in some regions.

Drought-resistant and delicious

Prickly pears are well designed for desert life. Water is stored in their flattened stems (cladodes) – sometimes defended by spines – and leaves are largely absent, which reduces evaporative water loss. The cactus's roots bind the soil, reducing erosion and encouraging organic matter to accumulate. This, in turn, improves soil fertility and water retention.

Both the fruits, known as *tuna* in Spanish, and the stem segments or "pads", known as *nopales*, are edible. This has encouraged cultivation in many arid areas, as has their potential to be used in farming. Spineless forms of prickly pear make excellent cattle food and also supplement the animals' moisture requirements, reducing their need for water during droughts. Spiny forms are used as fences around animal corrals.

Prickly pear stem segments can be eaten raw or cooked, often sliced as a side dish or taco filler. Spineless forms are preferred, but prickly pads can be peeled or rubbed to remove the spines. Alcoholic drinks such as the Italian *fico d'India*, Maltese *bajtra*, and Mexican *colonche* are based on prickly pear fruits. Eating the pads may lower blood sugar and insulin levels, while eating the fruit seems to reduce cholesterol levels. The fruit may also help prevent some forms of liver damage and reduce hangover symptoms.

➤ Flowering cactus
Prickly pear shrubs can grow up to 5 m (16 ½ ft) tall. Their drought-resistant, flattened stems are grey-green in colour, covered with a blue-tinged wax coating. Domesticated plants rarely have spines, whereas wild forms often do.

Similar herbs

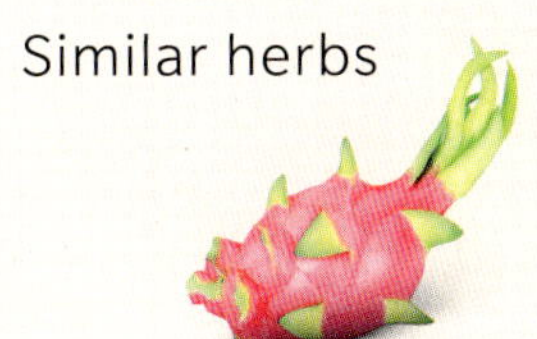

DRAGON FRUIT
Selenicereus undatus

This large vining cactus, from Mexico and Central America, has edible fruits that are rich in antioxidants and may reduce blood sugar levels.

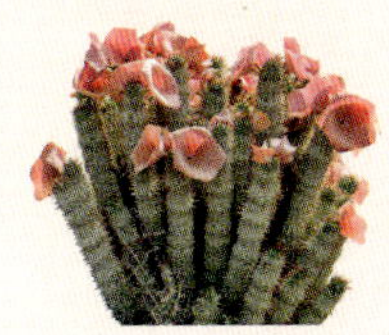

KALAHARI CACTUS
Hoodia gordonii

A succulent shrub from Namibia and South Africa, this plant is widely promoted as an appetite suppressant but is now endangered in the wild.

COLLECTING COCHINEAL

Carmine or cochineal is a naturally occurring dye derived from insects that feed as a parasite on prickly pear cacti. The insects are scraped off cactus stems and crushed to produce the pigment. Cochineal has been farmed for centuries to colour food, clothing, and cosmetics, although modern industrial pigments have replaced it in some applications.

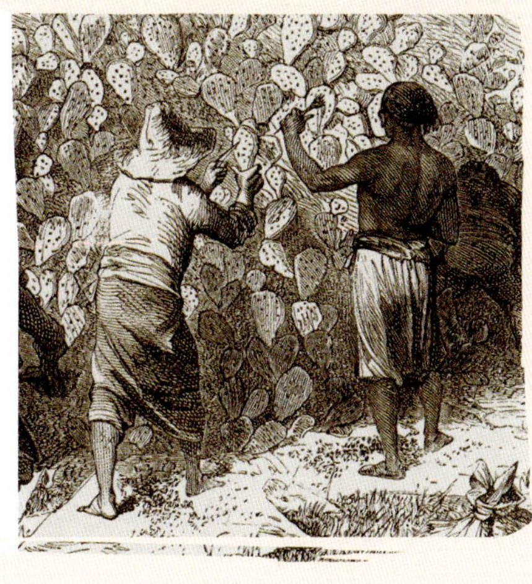

ALGERIAN COCHINEAL PRODUCERS

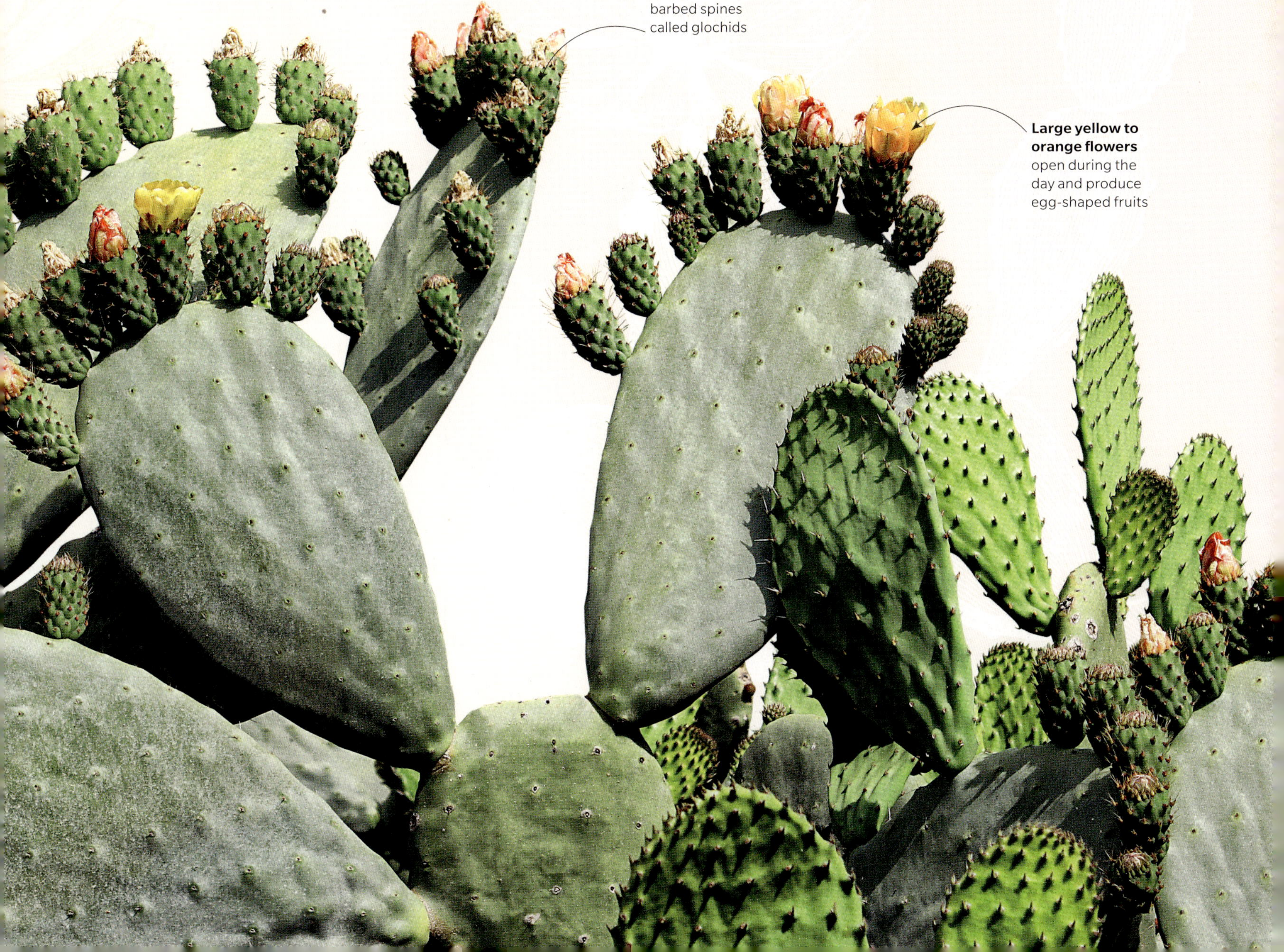

Fruits are covered in tiny, hair-like, barbed spines called glochids

Large yellow to orange flowers open during the day and produce egg-shaped fruits

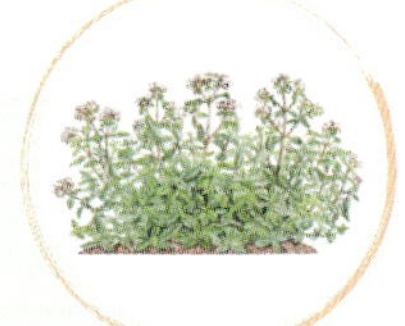

Uses Medicines; cooking; perfume; cosmetics; home

Parts used Leaves, stems, flowers

Active ingredients Carvacrol, thymol, terpinen-4-ol, p-cymene, terpinene, myrcene, caryophyllene, vitamins K and B, iron, manganese, magnesium, calcium

Habitat Chalky scrublands, well-drained soil and sunny, sheltered spots

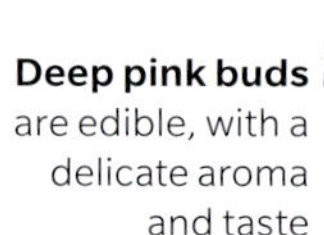

Deep pink buds are edible, with a delicate aroma and taste

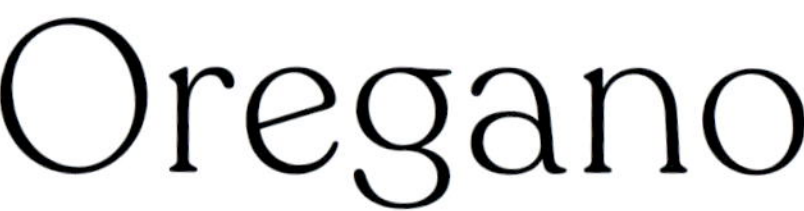

Oregano

Origanum vulgare

With its bushy form, small aromatic leaves, and clusters of pink flowers, this "herb of joy" delivers a pungent, pepper-citrus note to many Mediterranean dishes. It has long been used for its antioxidant, anti-bacterial, antifungal, and anti-inflammatory benefits.

Native to Europe, the Middle East, parts of Central Asia, and North Africa, oregano was probably introduced to the Americas by European colonists. The genus *Origanum* includes several herbs that have been used since antiquity for culinary, cosmetic, medicinal, and ritualistic purposes. Grouped together for their strongly aromatic leaves, prolific tubular flowers, and decorative bracts, are *O. vulgare* – also known as oregano and wild marjoram – and *O. majorana* – referred to as marjoram or sweet marjoram. Both have flavourful leaves, square stems, and clustered flower formations. However, oregano has a strong peppery scent and taste, while marjoram is much sweeter. Oregano's blooms are a deep pink-purple, as opposed to marjoram's white. When observed in their native habitat – on dry, infertile, alkaline soils – oreganos in flower can swathe whole fields, hedge banks, or mountainsides in colour.

◄ Flavourful leaves
Leaves of oregano such as *O. v.* subsp. *hirtum* have a bold, slightly bitter taste that can be subdued by cooking or drying. Steam-distillation releases their medicinal compounds.

Dried leaves are commonly used on pizza and in pasta sauces

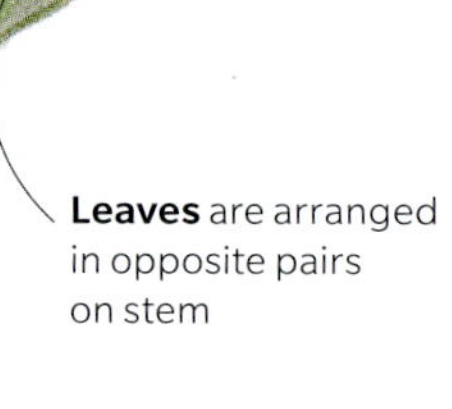

Leaves are arranged in opposite pairs on stem

The terms *Origanum* and oregano stem from the Greek word *oros* for "mountain" and *ganos* meaning "joy", together denoting a "herb of joy". *Vulgare* refers to a commonly found plant.

Holistic healing

Oregano is used to treat ailments of the digestive system including indigestion, diarrhoea, stomach ache, and nausea. It has antiflatulent and antispasmodic properties. It has also been traditionally used to heal wounds, treat bacterial or viral infections, and provide relief from symptoms of certain respiratory conditions such as coughs, colds, and congestion. These antibacterial and antiviral benefits are thought to stem from oregano's key active ingredients thymol (see p.102) and carvacrol, common bioactive components in the essential oils of the Lamiaceae or mint family. In addition, these ingredients act as powerful antioxidants that help to fight damage from harmful free radicals (highly unstable and reactive molecules) in the body and reduce inflammation.

A culinary favourite

Oregano was cultivated as food by the ancient Greeks and then the Romans, who spread the herb across their empire and trade routes. Today, it is a well-known culinary herb, synonymous with Mediterranean Greek and Italian cuisines. The fresh leaves are peppery, and sometimes bitter in aroma and flavour, with only a small

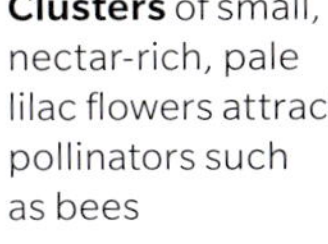

Clusters of small, nectar-rich, pale lilac flowers attract pollinators such as bees

◄ Tubular flower
This bushy, woody perennial has creeping roots and small, aromatic, ovate leaves. It bears clusters of small, tubular pale pink flowers in summer and early autumn.

HERB OF JOY

This ancient drinking vessel dating back to c.475 BCE depicts the Greek goddess of love and beauty, Aphrodite, sitting on a swan. In Greek mythology, oregano is said to have been created by Aphrodite, who was believed to have grown the herb in her garden on Mount Olympus, as a symbol of happiness and joy for all around. This symbolism inspired the herb's use in wedding crowns.

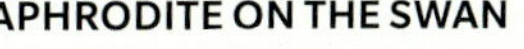

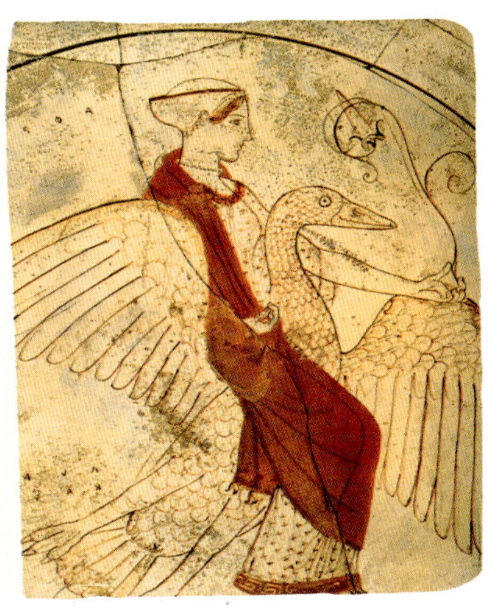

APHRODITE ON THE SWAN

> " There is scarcely a better herb growing for relieving a sour stomach, loss of appetite, cough, consumption of the lungs. "
>
> NICHOLAS CULPEPER, *Complete Herbal*, 1653

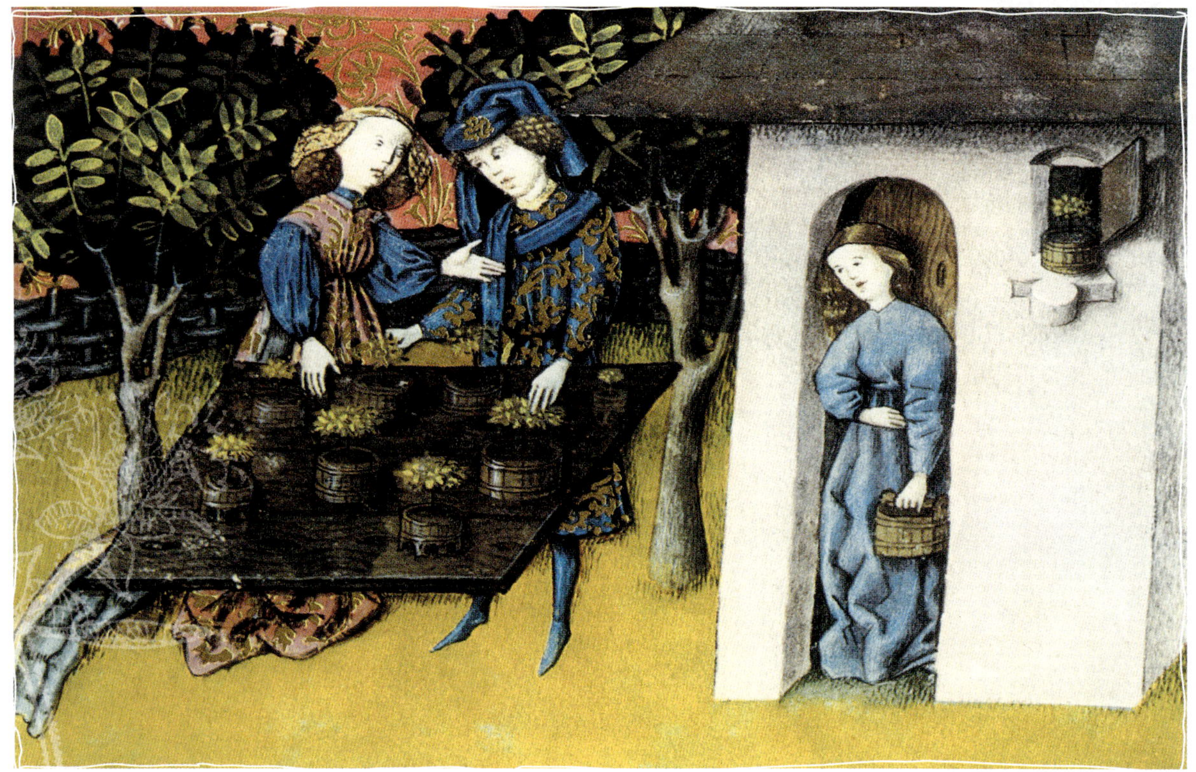

◄ **Harvesting oregano**
This illustration from the 13th-century medical codex *Tacuinum Sanitatis* shows an oregano harvest. Its leaves were chewed or applied as a compress to help combat rheumatism, toothache, coughs, and digestive issues.

Similar herb

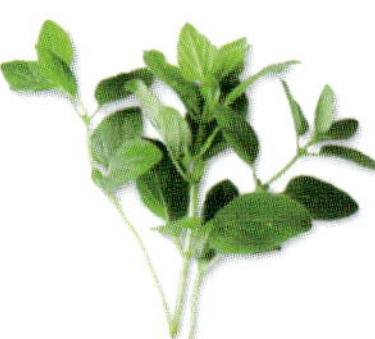

MAJORUM
Origanum majorana
With a sweet, floral, and woody taste and aroma, it is part of the culinary spice mix *za'atar*. Its oil is used for muscle relief.

" The whole plant [oregano] is a warm aromatic... "

WILLIAM MEYRICK, *The New Family Herbal ; Or, Domestic Physician*, 1790

amount needed to elevate a dish with a pungent, herbaceous note. The leaves can be added towards the end of cooking to ensure they do not overpower the dish. Alternatively, they can be used dried, either as dehydrated leaves or crushed flakes, to sprinkle in pasta, sauces, soups, salads, stuffing, or dressings, or on pizza, breads, meat, fish, or roasted vegetables. Greek oregano (*O. v.* subsp. *hirtum*) is an integral part of the typical Greek condiment *ladolemono* dressing made with olive oil, lemon juice, and garlic. This subspecies has a slightly earthier taste. Oregano flowers can also be used for culinary purposes, as a pretty garnish in food or drinks, or as a mellow alternative to the leaves. When combined with complementary flavours, such as citrus fruits or sweet almonds, oregano is a tasty addition to cakes and bakes.

Treat for the senses

Oregano's essential oil can be used in perfume. Its woody, balsamic scent was thought to have been a particular favourite of the Ancient Greeks. Oregano stalks and flowering tops can be used to create a reddish brown natural dye for wool, silk, or linen.

Leaves hold the most volatile oil and are small, olive-green and spade shaped

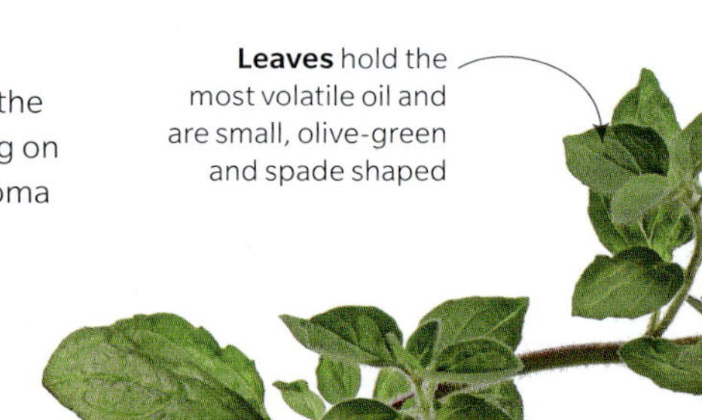

► **Oregano sprig**
Sprigs of oregano can be used whole or the leaves plucked off as needed. Depending on climate and cultivation, the taste and aroma can be earthy and warm or camphorous enough to numb the tongue.

Winter Savory

Satureja montana

Uses Medicines for digestive ailments; cooking

Parts used Leaves, stems, flowers

Active ingredients Carvacrol, thymol terpinenes, p-cymene

Habitat Rocky hillsides; well-drained, alkaline soil and dry, sunny climates

Similar in appearance to rosemary, winter savory is highly aromatic and is traditionally used as a strewing herb. It also helps dispel wind, treat insect bites and stings, and is considered an aphrodisiac.

The genus name *Satureja* is thought to have links to the Ancient Greek word *satyr*, which refers to a notoriously lustful woodland god who used the herb as an aphrodisiac. The genus comprises winter savory (*S. montana*) and summer savory (*S. hortensis*), both of which have aromatic properties and are used for culinary and medicinal purposes. Winter savory is a darker leaved perennial with a sharper, peppery taste; summer savory is an annual, has lighter bronze-green leaves, and is more delicately flavoured.

A complementary digestive

Winter savory is native to the warm, temperate regions of southern Europe and the Mediterranean. Both herbs have been historically used to enhance the flavour of bean stews. They have the added advantage of counteracting wind that may build up in the digestive system as a result of the slow breakdown of gas-producing sugars. Both are known to be carminative, emmenagogic (stimulate menstrual flow), antispasmodic, expectorant, antioxidant, and aphrodisiac. They contain significant levels of the compounds thymol and carvacrol, which have antibacterial and antifungal properties. Naturally antiseptic and anti-inflammatory, the two savories can also be used to provide relief from insect bites by placing a sprig or soothing poultice of their crushed leaves directly on the affected area.

Narrow lance-shaped leaves can be used fresh or dried

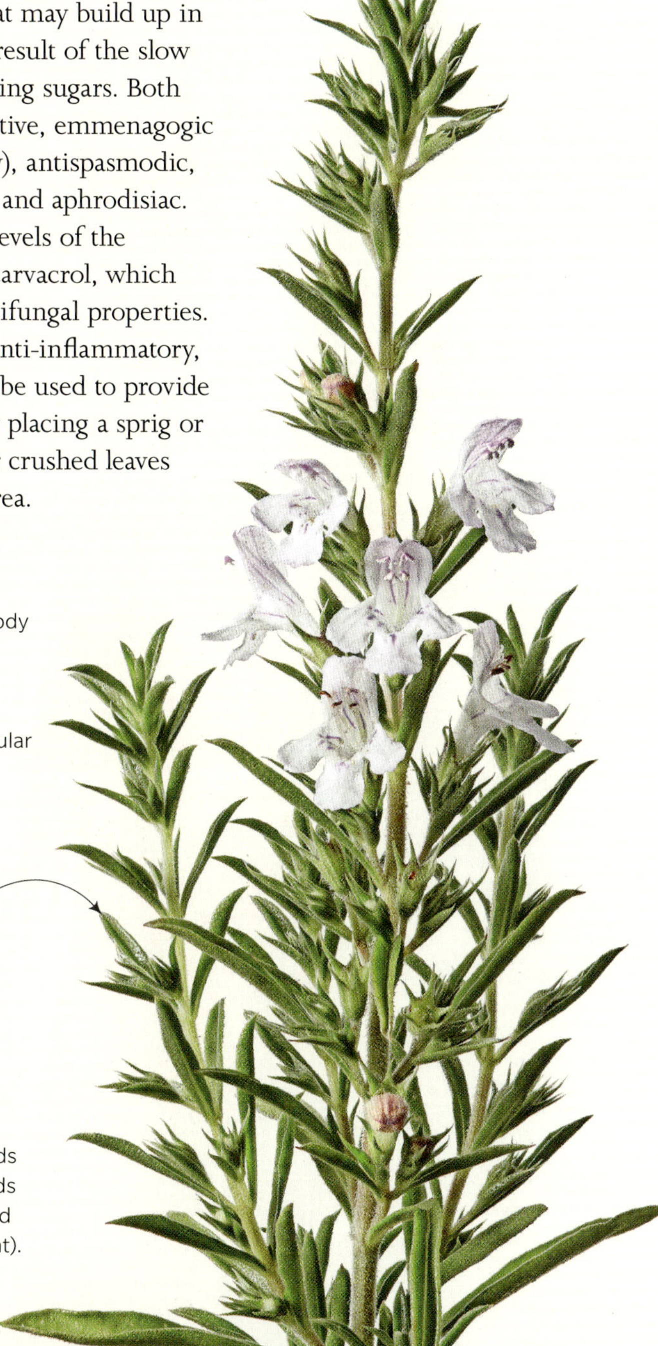

➤ Elegant stems
Winter savory's thin, semi-woody stems support an abundance of low-growing, dark green, aromatic foliage, and delicate, palest purple, nectar-rich, tubular flowers that are also edible.

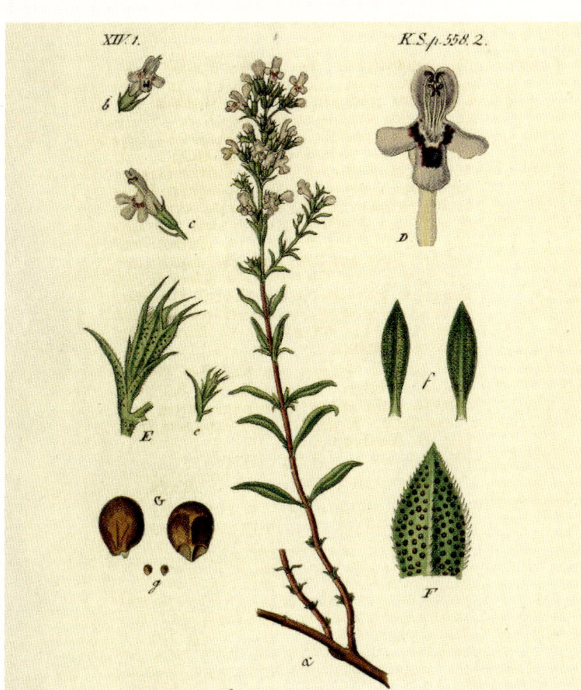

◄ Through the seasons
This engraving shows winter savory's parts including its buds (centre left), flowers (top), seeds (bottom left), and gland-dotted leaves (centre and bottom right).

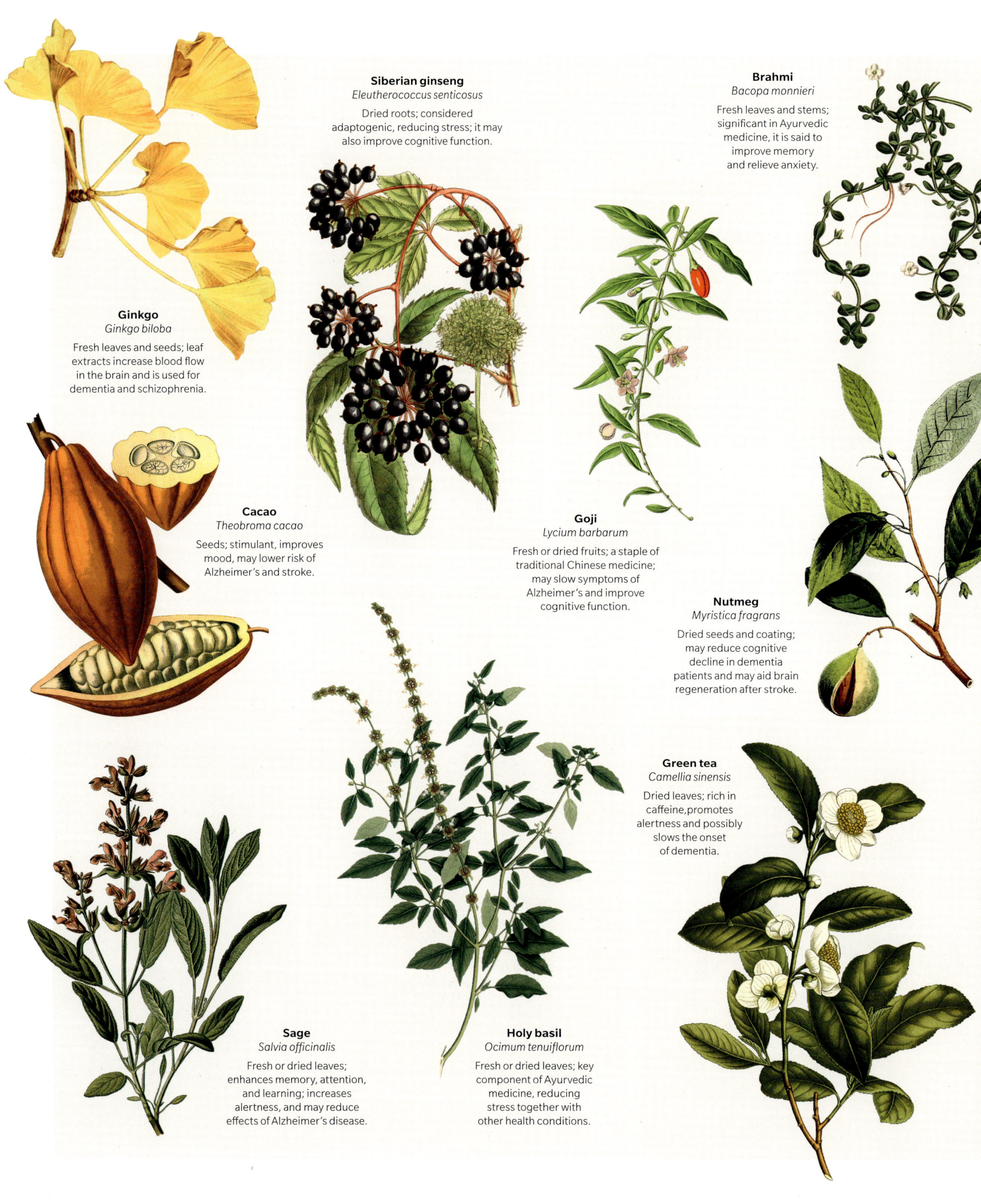

Ginkgo
Ginkgo biloba
Fresh leaves and seeds; leaf extracts increase blood flow in the brain and is used for dementia and schizophrenia.

Siberian ginseng
Eleutherococcus senticosus
Dried roots; considered adaptogenic, reducing stress; it may also improve cognitive function.

Brahmi
Bacopa monnieri
Fresh leaves and stems; significant in Ayurvedic medicine, it is said to improve memory and relieve anxiety.

Cacao
Theobroma cacao
Seeds; stimulant, improves mood, may lower risk of Alzheimer's and stroke.

Goji
Lycium barbarum
Fresh or dried fruits; a staple of traditional Chinese medicine; may slow symptoms of Alzheimer's and improve cognitive function.

Nutmeg
Myristica fragrans
Dried seeds and coating; may reduce cognitive decline in dementia patients and may aid brain regeneration after stroke.

Green tea
Camellia sinensis
Dried leaves; rich in caffeine,promotes alertness and possibly slows the onset of dementia.

Sage
Salvia officinalis
Fresh or dried leaves; enhances memory, attention, and learning; increases alertness, and may reduce effects of Alzheimer's disease.

Holy basil
Ocimum tenuiflorum
Fresh or dried leaves; key component of Ayurvedic medicine, reducing stress together with other health conditions.

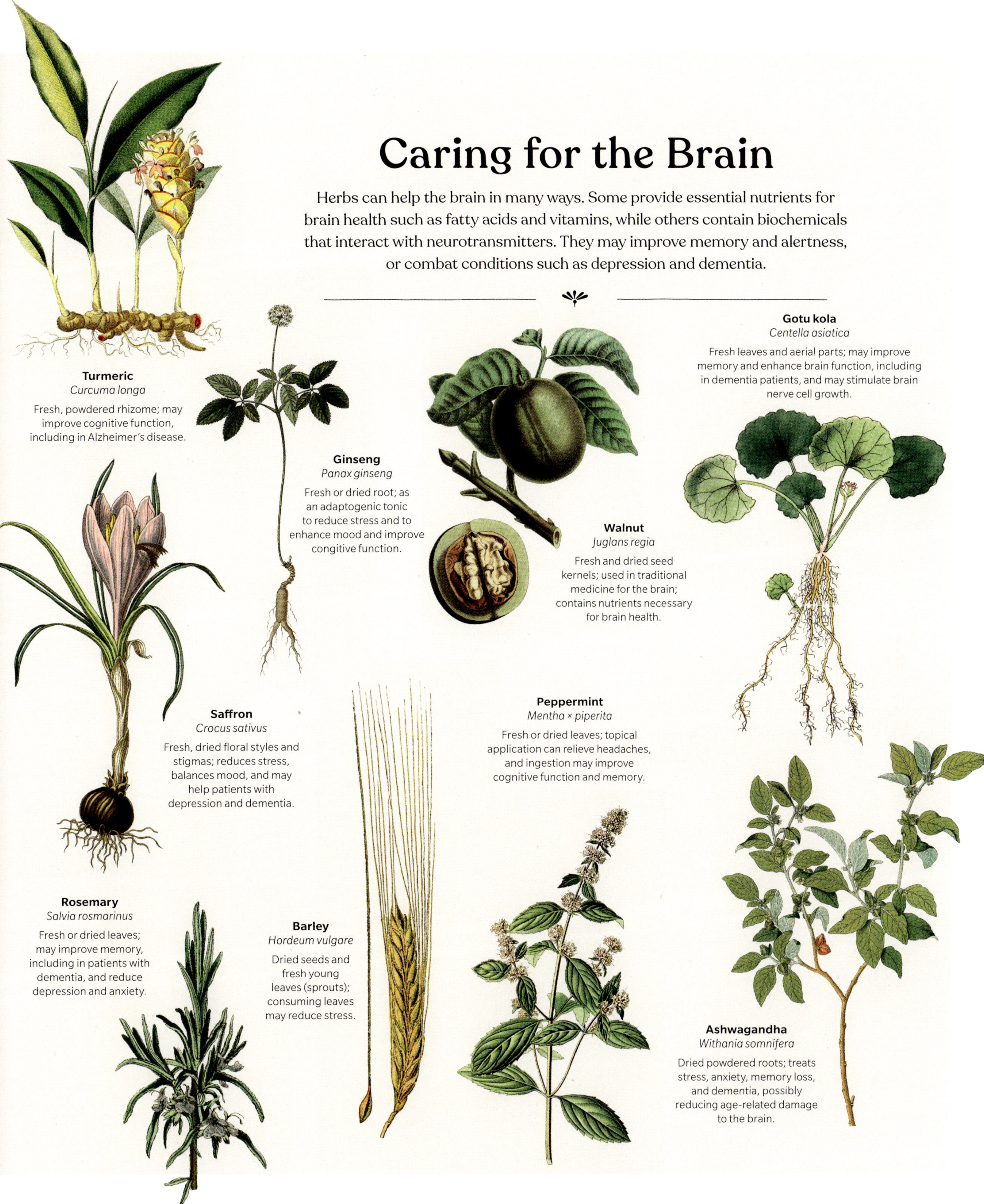

Caring for the Brain

Herbs can help the brain in many ways. Some provide essential nutrients for brain health such as fatty acids and vitamins, while others contain biochemicals that interact with neurotransmitters. They may improve memory and alertness, or combat conditions such as depression and dementia.

Turmeric
Curcuma longa
Fresh, powdered rhizome; may improve cognitive function, including in Alzheimer's disease.

Ginseng
Panax ginseng
Fresh or dried root; as an adaptogenic tonic to reduce stress and to enhance mood and improve congitive function.

Walnut
Juglans regia
Fresh and dried seed kernels; used in traditional medicine for the brain; contains nutrients necessary for brain health.

Gotu kola
Centella asiatica
Fresh leaves and aerial parts; may improve memory and enhance brain function, including in dementia patients, and may stimulate brain nerve cell growth.

Saffron
Crocus sativus
Fresh, dried floral styles and stigmas; reduces stress, balances mood, and may help patients with depression and dementia.

Peppermint
Mentha × piperita
Fresh or dried leaves; topical application can relieve headaches, and ingestion may improve cognitive function and memory.

Rosemary
Salvia rosmarinus
Fresh or dried leaves; may improve memory, including in patients with dementia, and reduce depression and anxiety.

Barley
Hordeum vulgare
Dried seeds and fresh young leaves (sprouts); consuming leaves may reduce stress.

Ashwagandha
Withania somnifera
Dried powdered roots; treats stress, anxiety, memory loss, and dementia, possibly reducing age-related damage to the brain.

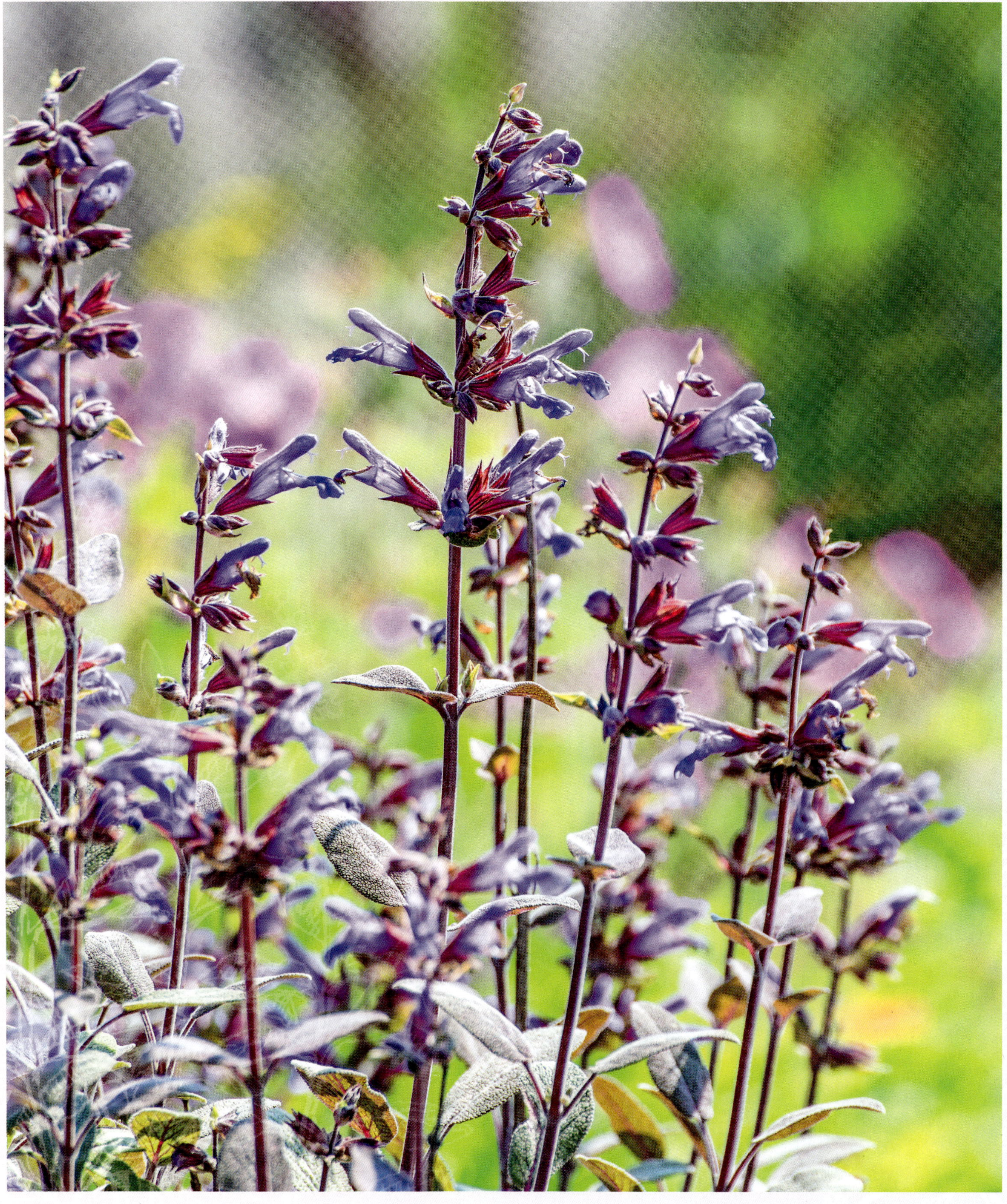

Uses Medicines, cooking, perfume, cosmetics

Parts used Leaves, flowers

Active ingredients Thujone, camphor, cineole, humulene, caryophyllene, linolenic acid, vitamin k, magnesium, zinc, copper

Habitat Limestone or shallow, dry, rocky soil

◄ Sun-loving sage
In early to mid summer, sage sends up short whorled spikes of lavender-purple flowers. Pinching off blooms encourages the plant to put its energy into fresh leaves.

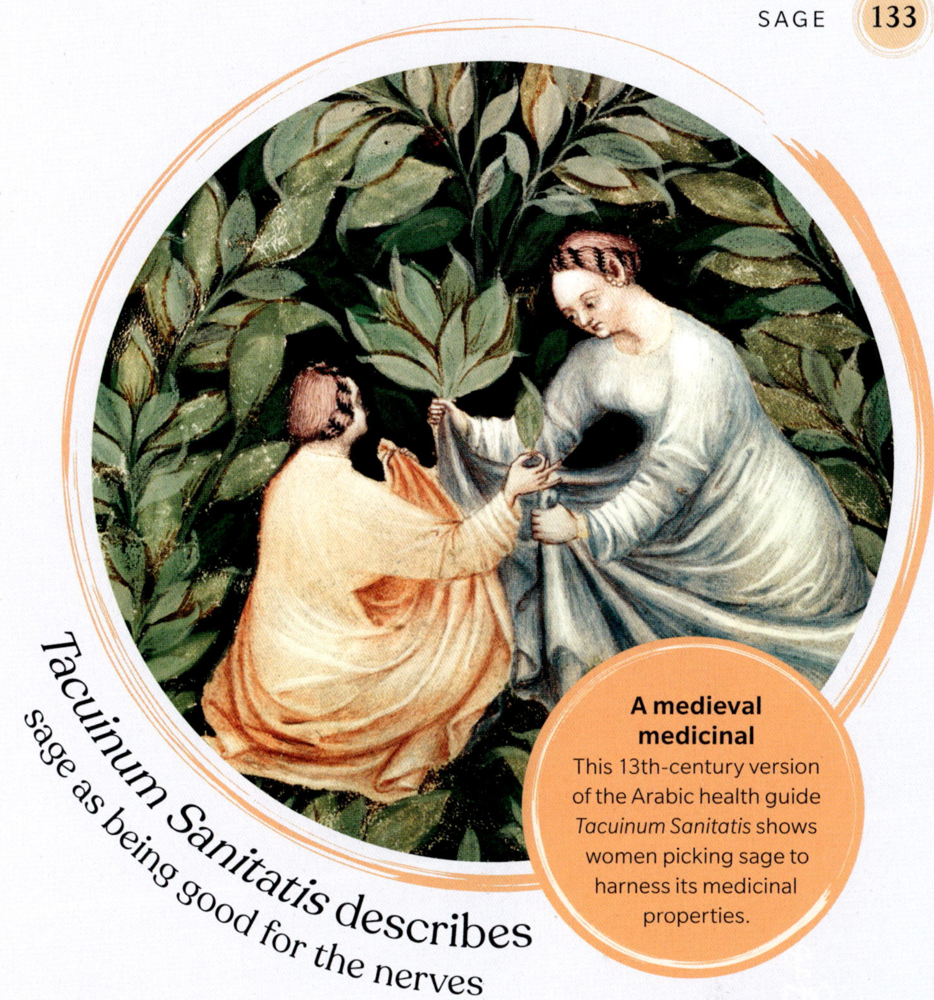

Tacuinum Sanitatis describes sage as being good for the nerves

A medieval medicinal
This 13th-century version of the Arabic health guide *Tacuinum Sanitatis* shows women picking sage to harness its medicinal properties.

Sage

Salvia officinalis

A well-known ingredient in sauces and stuffing, pungent, grey-green sage leaves have also been used for medicinal and ritualistic purposes since antiquity.

Hailing from the largest genus of the mint family (Lamiaceae), sage is native to parts of Western Europe and the Mediterranean and naturalized elsewhere. It is one of more than 1,000 species of *Salvia* and a relative of herbs such as clary sage (*S. sclarea*) and more recently rosemary (*S. rosmarinus*, formerly *Rosmarinus officinalis*).

Herbal medicine chest

Sage was first named as *Salvia* by Roman scholar Pliny the Elder in *Naturae Historiae* (77–79 CE), from the Latin *salvare* meaning "to save, or to heal". He describes a herb "similar in appearance to mint, white and aromatic" that appears to have potentially emmenagogic (stimulates menstrual flow) and antifungal properties. Common sage is now known to provide these benefits and numerous others. It is antibacterial, antiviral, anti-inflammatory, antioxidant, carminative (relieves flatulence), styptic (stops bleeding), astringent, diuretic (increases urine production), and

► Sacred sage
Some Indigenous American peoples traditionally burn bundles of sage as part of a ceremonial smudging ritual to help purify or bless certain people or places.

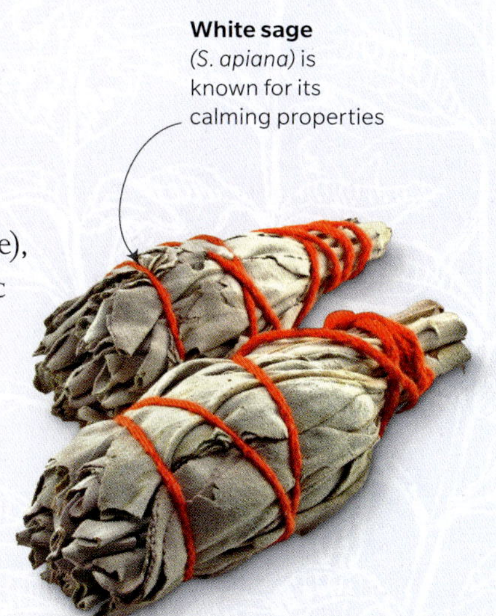

White sage (*S. apiana*) is known for its calming properties

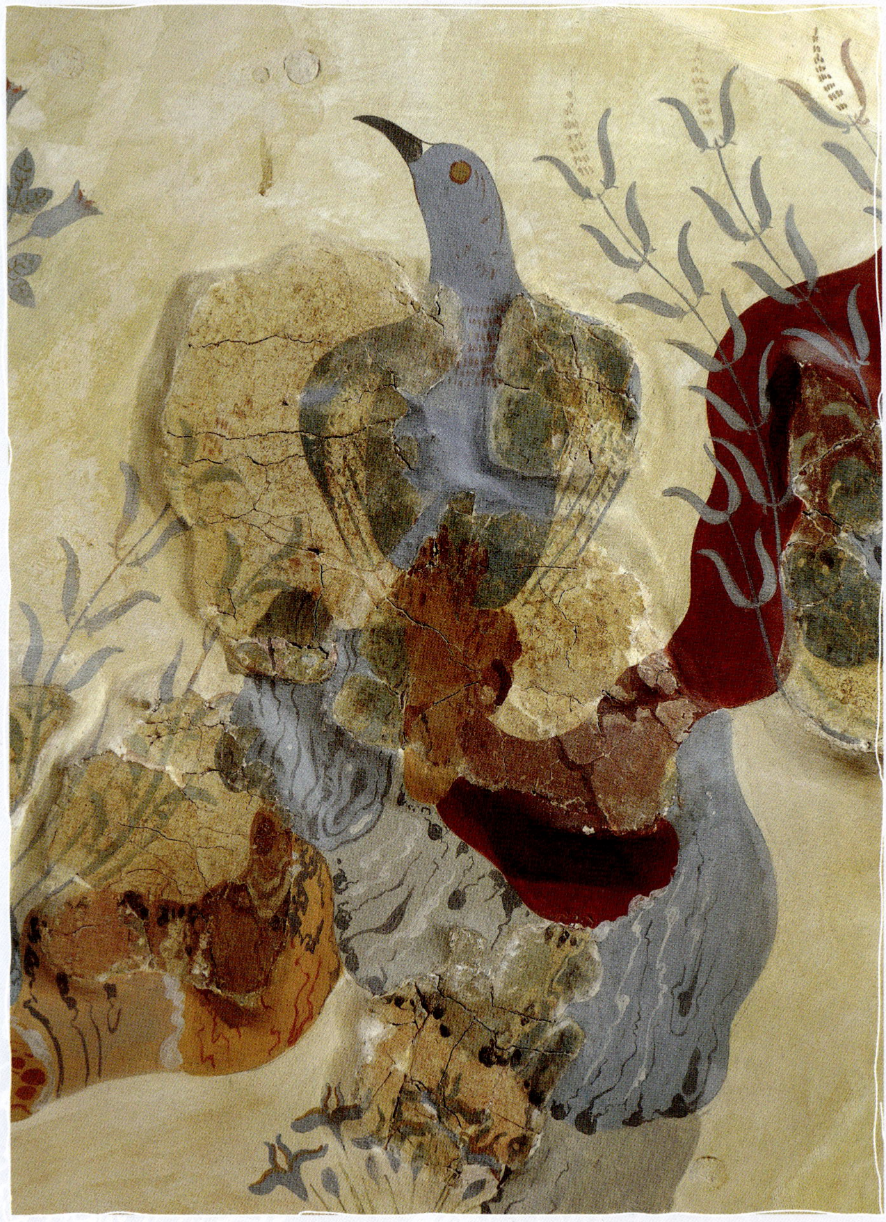

◄ Greek sage
One of the first purported images of sage – possibly locally found Greek sage (*S. fruticosa*) – is the Minoan "Blue Bird" fresco (c.1500 BCE) from Knossos palace in Crete.

antispasmodic. The herb is rich in phytoestrogens, which mimic the effects of oestrogen, and it is also a nervine tonic, used to relieve stress and promote wellbeing. Consequently, sage was seen as a cure-all by many ancient civilizations, who used it as a remedy for infertility and to fight disease. The Greeks referred to sage as *elelisphakos* (thought to be a cultivated version of the wild sage-like shrub *sphakos*, as described by Greek philosopher Theophrastus) and harnessed its many medicinal applications. According to physician Dioscorides in *De Materia Medica* (50–70 CE), they used it to induce the flow of urine and menstrual blood, dye the hair black, staunch wounds, cleanse ulcers, treat coughs and chills, combat dysentery, prevent genital itching, and trigger abortion. Sage's antimicrobial properties also made it useful as a meat preservative and to treat infectious diseases such as the plague, including the 14th-century Black Death.

A holy herb

The Greeks considered sage to be a sacred herb, dedicated to the sky god Zeus, and the Romans associated it with their equivalent deity Jupiter. They both included it in religious rituals: to honour the gods, communicate desired outcomes, quicken the senses, and cultivate wisdom. Sage continued to be revered in the Middle Ages, when it was not only used to treat maladies but also to boost the brain and improve the memory. (Its potential in this field is currently being studied for the treatment of Alzheimer's.) This association with memory and mental function ties in with the word "sage" being used to describe an older wise person, and links to the general idea of longevity. The latter was much sought after in medieval times, and both *S. officinalis* and the less hardy three-lobed sage (*S. fruticosa*) – also native to Mediterranean Europe, the Middle East, and North Africa – were

KING OF THE HERBS

Charlemagne, king of the Franks from 768 to 814 CE and first emperor of the Holy Roman Empire from 800 to 814 CE, ordered by way of his capitularies (a series of legislative, administrative, or religious instructions) that certain plants be grown on his various Roman-inspired estates in Western Europe, with two-thirds retained for the crown's use. These included highly regarded culinary and medicinal herbs such as sage, rosemary, fennel, and coriander.

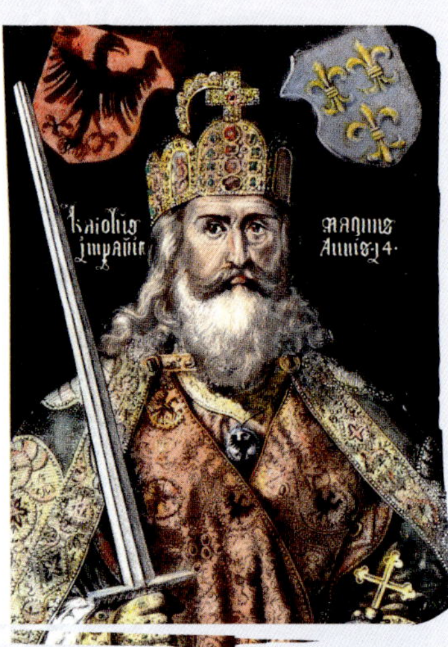

ENGRAVING OF CHARLEMAGNE, c.1500s

thought to extend life expectancy. In medieval monastic herb gardens, sage was grown for its medicinal and culinary benefits as well as for ceremonial use.

Food for thought

Traditionally, sage was drunk as a tea to help combat symptoms of menopause, including night sweats and hot flashes. Sage tea was also popular in China, where the dried herb was traded for black tea (*Camellia sinensis*) by 17th-century Dutch merchants. Today, the herb is a well-known ingredient in cooking, bringing a warm, earthy, pungent note to soups, stews, cured meats, and pasta, even among other strong flavours. Sage and onion stuffing is a particularly popular accompaniment to roasts and thanksgiving meals. It is a much-loved flavour combination that can also help the digestion of fatty ingredients such as meat.

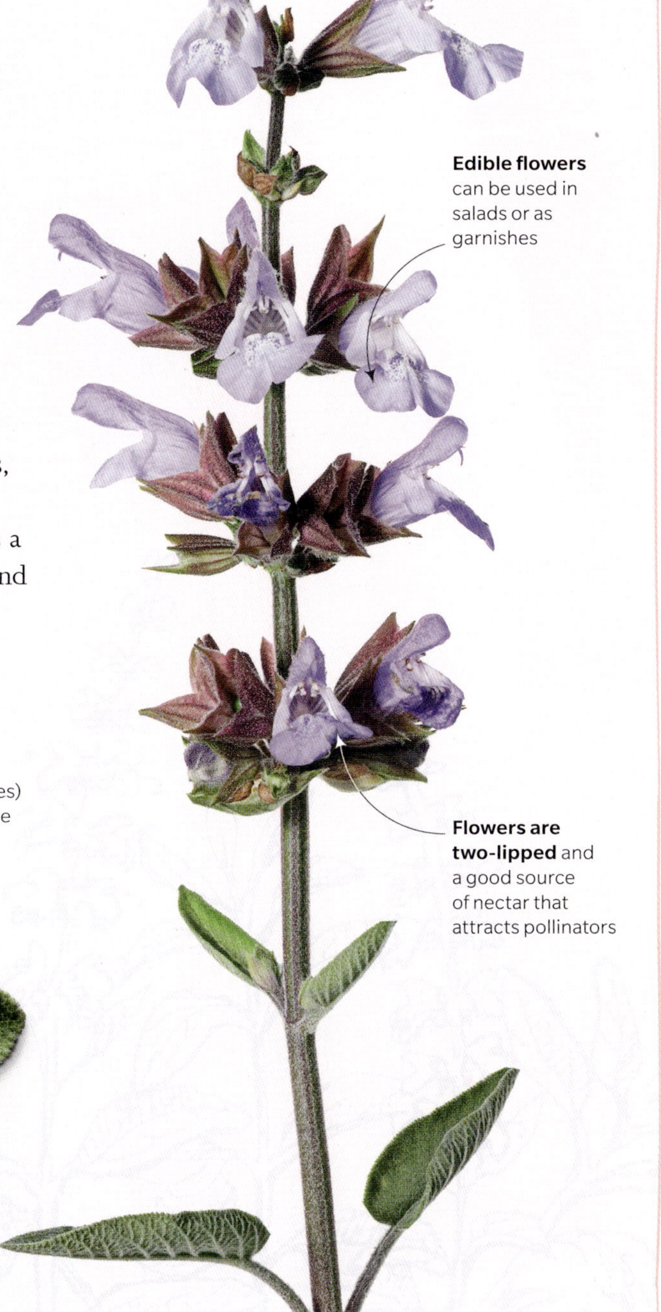

Edible flowers can be used in salads or as garnishes

Flowers are two-lipped and a good source of nectar that attracts pollinators

Tiny hairs (trichomes) help the plant reduce water loss

DOWNY LEAF

Similar herbs

PURPLE SAGE
Salvia officinalis 'Purpurascens'
Purple sage is mainly grown as a culinary and ornamental herb but also has medicinal uses. Young purplish leaves become grey-green at maturity.

TRICOLOR SAGE
Salvia officinalis 'Tricolor'
The pink, white, and purple variegation on the young leaves and violet-blue flowers of this cultivar make it ideal for culinary, cake, or cocktail garnishes.

WHITE SAGE
Salvia apiana
This white-flowered sage, common to California and parts of Mexico, is used by some Indigenous American cultures in rituals, cooking, and medicine.

➤ Sage plant
Prized for their aromatic scent and flavour, the leaves are the most used part of the sage plant, which can grow to around 60 cm (2 ft) tall and provides an abundance of grey-green foliage.

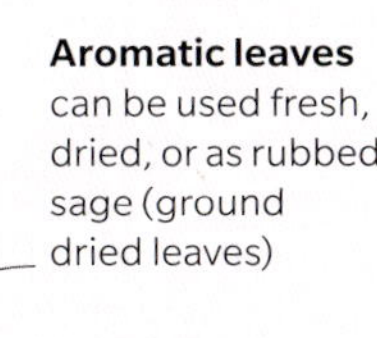

Aromatic leaves can be used fresh, dried, or as rubbed sage (ground dried leaves)

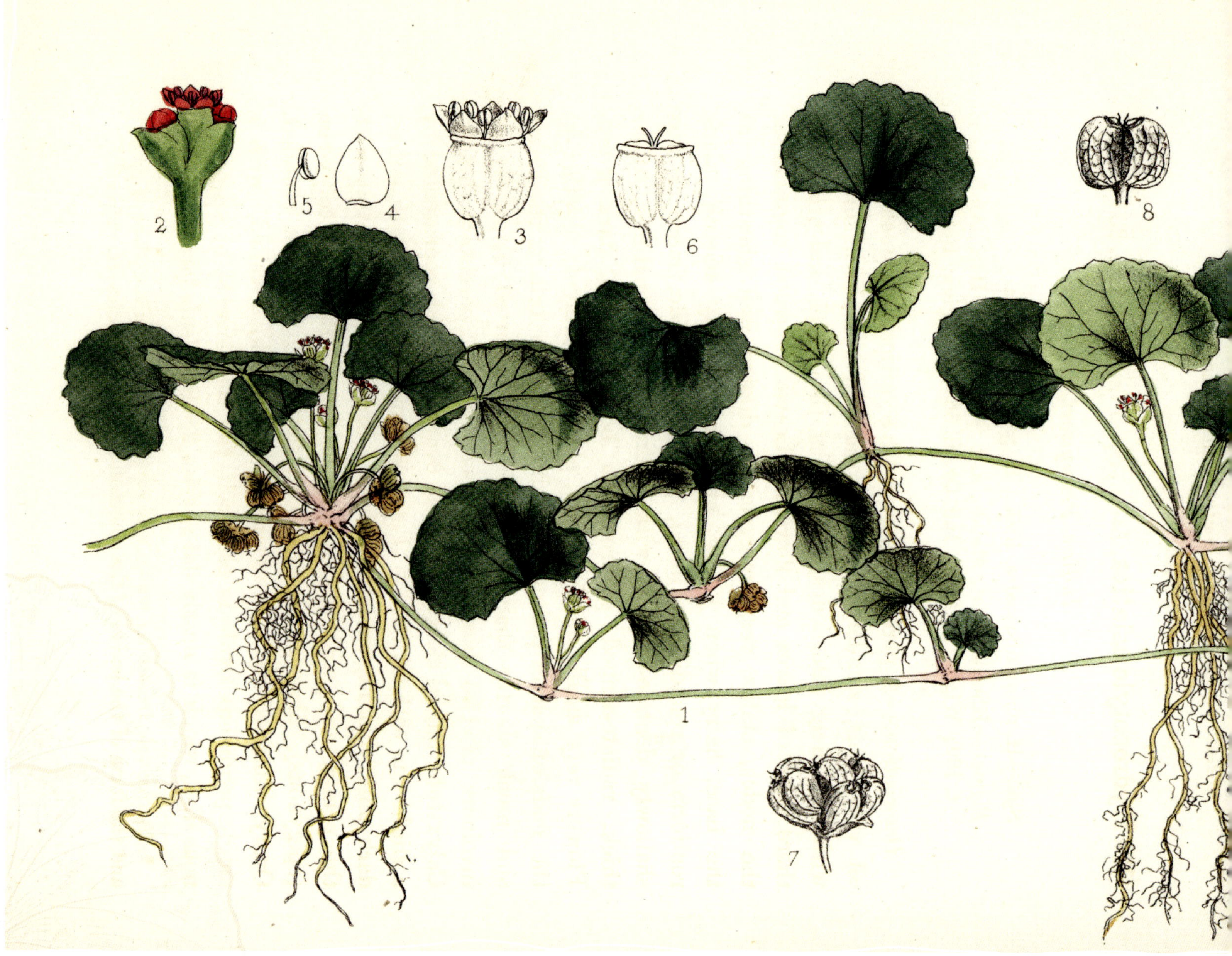

▲ Stems and roots
Gotu kola produces horizontal stems that root at each node, allowing it to quickly colonize open ground and form a dense carpet that suppresses competing plants.

Gotu Kola

Centella asiatica

Gotu kola is an important component of traditional medicine, especially in Southeast Asia, treating wounds and poor circulation and improving memory. Its healing properties extend to the environment, as the plant can be used to help clean up pollution.

Uses Medicines, cooking, cosmetics

Parts used Leaves, stems

Active ingredients Triterpenoids, including asiatic acid and madecassic acid, triterpenoid glycosides

Habitat Damp environments in tropical and sub-tropical areas

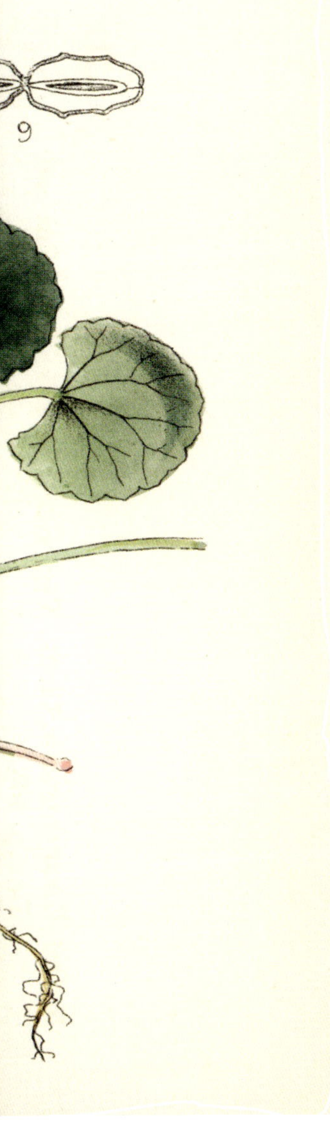

With a widespread distribution in sub-Saharan Africa and southern Asia, east to Japan and New Zealand, gotu kola has amassed many common names, including Indian pennywort, mandukparni, cica (a contraction of its scientific name *Centella asiatica*), and tiger grass. According to legend, it earned the latter name when wounded tigers were observed rolling in gotu kola to heal themselves. The story states that this is how humans first learned of the herb's medicinal properties.

From salads to skin complaints

Gotu kola has an extensive history among the traditional medicines of China, India, Indonesia, and elsewhere. It is used as a memory enhancer and may prove valuable in the treatment of Alzheimer's, stroke, and depression. On the skin, gotu kola accelerates wound healing by increasing cell growth and collagen production. These properties make it a popular component of anti-ageing cosmetics. They also contribute to its ability to improve circulation and reduce varicose veins and ankle swelling during flights. Beyond the medicine cabinet, the bittersweet leaves of gotu kola are an important component of salads, such as Sri Lankan *mallung* and Malaysian *ulam*.

Stems and leaves contain active ingredients

◄ Dried gotu kola
Dried leaves can be steeped and served as tea. They do not contain caffeine and do not act as a stimulant.

In contrast, the flowers and fruits have a strong bitter flavour and are, therefore, discarded during preparation.

Native to wetlands, plant stems grow horizontally along the soil surface, rooting as they go and producing mats of foliage that extend out across the water. Gotu kola roots can absorb toxic heavy metals such as zinc, copper, and lead directly from the soil. Consequently, the plant has been employed in Asia to clean contaminated sites in a process known as bioremediation. With its affinity for water, gotu kola is also able to extract metals from effluent, and can be used to clean polluted water. Bioremediation does not work everywhere, because very high concentrations of metal will ultimately retard plant growth, but the process is inexpensive and low intensity, and does not damage existing soils.

> “Improves memory, intellect, and imparts a celestial glow to the complexion.”
>
> *Sushruta Samhita* aka *Compendium of Suśruta*, date unknown

Similar herbs

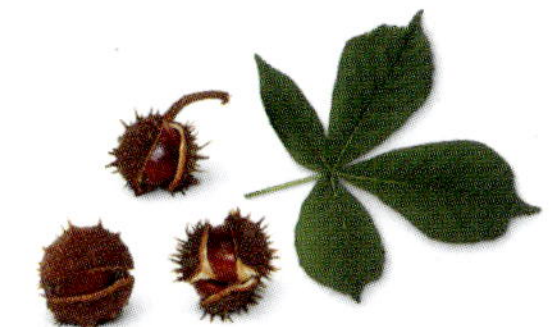

HORSE CHESTNUT
Aesculus hippocastanum
Seeds of this European deciduous tree are used to treat chronic venous insufficiency and sports injuries.

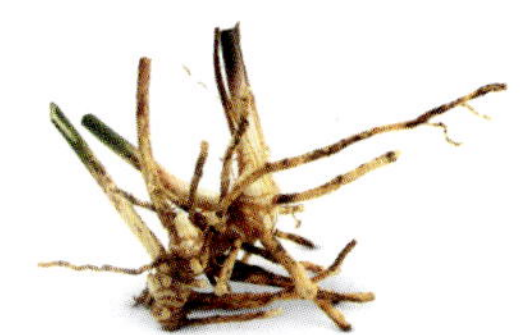

BUTCHER'S BROOM
Ruscus aculeatus
The rhizomes of this evergreen perennial from the Mediterranean are used to treat circulatory issues, such as varicose veins, and haemorrhoids.

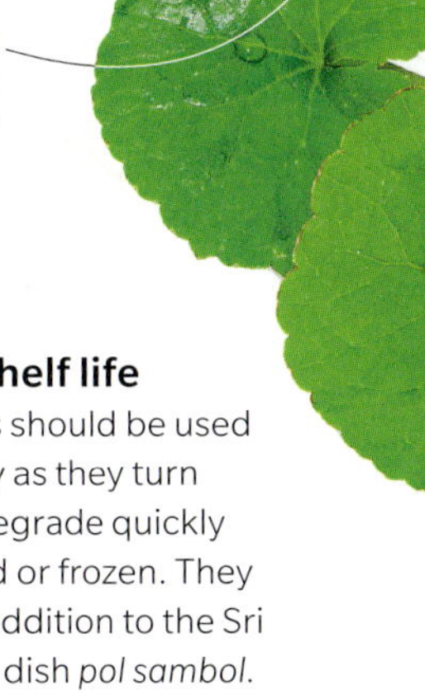

A deep cleft distinguishes it from similar leaves

► Short shelf life
Fresh leaves should be used immediately as they turn black and degrade quickly when chilled or frozen. They are a great addition to the Sri Lankan side dish *pol sambol*.

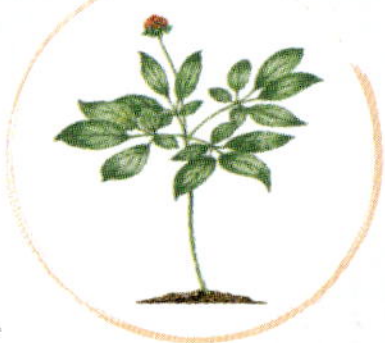

Uses Medicines to treat stress, fatigue, poor memory, culinary as tea

Parts used Roots, rarely leaves and stems

Active ingredients Ginsenosides (up to 40 different types), gintonin

Habitat Temperate montane forests

Fine root hairs contain more ginsenosides than the main tap root

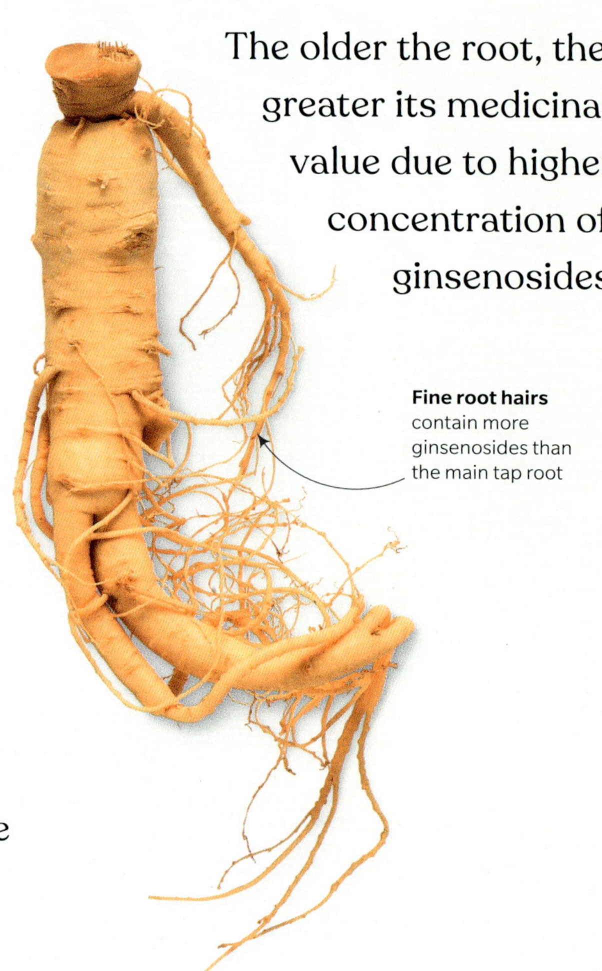

The older the root, the greater its medicinal value due to higher concentration of ginsenosides

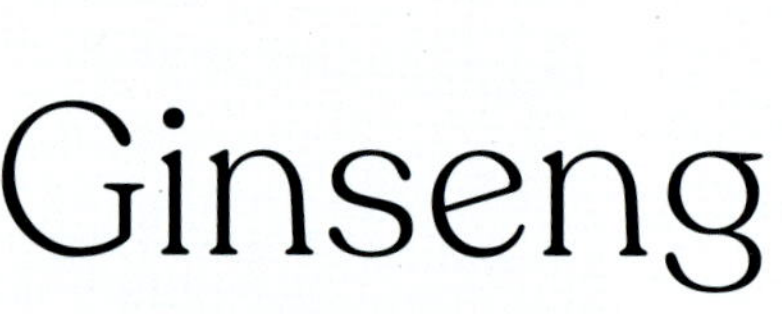

Ginseng

Panax ginseng

Ginseng's genus name *panax* – the Latin word for "cure all" – reflects its importance in traditional Chinese medicine, which uses this versatile herb is used to treat everything from stress to diabetes.

Panax occurs naturally in North America and Asia, but of its 14 species, only two occur in the former, with American ginseng (*P. quinquefolius*) being widely used as a medicine. *P. ginseng* is native to north-east China, Korea, and south-east Russia. Also known as Asian ginseng, it is hugely significant in the medical practices of many Asian nations and over-collection of wild plants poses a threat to their natural populations. While ginseng is easily farmed, Chinese buyers show a marked preference for the wild plant, which is considered to have better medicinal properties and thus fetches higher prices. Some farmers now plant ginseng in suitable wild habitats so it develops the wild characteristics desired by the herbal market. As ginseng plants become rarer in the wild, their monetary value increases. Several countries now monitor and control the harvest in order to protect wild populations, but poaching persists.

Ginseng plants should only be collected in the autumn, when the fruits are red, and only from plants with at least three leaves, each with five leaflets. These are indicative of a mature plant with a developed root.

WHAT IS AN ADAPTOGEN?

Today, stress is a major cause of unhappiness and ill health, and practitioners of herbal medicine recommend adaptogens as a treatment. Adaptogenic herbs like ginseng are said to interact with the body's glandular system, particularly the hypothalamic-pituitary-adrenal (HPA) axis, to restore hormonal balance. Popularized during World War II to aid soldiers, adaptogens continue to be utilized by herbalists and traditional medicine practitioners, though supporting clinical trials are few.

Healthy choices

Due to the popularity of ginseng, the name is applied to several other plants, not all of which have the same properties. Ginseng is part of the ivy family (Araliaceae), as is Siberian ginseng (*Eleutherococcus senticosus*), while Indian ginseng

▲ **Ginseng root**
Herbal ginseng products are made from roots, collected in the wild or farmed. However, the leaves contain up to 12 times the concentration of active ingredients (ginsenosides) as compared to the root.

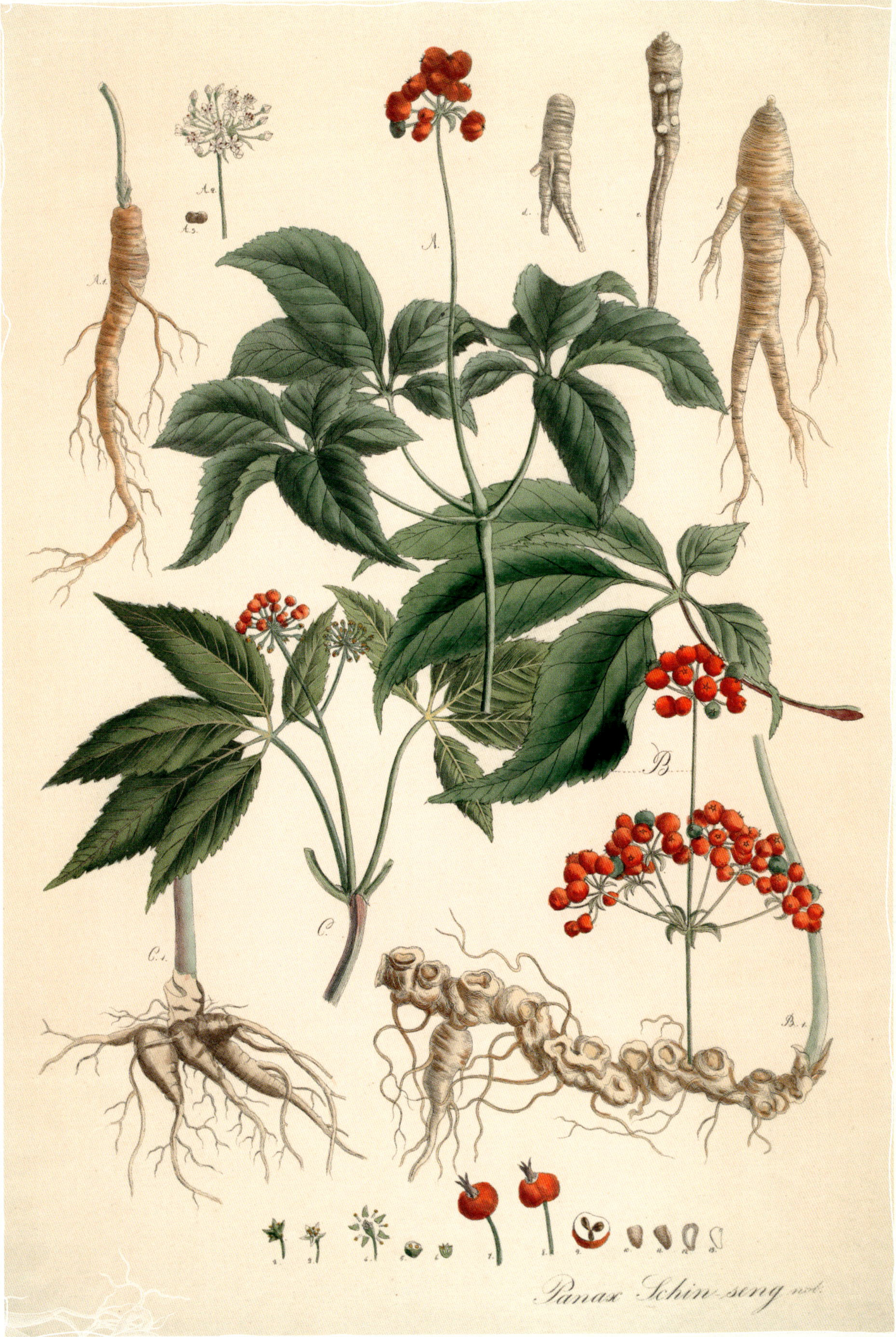

◄ Botanical illustration
Ginseng is an herbaceous perennial growing from an elongated underground rootstock. The stems bear palm-like compound leaves and clusters of small green flowers, followed by red fleshy fruits.

Similar herbs

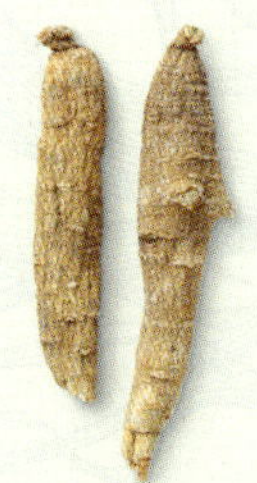

AMERICAN GINSENG
Panax quinquefolius
Native to eastern Canada and the US, this species was used medicinally by some Indigenous Americans and is now farmed.

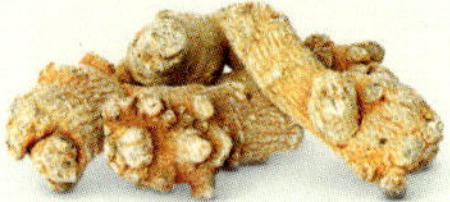

CHINESE GINSENG
Panax notoginseng
One of the few ginseng species from subtropical regions, this plant occurs in southern China and Vietnam, where it is collected from the wild.

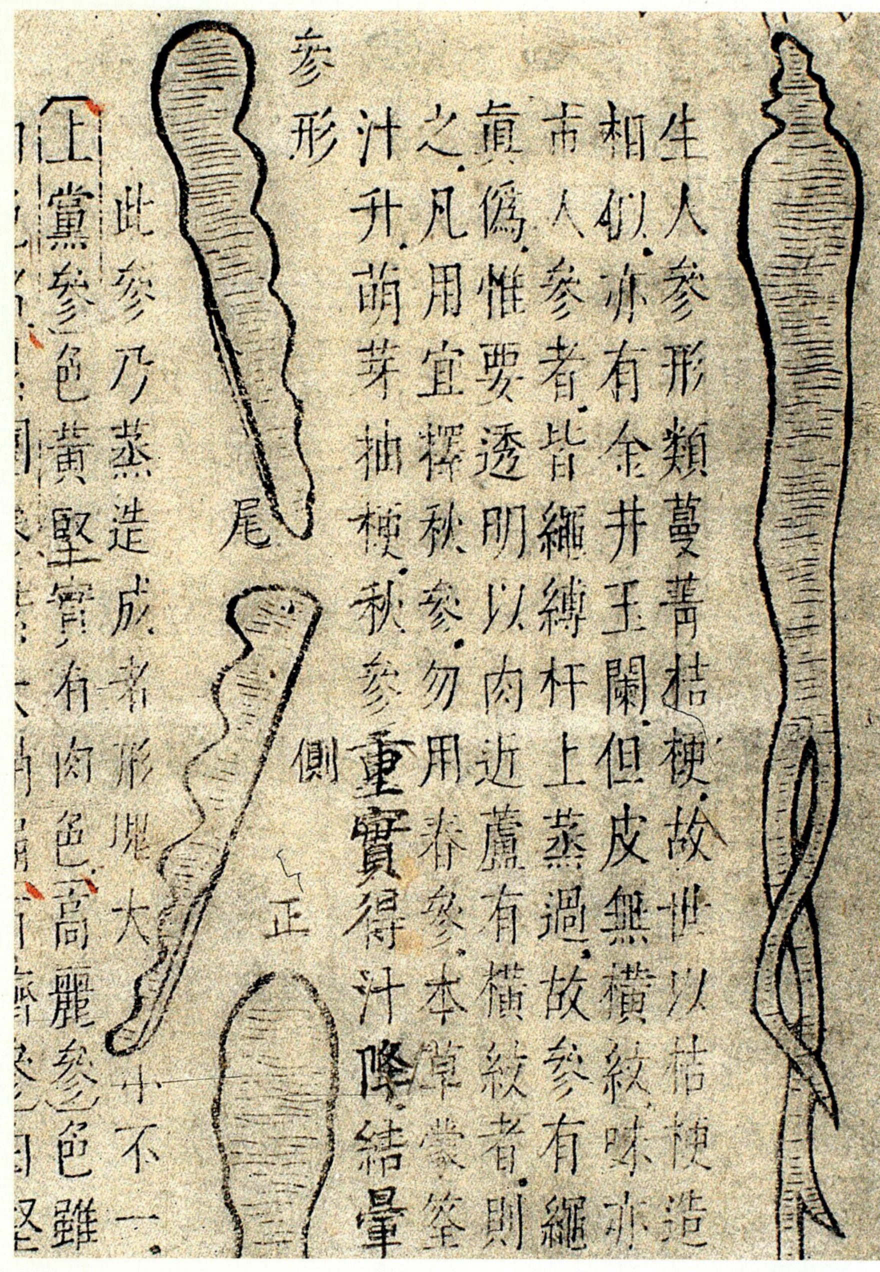

生人參形類蔓菁桔梗故世以桔梗造
相似亦有金井玉闌但皮無橫紋味亦
市人參者皆纏縛杆上蒸過故參有纏
眞僞惟要透明以肉近蘆有橫紋者則
之凡用宜擇秋參勿用春參本草蒙筌
汁升萌芽抽梗秋參重實得汁降結暈

參形

尾

側

正

此參乃蒸造成者形塊大小不一

上黨參色黃堅實有肉色高麗參色雖

(*Withania somnifera*) is in the potato family (Solanaceae) and Amazon or Brazilian ginseng (*Hebanthe erianthos*) is in the spinach family (Amaranthaceae). Only members of the Panax genus are true ginseng and care should be taken to identify the source when using it medicinally.

An adaptogen, ginseng is said to help reduce stress, increase energy, boost the immune system, reduce the risk of cancer, and lower blood sugar levels in people with type 2 diabetes. Other areas where ginseng may hold promise include lowering the risks of catching colds and influenza, improving memory, and reducing the symptoms of menopause. As is often the case with traditional herbal remedies, only limited clinical evidence supports its effectiveness. Ginseng may also interact with some prescribed medications, such as warfarin and aspirin.

Food and drink

Ginseng root, and to a lesser extent its leaves, are popular ingredients in Korean cuisine. *Insam-ju* is an alcoholic beverage flavoured with ginseng and *samgye-tang* is a soup made from a whole chicken with ginseng added. The bitter and earthy flavour of ginseng can be off-putting and sweeteners are typically added to energy drinks that feature this herb.

◄ ***Bencao yuanshi***
Translated as *Origins of Materia Medica*, this 17-century book by Chinese botanist Li Zhongli describes various medicinal substances, their origins, and characteristics. On this page, a ginseng root features prominently (right).

GINSENG TEA

Ginseng root is consumed in a variety of ways, but often as a tea and particularly in China and Korea. Ginseng tea can be made either by soaking fresh roots in hot water, or by adding ground or powdered root to boiling water. In Korea, chestnuts and jujube fruits are often added to the tea, which can be sweetened with honey.

Sold loose or in tea bags, ginseng tea has a bitter, earthy flavour

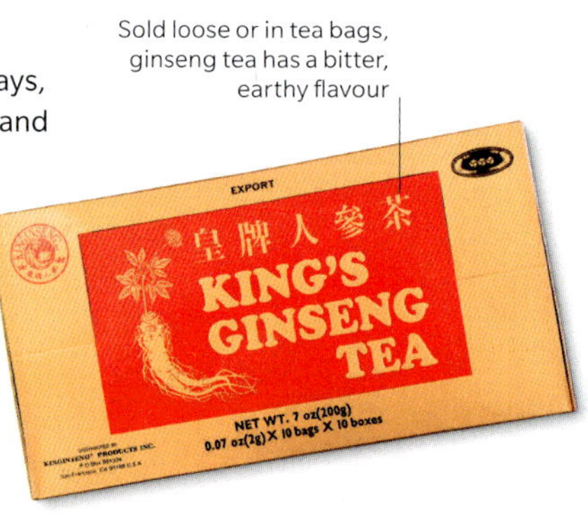

GINSENG TEA

Red and white ginseng are the **same species** – red roots have been steamed, while white roots have not

Black Cohosh

Actaea racemosa

Black cohosh is one of several significant herbs native to North America that was utilized as a medicine by Indigenous peoples before colonization, then adopted by the new arrivals. It is now in use around the world.

Uses Medicines for menopause symptoms, gynaecological problems, snakebites

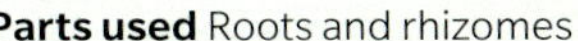

Parts used Roots and rhizomes

Active ingredients Actein, cimicifugoside, caffeic acid, isoferulic acid

Habitat Temperate woodlands

Wild across much of eastern North America, black cohosh ranges from Ontario, in Canada, south to Georgia and west to Missouri, in the US. It should not be confused with blue cohosh (*Caulophyllum thalictroides*), another medicinal herb used by Indigenous Americans. Black cohosh flowers in late summer, bears dry capsule fruits, and is a member of the buttercup family (Ranunculaceae). Blue cohosh flowers in spring with yellow, green or brown blooms, has blue fleshy berries, and is a member of the barberry family (Berberidaceae) Traditionally, both cohoshes have been used in the treatment of obstetric and gynaecological conditions, though their specific actions and side effects are different.

Hot topic

Black cohosh is now used in treating symptoms of menopause, in particular, hot flushes, night sweats, and sleep disturbance. It may alleviate flushes related to breast cancer treatment and even reduce the risk of developing breast cancer.

▼ Flowering spires
Borne in tall racemes, black cohosh flowers have a distinctive fragrance that is described as sweet, cloying, or even putrid. It has been used as an insect repellent, earning it the common name "black bugbane".

Small flowers have dense clusters of white, pollen-bearing stamens

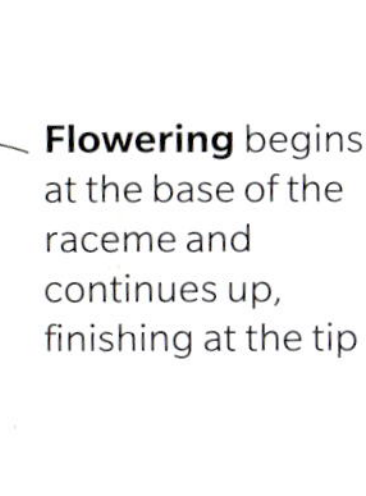

Flowering begins at the base of the raceme and continues up, finishing at the tip

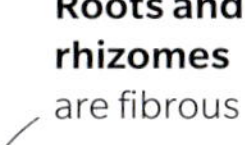

Roots and rhizomes are fibrous

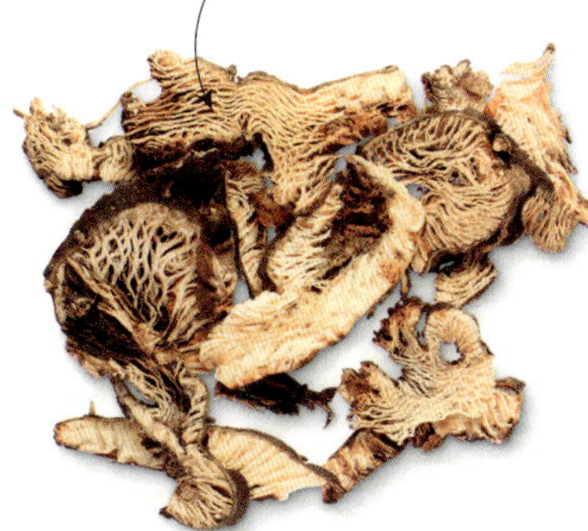

▲ Dried roots
Black cohosh roots are harvested in autumn, when they are at their peak weight and medicinal potency. These can be used fresh, or dried to make tablets, tinctures, and teas.

> " Cohosh root... is a common medicine for kidney trouble... or, as [the Penobscots] describe it, 'feeling all played out'. "
>
> FRANK SPECK, *Medicine Practices of the Northeastern Algonquians*, 1917

Similar herbs

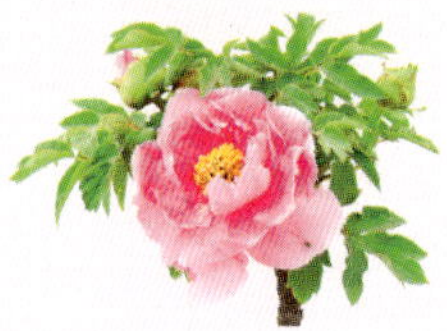

MOUTAN PEONY
Paeonia x suffruticosa
This cultivated tree peony from China is grown as an ornamental and for its root bark, to treat inflammatory bowel conditions such as Crohn's disease.

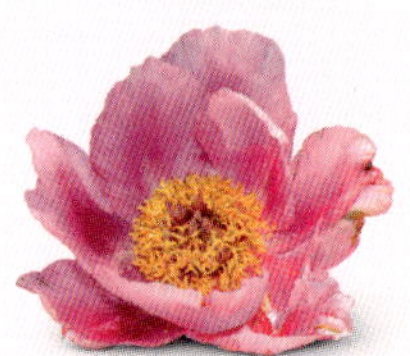

COMMON PEONY
Paeonia officinalis
Native to southern Europe, this herbaceous peony has a long history as a medicinal and ornamental plant. The roots are used to treat epilepsy and ulcers.

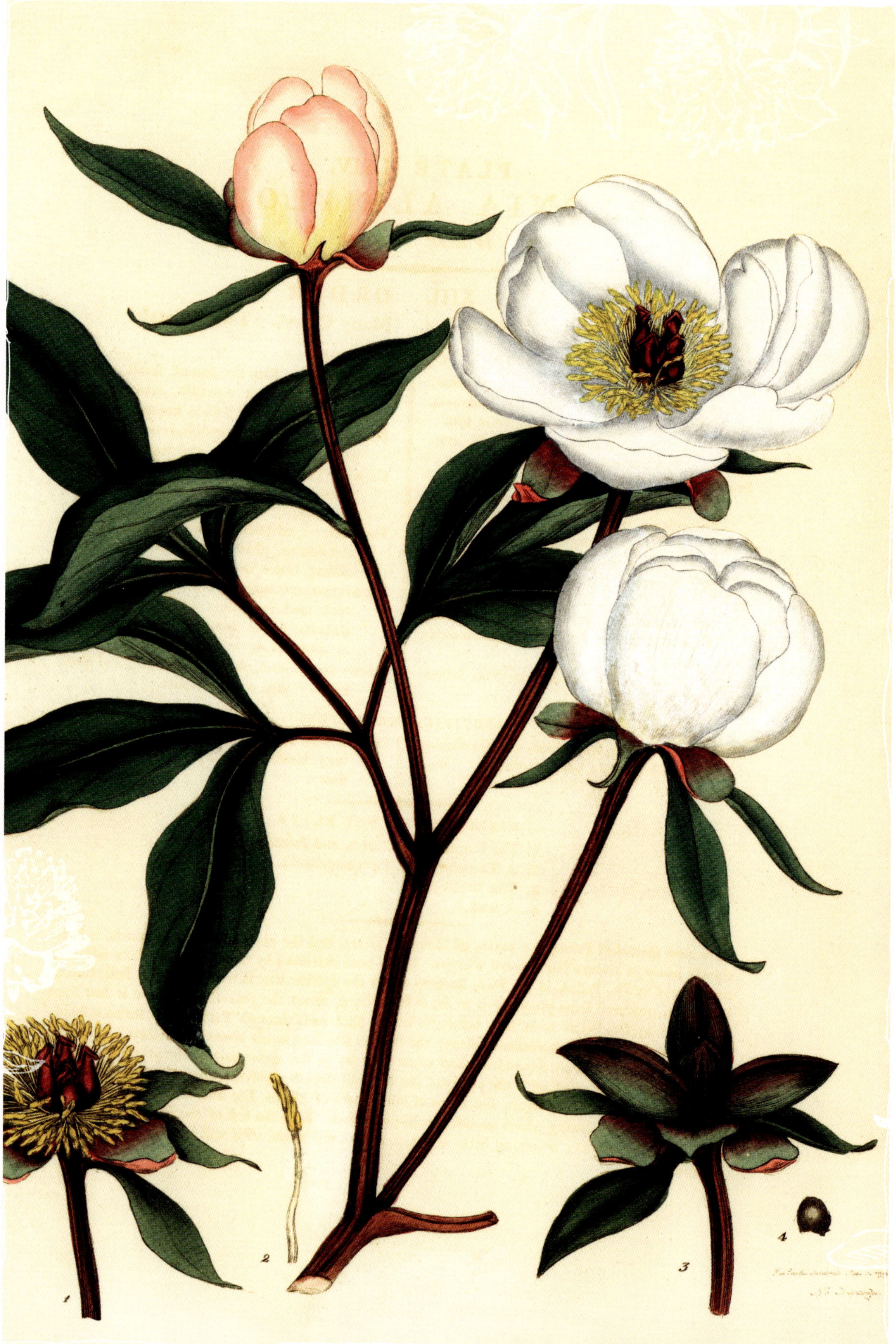

➤ **Classic peony**
One of 15 peony species native to China, white peony has single, fragrant, white or pink flowers and a central boss of yellow stamens.

White Peony

Paeonia lactiflora

Uses Medicines

Parts used Roots

Active ingredients Paeoniflorin, albiflorin, lactiflorin

Habitat Dry woodland edges, stony slopes and riverbanks, mainly in temperate regions

One of the first Chinese peony species to arrive in Europe, this plant is the parent of many popular ornamental varieties and remains a common garden plant around the world. In China, it is also significant for its medicinal uses.

The medicinal use of white peony has been documented for almost 2,000 years in China, where it is known as *shao yao*. White peony root, or *bai shao*, refers to the peeled, prepared tuberous root. Red peony root, or *chi shao*, is the unpeeled root from the same peony species. The two root preparations have different medicinal uses: white peony root tonifies the liver; the red encourages blood flow.

Modern Chinese herbalists (together with those in Korea and Japan) use white peony root to treat rheumatoid arthritis, hepatitis, and abdominal cramps or spasms. A common white peony extract is total glucosides of peony (TGP), produced from the roots using water and ethanol; the chemical compound paeoniflorin makes up to 90 per cent of the product. TGP is used to treat autoimmune conditions such as lupus and psoriasis.

Floral favourite

White peony is a significant species in breeding ornamental peonies. The first plants introduced to Europe had white flowers, thus the Latin name *lactiflora*, meaning "flower the colour of milk". However, wild forms can have pink blooms too and modern cultivars derived from white peony may have white, pale or dark pink flowers varying in size and number of petals.

Peonies are considered classic cottage-garden plants, whether herbaceous perennials such as *Paeonia lactiflora* or, more recently, the larger-flowered shrubs (tree peonies). They have inspired many artists, including European painters Pierre-Auguste Renoir, Vincent van Gogh, and Édouard Manet.

▼ Cultivated charm
White peony is the parent of many garden hybrids, including those with double flowers, where the pollen-bearing stamens are converted into additional frilly petals, as in this form.

Carpel, or female part, ends in stigma, which receives pollen

Large, outer petals are known as guard petals

White peony root has been cleaned, boiled, peeled of its red skin, dried, and then sliced

◄ Healing root
After being harvested from four- or five-year-old plants and prepared, white peony roots can be used to make a tea or tincture or ground into a powder.

" White peonies... send out light while the rest of the yard grows dim. "

JANE KENYON
"Peonies at Dusk", *Constance: Poems,* 1993

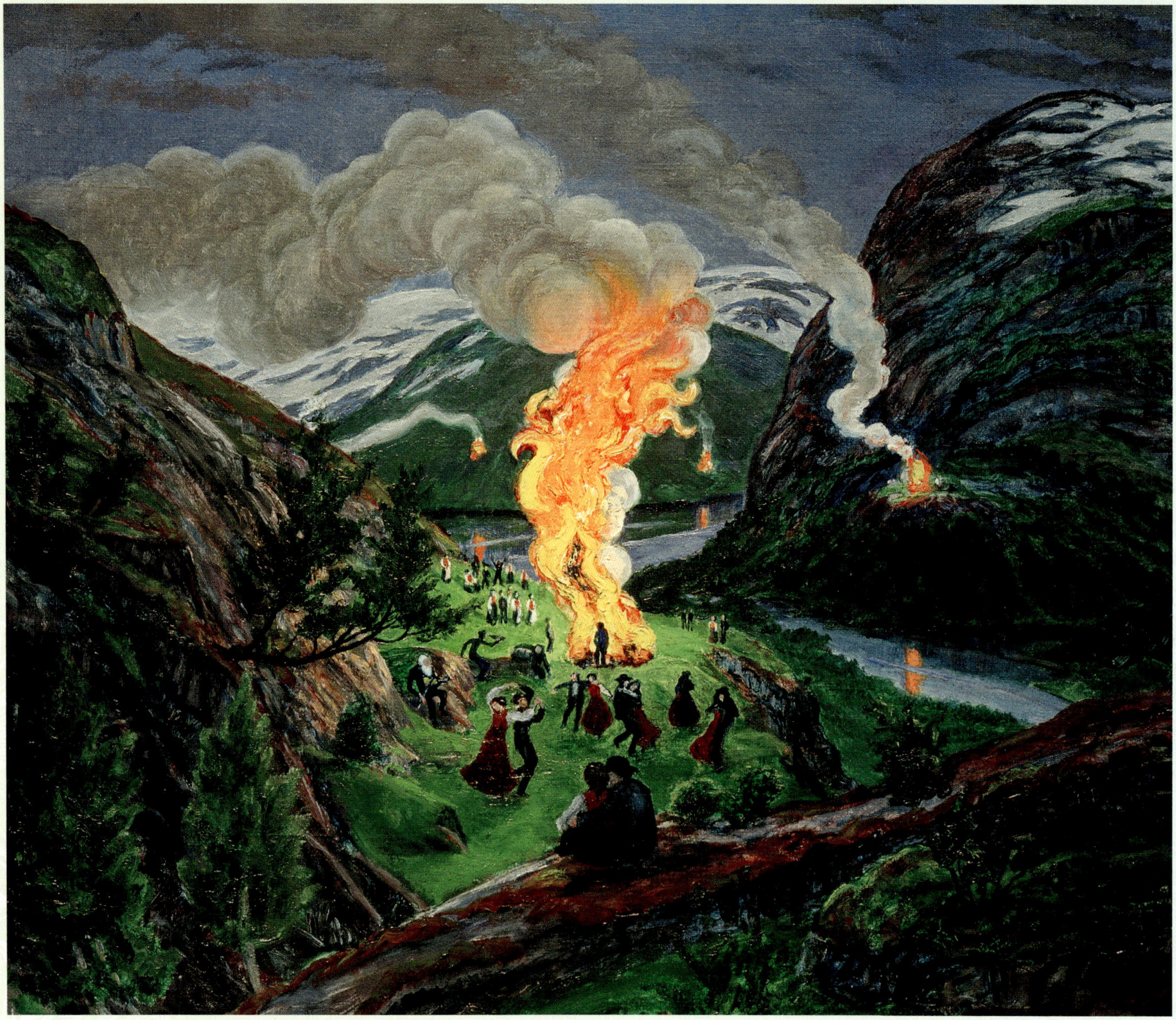

St John's Wort

Hypericum perforatum

Used in traditional medicine since ancient times, St John's wort is still an over-the-counter remedy for mild cases of depression. An oil infusion is used topically to treat burns, wounds, and sore muscles.

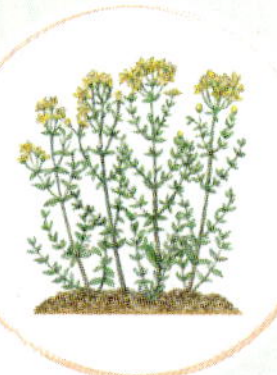

Uses Medicines for depression, inflammation, and skin ailments; tea

Parts used Flowers, leaves

Active ingredients Hypericin, pseudohypericin, hyperforin, volatile oils

Habitat Grassland, banks, and open woodland in temperate regions

Common St John's wort (*Hypericum perforatum*) belongs to a close-knit genus of plants, which usually have clusters of bright yellow flowers. An attractive garden plant, it grows up to 1 m (3 ft) in height and has tiny, translucent dots, or "perforations", in its leaves.

The genus name *Hypericum*, which means "above picture", is derived from the ancient Greek practice of hanging bunches of these flowers above shrines to ward off evil spirits. The plant is named after St John the Baptist as it blooms around Midsummer, 24 June, the traditional feast day celebrating the saint's birth.

St John's wort has long been seen as providing protection against witchcraft and enchantment. It was also believed to bring good luck, ensure peace and prosperity at home, and improve crop yield. To this end, people would hang sprigs over their doors and windows, or slip a few into their clothes or under pillows.

Medicinal properties

In the past, some herbalists believed that plants' visual characteristics indicated their medicinal uses (see p.14). So, the translucent dots in its leaves were seen as a sign that St John's wort could be used to heal wounds. When crushed, its buds, flowers, and fresh seed capsules release a red liquid, which prompted the idea that it may be used to cure blood disorders. It is now known that this liquid does indeed have pharmaceutical properties. It contains the red pigment hypericin – a substance that can affect moods – and is widely marketed as a herbal antidepressant. As "Hypericum oil", it is available either in pure form or mixed with other scented oils such almond or calendula. It is also sold as a balm for aches and pains, or as a dietary supplement. A second biochemical, hyperforin, is under active research for its potential antibiotic properties. These supplements can adversely react with other medication; it is advisable to consult with a doctor before taking.

◄ *Midsummer Eve Bonfire*, 1910
In this painting, Norwegian artist Nikolai Astrup depicts a Midsummer's eve celebration, which involves people adding herbs such as St John's wort to huge bonfires for protection against evil spirits.

► Sun-like blooms
This hairless plant bears buds that bloom into five-petalled flowers. A spray of pollen-bearing stamens at the centre of the flower resemble a sunburst.

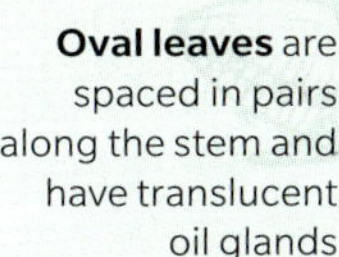

Oval leaves are spaced in pairs along the stem and have translucent oil glands

Golden yellow flowers are fringed with a few black oil glands

St John's wort was used as a herb for healing wounds in the Crusades (1095–1291)

Similar herbs

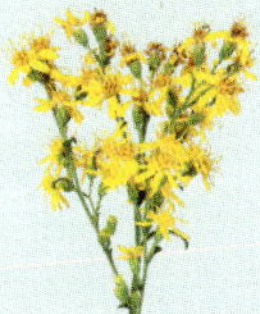

EUROPEAN GOLDENROD
Solidago virgaurea
Found growing in waysides and open woodlands, this plant has traditionally been used to treat urinary tract disorders and ulcers.

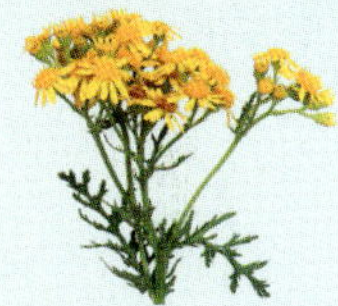

COMMON RAGWORT
Jacobaea vulgaris
Also known as St James' wort as it blooms around St James' Day. This flower is used externally to relieve rheumatism.

▲ Dried flowers
St John's wort flowering tops can be dried to use as a herbal tea. They can also be infused with oil to make a healing concoction for topical application.

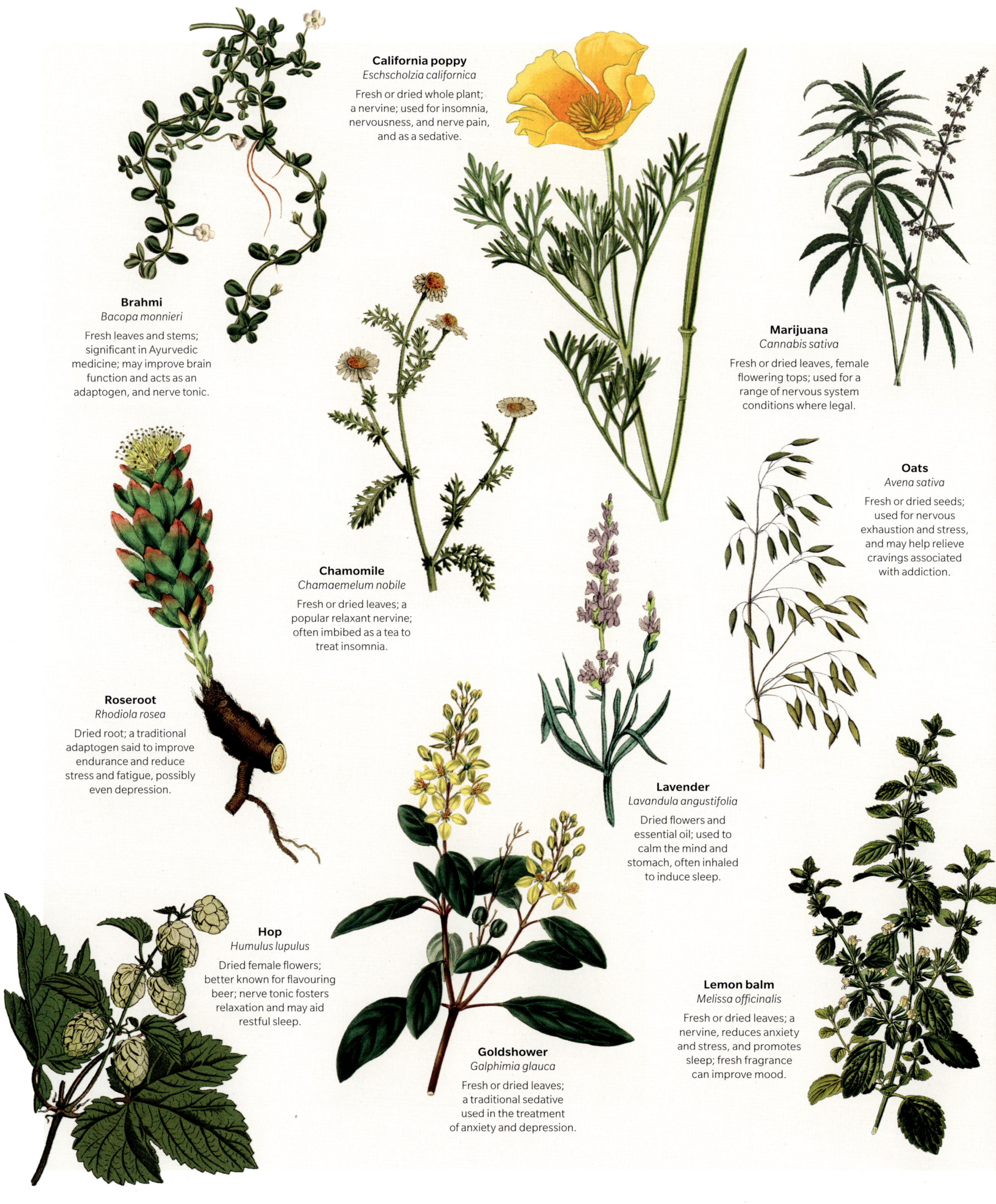

California poppy
Eschscholzia californica
Fresh or dried whole plant; a nervine; used for insomnia, nervousness, and nerve pain, and as a sedative.

Brahmi
Bacopa monnieri
Fresh leaves and stems; significant in Ayurvedic medicine; may improve brain function and acts as an adaptogen, and nerve tonic.

Marijuana
Cannabis sativa
Fresh or dried leaves, female flowering tops; used for a range of nervous system conditions where legal.

Oats
Avena sativa
Fresh or dried seeds; used for nervous exhaustion and stress, and may help relieve cravings associated with addiction.

Chamomile
Chamaemelum nobile
Fresh or dried leaves; a popular relaxant nervine; often imbibed as a tea to treat insomnia.

Roseroot
Rhodiola rosea
Dried root; a traditional adaptogen said to improve endurance and reduce stress and fatigue, possibly even depression.

Lavender
Lavandula angustifolia
Dried flowers and essential oil; used to calm the mind and stomach, often inhaled to induce sleep.

Hop
Humulus lupulus
Dried female flowers; better known for flavouring beer; nerve tonic fosters relaxation and may aid restful sleep.

Lemon balm
Melissa officinalis
Fresh or dried leaves; a nervine, reduces anxiety and stress, and promotes sleep; fresh fragrance can improve mood.

Goldshower
Galphimia glauca
Fresh or dried leaves; a traditional sedative used in the treatment of anxiety and depression.

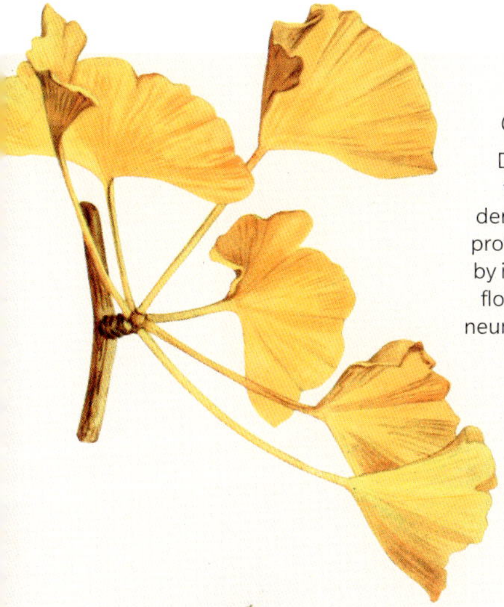

Ginkgo
Ginkgo biloba
Dried leaves; a treatment for dementia, possibly protecting the brain by improving blood flow or promoting neuron regeneration.

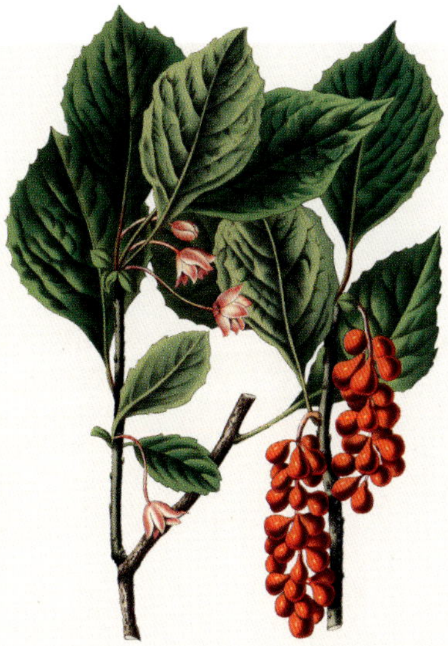

Schisandra
Schisandra chinensis
Fresh or dried fruits; an alleged adaptogen reducing stress and anxiety; may improve depression and cognitive function.

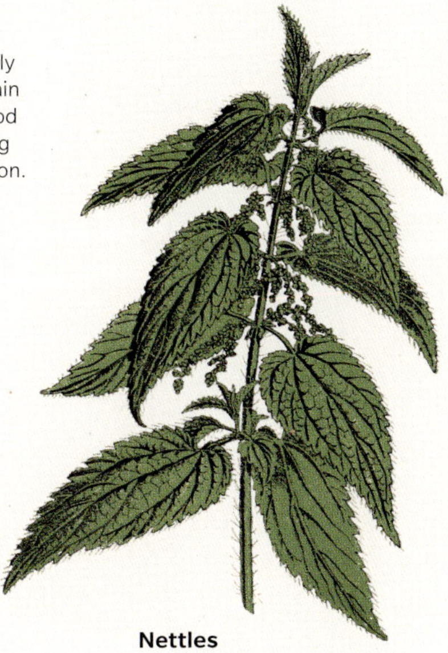

Nettles
Urtica dioica
Fresh or dried leaves; may help repair peripheral nerve damage (neuropathy) from diabetes.

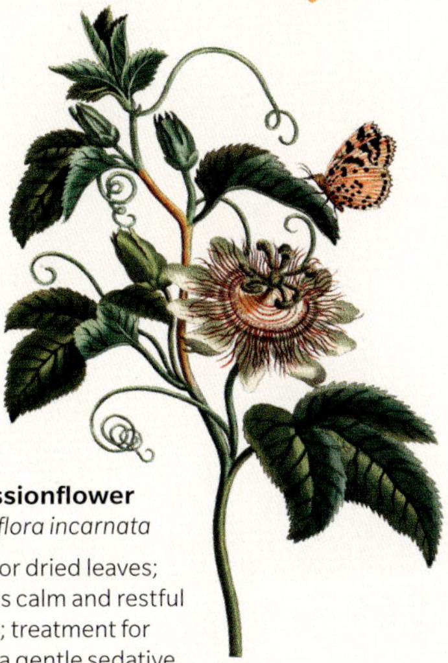

Passionflower
Passiflora incarnata
Fresh or dried leaves; promotes calm and restful sleep; treatment for anxiety, a gentle sedative.

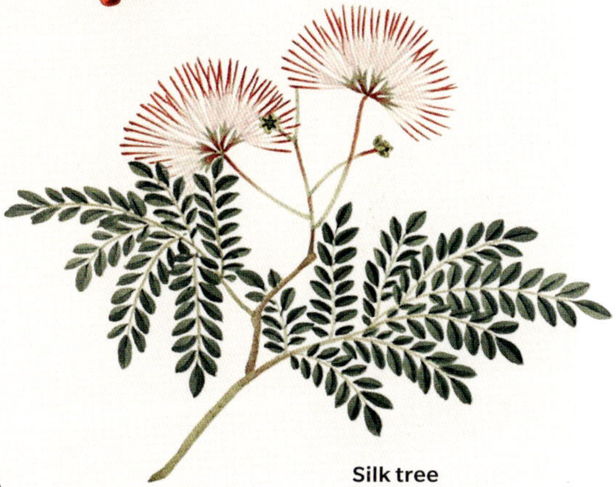

Helping the Nervous System

The nervous system, made up of the brain, spinal cord, and sensory and motor neurones around the body, detects and reacts to stimuli. Herbal remedies known as nervines specifically support the nervous system, while adaptogens protect the nervous system by helping the body respond to stress.

Silk tree
Albizia julibrissin
Dried bark, flowers; a nervine inducing calm and reducing insomnia; used as a mild sedative and treatment for depression.

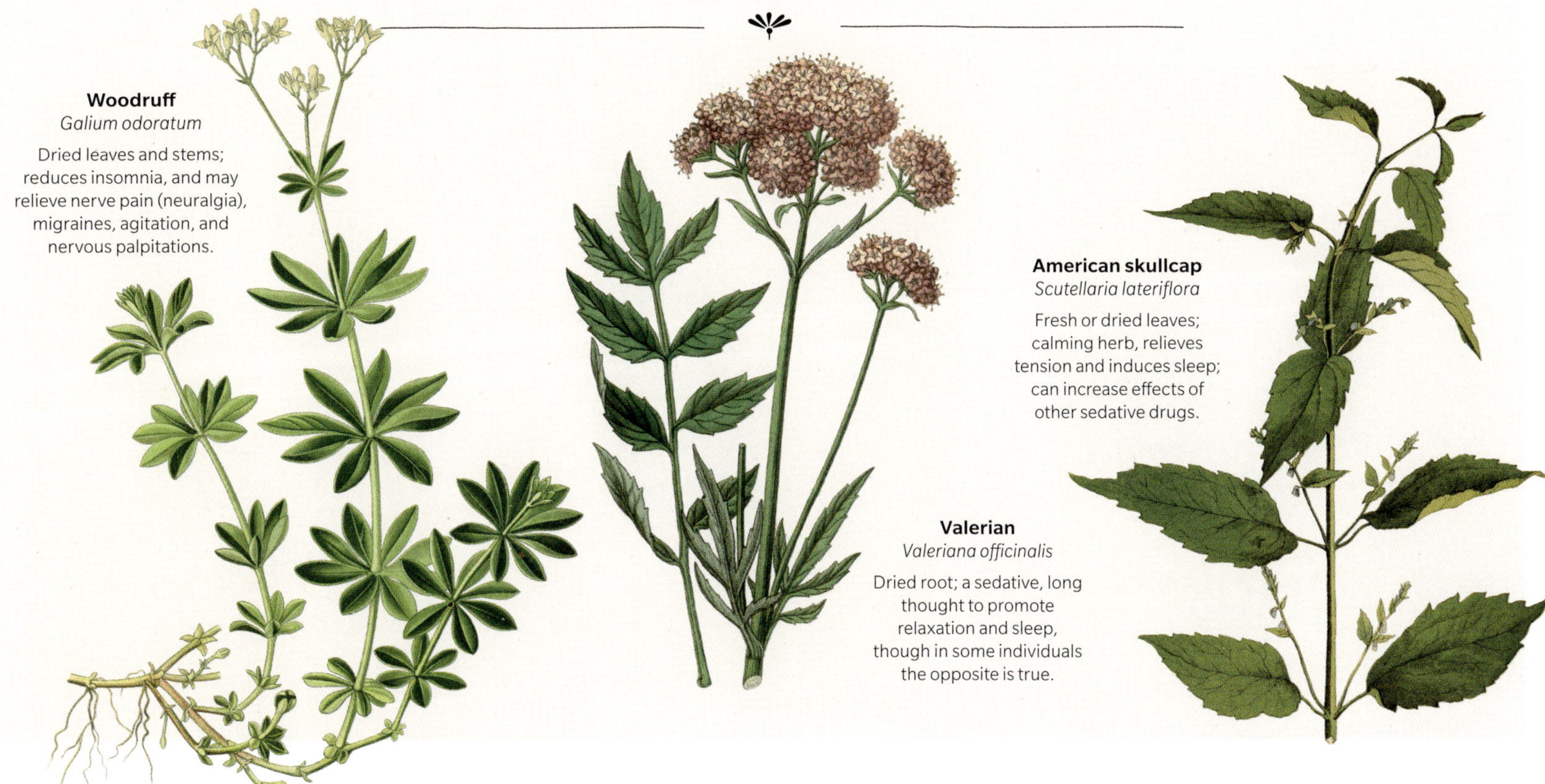

Woodruff
Galium odoratum
Dried leaves and stems; reduces insomnia, and may relieve nerve pain (neuralgia), migraines, agitation, and nervous palpitations.

American skullcap
Scutellaria lateriflora
Fresh or dried leaves; calming herb, relieves tension and induces sleep; can increase effects of other sedative drugs.

Valerian
Valeriana officinalis
Dried root; a sedative, long thought to promote relaxation and sleep, though in some individuals the opposite is true.

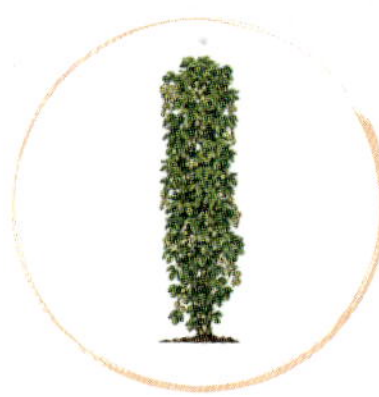

Uses Medicines, brewing, cooking, perfumes, and skincare

Parts used Female flowers, leaves, shoots, stems

Active ingredients Humulone and lupulone; xanthohumol; terpenes

Habitat Northern temperate regions; edges of woodland and fields, hedgerows, and scrubland

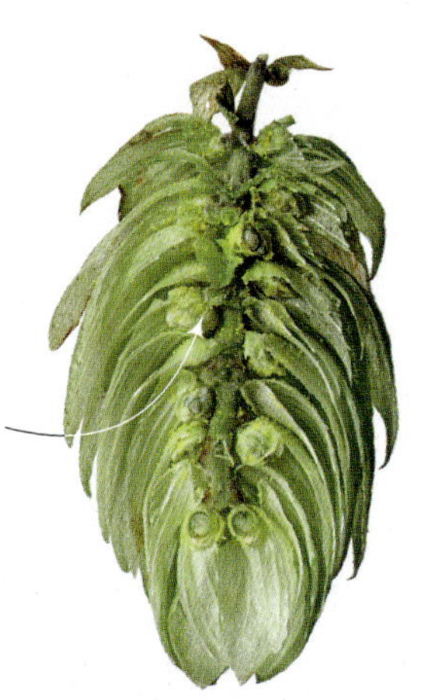

Lupulin glands contain the active resins, bitter acids, and volatile compounds, which give hops their characteristic bitter flavour

INSIDE A STROBILE

Leaves yield dye and young shoots can can be blanched for soups

Papery bracts and bracteoles protect female flowers and form cone-like structures

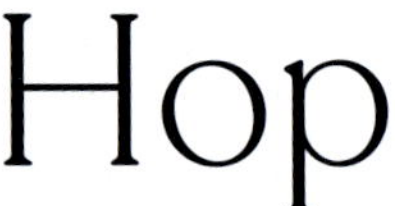

Hop

Humulus lupulus

Now synonymous with the brewing of beer, the bitter-tasting, vining hop plant has also been traditionally used for its calming effects and for making a fabric.

"The manifolde vertues of Hops do manifest argue the wholesomenesse of beere above ale; for the hops rather make it a physical drinke to keepe the body in health, than an ordinary drinke for the quenching of our thirst". So wrote English herbalist John Gerard in his *The Herball, or Generall Historie of Plantes* (1597). What he was referring to was the practice of adding of hops to traditional English ale – a sweet, rudimentary brew made with malted barley – harnessing organic acids and volatile compounds in the lupulin glands of female hop flowers to balance the sweetness with natural bitterness and a fruity, citrus flavour. The addition of hops preserved ale for longer, due to what are now known to be its antimicrobial properties. Its bitter agents also promoted a longer-lasting head of foam.

A natural sedative

Hops were also historically used for their medicinal properties, to treat venereal and skin diseases, tackle sluggish livers, improve appetite, and combat hysteria. Its young shoots or sprouts were cooked up as a nutritious, asparagus-like vegetable, and the long, strong fibres were used to make fabric. As with fellow hemp family member cannabis (see pp.234–37), it is naturally sedative and anxiolytic (anxiety reducing). Hops are still used today – as a tea or stuffed in pillows – to help soothe the nerves and combat insomnia.

▲ **Hop "flowers"**
Cone-like female hop "flowers", or strobiles, are used in brewing and medicine. Known as hops, they have numerous lupulin glands.

> " A pillow of warm Hops will often relieve toothache and earache and allay nervous irritation. "
>
> MRS M. GRIEVE, *A Modern Herbal*, 1931

HOLY HOPS

In the Middle Ages, several European religious establishments undertook beer production. In keeping with the Benedictine philosophy of "live by the work of your own hands", many monasteries sustained themselves by making beer for distribution and personal consumption. The monks improved the brewing process by adding hops for a better-tasting beer that lasted longer.

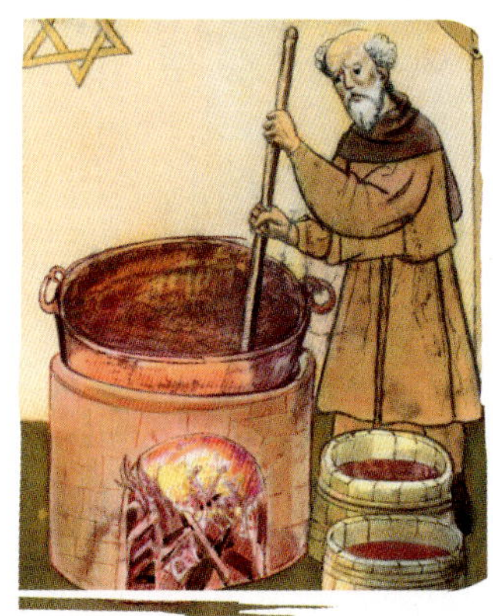

GERMAN ILLUSTRATION OF A BREWER

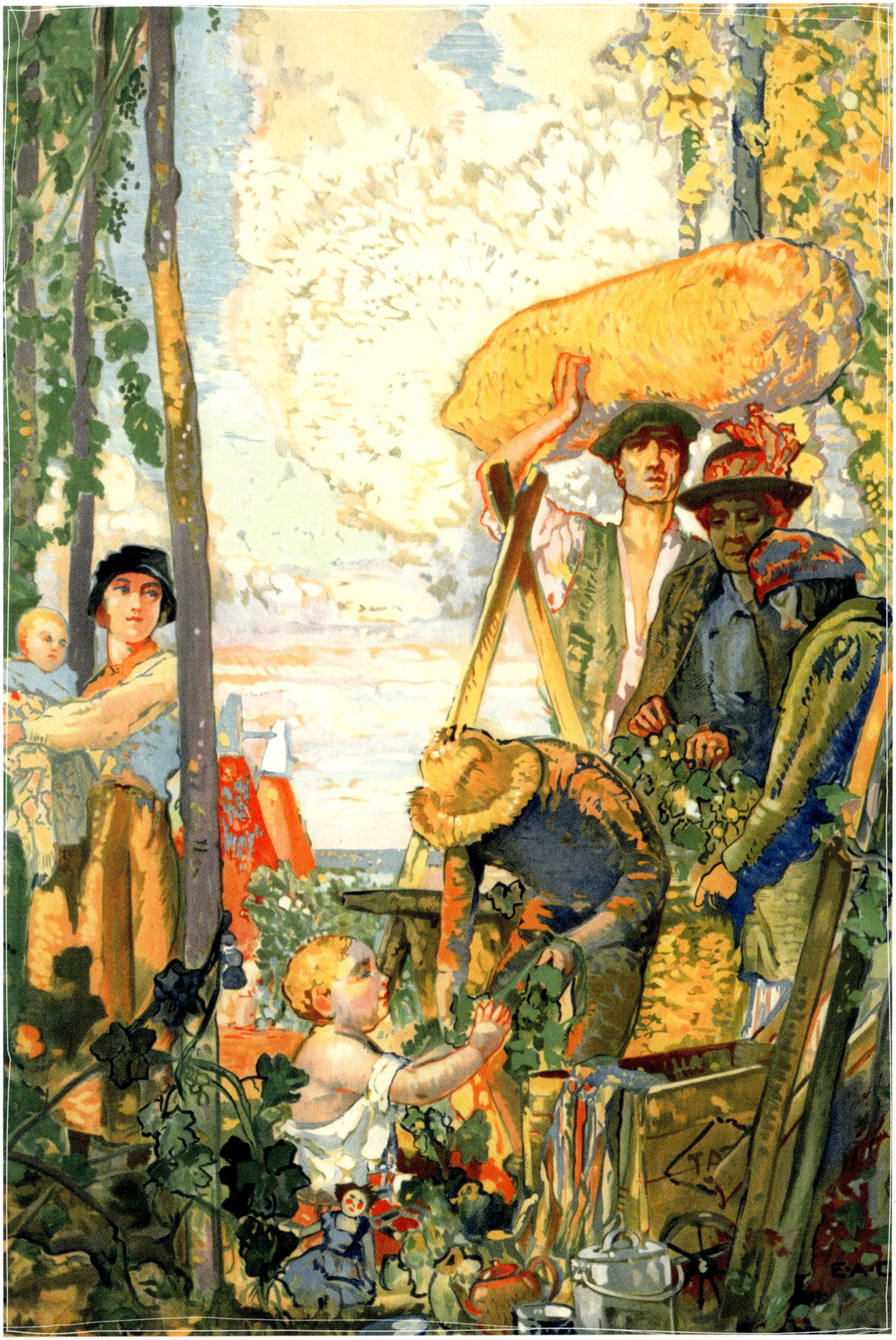

◄ "Taming the bine"
In the UK, the practice of growing hop bines (flexible, climbing stems) in mounds was replaced by the poles and stringing method in the late 1800s, as illustrated by English painter Elijah Albert Cox in his 1924 poster *Hop pickers in Kent*. This involved training hop bines to climb poles.

Similar herbs

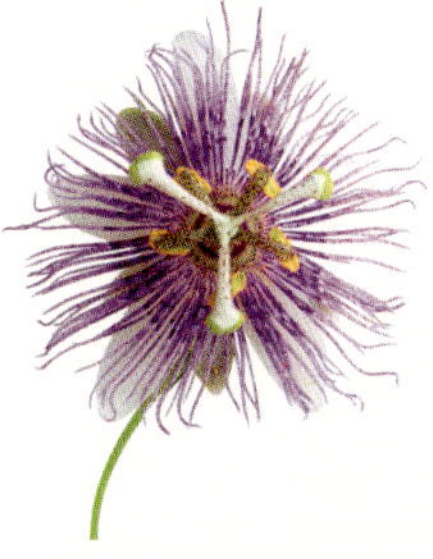

PURPLE PASSIONFLOWER
Passiflora incarnata
Native to the southern US, this plant, like hop, has sedative and anxiolytic properties. It is one of the "three sisters of sleep", along with hops and valerian.

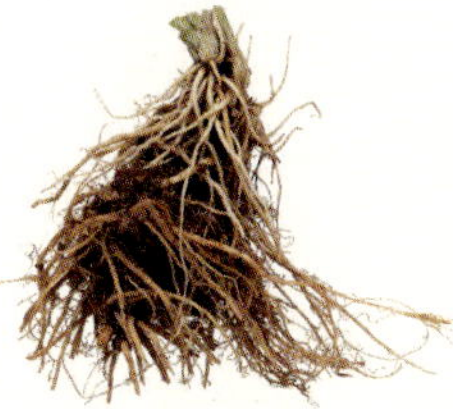

VALERIAN
Valeriana officinalis
The root of this pale pink-flowered herbaceous perennial, native to parts of Europe and Asia, can be used to relieve nervous tension and aid sleep.

Lemon Balm

Melissa officinalis

The leaves of this herb have a lemony fragrance and taste that is popular as a tea and culinary flavour. It also possesses soothing, healing, and restorative properties for the body and mind.

Uses Medicines, cooking, cosmetics, perfumes

Parts used Leaves, stems, flowers

Active ingredients Citral, citronellal, linalool, geraniol, rosmarinic acid, caffeic acids, and tannins

Habitat Meadows and fields; rich, moist, well-drained soils in full sun or partial shade; temperate climates

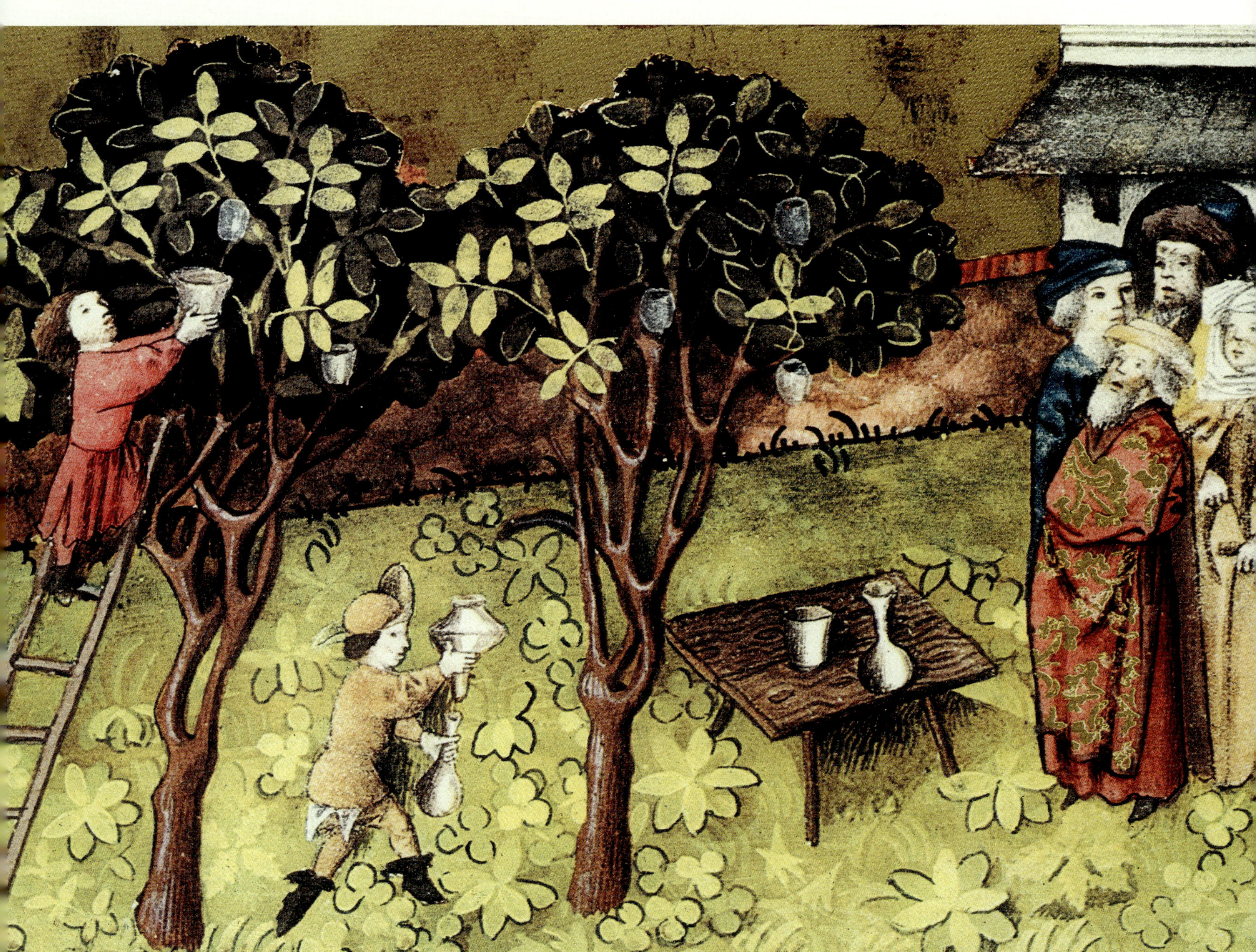

The **antiviral properties** of lemon balm may **speed healing** of *herpes simplex* **cold sores**

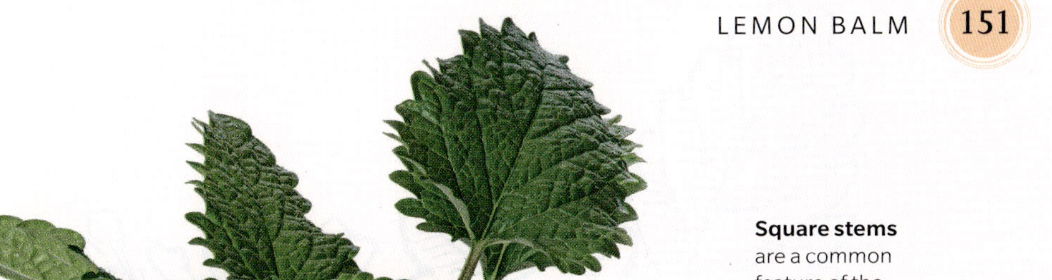

Square stems are a common feature of the mint family

Leaves have softly serrated margins and fine hairs

A member of the mint family Lamiaceae, which includes many aromatic herbs such as basil and marjoram, lemon balm is native to the Mediterranean, Iran, north-west Africa, and Central Asia. The distinctive flavour and bouquet of bruised lemon balm leaves has a mild lemon aroma, largely due to the presence of citral and citronellal, with minor notes from rose-scented geraniol and lavender-scented linalool.

Melissa essential oil, which is distilled from the leaves for commercial use, has been found to exhibit antimicrobial, antioxidant, and anti-inflammatory properties; it may help to reduce anxiety, relax muscles, and promote sleep; and it provides an anti-viral line of defence against common ailments such as cold sores. The oil can also be an effective repellent of insect pests.

A heart-felt herb

Lemon balm's medicinal applications are supported by thousands of years of use by various cultures and practices, from the Ancient Greeks, Romans, and Persians to Ayurvedic herbal medicine. The herb featured in many early written herbals, such as Theophrastus' *Historia Plantarum* in the 3rd century BCE and Dioscorides' *De Materia Medica* in the 1st century BCE, as well as later landmark medical works. John Gerard, in his *Herball*, cites the 11th-century Persian polymath Ibn Sina (also known as Avicenna), writing in his book of "the infirmities of the heart" that lemon balm makes the heart merry and joyful, and strengthens the vital spirits. This mood-enhancing effect is also mentioned in the herbals of Nicholas Culpeper and John Parkinson. The latter wrote in his *Paradisi in Sole Paradisus Terrestris* (1629) that lemon balm eases "suddaine qualmes or passions of the heart", whether they be "rife from melancholy" or from illness.

▲ Lemon balm foliage
The green parts of this close relative of mint contain medicinal properties. Cut the plant back hard in summer for a new, lush crop of fresh leaves.

> " Bawme drunke in wine... comforts the heart, and driveth away all melancholy and sadnesse. "
>
> JOHN GERARD, *The Herball, or Generall Historie of Plantes*, 1597

BEE MAGNET

Lemon balm's small flowers have a high nectar content and the scent of the leaves attracts and calms bees, so the herb is also known as bee balm. Pliny the Elder in his *Natural History* (77–79 CE) declared that "bees do find their way home by it". In fact, herbal tradition recommended rubbing a few leaves of lemon balm on the inside walls of a new hive to encourage a swarm to move in.

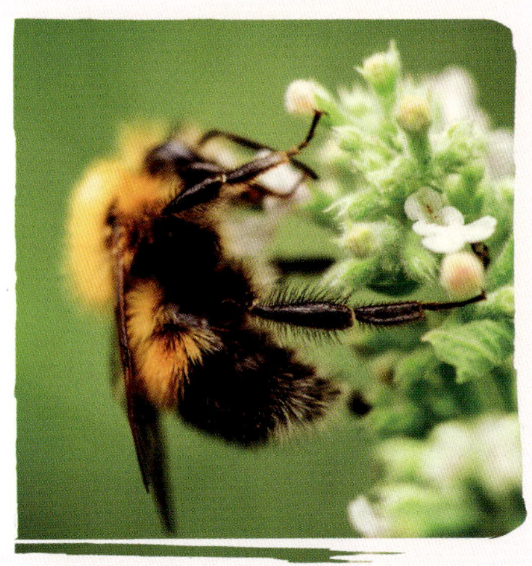

BEE DRINKING NECTAR

◄ Origins of the name
Beekeepers, seen in this 15th-century illustration, used lemon balm to attract bees. In fact, the genus name *Melissa* derives from the Ancient Greek word for a honeybee, or from the name of a nymph who fed honey to the infant Greek god Zeus.

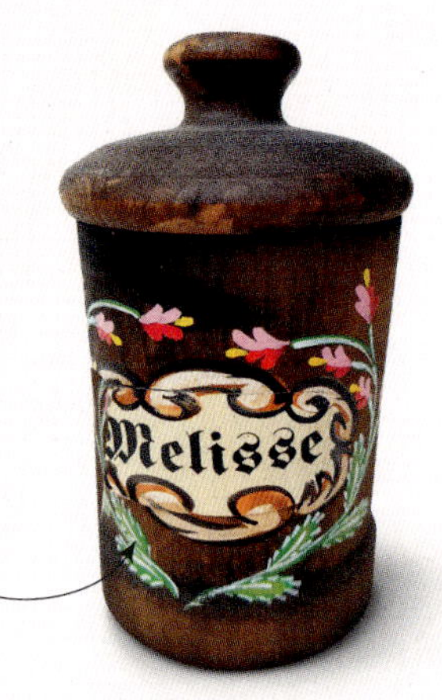

➤ Lemon balm tea
This vintage German *teedose* (tea caddy) is designed to hold lemon balm or melissa tea, helpful for soothing anxiety, sleep disorders, and indigestion.

Tea caddies for storing dried herbal teas were made from wood or tin

WHAT IS A NERVINE?

Nervines are herbs that are thought to support our central nervous system, which is responsible for conveying messages between the brain and body. Nervine tonics are said to nourish and protect nerve cells; nervine relaxants promote calm and reduce anxiety; and nervine stimulants are used to energize and boost stamina. Examples of nervines include lemon balm, German chamomile (see pp.244–47), and St John's wort (see pp.144–45).

Today, studies have shown that lemon balm could be mood-boosting and anxiety-reducing, by raising levels in the brain of a neurotransmitter called gamma-aminobutyric acid (GABA) that blocks impulses between brain nerve cells to help promote calm. Lemon balm is thought to do this by inhibiting an enzyme, GABA-transaminase, which effectively works to break GABA down. Similar effects may be gained simply by tearing up lemon balm leaves to inhale their aroma, or leaving bouquets or pots of the herb around the home or under doors and windows – lemon balm can also repel mosquitoes.

A traditional melissa-based elixir, extract, or tincture taken orally is a more direct and popular way to access its benefits, as is a few drops of melissa essential oil released via a home diffuser.

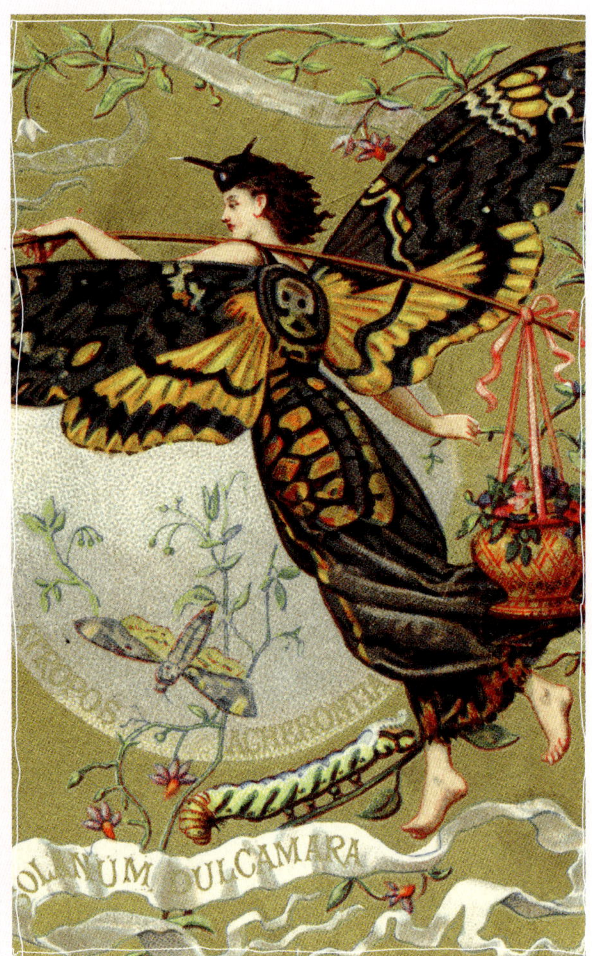

➤ French tonic
This trade card was issued in 19th-century France to advertise *Eau de Mélisse des Carmes*, a tonic invented by 17th-century Carmelite monks that mixed herbs and spices with lemon balm as the main ingredient.

Soothing and refreshing

Lemon balm has a long history as a herbal tea, made with fresh or dried leaves infused in just-boiled water. The tea is uplifting and calming for the senses, with similarly soothing effects on the digestive system. It may also relieve tension headaches and induce sweating, which could be helpful in reducing fevers.

Lemon balm tea is refreshing when served cold, or even iced, on a hot day. The lemony flavour is also delicious in cocktails and cordials and in liqueurs such as Bénédictine and Chartreuse, which were developed by French monks in the 16th and 18th centuries. Lemon balm's flavour translates well if infused in a culinary syrup, vinegar, or oil. The fresh leaves bring a zing to salads, ice-creams, and meat stuffings and the edible flowers can be candied or used to garnish fruit, salads, or drinks.

Scent and salve

A lemon balm infusion can be used to create a circulation-boosting facial steam or astringent skin toner and, if mixed with beeswax and olive oil, as a skin salve, ointment, or balm. *Melissa* is also a popular perfume note, providing a minty, lightly spicy alternative to lemon, while its fresh scent and anti-viral properties make it an ideal ingredient for natural home cleaners.

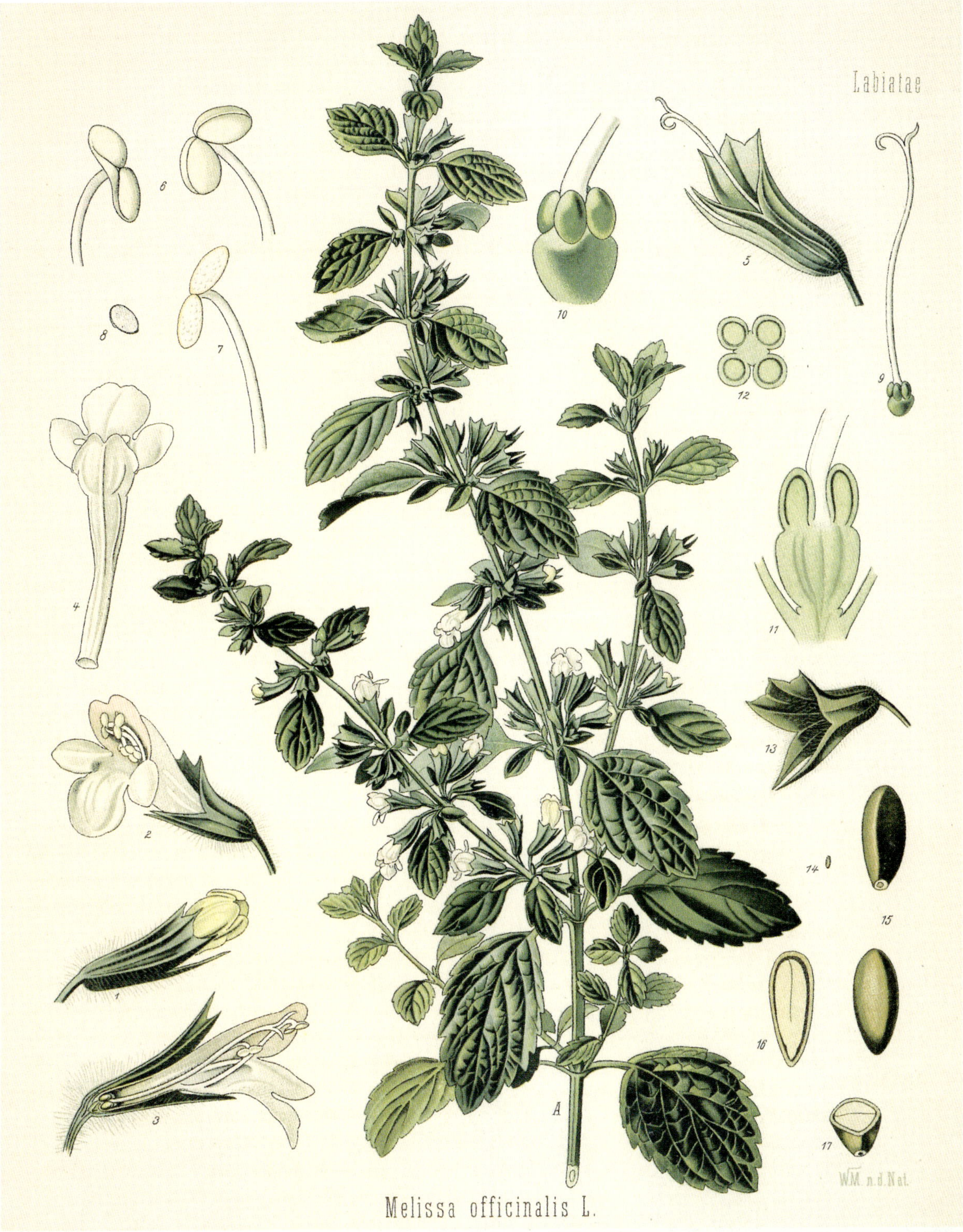

◄ Lemon balm flowers
The herb blooms from early summer through to early autumn. The double-lipped flowers are small, white, pale yellow, or pale purple, and are borne in whorls in the upper leaf axils.

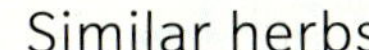

Similar herbs

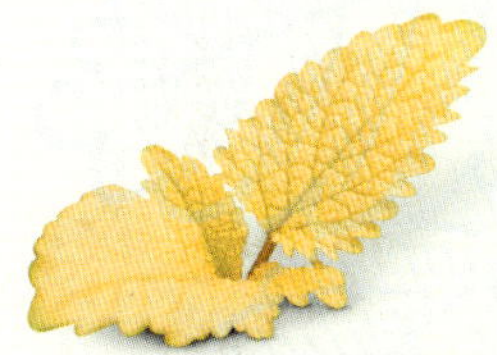

BALM 'ALL GOLD'
Melissa officinalis 'All Gold'

This lemon balm creates a splash of colour in the garden, but scorches easily so grow it in part shade. It can be used medicinally, in a tea, or as a garnish.

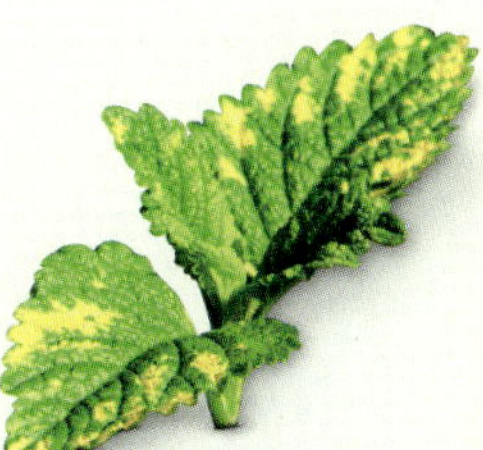

YELLOW-LEAVED LEMON BALM
Melissa officinalis 'Aurea'

The attractive, golden variegation of yellow-leaved lemon balm can spread to a large part of the leaf. This cultivar also possesses lemon balm's herbal properties.

King Charles V of France (1338–80) is said to have taken a cup of lemon balm tea every day as a health tonic

Deadly Nightshade

Atropa bella-donna

The most distinctive feature of this tall, herbaceous plant is its large, glossy, poisonous black berries, which have secured its macabre reputation. However, it also has benevolent herbal uses.

Uses Medicines for eye surgery, stomach disorders, drying up secretions

Parts used Whole plant, roots, berries

Active ingredients Atropine (hyoscyamine mixture), scopolamine (also known as hyoscine)

Habitat Open ground on banks and woodland glades, chalk or limestone soil

Found across Europe, North Africa, and Asia, and also naturalized in North America, deadly nightshade, or belladonna, is rich in tropane alkaloids, especially atropine, which is named after the plant's genus *Atropa*. These alkaloids block the neurotransmitter acetylcholine and inhibit the body's nervous system at high doses causing altered heart rate, delirium, and respiratory paralysis, ultimately leading to death. Deadly nightshade is said to have been a favourite of poisoners and there have been many accidental poisonings, especially from the attractive, shiny, sweet-tasting berries.

Despite its sinister reputation, the ancient Greek physician Theophrastus recommended cautious use of deadly nightshade for pain relief or sleeplessness, and even as part of a love potion. Juice from the plant has historically been used to treat upset stomachs and flatulence. In the 19th century, European pharmacies sold the powdered root for respiratory disorders and as a pain reliever, although there is no scientific evidence of its effectiveness. Deadly nightshade was also used around this time in skin creams and as eyedrops to dilate pupils and so beautify the eyes.

The plant has been used in homeopathy and as a recreational intoxicant, although this can be dangerous. Use of its natural extracts are no longer encouraged but prescription drugs include Donnatal, used to treat bowel disorders, irritable bowel syndrome, and intestinal cramps mixes deadly nightshade alkaloids with a sedative.

Similar herb

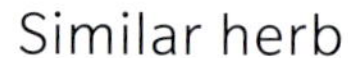

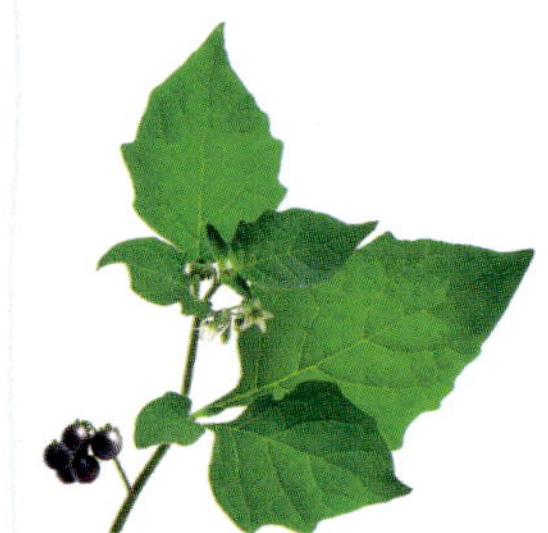

BLACK NIGHTSHADE
Solanum nigrum

Black nightshade varies in toxicity. Some strains are edible and its ripe berries and leaves have been used medicinally and for food. Others strains contain higher levels of solanine and are mildly poisonous.

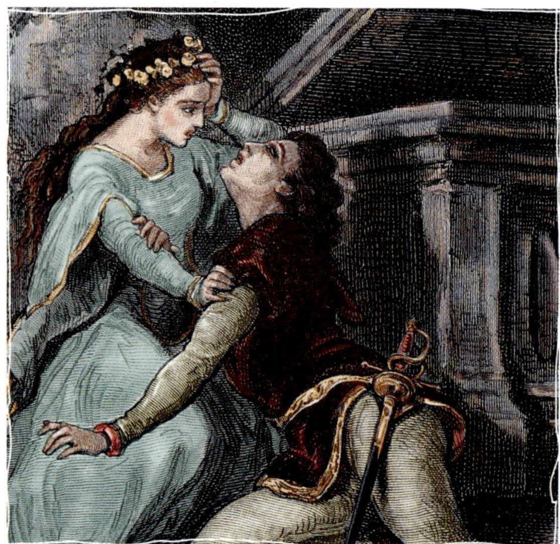

▲ **The death of Romeo**
Deadly nightshade may have been the inspiration for the unnamed poison featured in William Shakespeare's *Romeo and Juliet*.

“ His veins were dark with a vivid belladonna tincture, the essence of jealousy. ”

CHARLOTTE BRONTE, *Villette*, 1853

LEGENDARY POISON

Deadly nightshade is thought to have been behind a number of poisonings in ancient Rome. The most famous of these poisonings is of Emperor Claudius in 54 CE. According to legend, Agrippina the Younger appointed a servant to poison Claudius, her husband. Deadly nightshade juice was reputedly fed to Claudius soaked into a mushroom and more poison was later dripped down his throat with a feather.

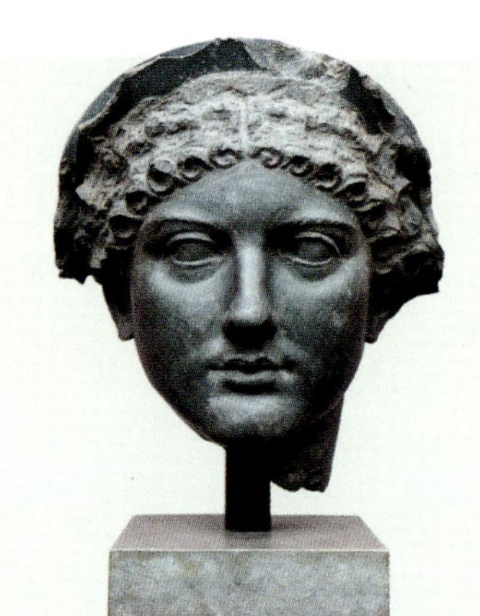

STATUE OF AGRIPPINA THE YOUNGER

Large oval, deep-veined leaves narrow to a point
Glossy, cherry-sized black berries are held on a persistent star-shaped calyx
Stout stems are sometimes hairless or bear short, glandular hairs
Drooping, bell-shaped flowers with a dusty-violet colour are clasped by a green calyx

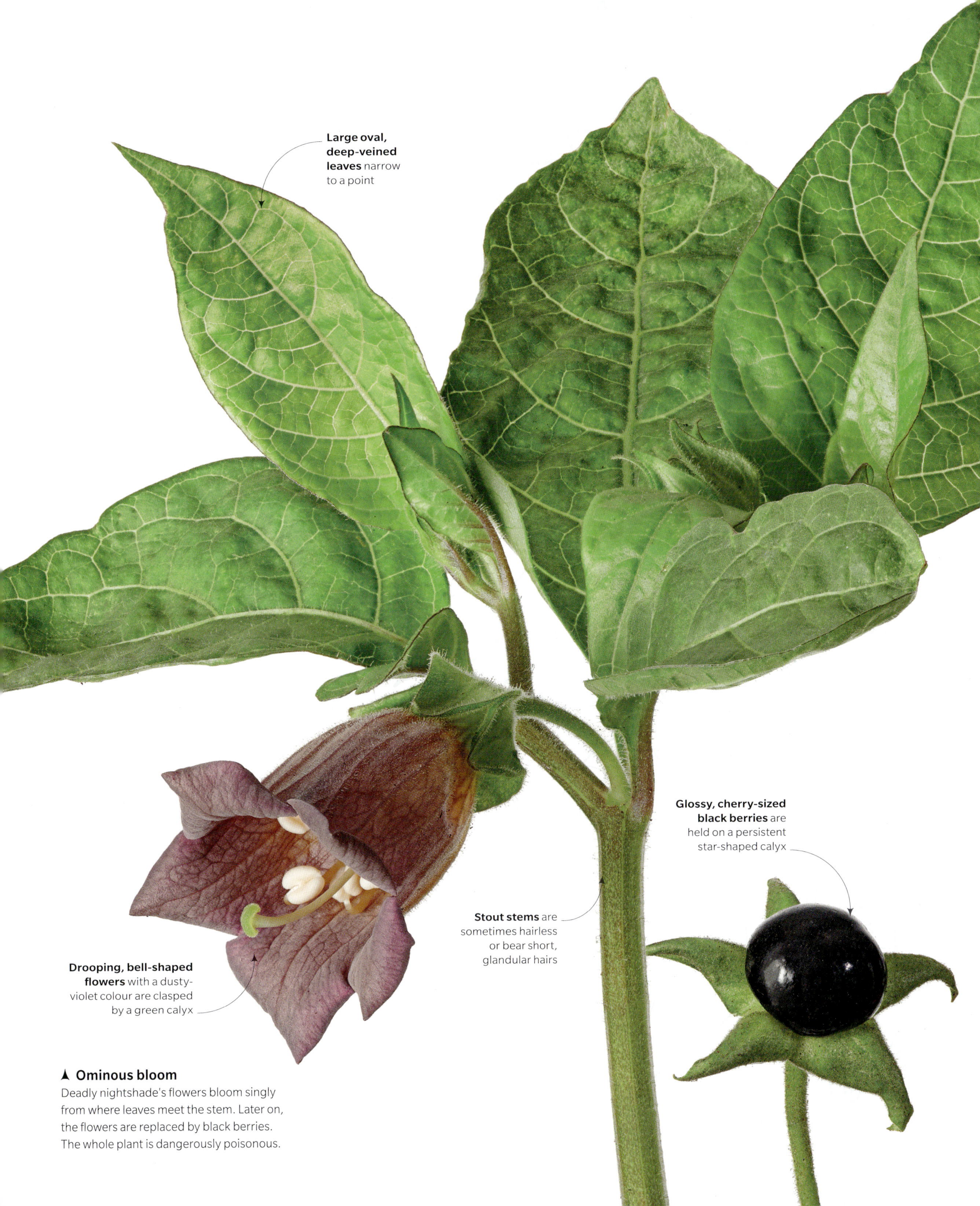

▲ **Ominous bloom**

Deadly nightshade's flowers bloom singly from where leaves meet the stem. Later on, the flowers are replaced by black berries. The whole plant is dangerously poisonous.

Feverfew

Tanacetum parthenium

Feverfew takes its name from the Latin *fabrifugia*, meaning "fever reducer". Although it is no longer used in the treatment of fevers, its reputation as a pain reliever remains.

British herbalist **Nicholas Culpeper** thought of feverfew as "a general **strengthener of the womb**" (1653)

Flowers measure 1–2 cm (3/8–3/4 in) across

White outer "petals", the ray florets, are short and broad, and surround the bright yellow disc florets

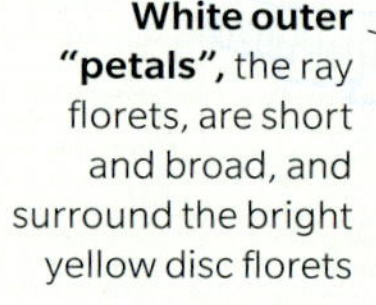

Uses Medicines for migraine, arthritis, tinnitus, and irregular menstruation

Parts used Leaves

Active ingredients Parthenolide, flavonoid glycosides, volatile oils including pinenes and camphor

Habitat Thrives in light, well-drained soil in full sunlight; widely naturalized on banks, walls, and waste ground

▼ Fragrant bunch
Closely related to tansy (*T. vulgare*) and oxeye daisy (*Leucanthemum vulgare*), feverfew is a strongly scented, perennial plant. It bears clusters of daisy-like flowers on long stalks, and grows up to 60 cm (2 ft) tall.

Often referred to as herbal aspirin, feverfew has been used to soothe headaches and relieve aches and pains through the ages. This plant smells of camphor, which acts as an insect-repellent. Although native to the Balkans and Central Asia, feverfew is widely naturalized, growing virtually worldwide, due, in part, to its use in traditional medicine. It is grown commercially as well as in gardens, with the double-flowered forms mainly cultivated as ornamentals.

The plant was known as an anti-inflammatory herb in Roman times. Its main active ingredient, and the one that delivers the most health benefits, is parthenolide, named after the plant's species name. In medical terms, parthenolide stops the production of prostaglandins, the molecules that cause inflammation in the human body. Feverfew has also proven to be effective against migraines. Recent research indicates that the phytochemicals present in the plant prevent the constriction of blood vessels in the brain that lead to severe headaches.

Over the ages, feverfew has gained the reputation of being a general pain reliever and an anti-depressant. Feverfew has also been touted as a remedy for toothaches, an antiseptic, and an insecticide, although there is little evidence for or against its effectiveness in such applications. Additionally, its possible anticancer benefits are under investigation. However, it contains allergens and sensitive individuals may experience contact dermatitis (skin inflammation), and fresh leaves or herbal tea can irritate the mouth.

Byzantine remedy
This drawing, thought to be of feverfew, appears in the earliest-surviving illustrated herbal, *Anicia Juliana Codex* (515 CE).

> " ... [Feverfew] purgeth by siege melancholy and phlegm; wherefore it is very good for them that are giddie in the head... "
>
> JOHN GERARD, *The Herball, or Generall Historie of Plantes*, 1597

Feathery leaves are divided and toothed, and partly covered in downy hairs

Similar herb

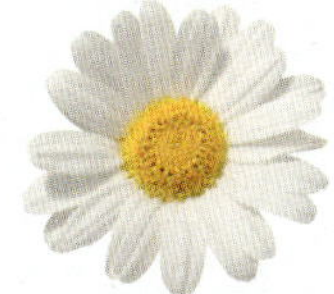

PYRETHRUM
Tanacetum cinerariifolium
Pyrethrum's flowers are cultivated for their showy, daisy-like blooms. Dried flower heads produce the natural insecticide, pyrethrin.

FEVERFEW IN FABLES

In floriography, or the language of flowers, feverfew is often referred to as bachelor's button for its round, button-like appearance. In Victorian England, it symbolized celibacy and could be worn by bachelors, indicating their single status. In the illustrated poem *A Flower Wedding* (1905), British illustrator Walter Crane depicts bachelor's button as a member of a wedding party.

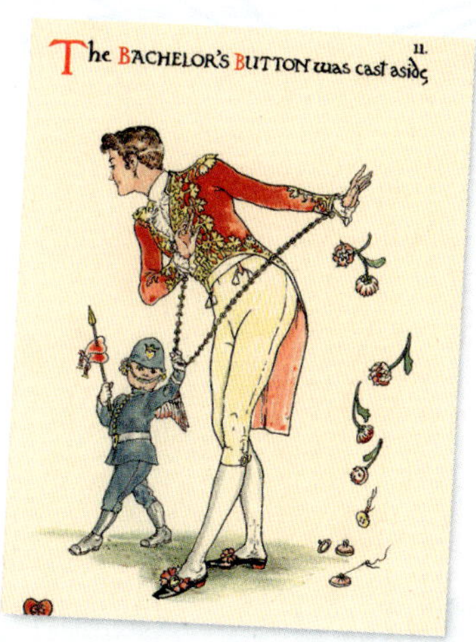

BACHELOR'S BUTTON

➤ *Echinacea purpurea*
A central "cone" of tiny tubular, bisexual flowers, or disc florets, is encircled by sterile, purple-pink ray florets upon a single stem. After pollination, the ray florets fall, leaving each disc floret in the cone to develop a single-seeded, dry fruit.

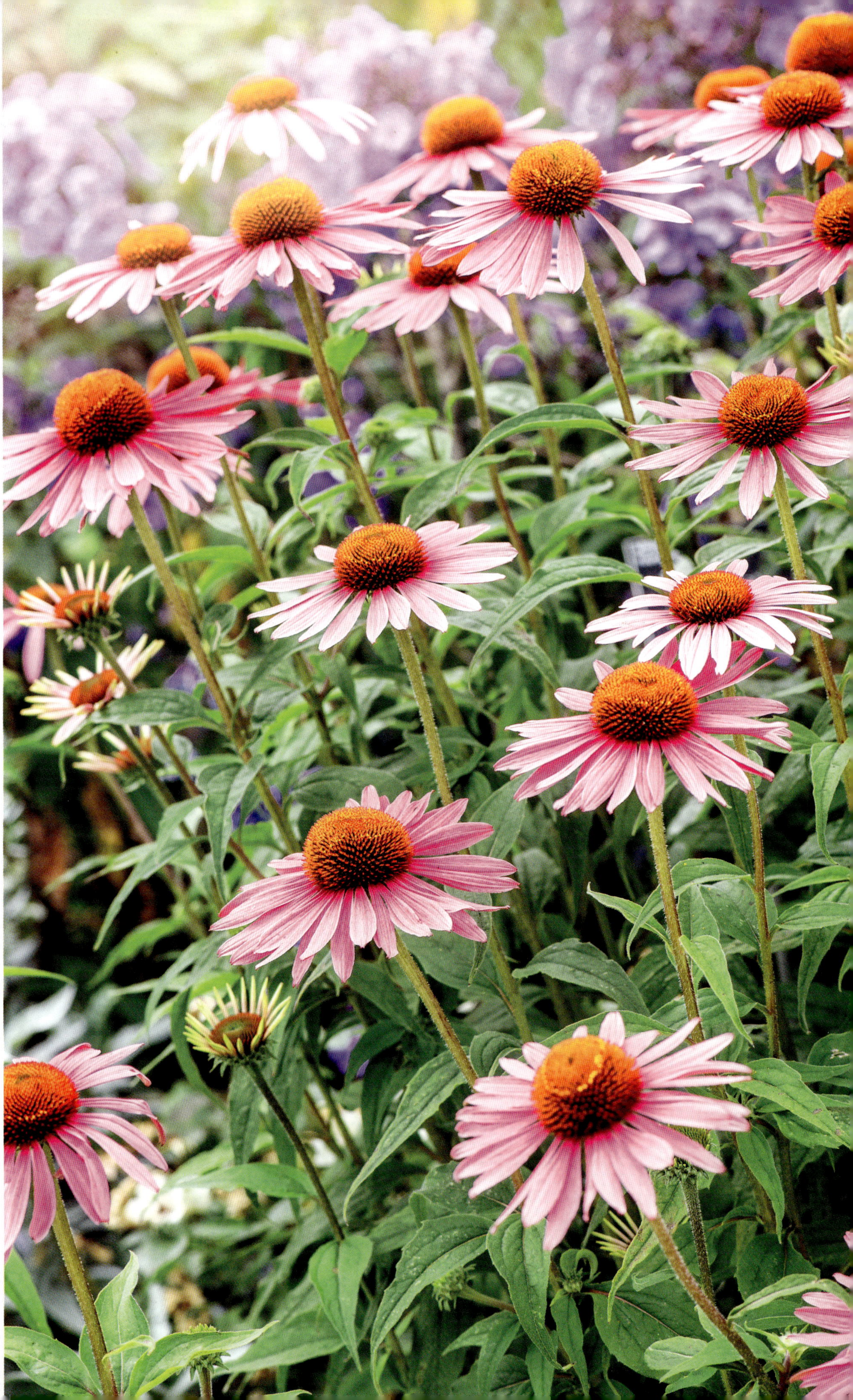

Similar herbs

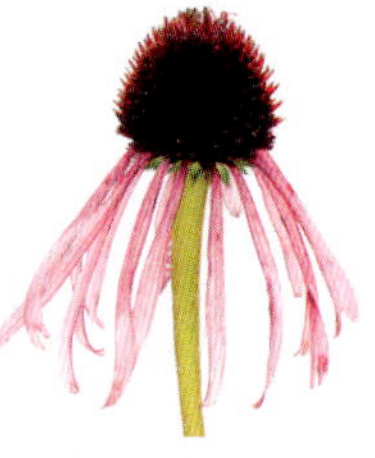

NARROW-LEAVED PURPLE CONEFLOWER
Echinacea angustifolia
This narrow-leaved species was widely used by Indigenous peoples of the North American central plains to treat a range of infections and diseases.

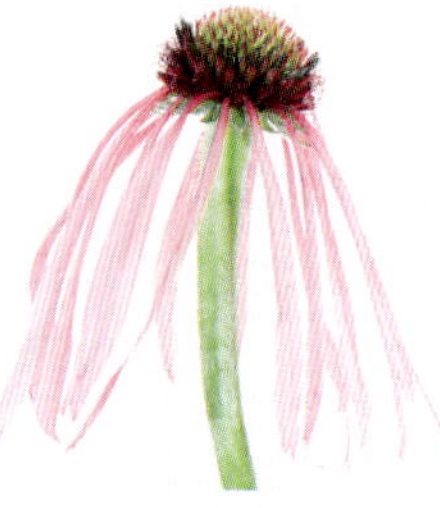

PALE PURPLE CONEFLOWER
Echinacea pallida
This coneflower has long, drooping, pale rose-purple or white ray florets; it is used in herbal preparations for colds and flu.

Uses Medicines for colds, flu, toothache, infection, inflammation, fever

Parts used Flower, leaf, root

Active ingredients Alkamides, caffeic acid, polysaccharides, glycoproteins, volatile oils, flavonoids

Habitat Full sun and free-draining soil of grasslands, open woodlands, and roadsides in temperate climates

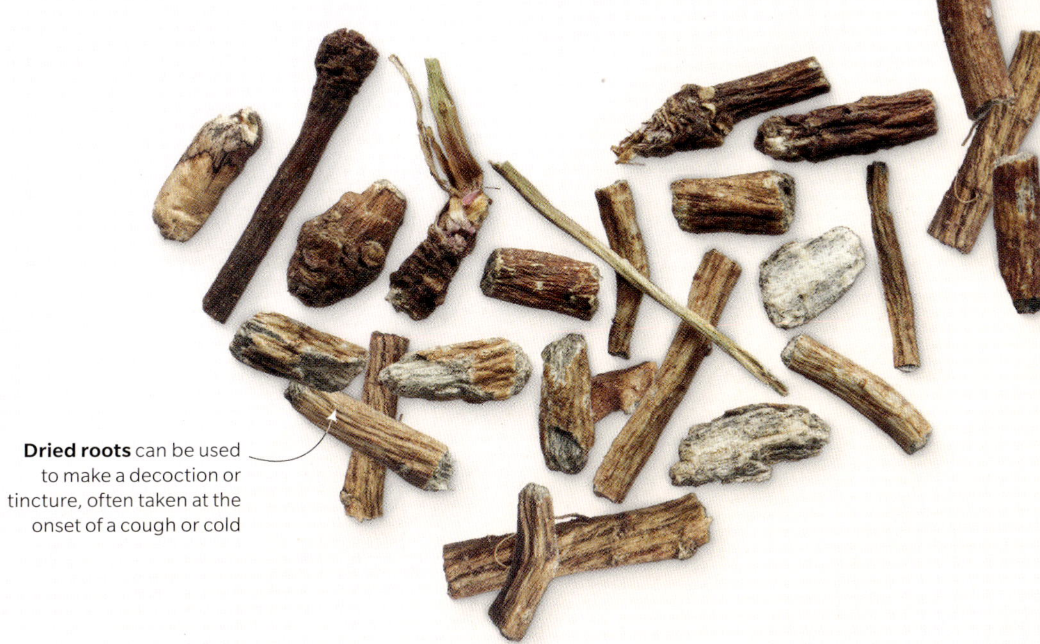

Dried roots can be used to make a decoction or tincture, often taken at the onset of a cough or cold

▲ **Echinacea roots** The long, thick taproots and other fleshy roots of *Echinacea purpurea*, *E. angustifolia*, or *E. pallida* are harvested in autumn in their second year of growth.

Echinacea

Echinacea purpurea

This wildflower of eastern and central North America gained notoriety in the 19th century as a remedy for rattlesnake bites. Today, it is most well known in Western herbal medicine as a curative for colds and flu.

This pretty prairie flower – now also a popular garden plant for its large, colourful, cone-centred, long-lasting flowers – is one of nine species of *Echinacea*, in the daisy family Asteraceae. *Echinacea purpurea* was previously named *Rudbeckia purpurea* by Swedish botanist Carl Linnaeus in 1753. It was moved to the new genus *Echinacea* by Conrad Moench in 1794, from the Greek word *ekhinos* meaning "spiny one" after its sea urchin-like central cluster of pointed bracts, or paleae, that remain after the flowers fade.

From snake bites to colds

E. purpurea's close cousin *E. angustifolia*, and less often *E. purpurea*, has been used for centuries by Indigenous peoples to treat stings, poisonous bites, inflammation, toothache, sore throats, and colds. This inspired colonizing Europeans to hail *E. angustifolia* as a healing cure-all, blood purifier, and rattlesnake bite remedy (see right). By 1898, *King's American Dispensatory* (third revision, by pharmacist John Uri Lloyd and doctor Harvey Wickes Felter) noted that echinacea was useful for blood infection, skin inflammation, syphilis, pain relief, fevers, and snake bites. The herb was dismissed by the American Medical Association in 1910, but gained popularity in 1930s Germany.

Today, several parts of *E. purpurea* are used together, mainly as a popular herbal remedy for coughs and colds: the flowers and leaves are high in immune-boosting polysaccharides, and the roots rich in volatile oils, antioxidant-enhancing alkamides, and antioxidant caffeic acid. Scientists are still pursuing solid reasons for its efficacy.

SNAKE OIL

In the early 1870s, a German physician from Nebraska created echinacea-based "Meyer's Blood Purifier", hailing it a cure-all for ailments from snake bites to typhoid. The term "snake oil" is now synonymous with false advertising, but Meyer's efforts did highlight the medicinal potential of echinacea.

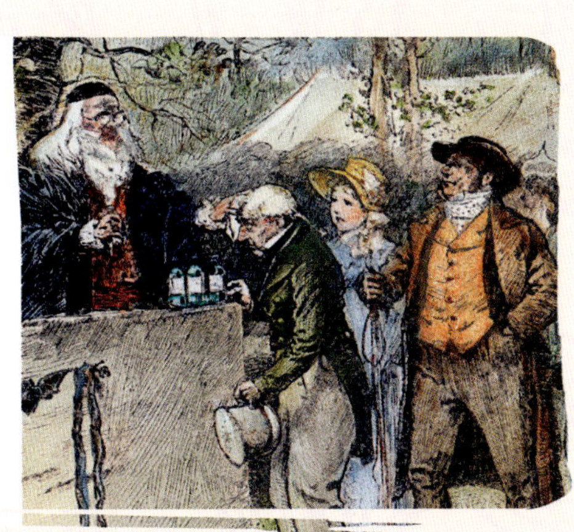

A QUACK DOCTOR SELLING TONICS

Wormwood leaves and oil have historically been used to repel moths and fleas

Universal remedy
Medieval physicians grew wormwood in medicinal gardens as it was widely used as a general remedy for all diseases.

Wormwood

Artemisia absinthium

Uses Medicines, flavouring

Parts used Flowers, leaves

Active ingredients Absinthin, artabsin, thujone, azulenes

Habitat Dry, uncultivated ground; in temperate regions

A bitter herb that grows across Europe, Asia, and North Africa, wormwood was used medicinally by the ancient Egyptians but is now best known for its use in alcoholic drinks such as vermouth, pernod, and absinthe.

Wormwood is an aromatic perennial with narrow, divided leaves, that are covered in greyish-green hairs on both surfaces. It is easily grown, and its attractive foliage makes this an interesting garden plant, often as cultivated varieties such as 'Lambrook Mist'. Its English name is one of the oldest plant names, and may refer to its former use as a tonic to dispel parasitic worms. The scientific name, *Artemisia*, was taken from Dioscorides, the ancient Greek physician, who named the plant after Artemis, the Greek goddess of the hunt and protectress of forests. This useful plant was "a gift from Artemis", and to this day dried wormwood is one of the herbs sold as Herb Artemisia.

The plant is best known for its strong aromatic scent when the leaves are crushed, and for its bitter but not unpleasant flavour. The natural

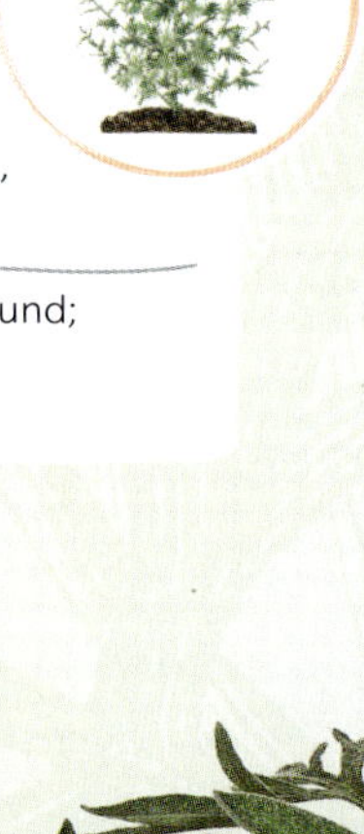

Small, pale-yellow, flowers are clustered in button-shaped heads (capitula) along the stalk
Narrow, silvery-green leaves are silky on both sides
Dried stems and leaves are used in tea
Lower leaflets divide deeply two or three times into narrow leaflets

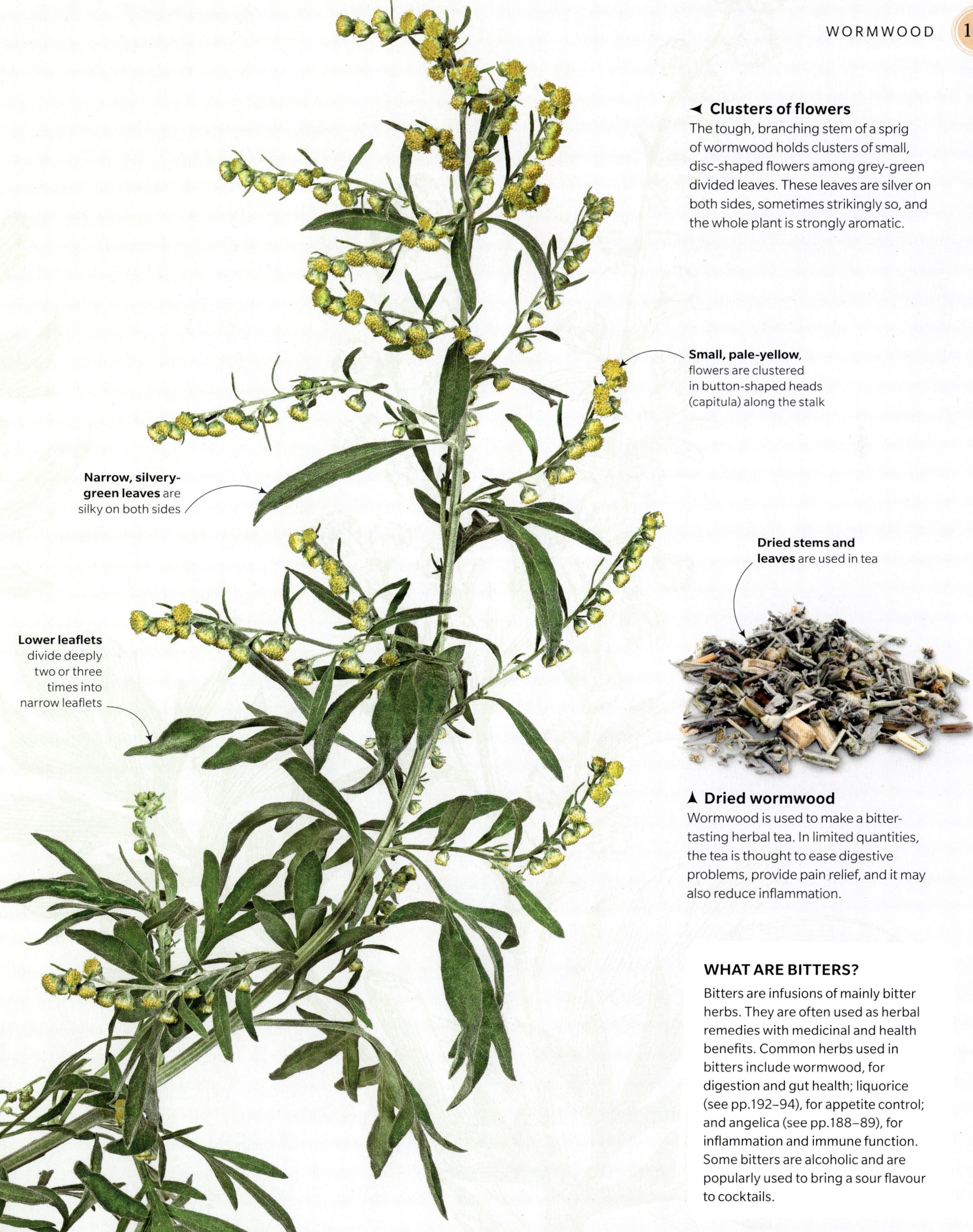

◄ Clusters of flowers
The tough, branching stem of a sprig of wormwood holds clusters of small, disc-shaped flowers among grey-green divided leaves. These leaves are silver on both sides, sometimes strikingly so, and the whole plant is strongly aromatic.

▲ Dried wormwood
Wormwood is used to make a bitter-tasting herbal tea. In limited quantities, the tea is thought to ease digestive problems, provide pain relief, and it may also reduce inflammation.

WHAT ARE BITTERS?

Bitters are infusions of mainly bitter herbs. They are often used as herbal remedies with medicinal and health benefits. Common herbs used in bitters include wormwood, for digestion and gut health; liquorice (see pp.192–94), for appetite control; and angelica (see pp.188–89), for inflammation and immune function. Some bitters are alcoholic and are popularly used to bring a sour flavour to cocktails.

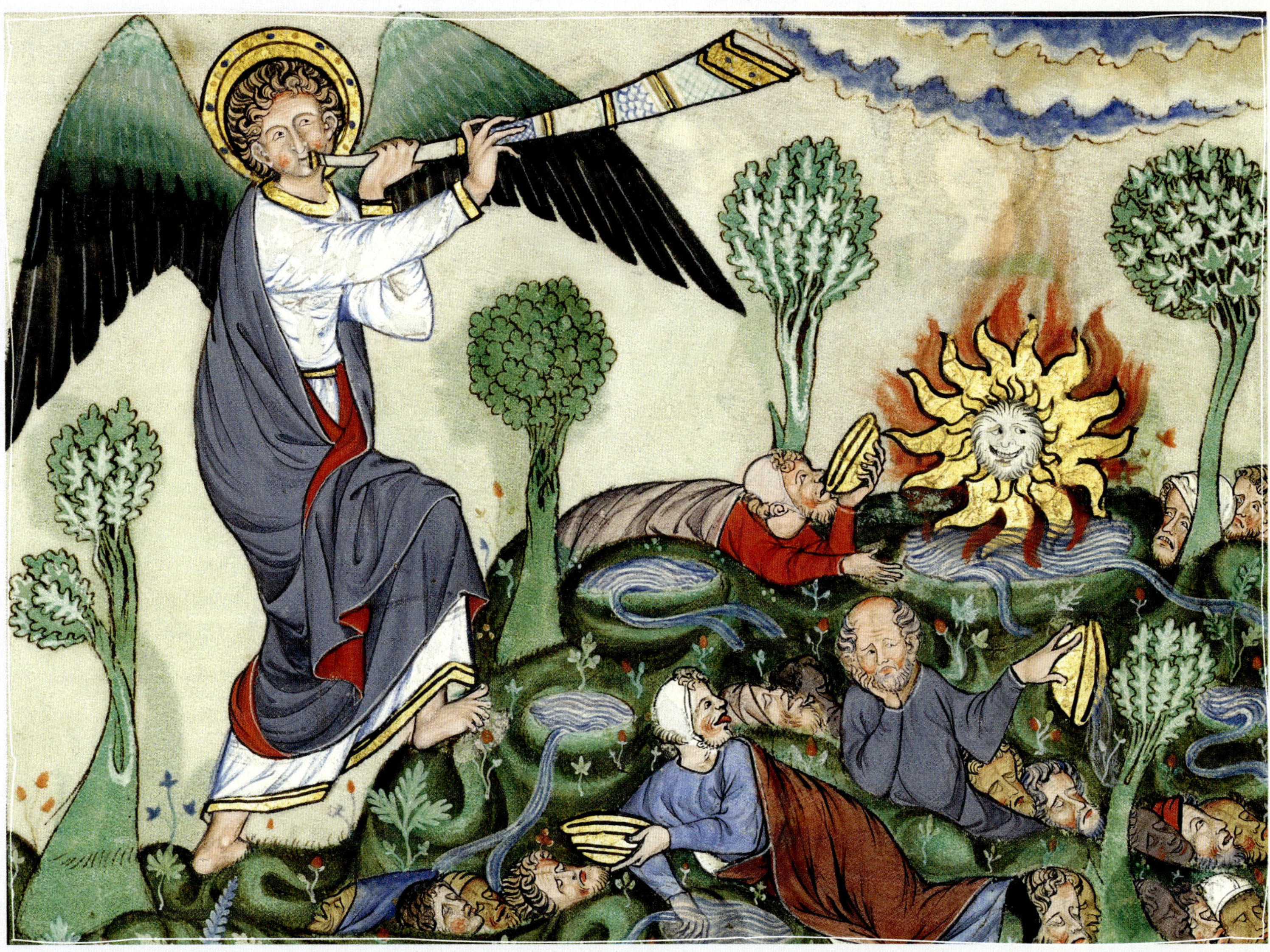

▲ Wormwood star
In the Christian Bible, wormwood is a metaphor for bitterness or an affliction. It appears in the *Book of Revelations* as a great star, called by an angel's trumpet, that falls blazing to Earth, poisoning water with a bitter taste. Wormwood is seen here as both a plant and a star above those who have died from drinking the water.

oils, whose biological function is likely to protect the plant from grazing animals, have been used medicinally as an antiparasitic since at least 1552 BCE when it was recorded in the ancient Egyptian medical text, Ebers papyrus.

Another early use of wormwood was as a deterrent to small pests. Freshly gathered and strewn on the floor, it repelled fleas, lice, and other pests. It was also added to chicken coops and nest boxes for the same purpose.

In medieval Europe, wormwood was used in the treatment of dyspepsia and other digestive problems, and to dispel internal parasites such as roundworms and tapeworms. More recently, extract of wormwood has shown promise in the treatment of Crohn's disease, and potential for some kinds of cancer treatment. However, the dosage needs to be carefully regulated due to the herb's toxicity. It is available in tablet form or as liquid tinctures, although medical advice is recommended first. Dried wormwood is also available over the counter as herbal tea, which is taken as a tonic or appetizer, or to aid digestion. Wormwood, and its relative mugwort, have historically been used as a seasoning in Scotland. The herbs have also been smoked, although with some danger of side-effects such as headaches and dizziness.

Powerful essence

Wormwood is sometimes used as fragrance in soap, cosmetics, and perfumes where it provides a strong bitter plant-like smell. By far the best-known use of wormwood, however, is as a

A WARNING TO DRINKERS

The perils of absinthe are depicted on this French poster from the turn of the 20th century, showing death himself serving at the bar, pouring out the dangerous green liquid. By 1915, "the green peril" had been banned in most countries in western Europe as well as the US. The sale of absinthe is now legal again in most countries, including France.

***LE PERIL VERT* BY T. BIANCO**

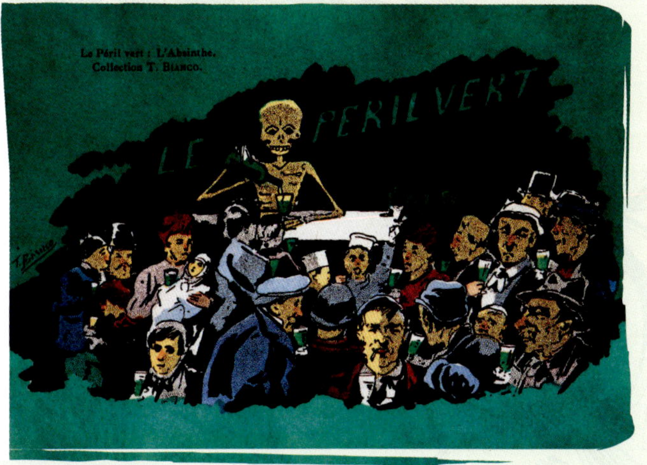

> The word **absinthe** is possibly derived from the Greek ***apsinthion*** meaning **"undrinkable"**

flavouring, especially for alcoholic drinks. In the 17th century, the English naturalist John Ray noted its use in brewing, removing the vinegary taste of bad beer. Even earlier, it was used to spice mead, and was sometimes used instead of hops as a bittering agent in beer. In Denmark it was used in home-brewed beer, while in Morocco wormwood is used in a warming tea called *sheeba* (or *shiba*). Wormwood is an ingredient of various bitter-tasting liqueurs, such as vermouth and the Balkan pelinkovac. It is also the key ingredient, along with anise and fennel, of the very strong alcoholic spirit known as absinthe, possibly named after the wormwood's species name, *absinthium*. Green in colour, and with a bitter, herbal taste, absinthe is traditionally drunk diluted with iced water strained through a cube of sugar. It was a popular drink in 19th century France, served in bars and cafes, and nicknamed the green muse or the green fairy.

> " Where [...] wormwood is strewne, no flea for his life dare abide to be knowne. "
>
> THOMAS TUSSER, *Five Hundred Pointes of Good Husbandrie*, 1580

One reason for its popularity in Bohemian circles was that, as well as being alcoholic, absinthe was also mildly mind-altering. Wormwood contains a chemical compound called thujone that excites the central nervous system. A couple of glasses of absinthe could result in euphoria, or deep introspection, and absinthe's dangerous reputation led to its prohibition in most European countries. Since the 1980s, absinthe is once again legally available to buy and drink, albeit with a lower, safer level of thujone.

Similar herbs

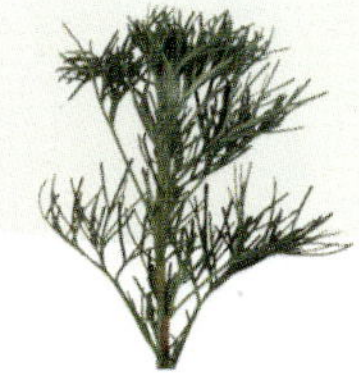

SOUTHERNWOOD

Artemisia abrotanum

This bushy herb, a native of Eurasia, has a camphor-like scent, and was used to fragrance homes. It is also grown in gardens.

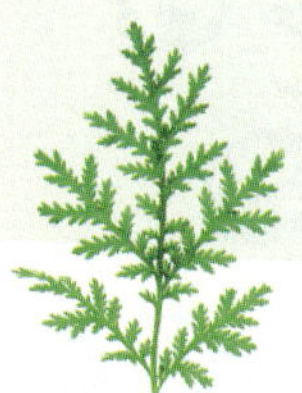

SWEET WORMWOOD

Artemisia annua

Long used in traditional Chinese medicine, extracts from this plant have more recently been used in the treatment of malaria.

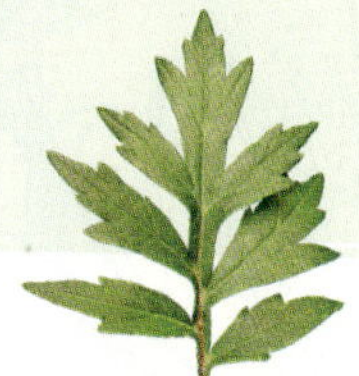

MUGWORT

Artemisia vulgaris

A scruffy plant common throughout Europe and Asia, it is used as a pot-herb and in a tea said to promote lucid dreaming.

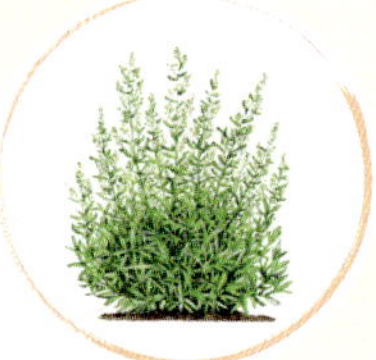

Uses Medicines for digestion and toothache, culinary, cosmetic, fragrance

Parts used Leaves, stems

Active ingredients Estragole (methyl chavicol), methyl eugenol, ocimene, pinenes, limonene

Habitat Temperate areas with well-drained soil and full sun, or dappled light

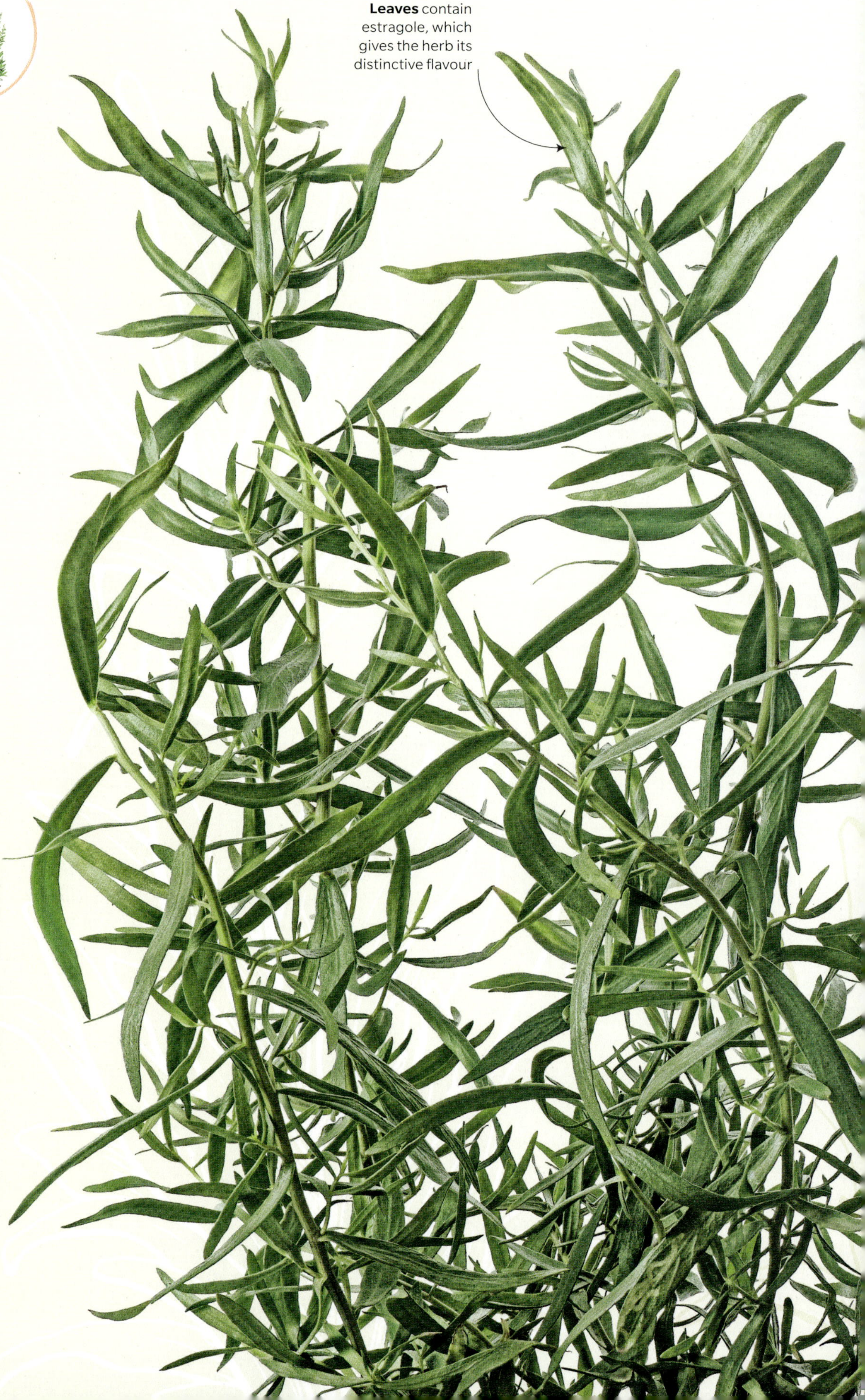

Leaves contain estragole, which gives the herb its distinctive flavour

➤ A culinary classic

French tarragon's slender stems and skinny leaves are best picked while young and eaten raw. In comparison, the closely related Russian tarragon has coarser, less aromatic leaves and a slightly bitter, pungent flavour.

ARTEMIS AND HERBS

Tarragon's genus name *Artemisia* stems from Artemis (known as Diana by the Romans), the Greek goddess of the hunt and the woods, as depicted in this ancient fresco in Naples, Italy. Legend has it that she gave species of *Artemisia* to Chiron the Centaur, famous for his wisdom and knowledge of medicine. Chiron is said to have developed medicines from the plants.

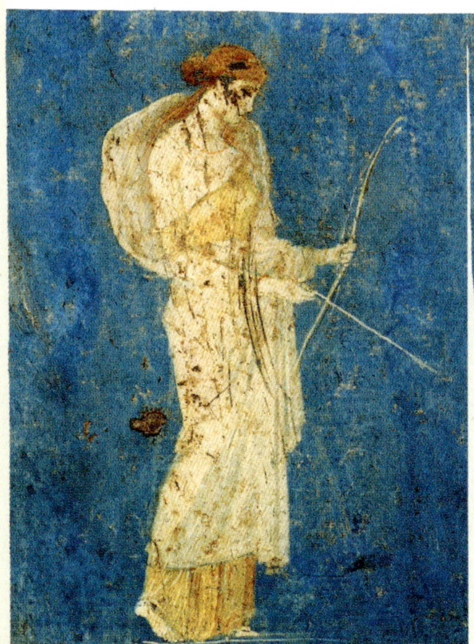

GODDESS ARTEMIS

French Tarragon

Artemisia dracunculus

This hardy and drought-resistant perennial herb is notable for its smooth, slender, aromatic leaves, and serpentine roots. It can be used to add a sweet, anise-like flavour to food, can aid digestion, and can also be used as a deodorizing essential oil.

Narrow, lance-shaped leaves curve out from a woody stem

Similar herb

COMMON SUNFLOWER
Helianthus annuus
The sunflower or daisy family Asteraceae, includes *Artemisia* and the common sunflower; a source of nutritious seeds and oil.

French tarragon is a cultivated form of tarragon, *Artemisia dracunculus*, a wild species in the Asteraceae family. As a culinary and medicinal herb, French tarragon is often referred to simply as tarragon. Its grey-green, lightly anise-flavoured leaves are widely used to season soups, sauces, meat, fish, and vegetables. Fresh tarragon leaves are added to béarnaise sauce just before serving to preserve their subtle flavour. Chopped tarragon is added to the Persian dish *sabzi khordan* and to the filling of the Slovenian dessert *potica*, while a tarragon-infused syrup is used to make the bright green Georgian sparkling soft drink *tarkhun*. Tarragon is also used alongside parsley, chives, and chervil in the French herb mix *fines herbes*.

A soothing standby

Besides its culinary uses, French tarragon also has many uses as a home remedy. Fresh or dried French tarragon leaves and stems can be infused into just-boiled water to make a digestive tea, helping to soothe stomach pain and bloating. Tarragon tea is known to be helpful as an appetite stimulant or to reduce stress, and may also ease insomnia. The ancient Greeks chewed sprigs of tarragon to treat tooth pain, drawing on the compound eugenol, which can have a numbing, naturally anaesthetic effect. Tarragon is still used for toothache but is less popular for this than clove oil, which is also rich in eugenol.

The main use of tarragon essential oil, which is extracted from the leaves, is in cosmetics or home fragrance. The oil is used to soothe the skin, while the sweet scent naturally deodorizes and can also act as an insect repellent.

Estragole, found in tarragon and basil, is named after *estragon*, the French name for Tarragon

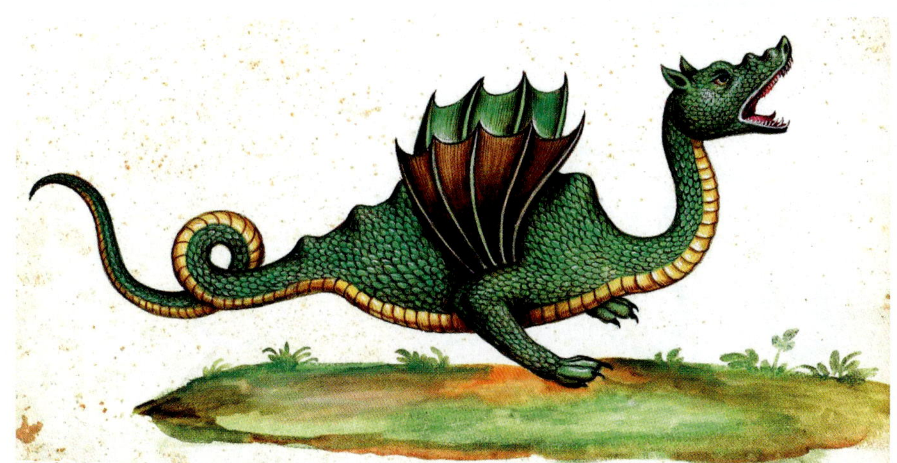

➤ Inspired by dragons
Tarragon's scientific species name *dracunculus* loosely translates as "little dragon" and relates to its serpentine shapes as the Latin word *Draco* is used to describe mythical serpents. Tarragon was also used as an ancient remedy for snakebites.

Aiding Digestion

Eating herbs can help to soothe our digestion, partly because plants generally take longer to digest. Millennia of informal human experimentation has identified species that are especially beneficial to our digestive health. This in turn helps support our nervous, immune, and hormonal systems.

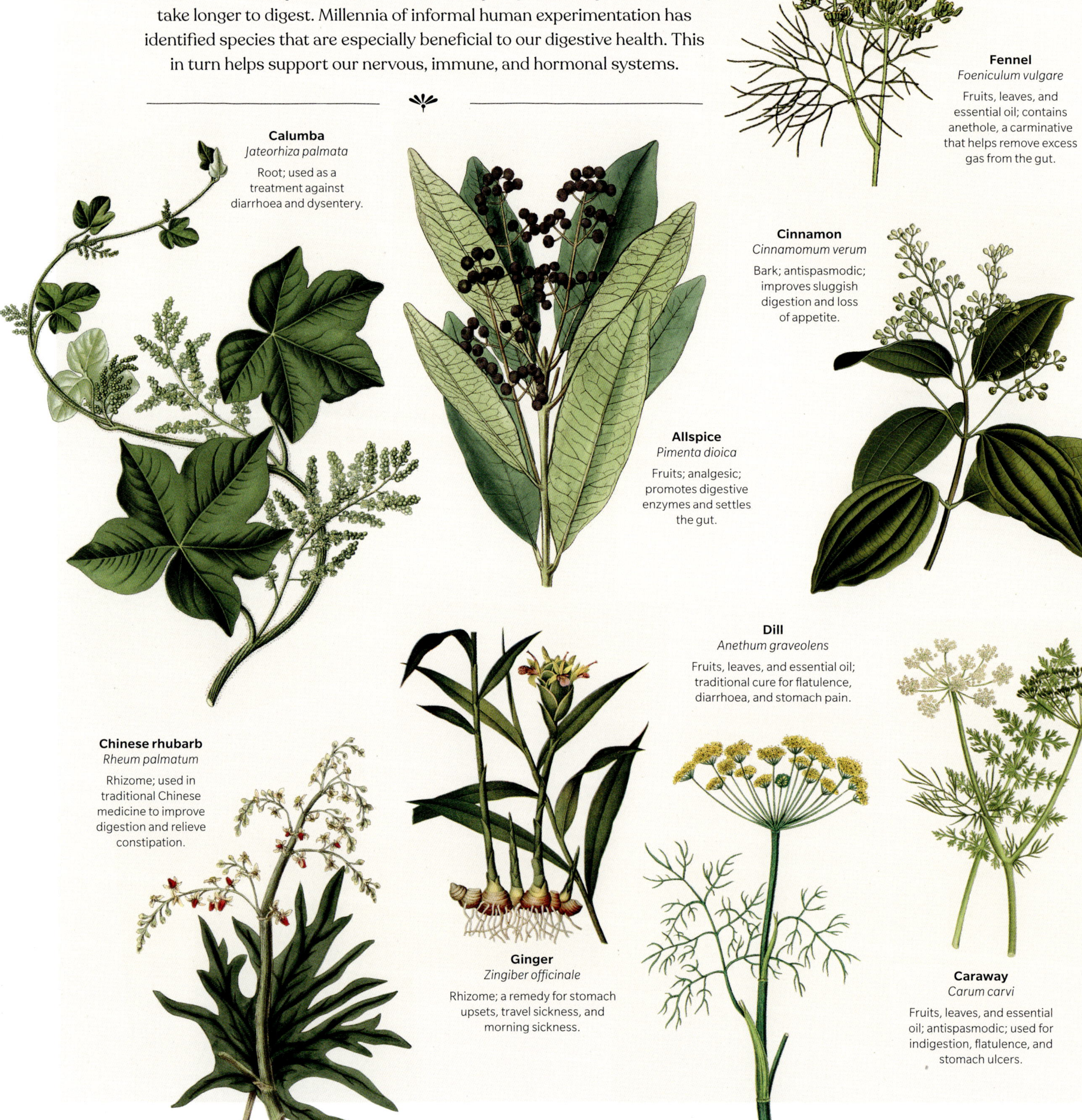

Fennel
Foeniculum vulgare
Fruits, leaves, and essential oil; contains anethole, a carminative that helps remove excess gas from the gut.

Calumba
Jateorhiza palmata
Root; used as a treatment against diarrhoea and dysentery.

Cinnamon
Cinnamomum verum
Bark; antispasmodic; improves sluggish digestion and loss of appetite.

Allspice
Pimenta dioica
Fruits; analgesic; promotes digestive enzymes and settles the gut.

Dill
Anethum graveolens
Fruits, leaves, and essential oil; traditional cure for flatulence, diarrhoea, and stomach pain.

Chinese rhubarb
Rheum palmatum
Rhizome; used in traditional Chinese medicine to improve digestion and relieve constipation.

Ginger
Zingiber officinale
Rhizome; a remedy for stomach upsets, travel sickness, and morning sickness.

Caraway
Carum carvi
Fruits, leaves, and essential oil; antispasmodic; used for indigestion, flatulence, and stomach ulcers.

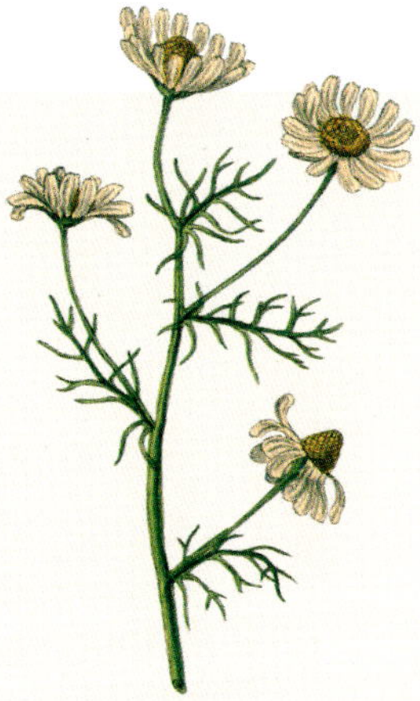

German chamomile
Matricaria chamomilla
Flowers; a tea is said to soothe nervous digestion, wind, and bloating.

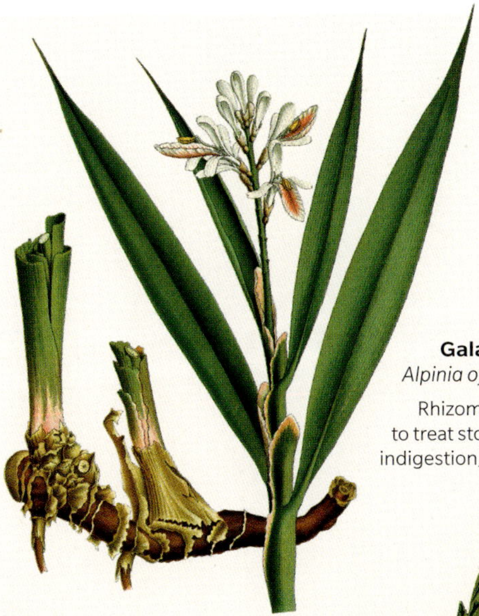

Galangal
Alpinia officinarum
Rhizomes; used to treat stomach pain, indigestion, and nausea.

Peppermint
Mentha piperita
Leaves and essential oil; eases stomach troubles, relaxes gut muscles, and stimulates digestive juices.

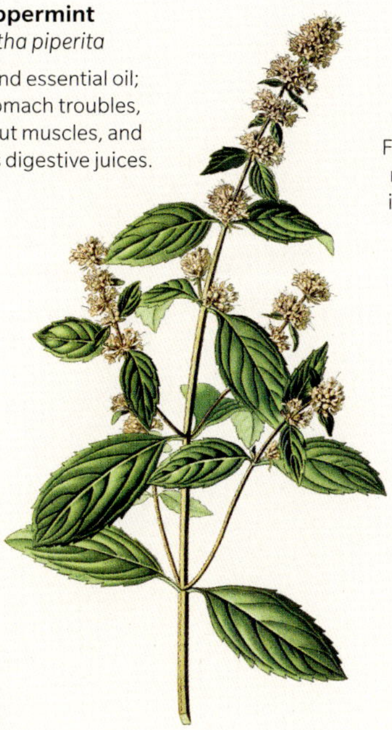

Pot marigold
Calendula officinalis
Flowers; tincture may help reduce gut inflammation in gastritis, peptic ulcers, and colitis.

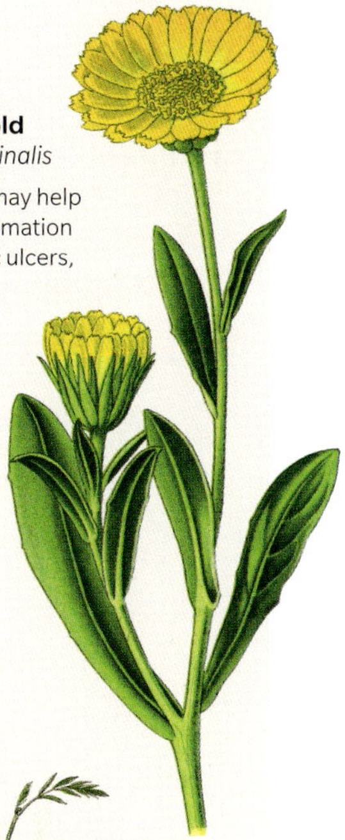

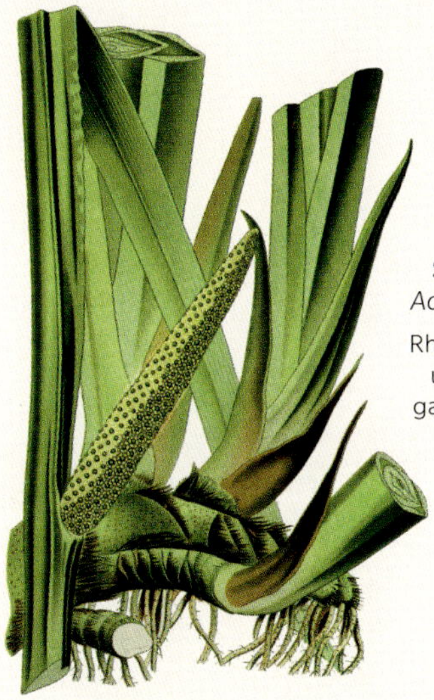

Sweet flag
Acorus calamus
Rhizome and oil; used to treat gastrointestinal ailments.

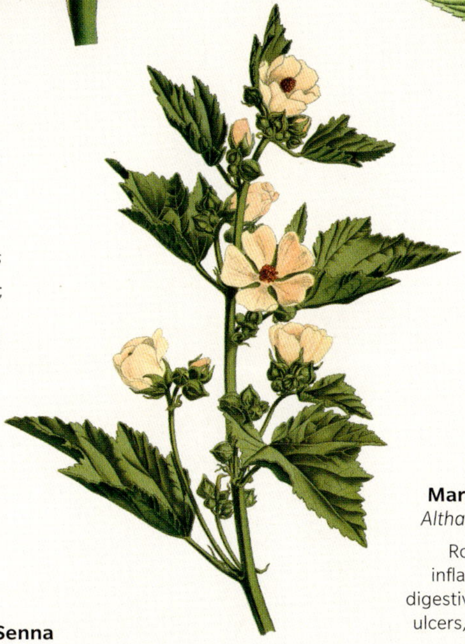

Liquorice
Glycyrrhiza glabra
Root and rhizomes; protects stomach lining; used in treatment of mouth and peptic ulcers.

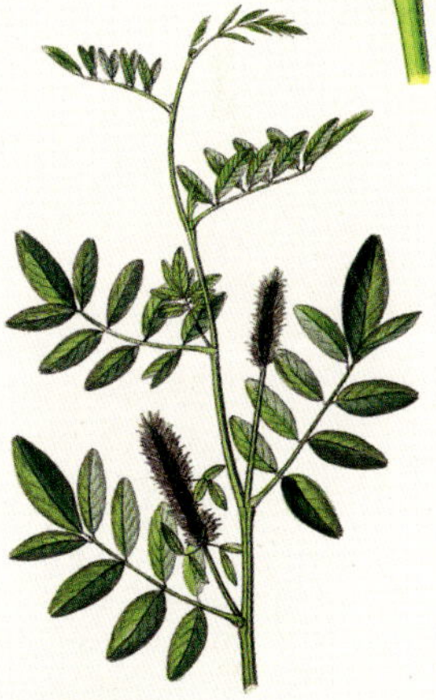

Marsh mallow
Althaea officinalis
Root; eases inflammation of digestive tract, peptic ulcers, and gastritis.

Senna
Senna spp.
Pods, leaves; a leaf tea acts as stimulant laxative against acute constipation.

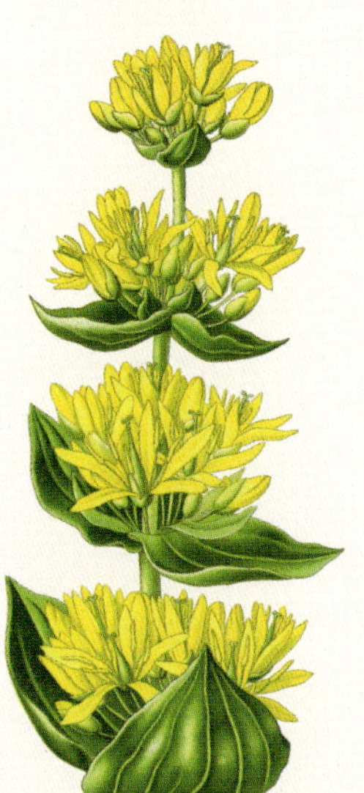

Yellow gentian
Gentiana lutea
Root and rhizome; drunk in a bitter aperitif; increases secretion of gastric juices and restores appetite.

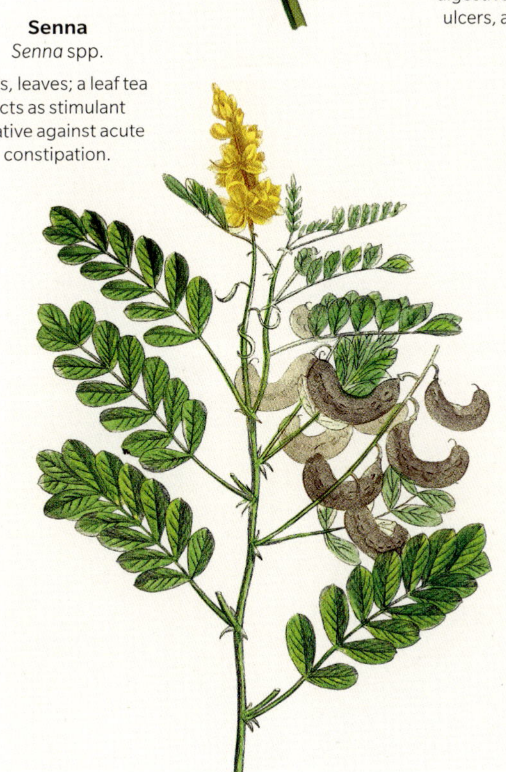

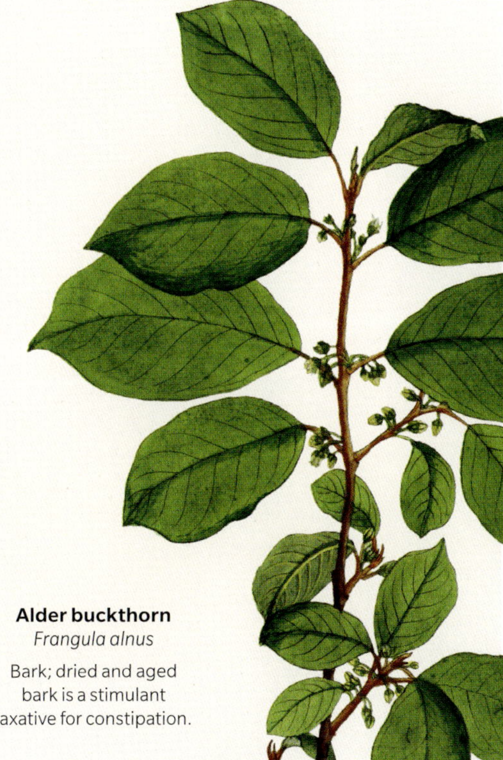

Alder buckthorn
Frangula alnus
Bark; dried and aged bark is a stimulant laxative for constipation.

➤ Lesser galangal
As this botanical drawing shows, lesser galangal produces leaves and flowers from a fleshy, underground stem, or rhizome, which is also the source of the spice.

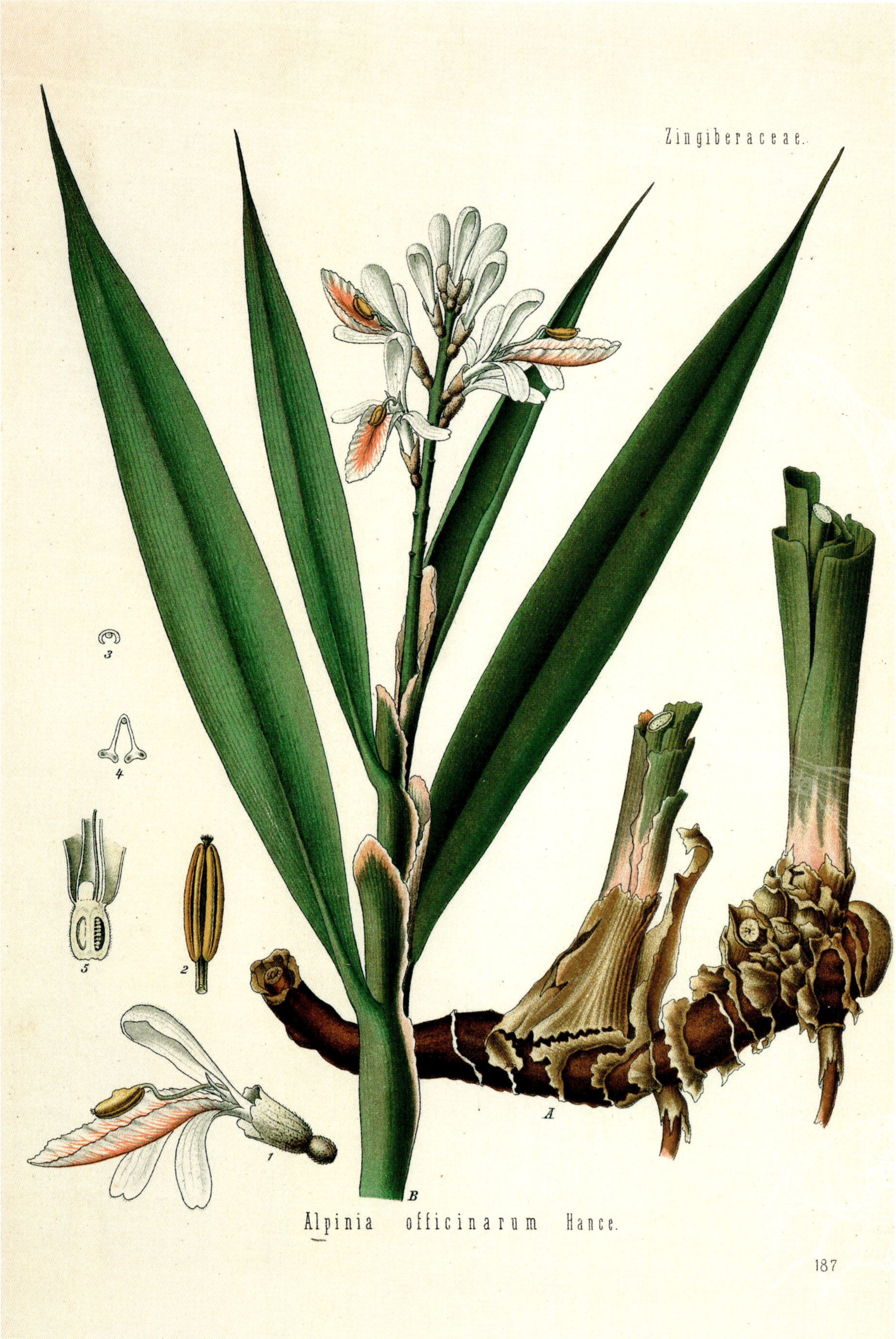

Similar herbs

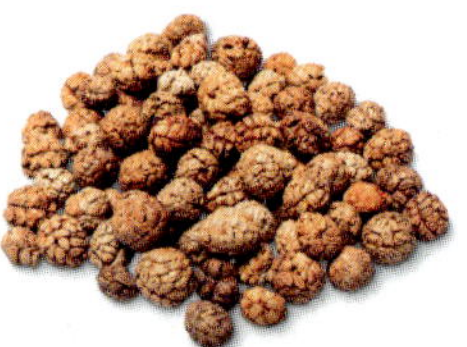

CAO DOU KOU
Alpinia hainanensis
This species is native from China to Vietnam and is grown as an ornamental and for medicinal use; the seedpods serve as a cardamom substitute.

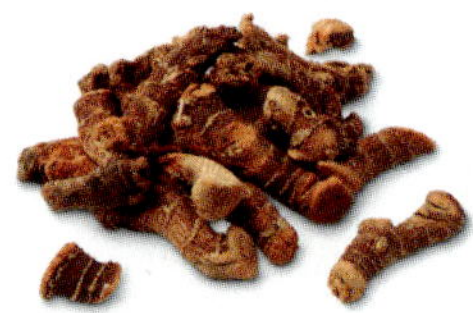

GREATER GALANGAL
Alpinia galanga
Native across much of Southeast Asia, the rhizome flavours Thai curries and Indonesian *rendang* and is also used to stimulate digestion and for inflammation.

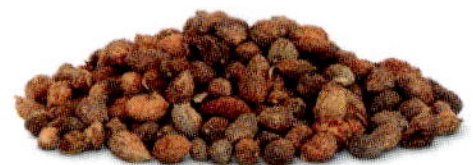

YI ZHI REN
Alpinia oxyphylla
The fruits and seeds of this Chinese and Vietnamese galangal are used in traditional Chinese medicine to treat excessive salivation, incontinence, and diarrhoea.

Zingiberaceae.

3
4
5
2
1
A
B

Alpinia officinarum Hance.

187

Uses Medicines; cooking; cosmetics; perfumery

Parts used Rhizomes

Active ingredients Flavonoids, including galangin, 1,8-cineole, and galangols

Habitat Mainly tropical rainforest, but also wetlands; rich soils and part shade

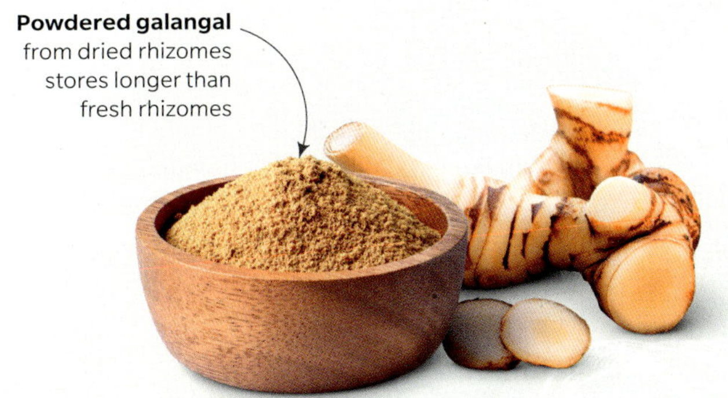

Powdered galangal from dried rhizomes stores longer than fresh rhizomes

◄ Galangal powder and rhizome
The fresh, peeled rhizome is preferred for most uses, but can be difficult to find in regions with climates unsuited to its cultivation. Powdered galangal is a common substitute.

Lesser Galangal

Alpinia officinarum

Alpinia is **named** for **Italian botanist** Prospero Alpini (1553–1617)

This herb is widely used, particularly in Southeast Asia, in medicine, cooking, and cosmetics. The common name galangal refers to several plants with similar, but not identical, uses and characteristics.

The word "galangal" and its global variants have a mysterious origin, possibly deriving from the Chinese name *gao liang jiang* or from Persian, via Arabic. Several *Alpinia* species bear the name; *A. officinarum* and *A. galanga* are most commonly utilized for their edible roots, while other species provide edible fruits and seeds.

Species of the related *Kaempferia*, and the unrelated sweet cyperus, or galingale (*Cyperus longus*) also use the name. All have fragrant roots or rhizomes that may be used medicinally, but they cannot be used interchangeably, so great care is needed to check that the correct species is used in preparations made from these herbs.

Food, fumigant, and fragrance

Lesser galangal is used as an antibacterial and an antiviral, to diminish inflammation and improve digestive health. Along with greater galangal (see opposite), it is best known as an ingredient in several cuisines, especially those of Southeast Asia. It flavours teas, and is a common part of curry pastes from Vietnam to Cambodia, and in Thai *tom yum* soup. Syrup spiced with galangal flavours several cocktails, and it is a traditional element of Polish spiced vodka, *Żołądkowa Gorzka*. Beyond the kitchen, the spicy balsam fragrance of lesser galangal is popular with perfumiers and, as a component of aromatherapy and massage oils, is said to improve mood and to banish depression.

In laboratory trials, lesser galangal essential oil has proven effective as a repellent for the cigarette beetle (*Lasioderma serricorne*), a pest of flour, tobacco, and other dried plant products. It is being investigated as a safe alternative to chemical insecticides for fumigating flour mills or as a coating on paper flour bags.

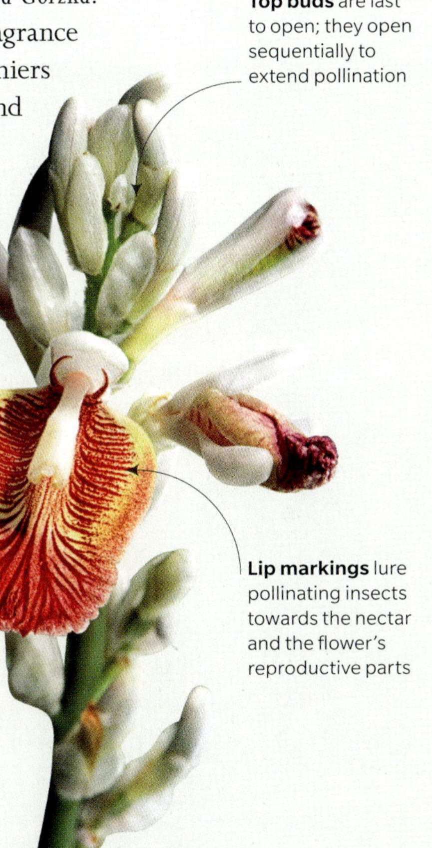

Top buds are last to open; they open sequentially to extend pollination

Lip markings lure pollinating insects towards the nectar and the flower's reproductive parts

► Galangal flower
Instead of producing pollen, two of the stamens fuse into an ornate lip, or labellum, to provide a landing pad for pollinating insects.

Long, narrow, pointed leaves are edible, with a milder flavour than that of the rhizome
Upright, reed-like stem bears alternate leaves in two rows
Rhizome has a thin, corky outer layer covering its useful yellow-white inside

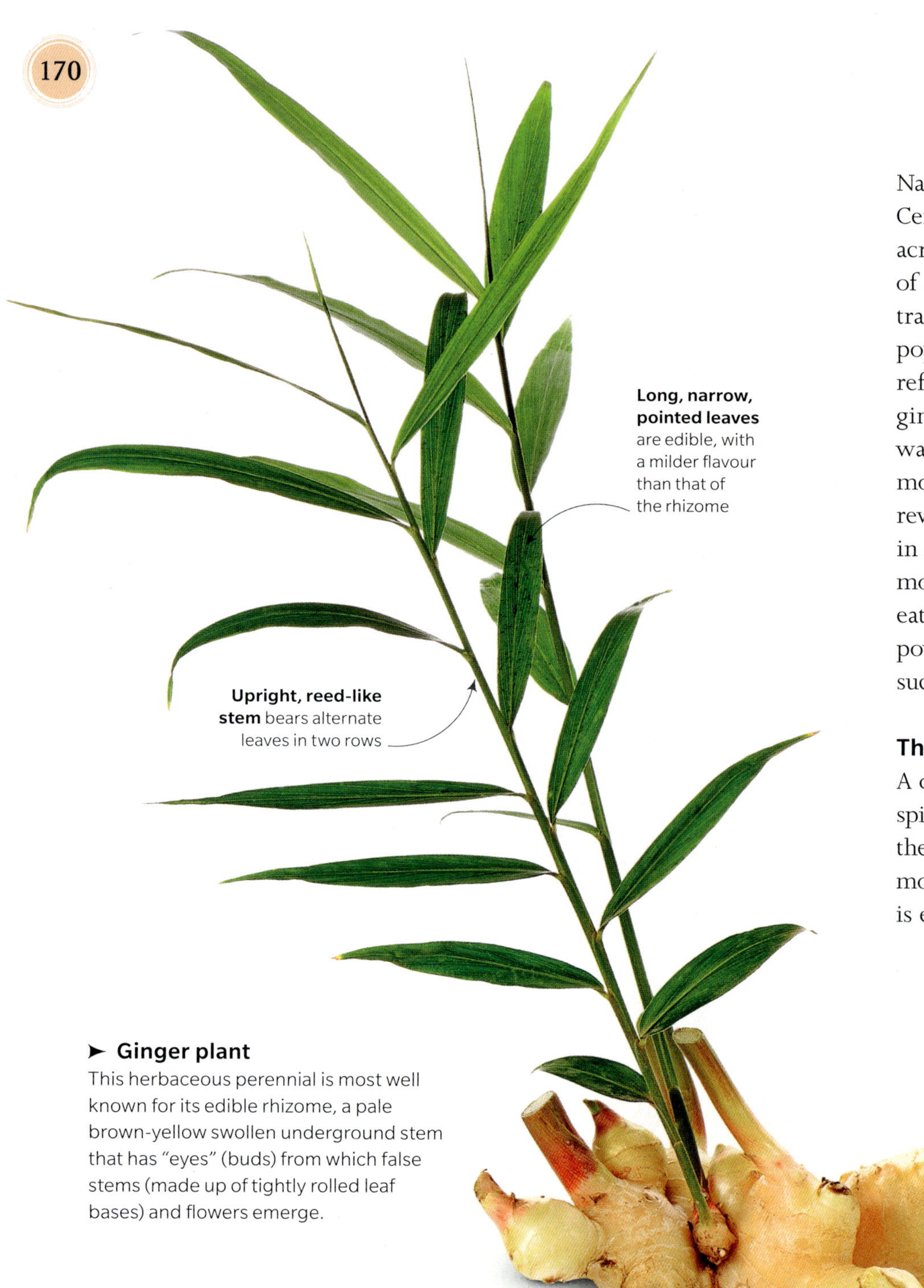

➤ **Ginger plant**
This herbaceous perennial is most well known for its edible rhizome, a pale brown-yellow swollen underground stem that has "eyes" (buds) from which false stems (made up of tightly rolled leaf bases) and flowers emerge.

Ginger

Zingiber officinale

Fresh or dried, powdered or crushed, as an oil or as a juice, the ginger rhizome packs a spicy punch in all its forms. Used to flavour food and drinks, it also has a warming, immune-boosting effect.

Uses Medicines; cooking; perfume; cosmetics

Parts used Rhizome, leaves, stem, flowers

Active ingredients Gingerols, shogaols, paradols, zingerone, terpenoids, flavonoids, vitamin C and B, magnesium, potassium, betacarotene

Habitat Humid, partly shaded tropical and subtropical forests

Native to tropical and subtropical regions of Central and East Asia and now widespread across the Pacific, ginger is an important part of Ayurveda (traditional Indian medicine) and traditional Chinese medicine, as well as being a popular culinary herb. A medicine chest herb – referring to its varied applications and benefits – ginger is commonly used to enhance digestion, warm the joints, boost circulation, and combat morning or motion sickness. The benefits of this revitalizing and energizing spice can be accessed in several ways. The rhizome, which contains the most potent active ingredients, can be juiced or eaten raw; it can also be used fresh, dried, or powdered in soups, curries, bakes, and drinks such as tea and fruit juice.

The gingerol effect

A delicious combination of pungent, sweet, and spicy, ginger is loaded with antioxidants from the group of compounds known as gingerols, the most potent of which is 6-gingerol. When ginger is eaten, this ingredient activates the spice receptors on the tongue to feel a "hot" sensation. In dried rhizomes, the gingerols are converted into the more pungent shogaols. When cooked, gingerols and shogaols transform into zingerone, providing sweet as well as spicy notes, as can be found in candied ginger, ginger biscuits, or pickles. Gingerols, shogaols, and zingerone have powerful anti-inflammatory, anti-emetic (combats nausea – see p.173), carminative (wind relieving), circulatory stimulant, and analgesic (pain reliever) effects. They can help ease arthritis, digestive upset, colds, period pains, toothache, fatigue, and migraines. While in perfume or scented cosmetics, ginger delivers a warm yet zingy fresh top note, which can act as an aphrodisiac.

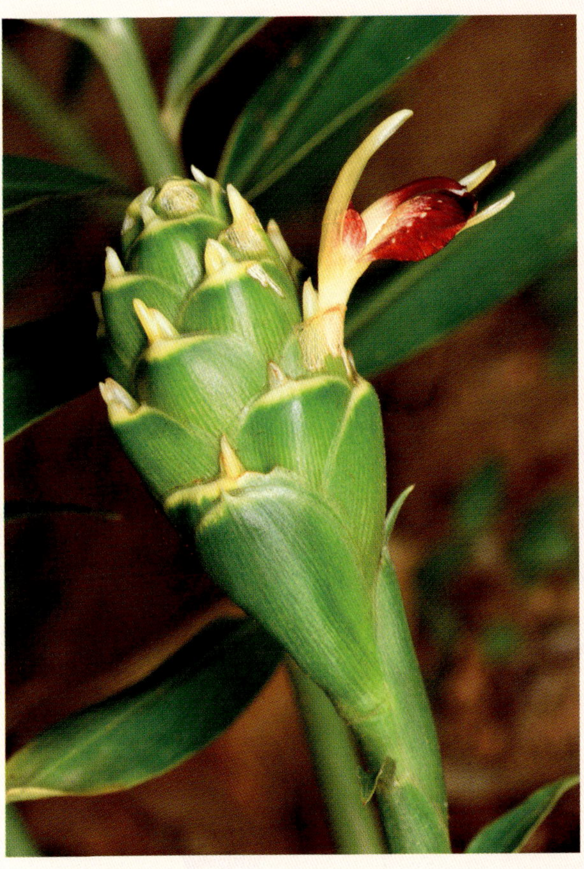

◄ Ginger flowers
The ginger genus includes several flowering species with red, pink, yellow, or purple flowers, some of which are grown as tropical outdoor ornamentals or houseplants. Common ginger (*Zingiber officinale*) produces cone-shaped spikes of pale yellow, purple-lipped flowers.

Spice routes

Records of ginger's use as a healing herb date back to more than 2,000 years. A compilation of the teachings of Chinese philosopher Confucius (551–479 BCE) made by his disciples and entitled *Analects* reports that he ate ginger with every meal to remove excess wind and dampness in the stomach. Its known use stretches back some 5,000 years, and it is thought to have featured in prehistoric cooking before being utilized for its medicinal properties.

> "Dioscorides reports that [Ginger] is right good with meat in sauces, or otherwise in conditures; for it is of a heating and digesting quality..."
>
> JOHN GERARD, *The Herball, or Generall Historie of Plantes*, 2nd edition, 1633

Ginger was exported via land and sea as part of the burgeoning spice trade. It made its way from India to the Middle East, from where it was exported across the Mediterranean region as a warming spice and an antidote to poison. Ancient Greeks and Romans embraced this expensive herb as a sign of wealth and status. Ginger was also transported by Austronesian peoples migrating from southern China to the

THE TALE OF GINGER ALE

In the 1850s, Irish apothecary Thomas Joseph Cantrell created a golden-style, fermented ginger ale using yeast, sugar, ginger root, and water. Schweppes – an established name in the aerated water industry – released a carbonated ginger ale for commercial consumption in the 1870s. In 1890, Canadian chemist and pharmacist John J. McLaughlin innovated further to produce a dry ginger ale, which was paler, lighter, and milder than its predecessors.

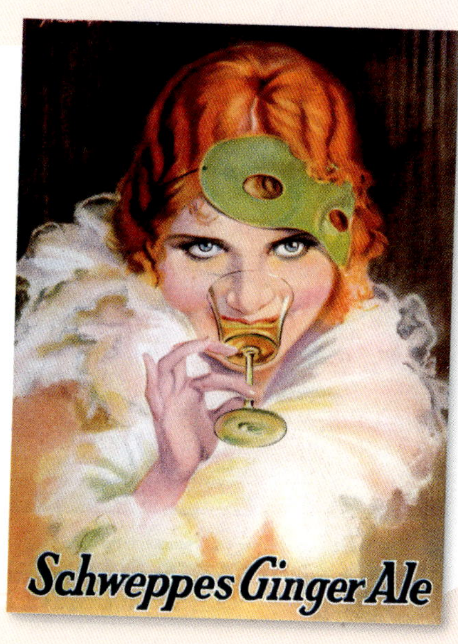

GINGER ALE ADVERTISEMENT, 1931

Similar herbs

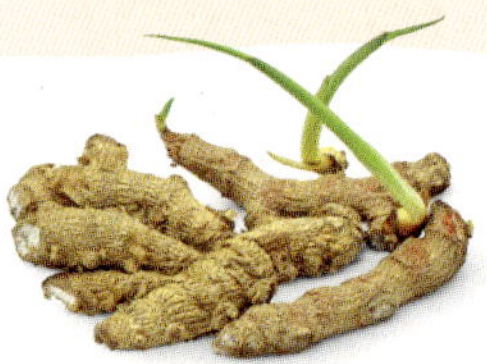

PLAI

Zingiber cassumunar 'Roxburgh'

The rhizome of ginger 'Roxburgh' is used in Thai massage. Its essential oil is believed to ease pain and inflammation.

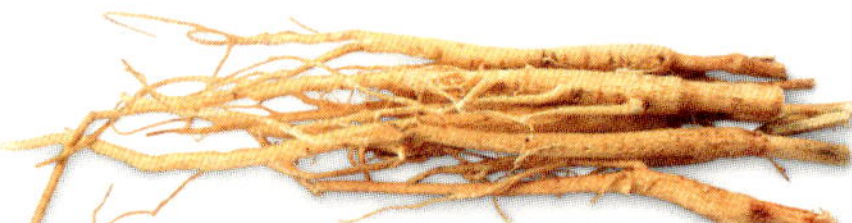

ASTRAGALUS

Astragalus membranaceus

The roots of this medicinal herb have warming and immune-boosting properties, and can be combined with ginger in a tea.

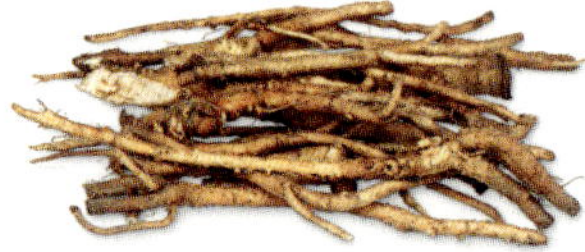

COMMON DANDELION

Taraxacum officinale

This plant's prominent taproots are rich in inulin, a type of soluble fibre that supports the growth and maintenance of healthy gut bacteria.

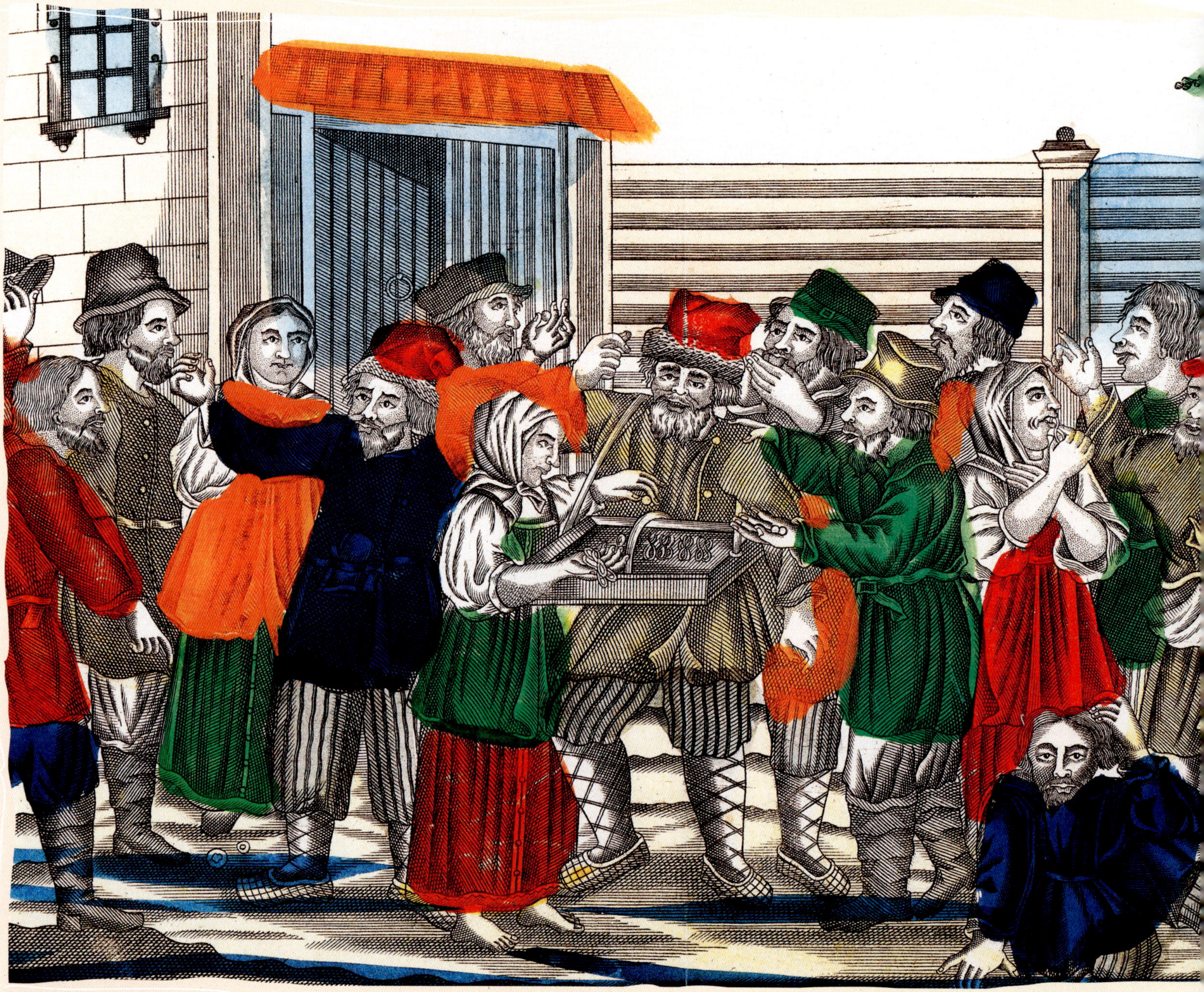

Philippines, Madagascar, and New Zealand. After the fall of the Roman Empire, it continued to be imported into Europe by sea, from India and Africa. It was carried as a potted plant or dried to preserve its shelf life over long voyages. Widespread European colonialism from the 11th century onwards expanded its reach further, as dominant European countries searched for gold and spices. Ginger also became one of the commodities that fuelled the trade of enslaved people.

Gingerbread

Although in Europe initially only the wealthy could afford exotic spices such as ginger and cinnamon, inspired new recipes trickled down to the masses, including that of the still popular festive mainstay, gingerbread. In medieval times, a similar sweetmeat – made using honey, pepper, saffron, and grated bread – was served at the end of a meal to aid digestion and sweeten the breath. These ingredients evolved to include cinnamon and then treacle, flour, and ginger root. This became a familiar treat at fairs and feasts. "Fairings" – gingerbreads moulded into different shapes and sometimes adorned with caraway seeds or candied angelica (see pp.188–89) – paved the way for the gingerbread people and houses (a German tradition) common today.

HOW DO ANTI-EMETIC HERBS WORK?

When the digestive tract is irritated by harmful substances, or a hormonal or physiological imbalance, neurotransmitter receptors in the brain can trigger nausea and vomiting by signalling stomach muscles to contract and expel unwanted contents. Volatile oils in anti-emetic herbs such as ginger and lemon balm (pp.150–53), help block such brain receptors and prevent sickness. Many anti-emetic herbs are also carminative, helping relieve trapped wind and soothe the digestive tract.

> " And I had but one penny in the world, thou should'st have it to buy gingerbread. "
>
> WILLIAM SHAKESPEARE, *Love's Labour's Lost*, c.1590

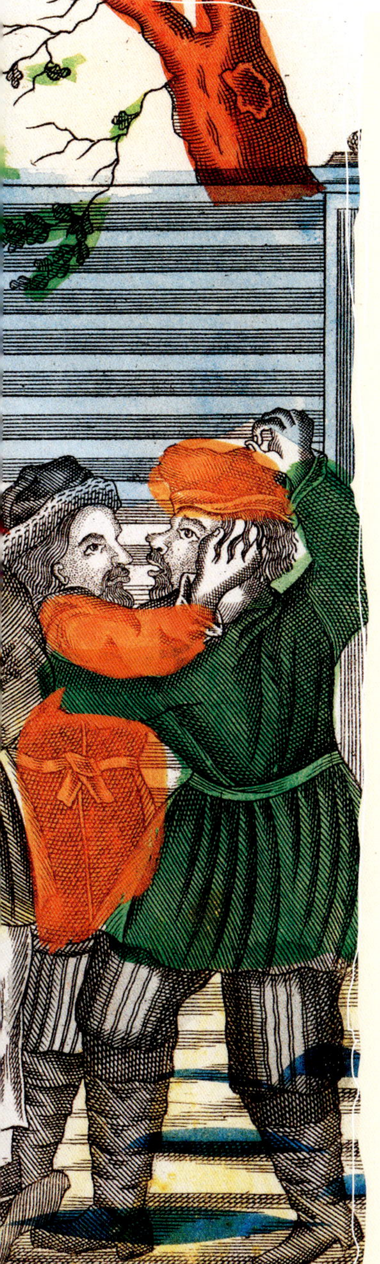

◄ *The song of the ginger syrup*, c.1858
In Russian folk medicine, a ginger infusion was prescribed as the treatment for asthma. The concoction was made by steeping fresh, grated ginger in warm alcohol and allowing it to infuse over a couple of weeks.

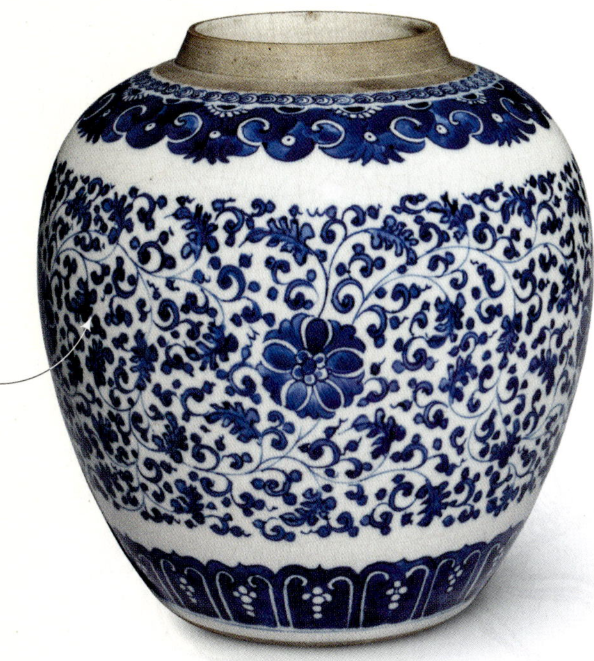

Floral motifs handpainted in cobalt blue on a white, high-shouldered, rounded porcelain jar

► Ginger jar
Ginger jars were originally used in ancient China to store and transport salt and oil, as well as spices including ginger. White and blue jars like this Qing dynasty specimen (1736–95) became popular decorative objects.

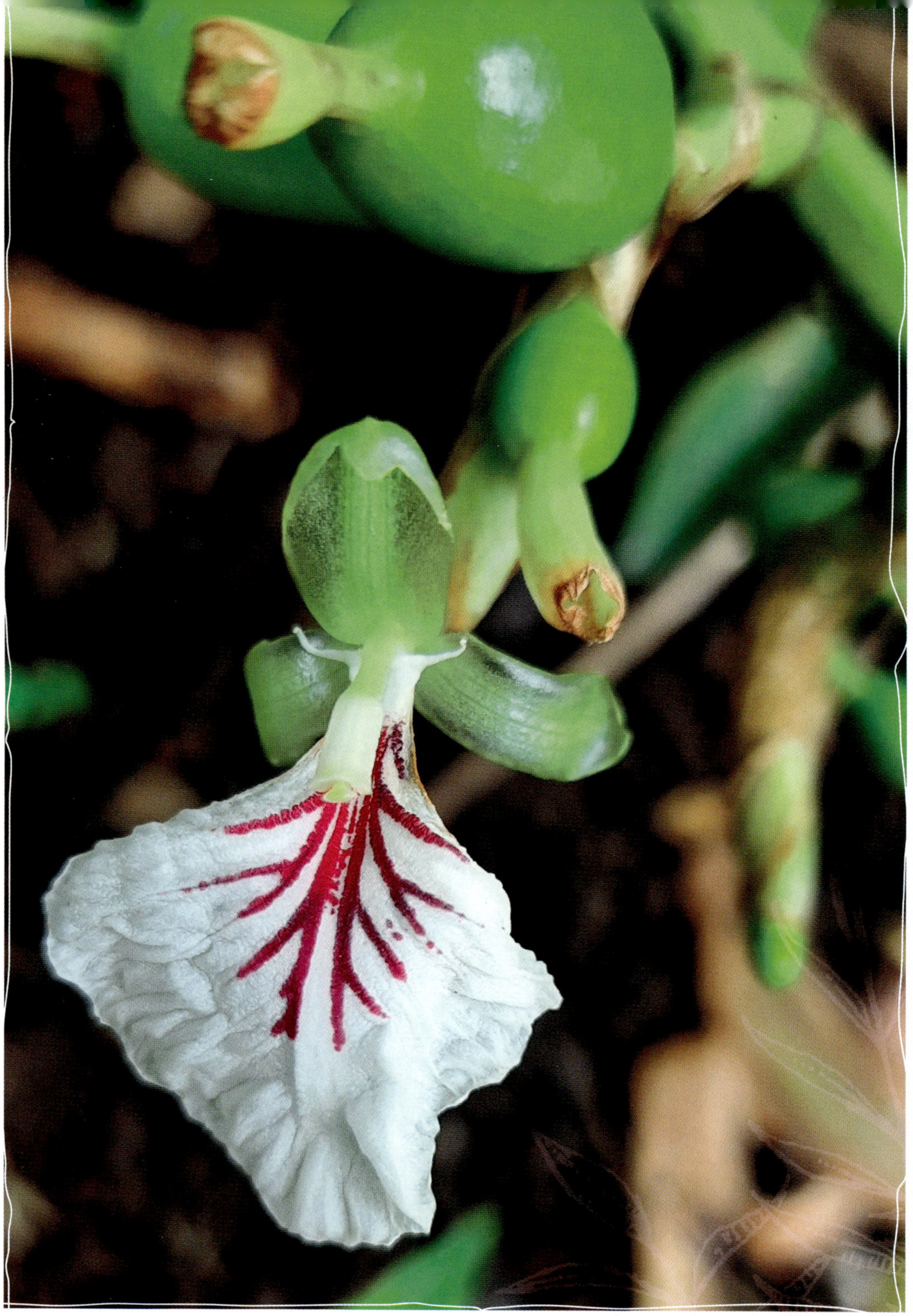

Prized for its flavour and aroma, cardamom is the **third most expensive spice**, after saffron and vanilla

◄ Decorated blooms
Orchid-like flowers bloom in loose heads. They have three green or white petals and a prominent, white lip (labellum) with pink or purple branched markings.

Cardamom

Elettaria cardamomum

Sometimes called the "queen of spices", cardamom is famous for its high price as well as its aromatic flavour. Its usage dates back to early Ayurvedic medicine, and ancient civilizations in Greece and Rome.

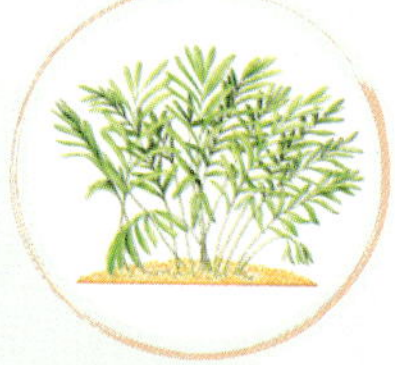

Uses Medicines for digestive and respiratory ailments; culinary, as a spice in savoury dishes, baking, hot drinks; cosmetics

Parts used Dried seed pods and seeds

Active ingredients 1,8-cineole, terpinyl acetate, limonene, sabinene

Habitat Tropical monsoon forests

The ginger family, Zingiberaceae, produces many important spices including ginger and turmeric, but both of these derive from rhizomes. Cardamom instead is produced from seeds, while the rhizome is rarely utilized. The best-known species is *Elettaria cardamomum*, also called green cardamom because of its green seed pods, which originated in the Western Ghats, India. This mountain range lines the west coast and includes the Yela Mala range, also known as the Cardamom Hills. Green cardamom has two common forms, Mysore and Malabar. Several other members of the family are also known as cardamom, but often have quite different flavour profiles. Today, India remains an important producer of the spice, though Indonesia and Guatemala are also significant producers.

Seeds keep their flavour when kept inside the pods

◄ Green fruits
Cardamom fruits (pods) are harvested when ripe and quickly dried to preserve the flavour. Whole pods and seeds are used in cooking.

Tropical seeds

In its natural habitat, cardamom grows beneath a canopy of tropical trees. In commercial cultivation, smaller trees, shrubs, and perennials are removed, retaining the forest canopy to protect the cardamom plants from the sun, while eradicating competition and ensuring maximum productivity of the spice. In many tropical countries, cardamom is a valuable cash crop, providing much-needed revenue for rural communities. However, this comes at a cost to biodiversity through the planting of a monoculture of cardamom and the disturbance of the habitat, which encourages the spread of non-native weedy plants.

As a spice, cardamom is widely utilized in many cuisines, including Scandinavia and its native India where whole pods are used to flavour rice, while ground seeds form part of many masalas (spice mixes). In the Middle East, cardamom seeds are added to ground coffee, and it flavours baklava, *halva*, and sweet rice puddings. Saudi Arabia is the world's largest importer of cardamom.

As a medicine, cardamom has long history in Ayurvedic practices. It is rich in antioxidants and is perhaps best known for the treatment of gastrointestinal problems such as heartburn, irritable bowel, and constipation. It may have antimicrobial and spasmolytic properties and has been used as a breath freshener, in chewing gum, and for cleaning teeth.

Similar herbs

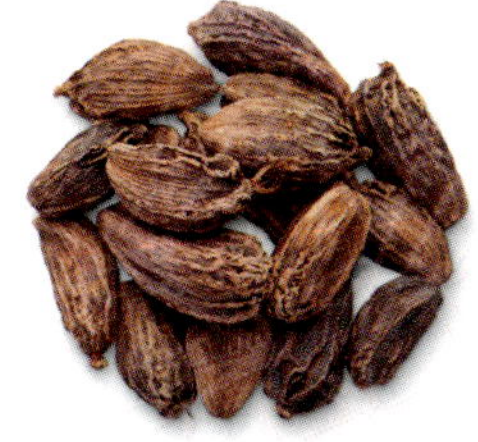

BLACK CARDAMOM
Amomum subulatum
Native from northern India to China, black cardamom has a smoky flavour and is favoured in savoury dishes. It is used to aid digestion and relieve congestion.

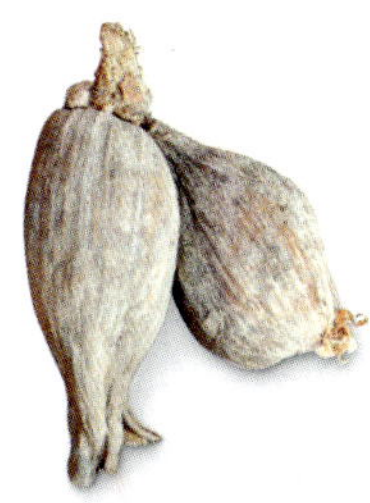

KORARIMA CARDAMOM
Aframomum corrorima
This East African species has a similar taste to green cardamom and is used in traditional medicine in Ethiopia as a carminative and a purgative.

► Sprawling shoots
Green cardamom grows from thick rhizomes. The tall shoots grow upright or sprawl across the forest floor with long, thin leaves.

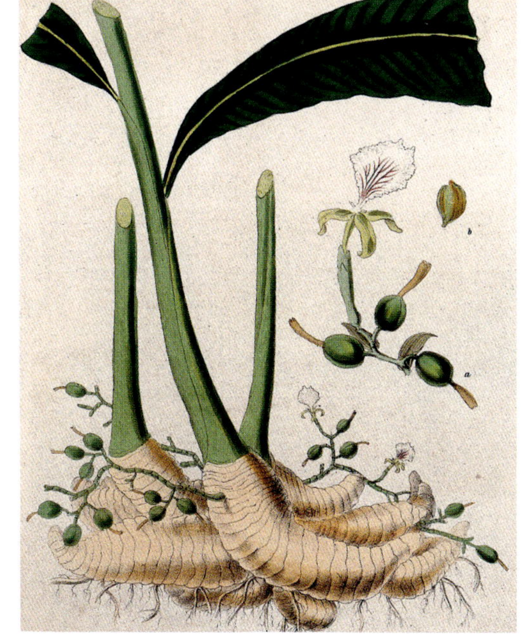

SPICE OF THE VIKINGS

Use of cardamom has a long history in Scandinavia. Many sources suggest the Vikings brought it to the north while trading in Turkey, but evidence is scant. However it arrived, its use is common throughout the region, especially at Christmas, where it flavours *glögg* (spiced wine) and enriched breads such as Finnish *pulla* and Swedish *kardemummabullar*.

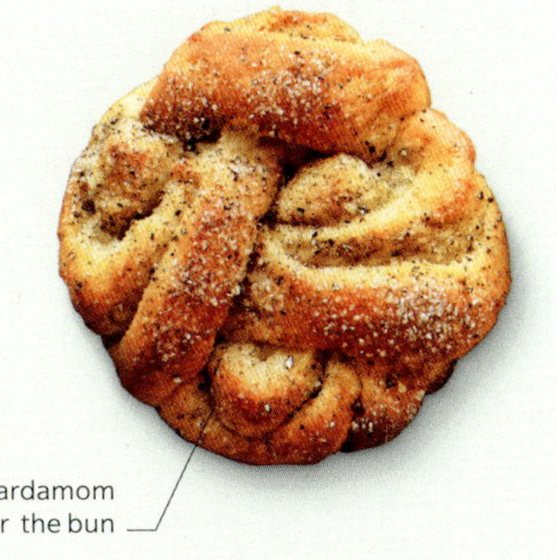

SWEDISH BUN WITH CARDAMOM

Ground cardamom seeds flavour the bun

Lemongrass

Cymbopogon citratus

The heady scent of lemongrass has long flavoured cuisines across Southeast Asia and its popularity has spread across the world. It is also a medicinal herb, cosmetic ingredient, and insect repellent; its fibres are even woven into fabric.

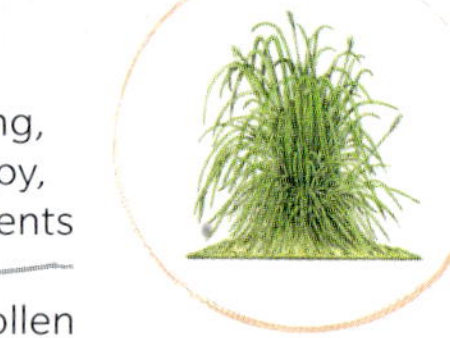

Uses Medicines, cooking, cosmetics, aromatherapy, perfumes, insect repellents

Parts used Leaves, swollen leaf bases, essential oil

Active ingredients Citral, citronellal, citronellol, geraniol, linalool, myrcene

Habitat Sun and moist, well-drained soils in tropical grasslands; also naturalized in some subtropical habitats

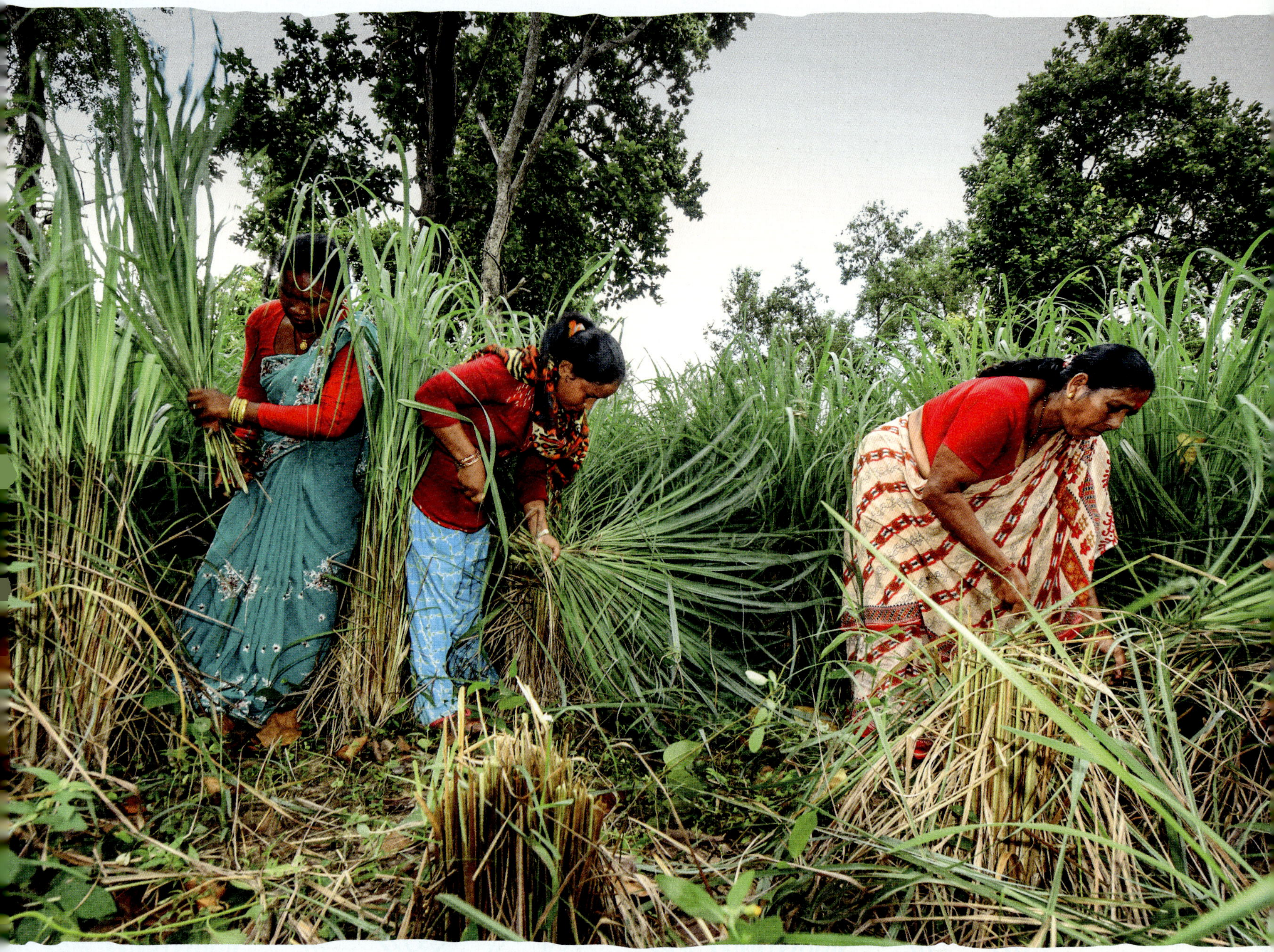

The likely origin of lemongrass is in India and Sri Lanka, but it has been widely grown across Southeast Asia for centuries and is now cultivated in tropical and subtropical regions of Africa and the Americas.

The taste and fragrance of lemongrass resemble that of lemon (see p.52) and the herb can serve as a substitute lemon flavouring. However, the two plants have slightly different flavour profiles. Lemongrass lacks the sourness of lemon and has earthier ginger and mint notes. Fresh lemongrass is superior in flavour to that of the dried grass in cooking, especially in stir fries.

Lemongrass is a common component of many cuisines, including Thai cooking; it is an essential ingredient, along with lesser galangal (see p.168) and lime leaves (see p.53), of *tom yum* soup. Cocktails, teas, and baked goods flavoured with this aromatic grass are increasingly common.

Lemongrass has a tough texture that quickly blunts knife blades, so the swollen leaf base must be grated, crushed, or finely sliced before adding it to food. If used whole in curries, soups, and stews, it is removed before eating.

Wax on leaf surface
Lemongrass's robust leaves are notable for their waxy surface, as seen here through a scanning electron microscope (SEM).

Lemongrass oil cells sit in between the green, photosynthesizing cells of the leaf and stem tissue

◄ Lemongrass stem and rhizome
This large, evergreen grass grows from a rhizome, or subterranean stem. The tough "stems" in fact consist of many, overlapping leaf bases (sheaths), with grassy leaf blades above up to 90 cm (36 in) long.

A bouquet of biochemicals

Lemongrass contains an array of biochemicals with uses in medicine, insecticides, cosmetics, and perfumery. An essential oil is extracted from the freshly gathered leaves and leaf bases by steam distillation.

In lemongrass oil, the main active component is citral, which possesses antimicrobial, sedative, and spasmolytic (spasm-easing) properties. Citral also occurs in significant quantities in herbs such as lemon verbena (*Aloysia citrodora*), lemon myrtle (*Backhousia citriodora*), lemon balm (*Melissa officinalis*, see p.150) and clove basil (*Ocimum gratissimum*). Medicinal uses for lemongrass include calming spasms in the digestive tract, treating colds and nervous conditions, such as stress and anxiety. In aromatherapy, it provides relief from muscle pain.

Natural pest control

Citronellol, a chemical component of lemongrass, acts as an insect repellent. Lemongrass pot plants are grown to drive away mosquitoes, but their effectiveness is equivocal beyond a few metres (yards). Lemongrass effectively repels stable flies (*Stomoxys calcitrans*), which bite livestock, pets, and humans, and disease-spreading houseflies (*Musca domestica*). In contrast, European honeybees (*Apis mellifera*) are attracted to the scent of lemongrass, so it is used as a lure to capture swarming bees.

◄ Aromatic harvest
Lemongrass forms clumps up to 1.5 m (5 ft) tall. It is harvested by hand, by cutting or pulling whole plants, above the rhizome, as done here in Nepal.

Uses Medicines for digestion; flavouring agent, and as a strewing herb

Parts used Rhizome, spadix, young stalks

Active ingredients Volatile oils like asarones (except in var. *americanus*), sesquiterpenes, bitter principles such as acorin

Habitat Edges of lakes, swamps, slow rivers and canals

➤ **Different scents**
Sweet flag has flat, sword-shaped leaves rising in tufts from a creeping stem, or rhizome. While its leaves have a pleasant citrus aroma with a whiff of vanilla, sweet flag's useful rhizome is said to smell like wet cake dough.

DNA evidence shows that sweet flag is among the **earliest monocots,** dating back to the **age of dinosaurs**

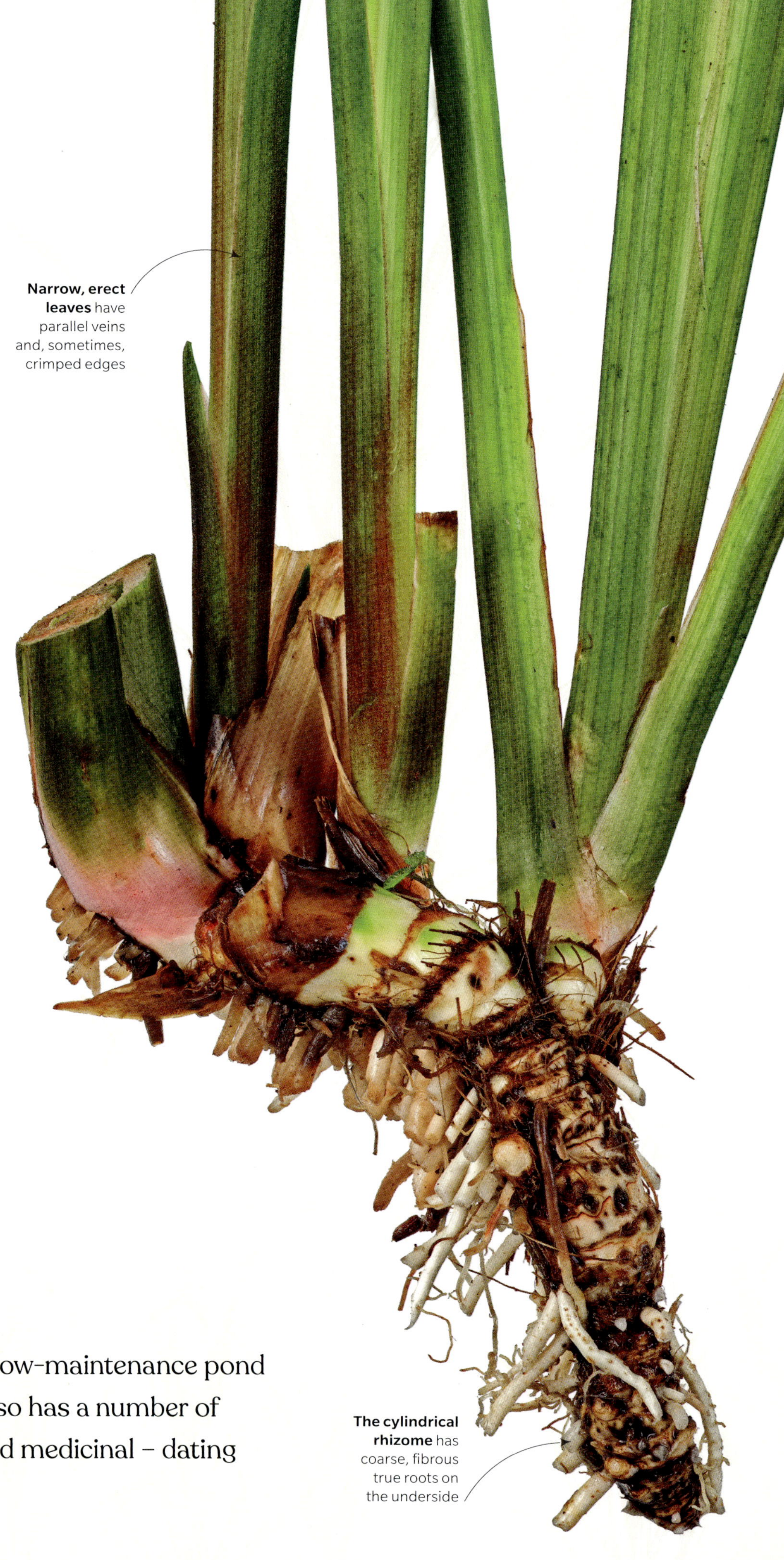

Narrow, erect leaves have parallel veins and, sometimes, crimped edges

The cylindrical rhizome has coarse, fibrous true roots on the underside

Sweet Flag

Acorus calamus

Notable for its sweet scent, this low-maintenance pond plant has decorative foliage. It also has a number of herbal applications – culinary and medicinal – dating back to ancient times.

Sweet flag has a long history of herbal use. In ancient times, the juice from this and related plants was used to treat eye infections. Its genus name, *Acorus*, is derived from the Greek word *akore*, which means "without pupil". In ancient Egypt, its oil was used in perfumes and for hair care. It was also said to help maintain healthy digestion, prevent stomach ailments and colitis, and was an antiflatulent. Chinese and Indian medical traditions consider this herb to be a source of strength and wellbeing, and believe it to be effective against respiratory conditions.

Sweet flag's scented but bitter-tasting "root", technically a rhizome, has more medicinal properties than its leaves. It is harvested in spring, before the leaves begin to grow. The roots can be dried and pulverized to be used as a pest-repellant. Sweet flag oil can also be used to treat head lice.

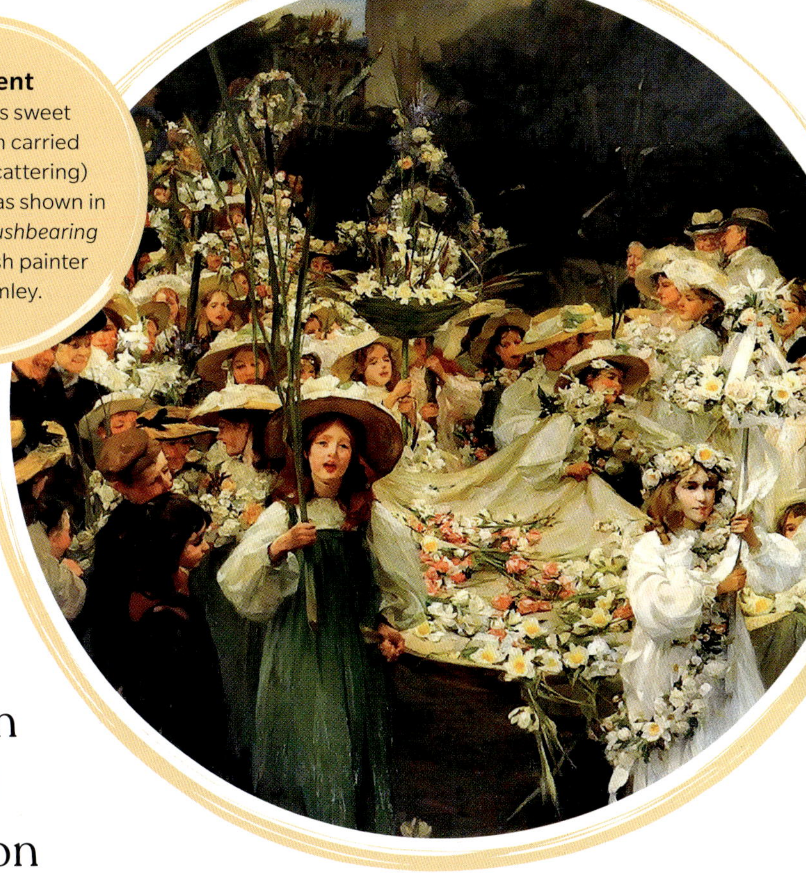

Holy scent
Plants such as sweet flag were often carried for strewing (scattering) in church aisles, as shown in *The Grasmere Rushbearing* (1905) by British painter Frank Bramley.

Sweet flag is also known as "singer's root" because chewing on its ginger-tasting "root" numbs vocal cords, allowing tired voices to go on

Extracts of the plant are used as a flavouring agent and as an ingredient in bitters – spirits infused with bitter plant extracts. In parts of North America, the roots of the native variety, var. *americanus*, have been used to make sweets called candied roots or calamus candy. While its sweet-tasting stalks can be peeled and eaten raw, its roots, once washed and peeled, can be chopped up and boiled as a kind of sweet vegetable, like yams.

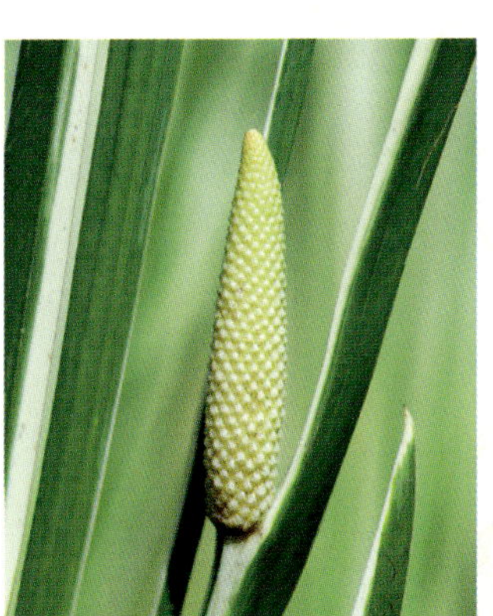

◄ Fragrant flower
Sweet flag only flowers when growing in water, producing a spadix – a spike of closely packed, yellow-green florets. Rising from the leaf axil, the spadix is 5–10 cm (2–4 in) long.

By any other name

Sweet flag grows in the temperate climates of North America and Eurasia, extending south to the Middle East, India, and Sri Lanka, and east to China. It has been cultivated in the Indian subcontinent and Europe. Generally known as calamus or cinnamon sedge, sweet flag is also called sway or sweet cane. It has many regional names as well, such as gladdon in Europe, *vacha* or *bach* in India, and *zhang chang pu* in China.

The species varies across its distribution and three varieties are recognized that differ in the quantity present of a volatile oil, beta-asarone, which is potentially carcinogenic. Highest concentrations are found in var. *angustatus*, from India and other parts of Asia, and it is absent from the North American variety. Some countries have restrictions on the level of beta-asarone permitted in foods containing sweet flag.

Similar herbs

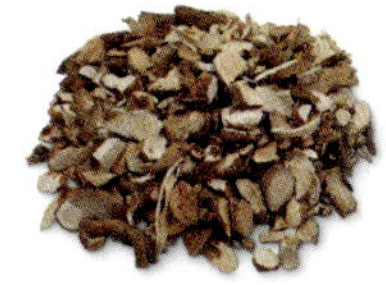

GRASS-LEAF SWEET FLAG
Acorus gramineus
This evergreen plant has narrower leaves than the sweet flag, and its roots are used to treat similar conditions as well.

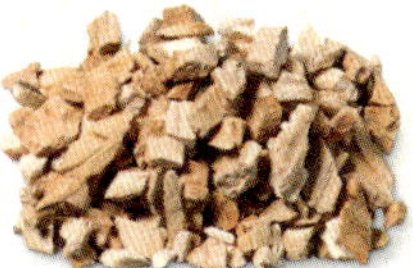

AMERICAN SWEET FLAG
Acorus calamus var. *americanus*
This North American variety was used by some Indigenous American tribes as medicine and in religious ceremonies.

Uses Medicines, cooking, perfume, cosmetics

Parts used Leaves, stems, flowers

Active ingredients Menthol, menthone, menthyl acetate, cineol, limonene, pulegone, caryophyllene, pinene

Habitat Moist, shaded areas such as stream sides

Margins are coarsely toothed
Aromatic foliage is dark green and slightly fuzzy, and often has reddish veins
Smooth stems are typically square in cross-section

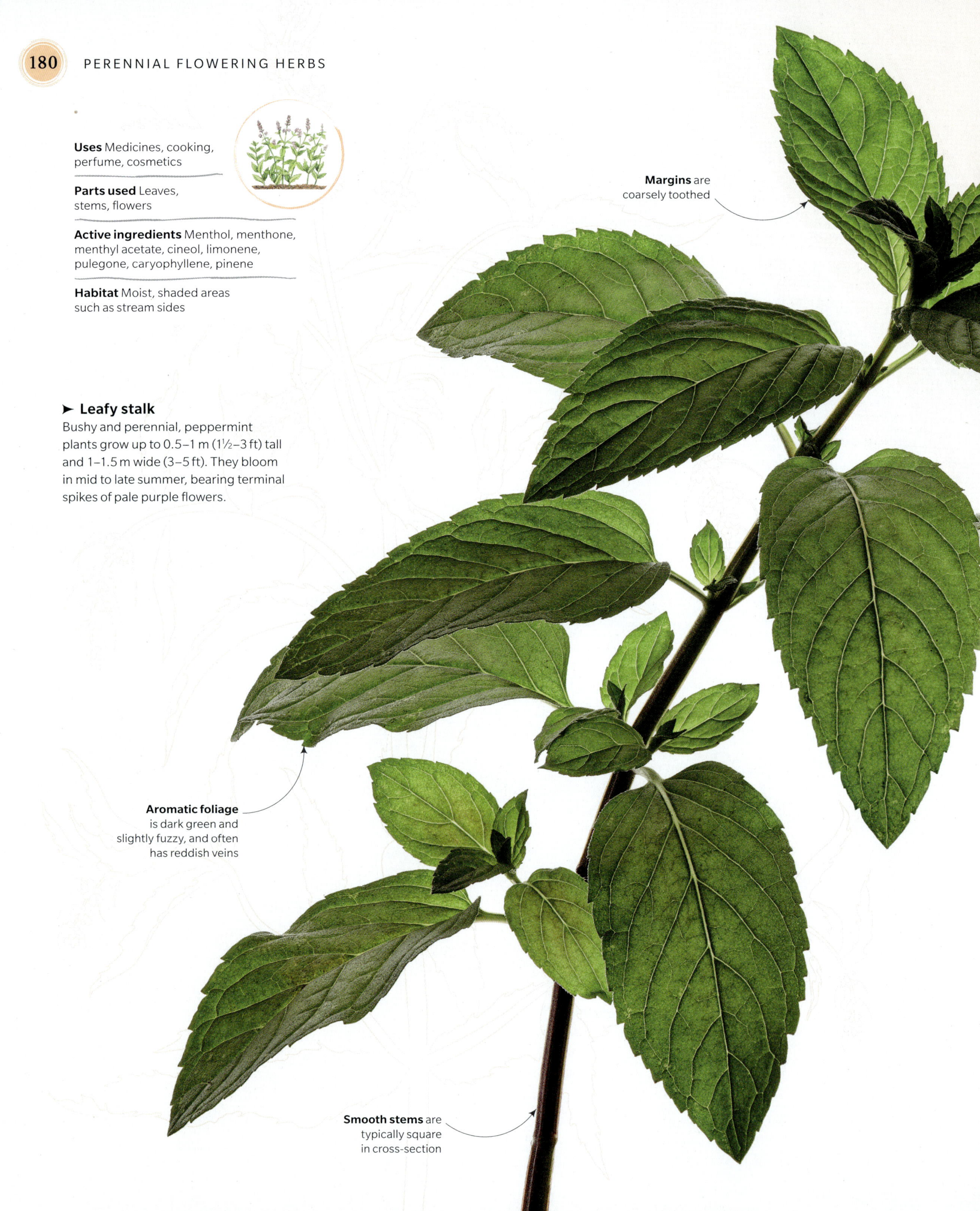

➤ Leafy stalk

Bushy and perennial, peppermint plants grow up to 0.5–1 m (1½–3 ft) tall and 1–1.5 m wide (3–5 ft). They bloom in mid to late summer, bearing terminal spikes of pale purple flowers.

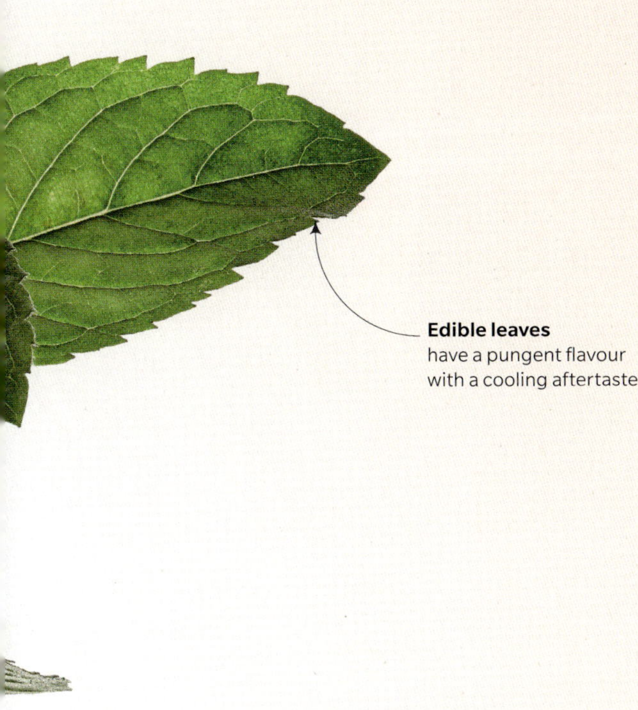

Edible leaves have a pungent flavour with a cooling aftertaste

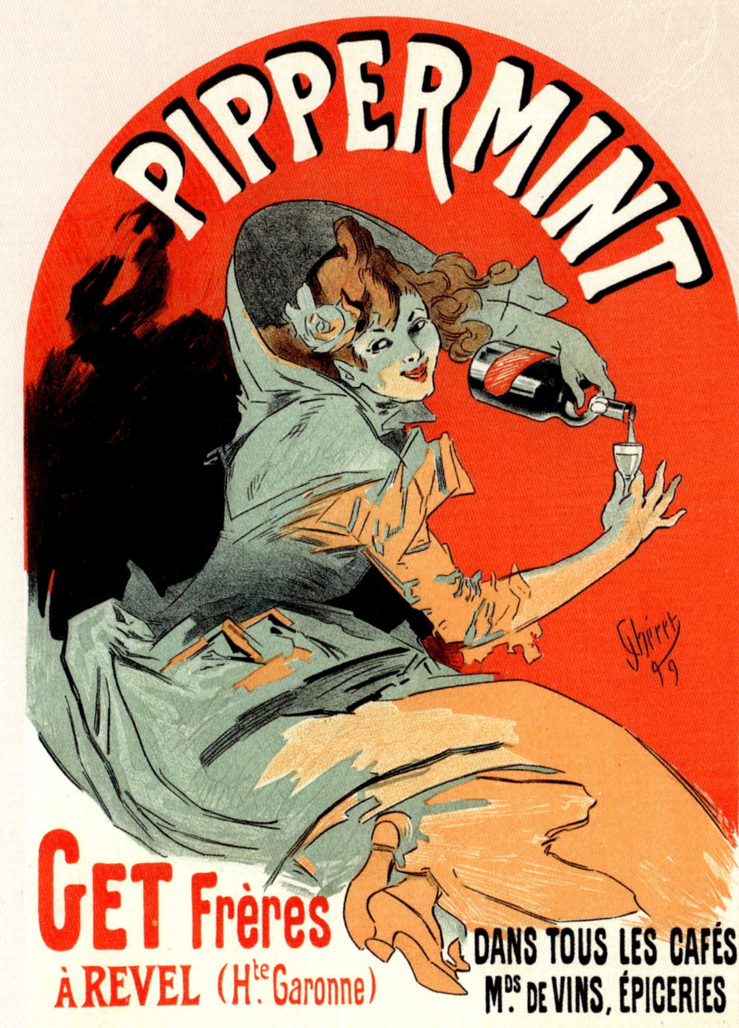

Peppermint

Mentha × piperita

▲ Crème de menthe
Pippermint (now marketed as Get 27) is a high-quality, crème de menthe liqueur. First manufactured in 1796, the popular beverage was later produced by the Get brothers, as seen in this 1899 poster by Jules Chéret.

This highly aromatic herb has been used for thousands of years to ease digestion, scent the body and home, enliven the senses, and as a refreshing ingredient in food and drinks.

As a naturally occurring hybrid species of mint (*Mentha*) – indigenous across Europe and the Middle East – peppermint found its way into many ancient civilizations, growing wild by riverbanks and in drainage ditches, and spreading vigorously above ground via stolons (runners) and underground via rhizomes.

In *A Modern Herbal* (1931), English herbalist Mrs M. Grieve describes "the several varieties of the Peppermint" as the most important of the mint family (Lamiaceae), and highlights commercial cultivars – 'Mitcham', 'Black', and 'White', for example – grown in England, France, Italy, Hungary, and the US for their volatile oils in particular. Peppermint is still widely cultivated today for its aromatic and flavoursome leaves and its essential oil, with large-scale producers including the US, Morocco, and Argentina.

Ancient worth

The ancient Egyptians are known to have used mint in many guises, including as a remedy for indigestion, for combatting unpleasant breath caused by poor nutrition and dental hygiene,

➤ Minty breath
"Curiously strong" Altoids were originally launched in the 1780s to relieve intestinal discomfort, but they are also used to freshen breath and to treat congestion and coughs.

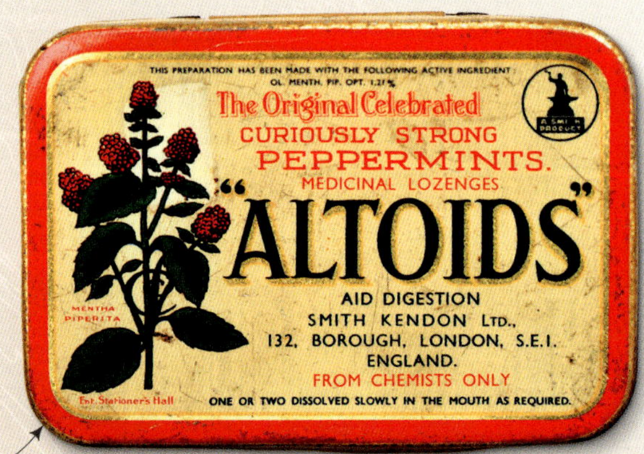

Lozenges are still packaged in distinctive metal tins

and as a ritual perfume. The ancient Greeks also advocated the use of mint for its scent, flavour, and invigorating properties. It was used in funerary rites, not only to mask bad aromas but also to encourage hope in the afterlife. The latter use is possibly linked with the genus name *Mentha*, which is thought to stem from the mythical story of the Greek nymph Minthe. Beloved by the god of the underworld, Hades, Minthe antagonized Hades' wife Persephone and was crushed into the earth, from which sprang a "mint" plant. The Romans also lauded mint, spreading its value and cultivation across their empire.

The mint plant was documented in various herbals as a popular culinary and medicinal herb, but the earliest record of the name "peppermint" is in English botanist John Ray's *Synopsis Methodica Stirpium Britannicarum* in 1696. There, he described its leaves as having a flavour of *fervido Piperis* or "hot pepper". Swedish botanist Carl Linnaeus fixed the herb's scientific name as *Mentha piperita* in 1753, and we now know peppermint to be a hybrid species – between water mint (*M. aquatica*) and spearmint (*M. spicata*) – which is indicated by the symbol "×".

Medicinal menthol

Peppermint was admitted into the *London Pharmacopoeia* – an official publication containing a list of medicinal drugs and directions for their use – in 1721. It has a sharp mint odour and taste, in contrast to less potent spearmint (*M. spicata*) or fruity mints, such as apple mint (*M. suaveolens*). The herb's strong aroma and flavour come largely from high levels of the compound menthol, which is known to trigger cold-sensitive receptors in the skin, thus providing a cooling or anaesthetic (painkilling) sensation. Menthol is a cholagogue (see p.185) and has choloretic and antispasmodic activities. It can help to relieve spasms in the stomach or other muscles, which is potentially beneficial in the treatment of irritable bowel syndrome and other digestive issues. In addition, peppermint has antibacterial, antiviral,

> " Both leaves and flowers have a pleasant scent, and a hot biting taste, like pepper. "
>
> NICHOLAS CULPEPER, *Complete Herbal*, 1653

Similar herbs

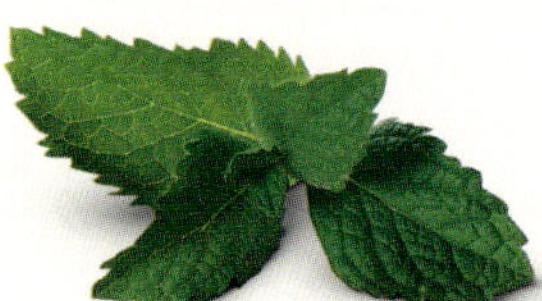

APPLE MINT
Mentha suaveolens
Rounded, softly hairy, grey-green leaves have a low menthol content and a fresh, fruity fragrance and flavour that works well in jellies, sauces, salads, and drinks.

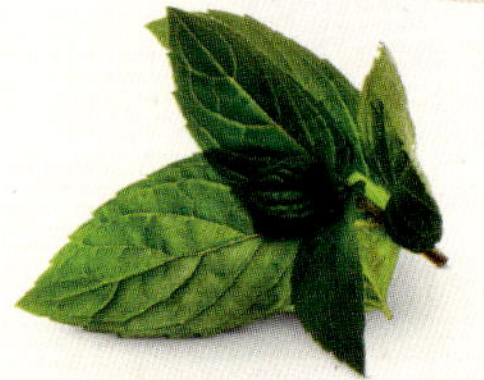

PENNYROYAL
Mentha pulegium
This traditional spearmint-scented folk remedy has been used to combat fleas and fight colds. The oil is highly toxic if ingested and can cause harm in pregnancy.

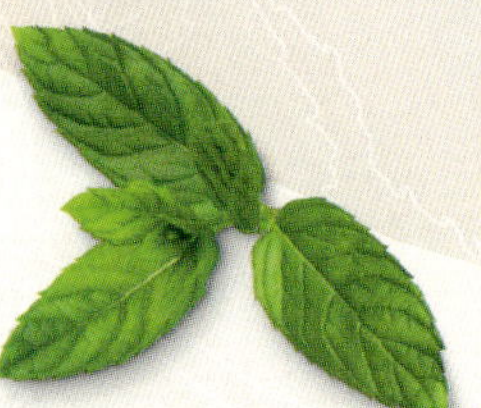

SPEARMINT
Mentha spicata
Spearmint has a high carvone content, which gives it a distinctive sweet smell. It is popularly used in toothpaste, Moroccan mint tea, chewing gum, and cosmetics.

In the Middle Ages, mint was used to treat insect bites, ease digestive problems, clean teeth, and freshen breath

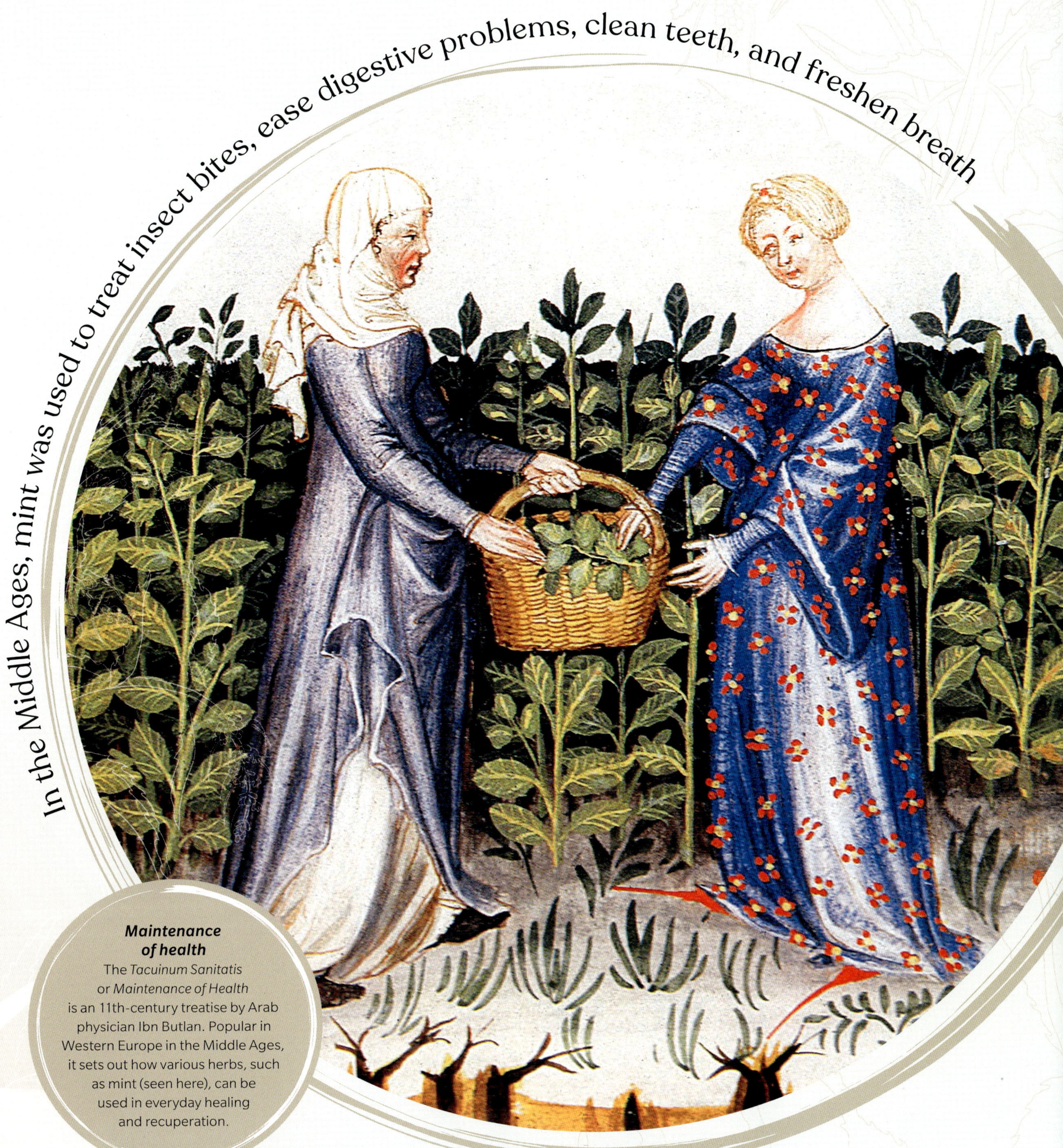

Maintenance of health
The *Tacuinum Sanitatis* or *Maintenance of Health* is an 11th-century treatise by Arab physician Ibn Butlan. Popular in Western Europe in the Middle Ages, it sets out how various herbs, such as mint (seen here), can be used in everyday healing and recuperation.

➤ Parts used
This detailed illustration from Dr Wilibald Artus's *Hand-Atlas* (1848) shows the various parts of peppermint, including the five-petalled, two-lipped flowers and the glandular-haired leaves from which the volatile oil is distilled.

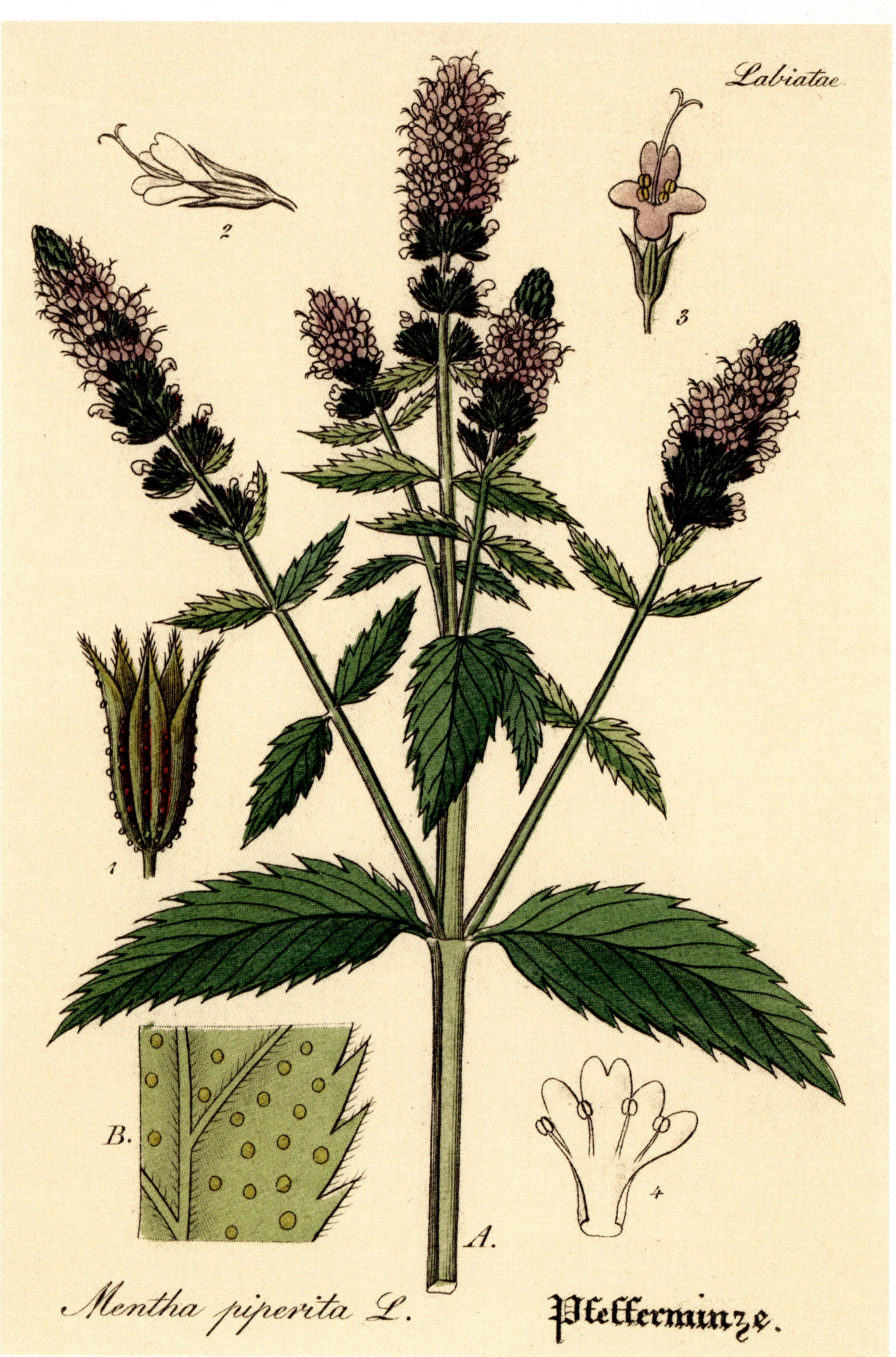

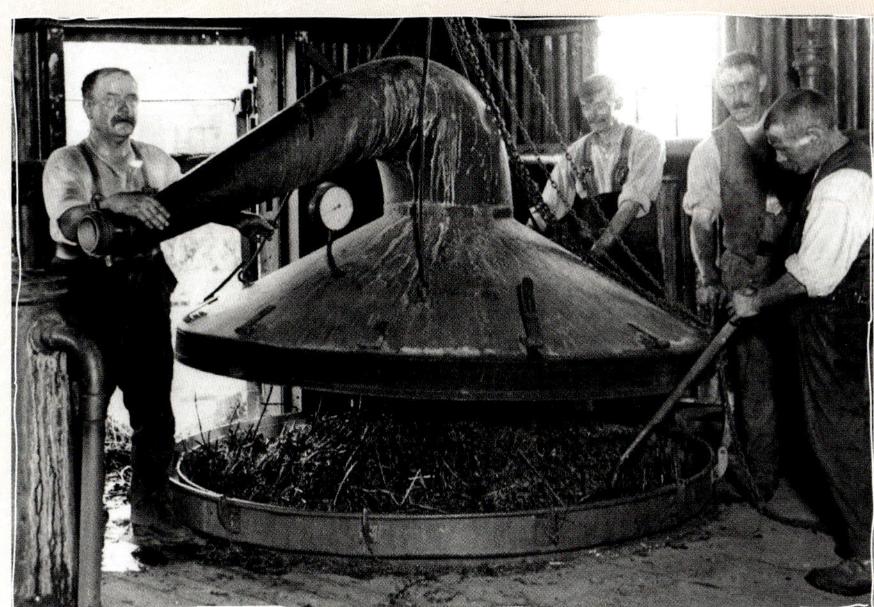

◄ Extracting oil
Peppermint essential oil is traditionally extracted from fresh or dried leaves using steam distillation, as practised at this distillery near Reigate, UK, in 1925. It can then be used to flavour food or in aromatherapy to treat various conditions.

The ancient Egyptians used mint as a digestive, as described in the Ebers Papyrus (c.1550 BCE)

and antiseptic properties, which are useful in the treatment of coughs, colds, throat infections, and flu. The benefits of the essential oil are often delivered through an inhalation or steam bath.

Minty fresh flavour and scent

Peppermint's clean fresh fragrance lends itself well to bath and body products. Its aromatherapeutic action reduces stress by simultaneously stimulating brain function and encouraging relaxation through the deeper intake of breath. This energizing calm can help create space for new ideas and foster optimism, without the potentially sedative effect of other nervines, such as lavender or chamomile. Peppermint oil can be used in perfumes, home scents, and cleaning products – the herb was traditionally strewn over floors to deodorize and freshen rooms – and works well with floral, citrus, or woody notes.

The scent of mint, most easily extracted by simply rubbing or crushing a leaf and holding it up to the nose, stimulates the taste buds. Popular refreshing treats include peppermint tea – drunk for its digestive, palate-cleansing, and energy-boosting effects, as well as for its pleasant flavour – and mint-flavoured cocktails (although spearmint provides a more subtle flavour for classics such as the mojito). Culinary favourites include mint sauce. Peppermint extract is used to create the defining taste of popular confectionery, for example chocolate mints, peppermint creams, and festive candy canes. Garden cultivars such as *M. × piperita* f. *citrata* 'Chocolate', reminiscent of the flavour of dark chocolate mints; *M. × piperita* f. *citrata* 'Lime', with fruity tones; and *M. × piperita* 'Lavender Mint', with a hint of lavender provide a suite of more niche flavours to use in food, drinks, and garnishes. Peppermint has also been a largely aromatic component of many oral hygiene products since the 19th century, with high levels of menthol providing minty fresh scent, flavour, and a clean cooling sensation in the mouth.

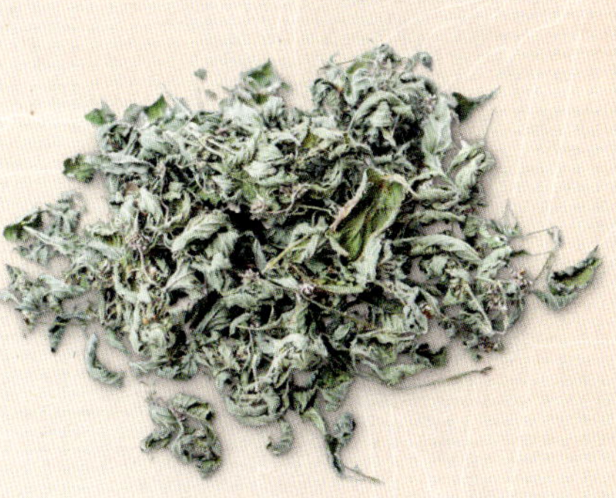

▲ Dried leaves
Peppermint's medicinal and culinary benefits can be preserved by drying its leaves. These can then be used whole or crushed.

WHAT ARE CHOLAGOGUES AND CHOLERETICS?

Choleretics help stimulate bile production in the liver, ready to flow into the gall bladder, while cholagogues help stimulate the flow of bile by assisting gall bladder contractions. Stored bile can then be used to break down fats into digestible fatty acids. It also helps flush the body of toxins. Herbs with choleretic-cholagogue properties include peppermint (*M.* x *piperita*), turmeric (*Curcuma longa*), mugwort (*Artemisia vulgaris*), and grapefruit (*Citrus* x *paradisi*).

Uses Medicines for digestive and respiratory conditions; galactagogue

Parts used Fruits (seeds), flowers (pollen), leaves, stalks

Active ingredients Trans-anethole, fenchone, limonene, pinene

Habitat Full sun and well drained soil; often near seacoasts

Golden pollen provides an intense, sweet, and earthy flavour in cooking

➤ Umbellated flowers
Fennel flower heads appear as umbrellas (umbels) of tiny flowers on slender stalks. The flowering stems are used as a flavouring agent in beverages and spirits, and their dried form is used in herbal teas.

Fennel

Foeniculum vulgare

Delicate stalks can be used to flavour soups and stews

Dark green, feathery leaves can be used as a garnish or to add flavour to food

This Mediterranean member of the carrot family (Apiaceae) can be found in the wild or grown as a garden herb. Its anise-flavoured flowers, fruits, and leaves are used in food and as a digestive.

Native to the Mediterranean, North Africa, the Middle East, and parts of Asia, fennel has been widely naturalized further afield. Its use as a herb can be traced as far back as ancient Egypt, where it was mentioned in the medical text Ebers Papyrus (c.1550 BCE). The ancient Greeks prized fennel, known as *marathos*, as a culinary and medicinal ingredient. The region of Marathon, where the Greeks defeated the Persians in battle in 490 BCE, was named for this herb, which grew in abundance there. It was recommended by Greek physicians Hippocrates and Dioscorides to increase breast milk production in nursing mothers. The Romans cultivated fennel to treat a number of maladies, including stomach ailments and the stings of scorpions and serpents. It is one

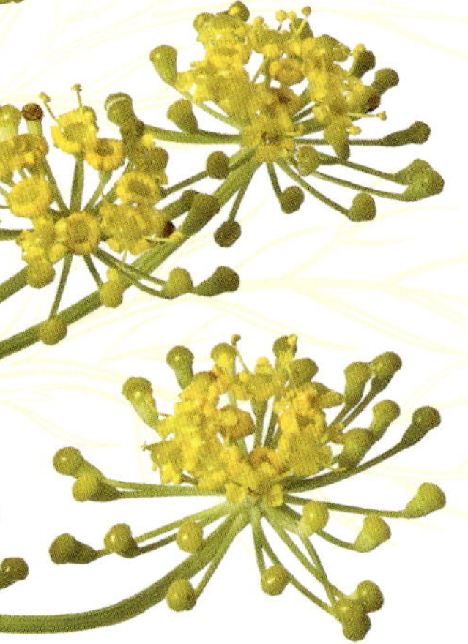

Yellow flowers bloom in mid to late summer, followed by fruits in late summer to early autumn

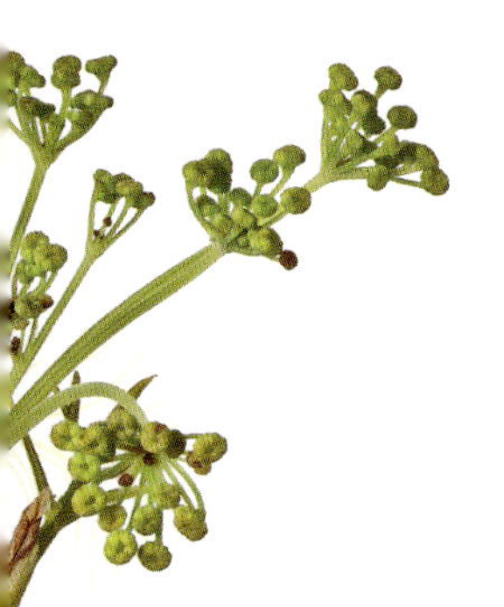

“The seed is carminative, expelling Wind, strengthening the Bowels and helping the Colic.”

ELIZABETH BLACKWELL, *A Curious Herbal*, 1737–39

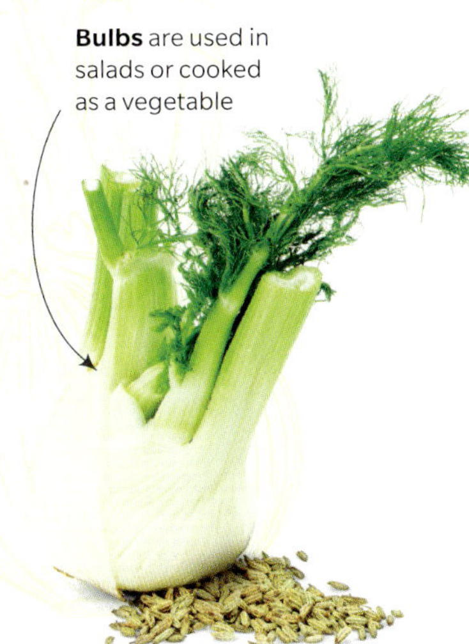

Bulbs are used in salads or cooked as a vegetable

of the herbs featured in the Saxons' Nine Herbs Charm – the recipe for a cure capable of warding off infection and poison. In his 10th-century *Canon of Medicine*, Persian polymath Ibn Sina (Avicenna) promoted the herb for treating eye conditions and as an anti-inflammatory.

➤ Florence fennel
Sometimes referred to as *F. v.* var. *azoricum*, Florence fennel is the group of cultivars grown for their edible "bulbs" or swollen leaf bases, which have a mild aniseed flavour.

Delivering health and flavour

Volatile compounds in fennel's essential oil include antibacterial and antiseptic agents. The compound anethole is being studied for its ability to suppress cell growth, with potential for use in anti-cancer applications. Evidence suggests fennel may have galactogenic (breast milk-increasing) and phytoestrogenic (estrogen-mimicking) properties to improve lactation in nursing mothers and regulate the menstrual cycle.

The two varieties most commonly used as herbs are bitter and sweet fennel. Bitter fennel (*F. v.* var. *vulgare*) is largely used medicinally and in Eastern European cooking. Sweet fennel (*F. v.* var. *dulce*) is more widely used in cooking.

As a culinary herb, fennel is used to flavour fish, breads, roasts, salads, sweet dishes, tea, and liqueurs. In India, fennel seeds (technically its fruits) are the core ingredient of the post-meal snack known as *mukhwas*, a naturally sweet, digestive aid and palate cleanser. It is also a key ingredient in Kashmiri and Gujarati cooking. In Chinese herbal medicine it is known as a cooling herb, while the ground seed is a component of Chinese five spice – a blend of sweet, bitter, salty, sour, and savoury spices for culinary use. The sweet, uplifting scent of this plant is also used in perfumes, bath and body products, and home fragrances.

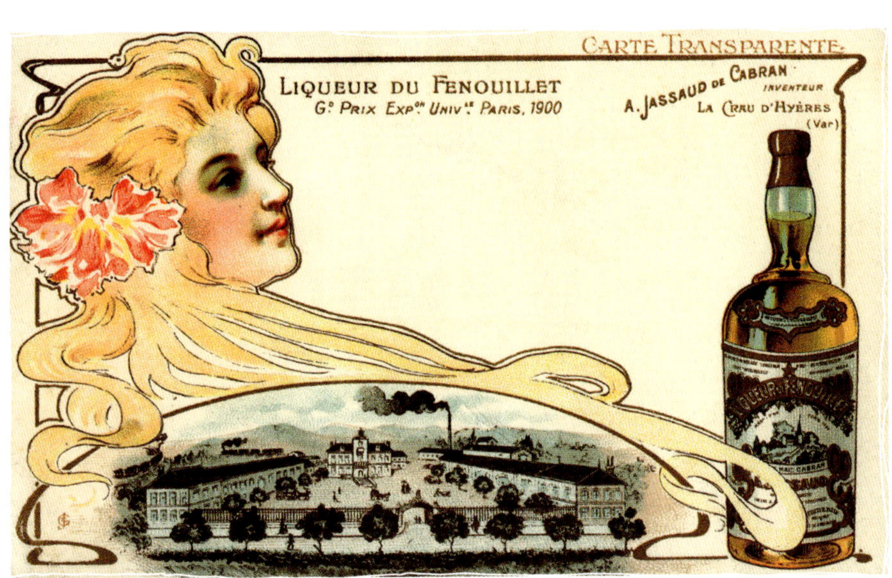

➤ Fennel-based digestive
Fennel is well known for its digestive qualities. The anti-inflammatory, antibacterial, and carminative (flatulence relieving) properties of its seeds help relax the gut. The early 19th-century French liqueur Fenouillet was one such remedy.

Similar herb

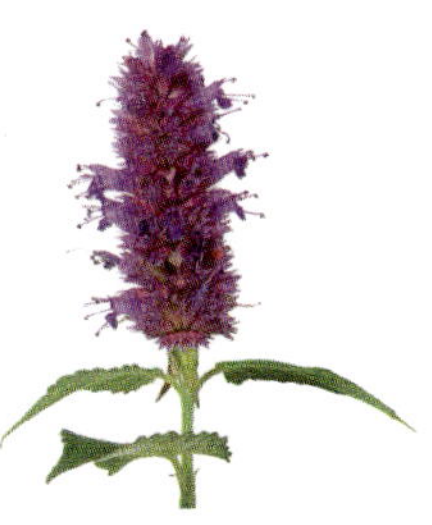

ANISE HYSSOP
Agastache foeniculum
As with fennel, this herb has an anise flavour, but with hints of mint, basil, and lemon. The leaves are traditionally used to treat coughs, sore throats, and fevers.

Angelica

Angelica archangelica

Uses Medicines for indigestion, rheumatism, colds; cooking; glue; perfume

Parts used Stalks, fruits (seeds), leaves, roots

Active ingredients Angelicin, pinene, phellandrene, terpenes, cyclopentadecanolide

Habitat Grows in damp soil and open spaces, such as marshes and riverbanks

From curing the plague and warding off evil spirits to flavouring liqueurs and garnishing cakes, this popular ornamental plant has an illustrious history, and its varied uses continue to the present day.

Native to northern Scandinavia, Russia, Iceland, Greenland, and the Faroe Islands, angelica is also known as the Viking herb. These Nordic seafaring warriors may have helped in the spread of the herb, carrying it with them as they colonized large parts of Western Europe, where it has been cultivated ever since. Angelica was likely an important herb at the time, not only as food and medicine, but also as a commodity for trade.

Heavenly herb

Angelica typically blooms around a Christian feast day associated with St Michael the Archangel (8 May). Legend has it that an archangel visited a monk in his dream and told him of the herb's virtues as a cure for the plague. It was also believed to provide protection against evil spirits, and was used as powder, syrup, poultice, or infusion to cure a wide range of ailments, including dog bites and ulcers. Angelica is now used for its carminative (preventing gas), expectorant (discharging mucus), and diaphoretic (inducing perspiration) properties.

The distinctive scent of its flowers and leaves has notes of earth, musk, celery, pepper, juniper, and a hint of citrus. This aroma can also be derived from its roots and is used in perfumes. Angelica fruits are used as a flavouring agent in liquors such as chartreuse, gin, and vermouth. Ironically, angelica root tea – to be avoided if pregnant or diabetic, or using blood-thinning drugs – has a bitter, warming, and invigorating taste that is thought to dispel the urge for alcohol. Perhaps the strongest-flavoured part of angelica, however, is its hollow stem, traditionally preserved by candying in sugar and used in slices on cakes or bakes, or as the emerald green component in tutti frutti ice cream. Stems can also be boiled up with sugar and lemon to make a gin-flavoured jam.

➤ Living large

This tall biennial puts down thick, brown tap roots to support its statuesque stalks, large leaves, and enormous umbels of flowers. It can be confused with its toxic relatives including water hemlock (*Cicuta virosa*) and giant hogweed (*Heracleum mantegazzianum*), so is best cultivated rather than foraged for use.

A "CURE" FOR THE PLAGUE

The bubonic plague swept through the medieval world leaving unprecedented death and disaster in its wake. With no medical cure or explanation in sight, people turned to religion and mysticism for respite. Nicknamed "the root of the Holy Ghost", angelica was seen as a possible cure. Plague doctors wore masks with beaks stuffed full of such fragrant herbs to afford them protection against the "bad air" thought to be responsible for the disease.

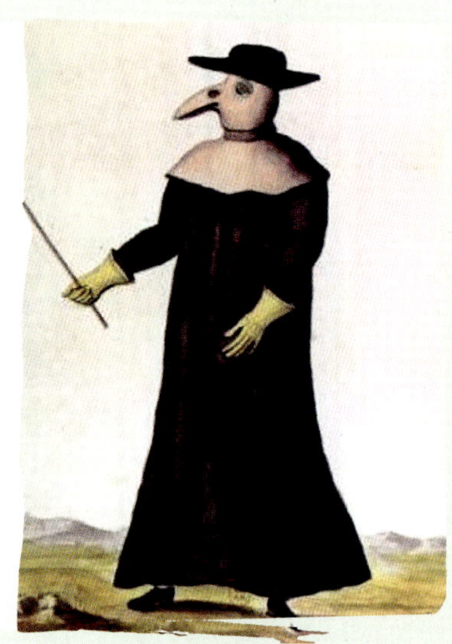

MEDIEVAL PLAGUE DOCTOR

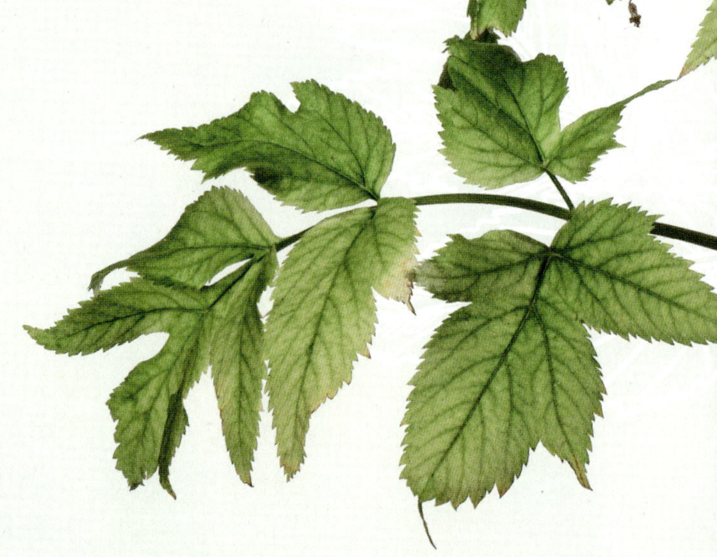

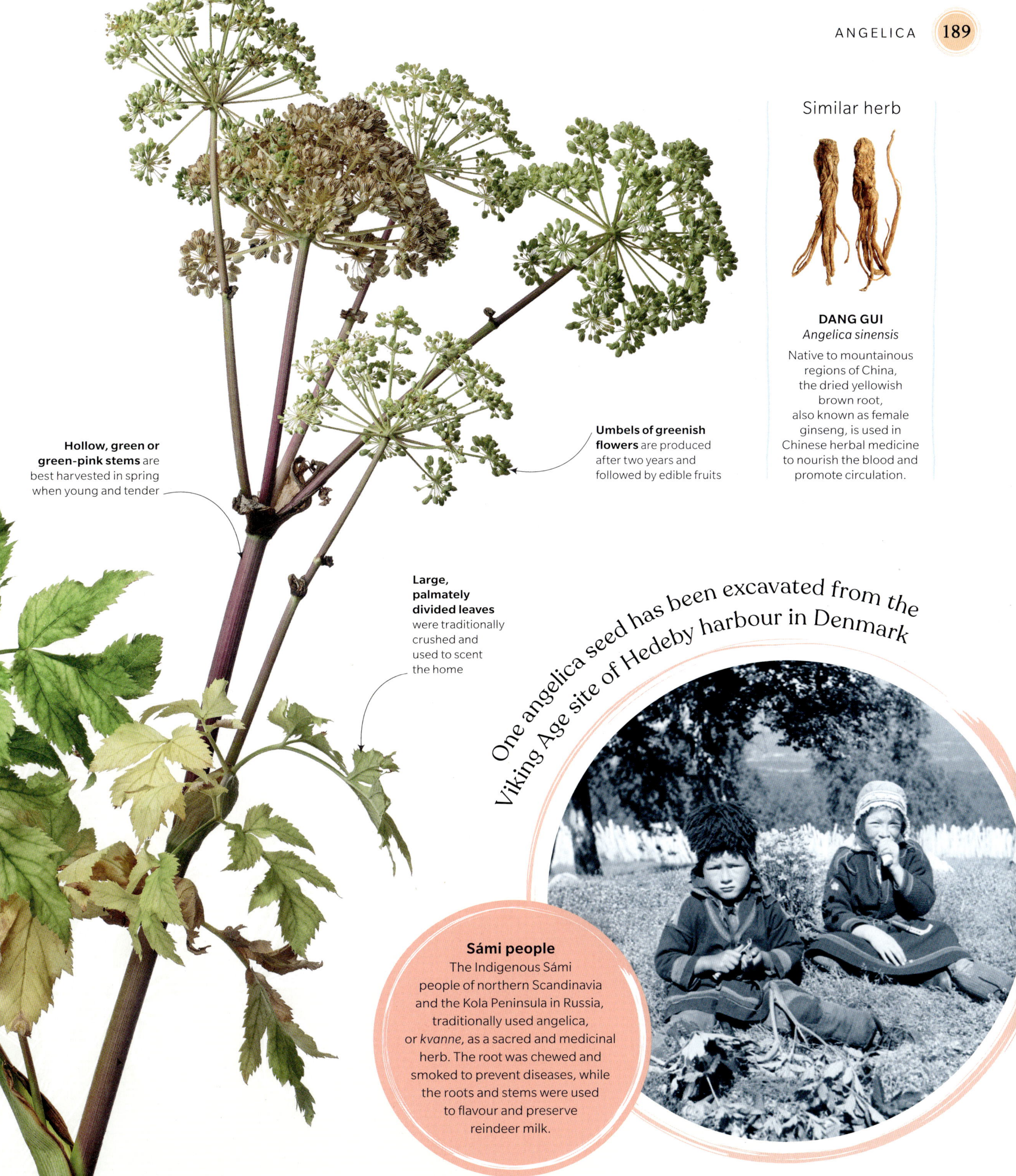

Hollow, green or green-pink stems are best harvested in spring when young and tender

Umbels of greenish flowers are produced after two years and followed by edible fruits

Large, palmately divided leaves were traditionally crushed and used to scent the home

Similar herb

DANG GUI
Angelica sinensis

Native to mountainous regions of China, the dried yellowish brown root, also known as female ginseng, is used in Chinese herbal medicine to nourish the blood and promote circulation.

One angelica seed has been excavated from the Viking Age site of Hedeby harbour in Denmark

Sámi people

The Indigenous Sámi people of northern Scandinavia and the Kola Peninsula in Russia, traditionally used angelica, or *kvanne*, as a sacred and medicinal herb. The root was chewed and smoked to prevent diseases, while the roots and stems were used to flavour and preserve reindeer milk.

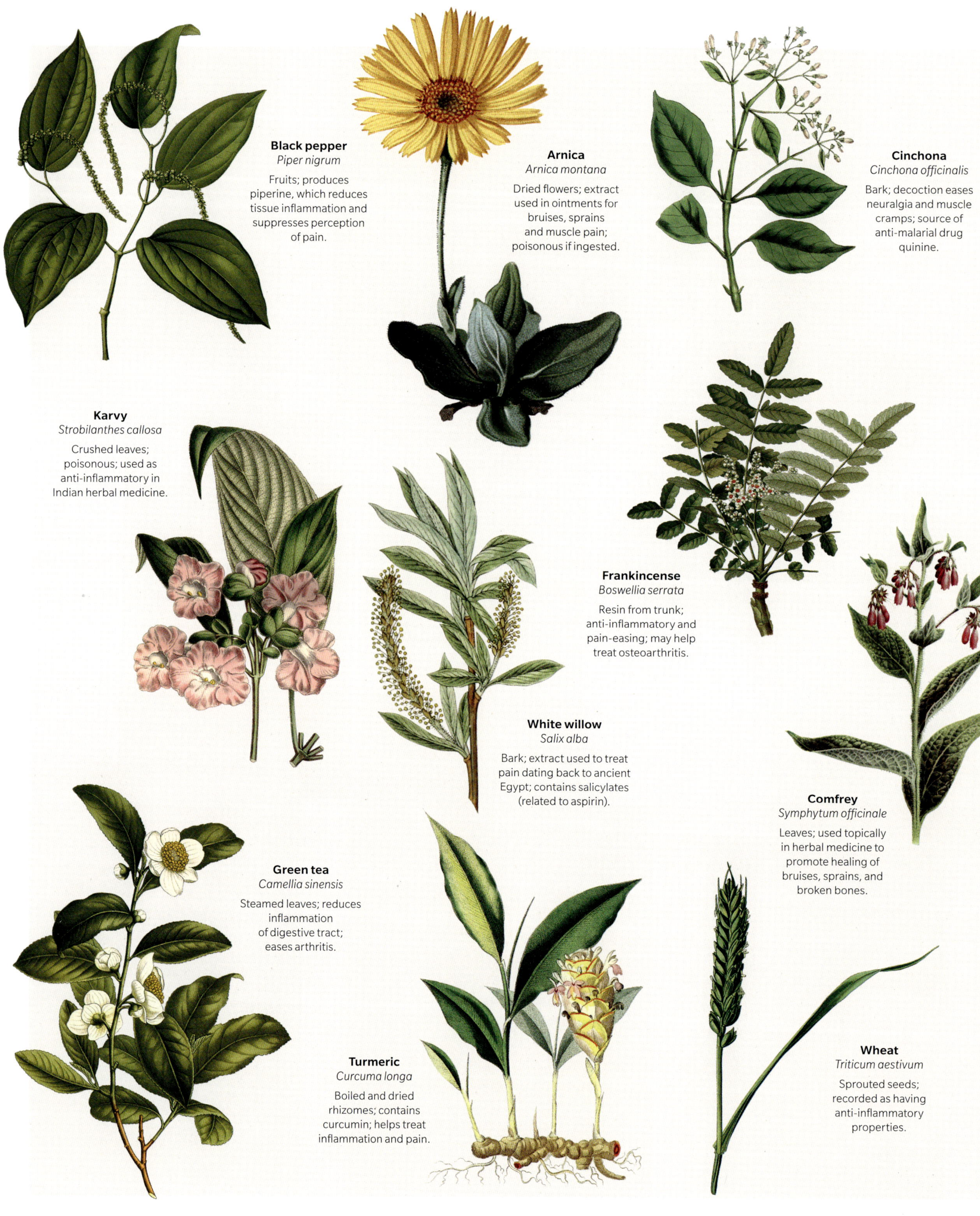
Black pepper
Piper nigrum
Fruits; produces piperine, which reduces tissue inflammation and suppresses perception of pain.
Arnica
Arnica montana
Dried flowers; extract used in ointments for bruises, sprains and muscle pain; poisonous if ingested.
Cinchona
Cinchona officinalis
Bark; decoction eases neuralgia and muscle cramps; source of anti-malarial drug quinine.
Karvy
Strobilanthes callosa
Crushed leaves; poisonous; used as anti-inflammatory in Indian herbal medicine.
Frankincense
Boswellia serrata
Resin from trunk; anti-inflammatory and pain-easing; may help treat osteoarthritis.
White willow
Salix alba
Bark; extract used to treat pain dating back to ancient Egypt; contains salicylates (related to aspirin).
Comfrey
Symphytum officinale
Leaves; used topically in herbal medicine to promote healing of bruises, sprains, and broken bones.
Green tea
Camellia sinensis
Steamed leaves; reduces inflammation of digestive tract; eases arthritis.
Turmeric
Curcuma longa
Boiled and dried rhizomes; contains curcumin; helps treat inflammation and pain.
Wheat
Triticum aestivum
Sprouted seeds; recorded as having anti-inflammatory properties.

Rosemary
Salvia rosmarinus
Leaves; rosmarinic acid protects against inflammatory diseases.
Lavender
Lavandula angustifolia
Flowers, leaves; oil of lavender helps heal burns and sores, and reduces inflammation; relieves pain of insect stings.
Magnolia
Magnolia officinalis
Flowers, bark; volatile oils soothe inflammation, muscle tension, and menstrual cramps.
Meadowsweet
Filipendula ulmaria
Leaves; salicylates (related to aspirin) ease arthritic, rheumatic, and joint pain, as well as headaches.
Clove
Syzygium aromaticum
Dried flower buds; oil treats wounds; reduces mouth inflammation and pain in toothache.
Ginseng
Panax ginseng
Root; extract used in traditional medicine against inflammatory diseases; adaptogenic tonic.
Jasmine
Jasminum officinale
Flowers; oil used in dermatology as an anti-inflammatory agent and antiseptic.
Japanese bitter orange
Citrus trifoliata
Fruit, flowers; valued in Asian medicine to treat digestive disorders, and as an anti-inflammatory including for allergic inflammation.

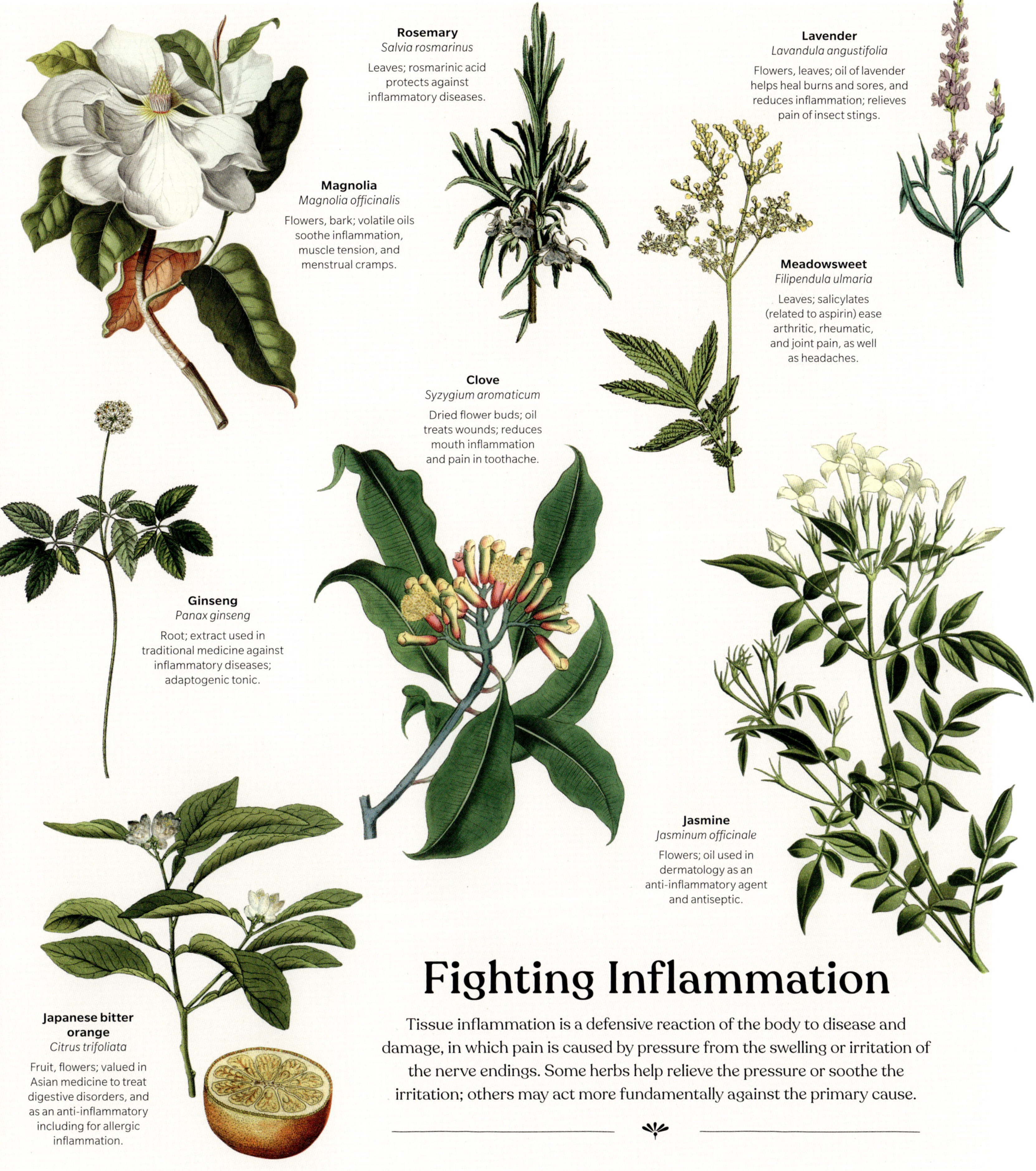

Fighting Inflammation

Tissue inflammation is a defensive reaction of the body to disease and damage, in which pain is caused by pressure from the swelling or irritation of the nerve endings. Some herbs help relieve the pressure or soothe the irritation; others may act more fundamentally against the primary cause.

Liquorice

Glycyrrhiza glabra

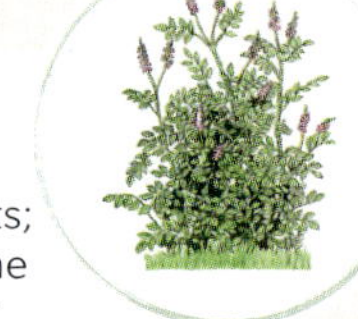

Uses Medicines for respiratory, digestive, and menopause-related ailments; cooking; cosmetics; perfume

Parts used Roots, rhizomes (stolons)

Active ingredients Glycyrrhizin, glabridin

Habitat Riverbanks, roadsides, field margins, in sandy soil, in warm temperate regions

Humans have used this naturally sweet herb since antiquity. Its roots and runners can be utilized as a culinary flavouring, in confectionary, and as a tea; they are also used to treat certain digestive and respiratory ailments.

The herbal extract and ingredient known as liquorice, or licorice, is made from dried roots and runners – low growing rooting stems – of the *Glycyrrhiza glabra* plant. Native to the Middle East, Asia, and the Mediterranean region of southern Europe, *G. glabra* is one of 17 accepted species in the genus including American liquorice (*G. lepidota*), hedgehog liquorice (*G. echinata*), and Chinese liquorice (*G. uralensis*).

A soothing herb

The name *Glycyrrhiza* stems from the Greek word *glukoriza*, as used by the physician Dioscorides in his book *De Materia Medica* (*On Medical Material*). In this five-volume pharmacopoeia, written from 50–70 CE, he describes the sweet (*glukos*) root (*riza*) of a small shrub that grows abundantly in the Mediterranean regions of Cappadocia and Pontus (now districts in Turkey). He states that these "bitter and sweetish" roots can be juiced, chewed, made into a decoction, or dried and ground. Dioscorides recommends its use for disorders of the arteries, chest, skin, and digestive system. He advocates taking it with a drink of raisin wine to quench thirst, rubbing it on to heal wounds, or applying it to growths on the membranes of the eyes. The book also chronicles the use of this herb by the Romans, who called it *dulcis radix*. It is thought that Romans issued this herb to their troops, who chewed on it to quench thirst and improve stamina.

In his book *Historia Naturalis* (77–79 CE), Roman scholar Pliny the Elder describes liquorice as a remedy for asthma, mouth ulcers, and throat conditions. Today, liquorice is known to have antioxidant, anti-inflammatory, and antimicrobial

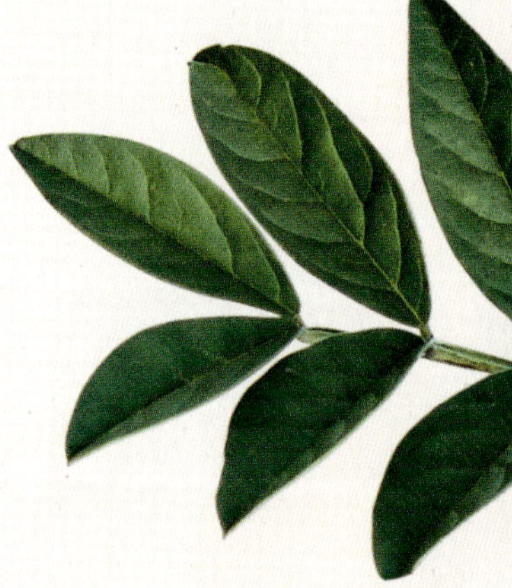

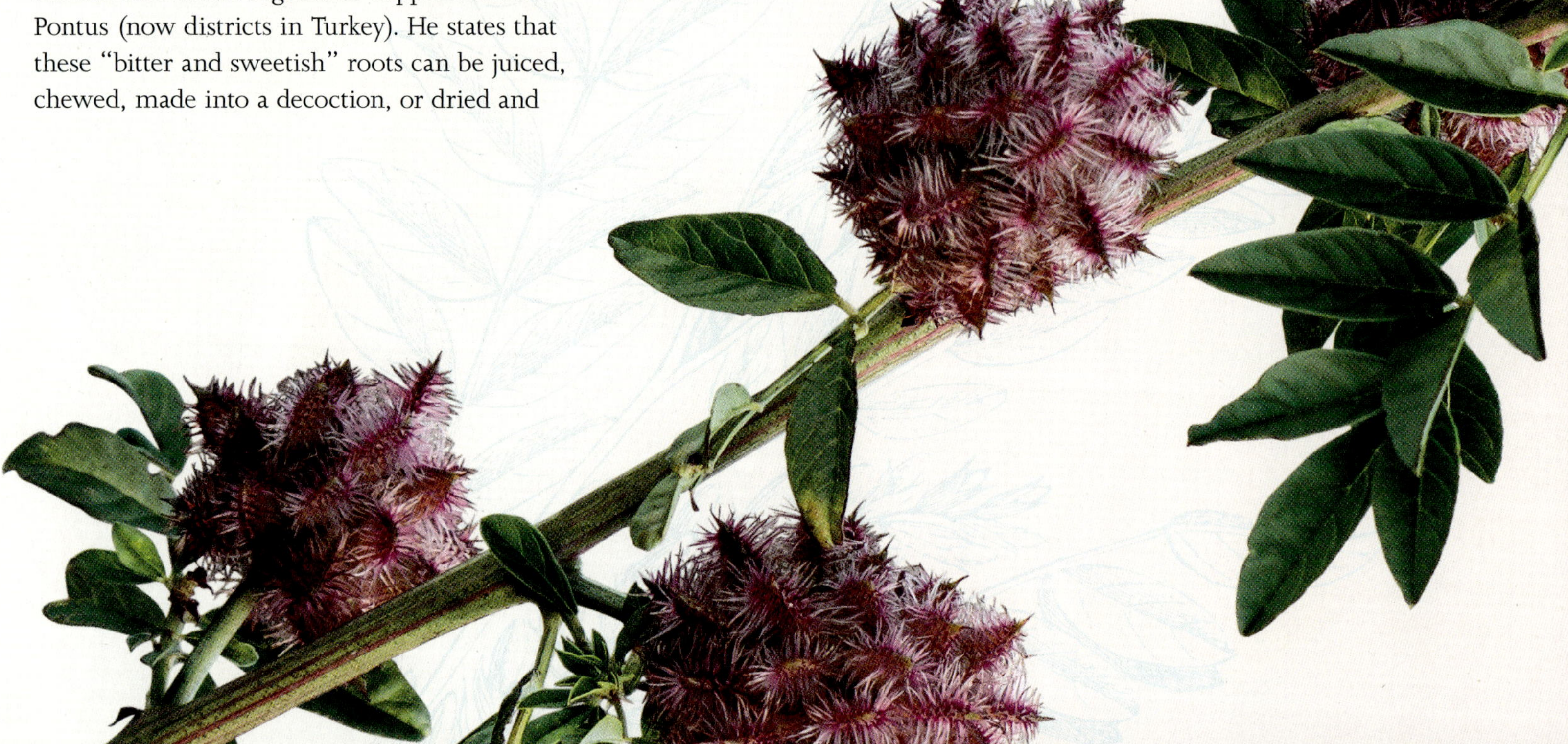

➤ Liquorice plant

Liquorice is a small, woody bush that grows to about 120 cm (47 in) tall. It bears sticky, pinnate leaves and upright spikes of flowers. Its fruit pods are smooth or sparsely hairy. Other species, such as the hedgehog liquorice (*G. echinata*), can have spiny fruit.

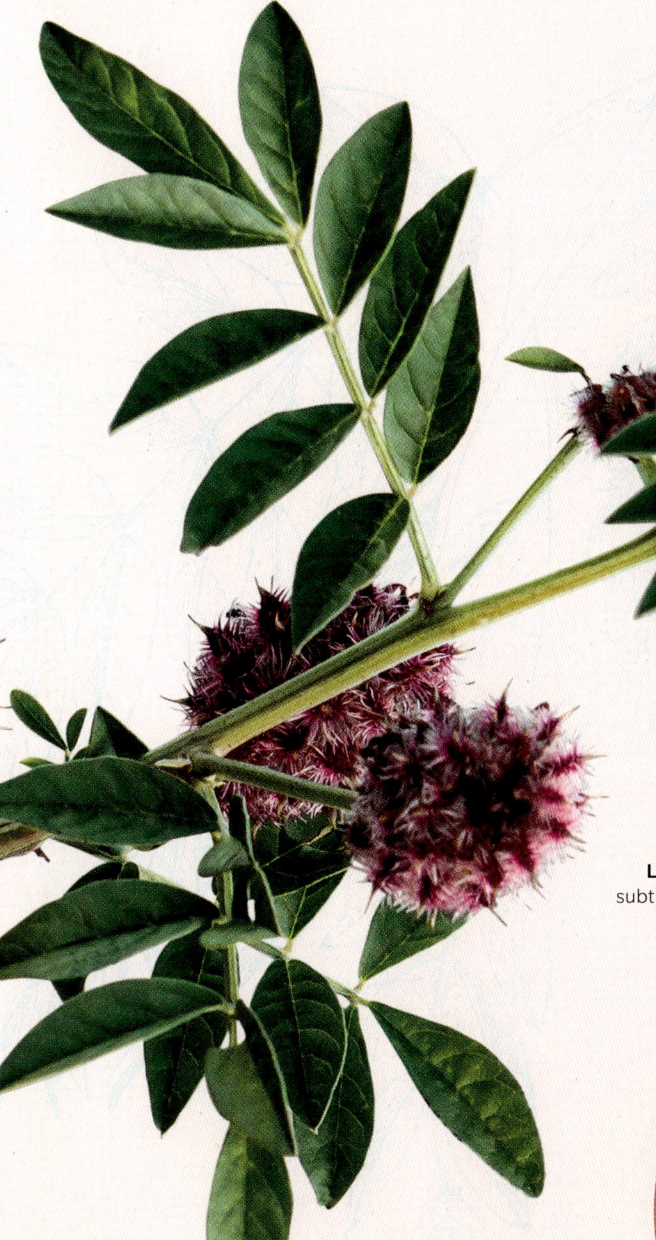

Leaflets give off a subtle liquorice scent

Spiny fruits appear after blooms in summer

The use of **liquorice** has been recorded on **Assyrian clay tablets** from around **2500** BCE

HOW DO LAXATIVES WORK?

Some plants work as laxatives to relieve constipation. These include husks from psyllium (*Plantago ovata*) seeds, which absorb water and are a bulk-forming laxative; senna from the pods or leaves of Alexandrian senna (*Senna alexandrina* syn. *Cassia angustifolia*), which stimulates bowel movements; and arachis oil from the peanut plant (*Arachis hypogaea*), which softens stools. Liquorice (*Glycyrrhiza* spp.) is a mild laxative and is added to other preparations for its sweet taste.

Wrinkled brown roots or "sticks" have a yellow stringy flesh inside

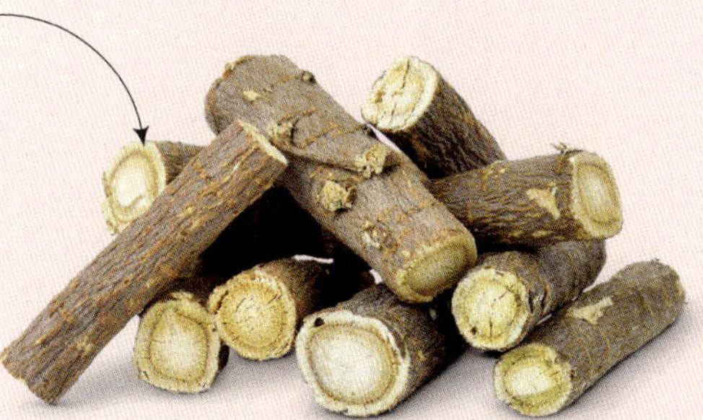

➤ Liquorice "sticks"

Liquorice has an extensive root system consisting of a tap root, root branches, and long horizontal stolons or runners, which can all be harvested in autumn to access their sweet, medicinal active ingredients.

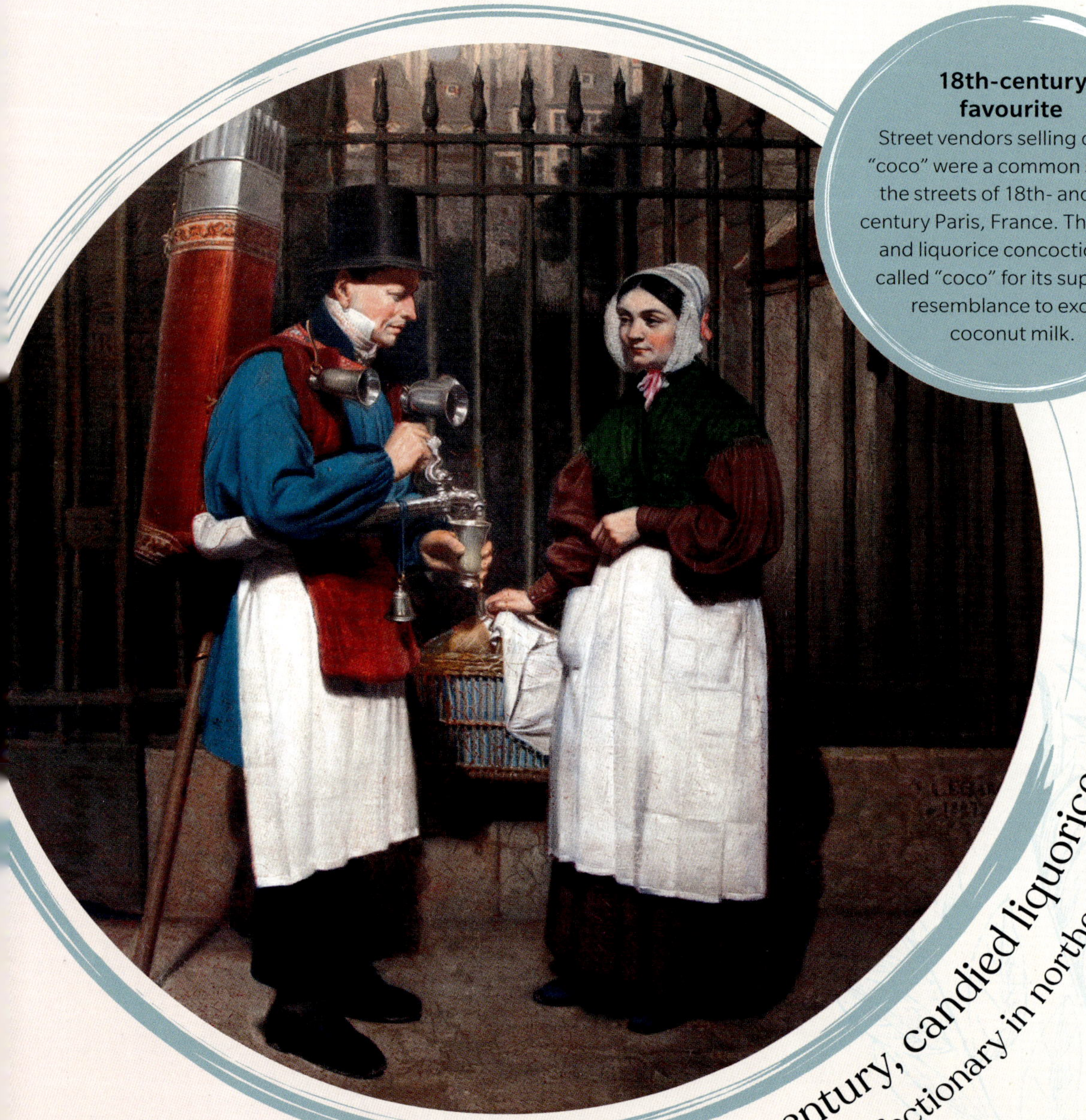

18th-century favourite

Street vendors selling cups of "coco" were a common sight on the streets of 18th- and 19th-century Paris, France. This lemon and liquorice concoction was called "coco" for its supposed resemblance to exotic coconut milk.

By the 19th century, candied liquorice was a popular form of confectionary in northern Europe

Similar herbs

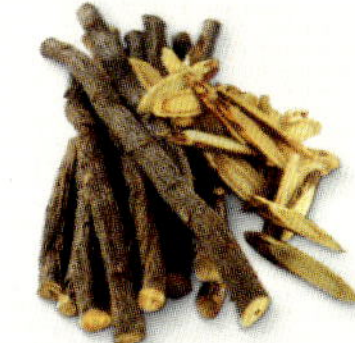

CHINESE LIQUORICE
Glycyrrhiza uralensis
Native to Asia, this is used in traditional Chinese medicine to regulate the immune system and potentially treat tumours.

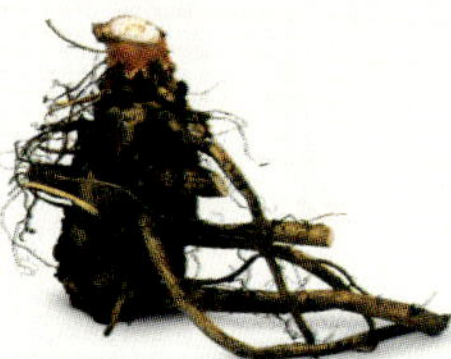

MARSH MALLOW
Althaea officinalis
Roots are useful for calming inflamed areas of the respiratory and digestive systems, treating skin conditions, and thickening food.

properties. It is used to soothe throats and the digestive system, treat bacterial and viral infections, and combat symptoms of menopause.

Naturally sweet

Many of liquorice's medicinal benefits relate to its key active ingredient glycyrrhizin, a compound that is 50 times sweeter than sugar (sucrose). This sweetness can be accessed simply by chewing the roots, but is more commonly extracted to be used as a flavouring and in confectionery. Liquorice has a strong flavour and can be used in sweet and savoury dishes, to make a soothing tea, or with other herbs in spice mixes, stocks, and marinades. The Dutch use it to make a salty candy called *drop* and the English to make sweet, colourful "allsorts". However, despite its pleasant taste, overconsumption of liquorice can be harmful.

➤ Liquorice candies
"Black" liquorice is a traditional, sugar-based candy that has been flavoured and dyed black using liquorice roots. Additional ingredients include starch/flour, gum Arabic, gelatine, and beeswax for shine.

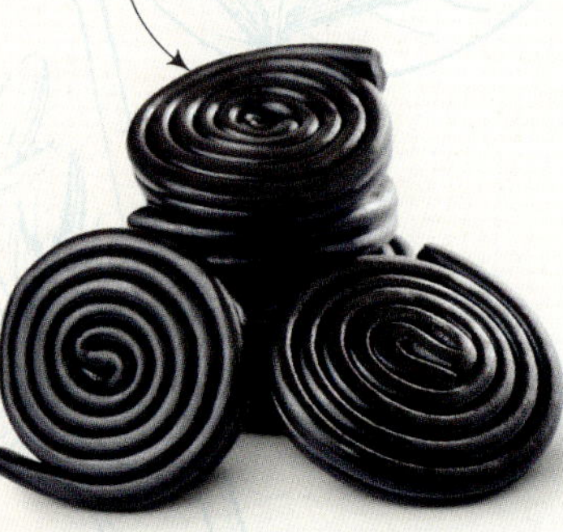

Liquorice wheels are made by rolling up still-warm candy ropes

Meadowsweet

Filipendula ulmaria

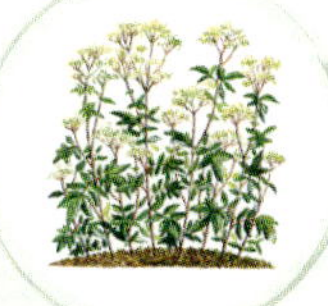

Uses Medicines for pain relief; cooking; cosmetics; perfume

Parts used Flowers, leaves

Active ingredients Salicylates including salicin, salicylaldehyde, and methyl salicylate; tannins; flavonoids; mucilage

Habitat Damp soil in grassland, heathland, meadows, and ditches

The flowers and leaves of this fragrant plant are traditionally used to scent the home and flavour food and drink. Meadowsweet also has gut-soothing, anti-inflammatory, and pain-relieving properties.

Borne in clusters, the creamy white flowers of this plant have an almond-like fragrance. In the past, it was used as an uplifting summer strewing herb and in bridal garlands. It was added to wine and beer as a sweetener – hence its common name meadowsweet, from meadwort (the mead or honey-wine herb). One of the sacred Druid herbs, it was also used to cure diarrhoea, to break a fever, and to treat joint and muscle pain.

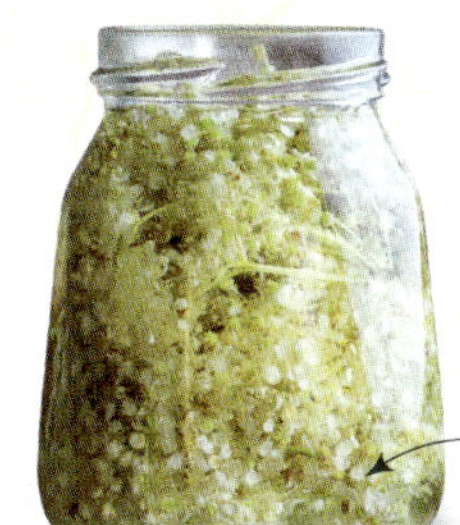

◄ Meadowsweet tincture
Meadowsweet flowers are combined with glycerine and alcohol to make a homemade remedy for inflammatory pain, headaches, and stomach ache.

Flowers soak, or macerate, for 4–6 weeks to create a healing tincture

The salicylic effect

Meadowsweet is now known to be gently astringent, diuretic, antimicrobial, analgesic, anti-inflammatory, and mucilaginous. It is used to treat gastric issues such as heartburn and stomach ulcers, and provide relief from osteoarthritic pain. Many of these benefits may be attributed to its high levels of salicylates – also found in willow (*Salix* spp.). The body oxidizes salicylates into salicylic acid, which provides pain relief. Both plants inspired the invention of the pain-relieving drug aspirin.

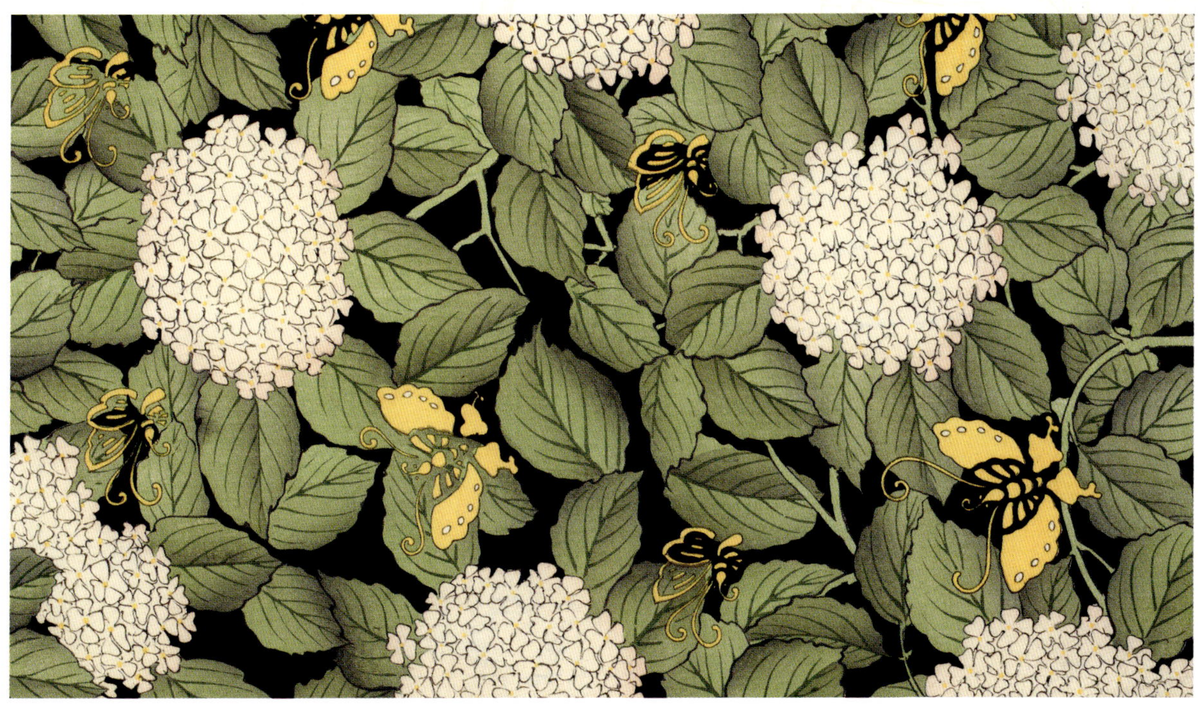

◄ Herbal inspiration
This woodblock print features stylized flowers and leaves inspired by the meadowsweet relative, germander meadowsweet (*Spiraea chamaedryfolia*). Both are in the rose family (Rosaceae).

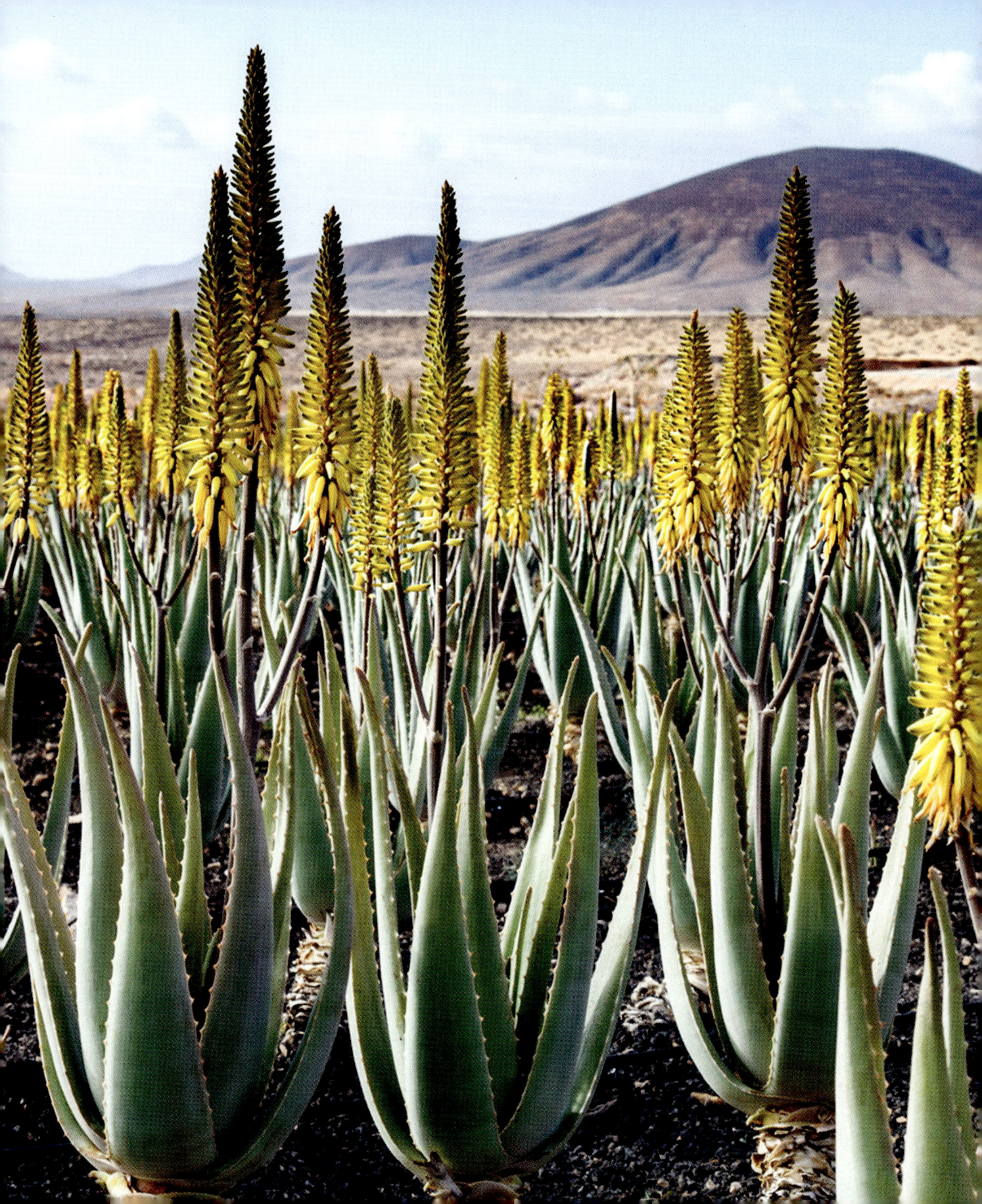

> “Romans call it aloa, and the Barbarians, aloe.”
>
> DIOSCORIDES, *De Materia Medica*, 50–70 CE

Uses Medicines for burns and wounds, cosmetics, cooking

Parts used Leaves

Active ingredients Salicylic acid, magnesium lactate, gel polysaccharides, folic acid, vitamins A, B, C, and E in gel; anthraquinones in leaf juice

Habitat Grows wild in rocky, exposed areas and arid climates

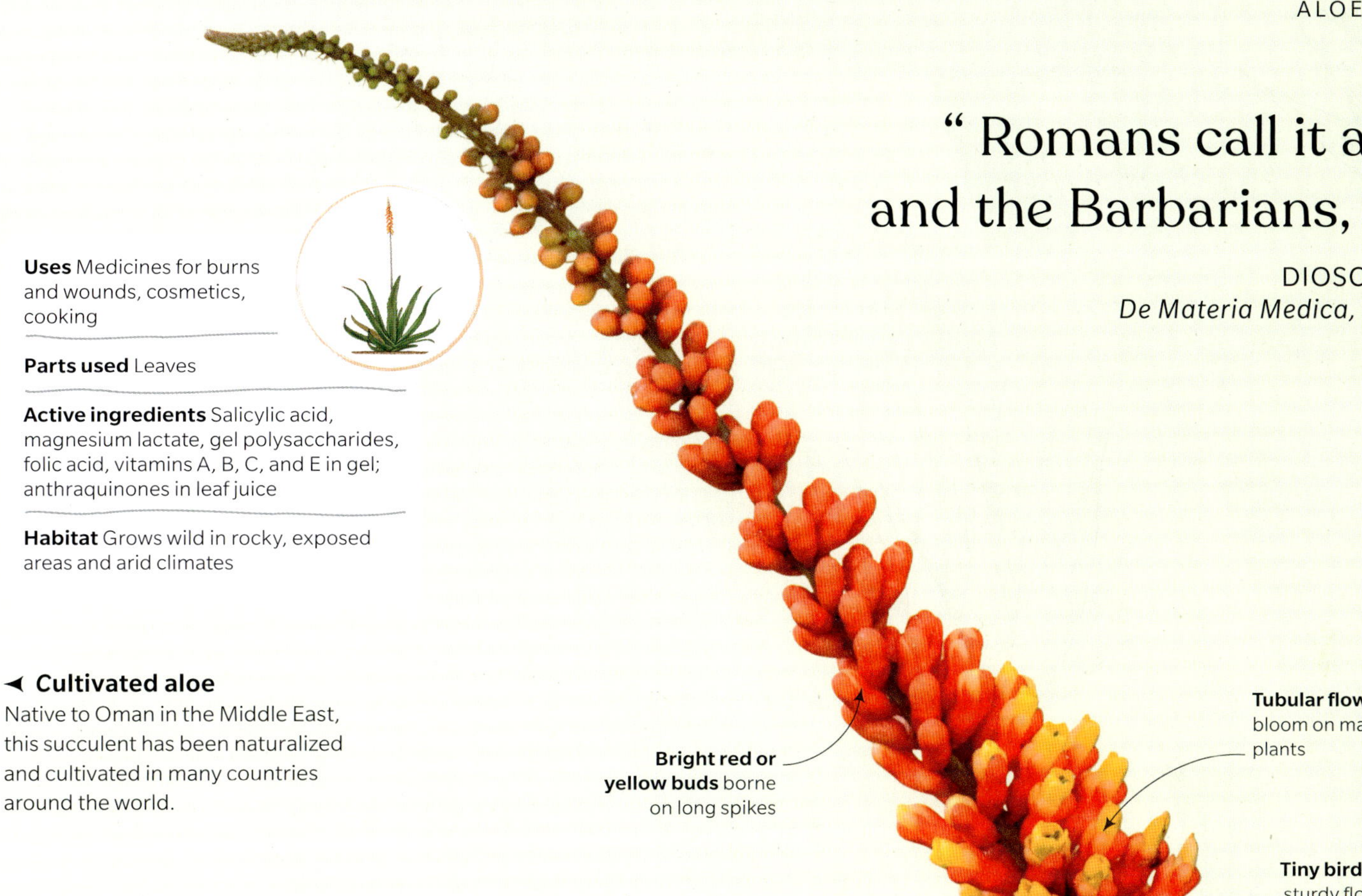

◄ **Cultivated aloe**
Native to Oman in the Middle East, this succulent has been naturalized and cultivated in many countries around the world.

Aloe Vera

Aloe vera

Aloe vera is among the world's most widely cultivated herbs. The gel from its leaves is commonly used to cool skin and maintain a healthy digestive system. However, as one of more than 500 members of the *Aloe* genus and with numerous synonyms, its history is less than straightforward.

Despite being so widely distributed and used around the world, *Aloe vera* is native only to the Arabian Peninsula, specifically Oman. Once the healing properties of this plant's gel became apparent, its popularity grew. Oman's proximity to early trade routes between Asia and the Mediterranean ensured that this hardy succulent travelled out and flourished wherever the conditions were suitable.

Its ability to store water in its thick, fleshy leaves not only helps aloe thrive in predominantly dry and arid climates, but is also the secret of its soothing gel. Stemless, green-grey aloe leaves have serrated, white-toothed edges and may have white flecks in some varieties. Its tubular buds transform into bright flowers, which are largely pollinated by birds. *Aloe* reproduces through either seeds or "pups" – cloned offsets that form at the base of a mature plant, which then grow into new plants.

Naming aloe

While more than 500 species of *Aloe* are accepted today, many are still referred to by synonyms or their botanic status remains unresolved. This is indicative of the confusion that abounds through

▲ **Summer-blooming flowers**
Aloe species are often pollinated by birds, such as this purple-rumped sunbird that feeds on the abundance of nectar found in the flowers.

➤ Barbados aloe
The German apothecary and botanist Basilius Besler (1561–1629) included several species of *Aloe* in his illustrated codex *Hortus Eystettensis* (1613) including Barbados aloe, an antiquated name for *Aloe vera*.

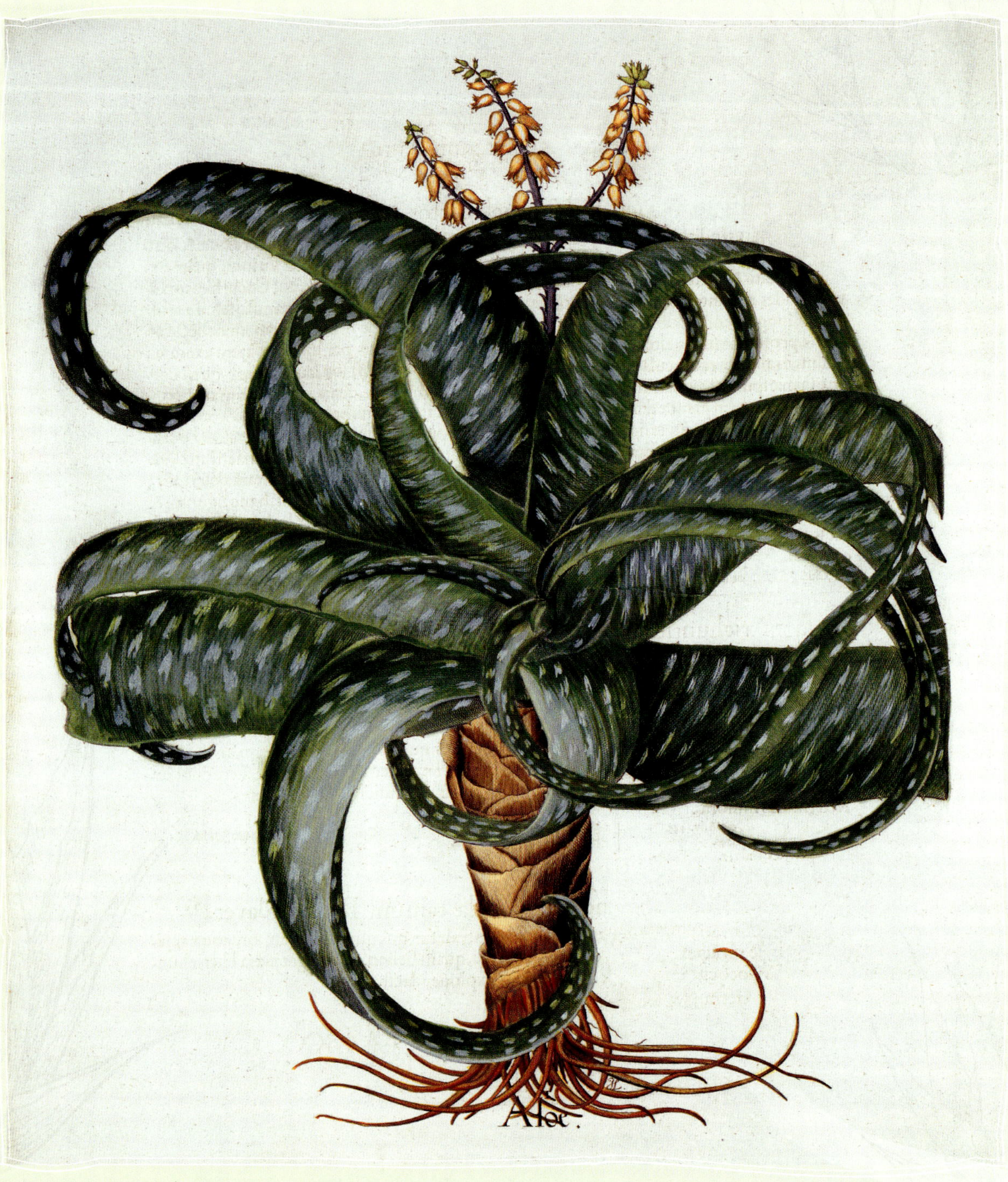

Regular intake of aloe sustained Indian leader **Mahatma Gandhi** during **long fasts**

the history of this herb as to what the "true" aloe really is. In 1753, Swedish botanist Carl Linnaeus first described this species, referring to it as *Aloe perfoliata* var. *vera*. Dutch botanist Nicolaas Laurens Burman wrote of *Aloe vera* in *Flora Indica* (1768), echoing the use of the Latin word *vera*, meaning "true". Those cultivated and then naturalized in Barbados were named *Aloe barbadensis*, as it was described by the English botanist Philip Miller in *The Gardener's Dictionary* (1768). This synonym is still used in the sale of *Aloe vera* as a popular houseplant, one of this attractive succulent's other main uses, alongside its benefits as a restorative and therapeutic herb.

The plant of immortality

The gel of this useful plant has been used for its healing properties for thousands of years. Aloe was known as "the plant of immortality" in Ancient Egypt, with a papyrus describing its pain-relieving and anti-inflammatory effects. Greco-Roman physicians, such as Aristotle, Hippocrates, and Dioscorides, hailed it as the cure for wounds, boils, eye infections, skin ailments, ulcerations, and hair loss. The Macedonian king Alexander the Great is said to have conquered the island of Socotra to secure a supply of aloe for his army. And so aloe's reputation grew. The 15th-century Italian explorer Christopher Columbus was said never to travel without it, reportedly proclaiming: "All is well, we have aloe on board". Its usefulness ensured that plantations of *Aloe* were eventually established in many tropical and subtropical parts of the world.

A CURE FOR POISON?

Throughout antiquity, people sought a universal antidote to all poisons. In the 1st century BCE such a cure-all antitode was referred to as theriac, from *theria*, a Greek word for "beast", alluding to the very real danger of venomous bites by wild animals. A page from the *Treatise on the Theriac*, an Arabic manuscript from the 13th century describing such explorations, features six potential theriacs, one of which (top left) appears to be a species of *Aloe*.

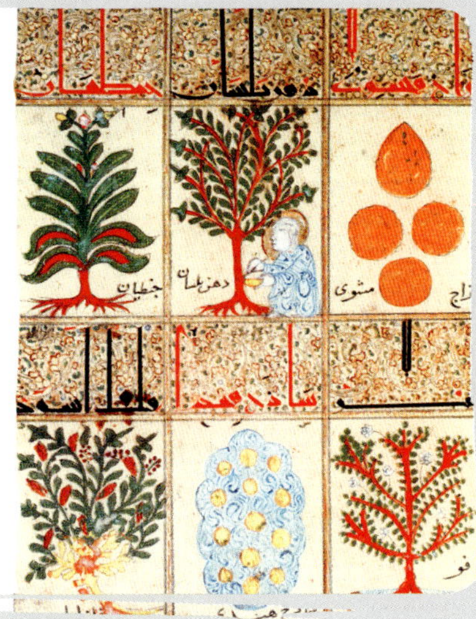

POTENTIAL ANTIDOTES AGAINST POISON

Healing herb

Although no one has proved its prowess as "the plant of immortality" quite yet, *Aloe vera*'s reputation as a healing herb persists. It is known as *kumari* in Ayurvedic medicine, meaning "young girl", alluding to its anti-ageing properties. Scientific studies suggest that *Aloe vera* gel has anti-inflammatory, antibacterial, antiviral, antiseptic, and cooling qualities, and can help revitalize skin and heal wounds. It can also be ingested to aid digestion and help to alleviate gut problems. Scraping an aloe leaf releases aloin, a bitter yellow juice found just beneath the epidermis. Historically, aloin was used as a strong laxative, but is no longer recommended, as it may be carcinogenic. Organizations such as the Royal Botanic Gardens, Kew, in the UK are conducting trials to establish if any other species of *Aloe* or related succulents, found wild in the Arabian Peninsula, Madagascar, and Africa, might also be of medicinal, cosmetic, or culinary benefit.

Egyptian queen Cleopatra is said to have used aloe as part of her daily skincare routine

Water storage cells
Veins dotted along inside edge of green, photosynthetic layer

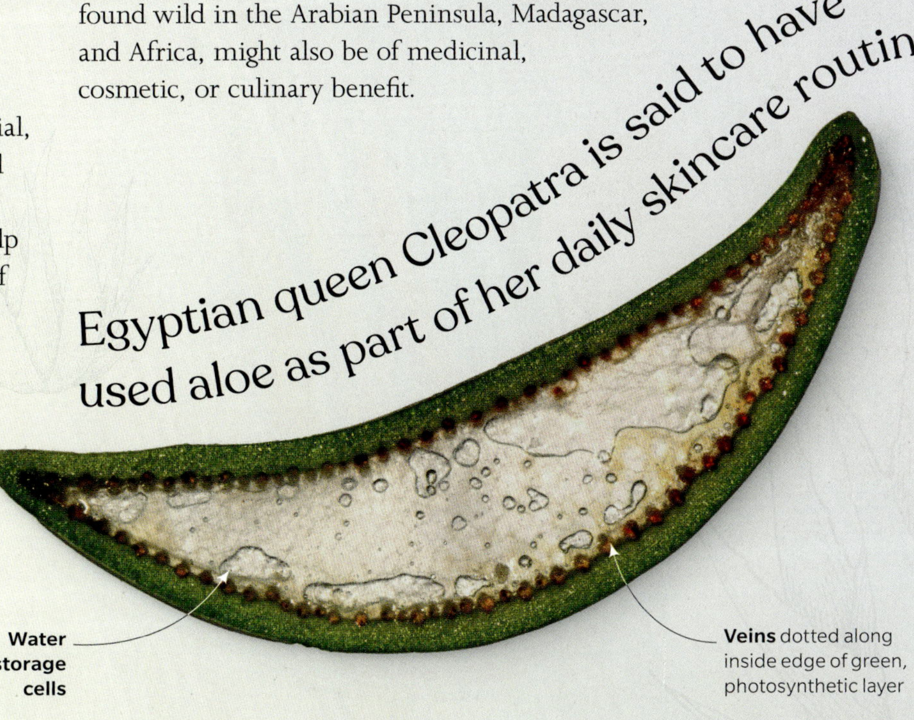

➤ **Sliced leaf of aloe**
The water stored in the inner parts of *Aloe vera* leaves make up for 99.5 per cent of the clear, sticky gel, with the remaining 0.5 per cent being soluble vitamins, minerals, phenolic compounds, and organic acids.

Similar herbs

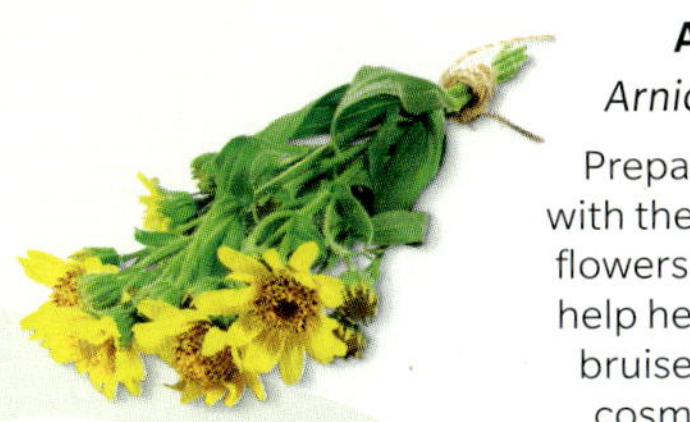

ARNICA
Arnica montana
Preparations made with the orange-yellow flowers are thought to help heal wounds and bruises. It is used in cosmetics as well.

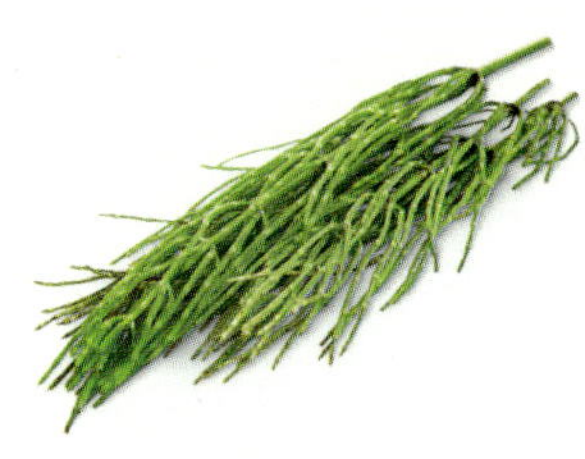

HORSETAIL
Equisetum arvense
A tea or tincture made from this antioxidant- and silica-rich living fossil is said to promote skin, hair, and bone health.

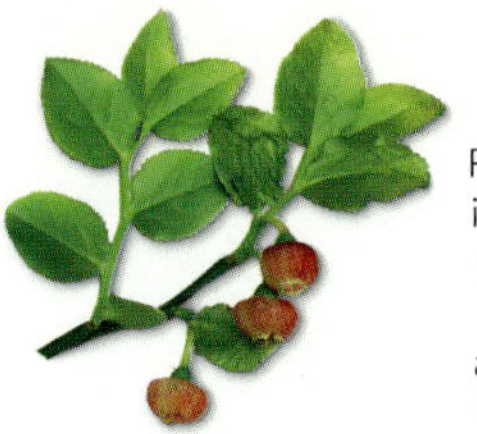

BILBERRY
Vaccinium myrtillus
Rich in antioxidants, it is used in skincare; its extract is thought to lower blood sugar; and berries are made into jams and jellies.

Uses Medicines; cooking; fibre; fertilizer

Parts used Leaves, roots, stems, seeds

Active ingredients Carotenoids, polyphenols, linolenic acid, flavonoids

Habitat Moist woodland and meadows, human habitations on phosphate-rich soil

➤ **Magnified hairs**
The cocktail of chemicals for the sting is contained in the bulb at the base of the long, brittle, syringe-like hairs. The shorter, more flexible hairs are non-stinging.

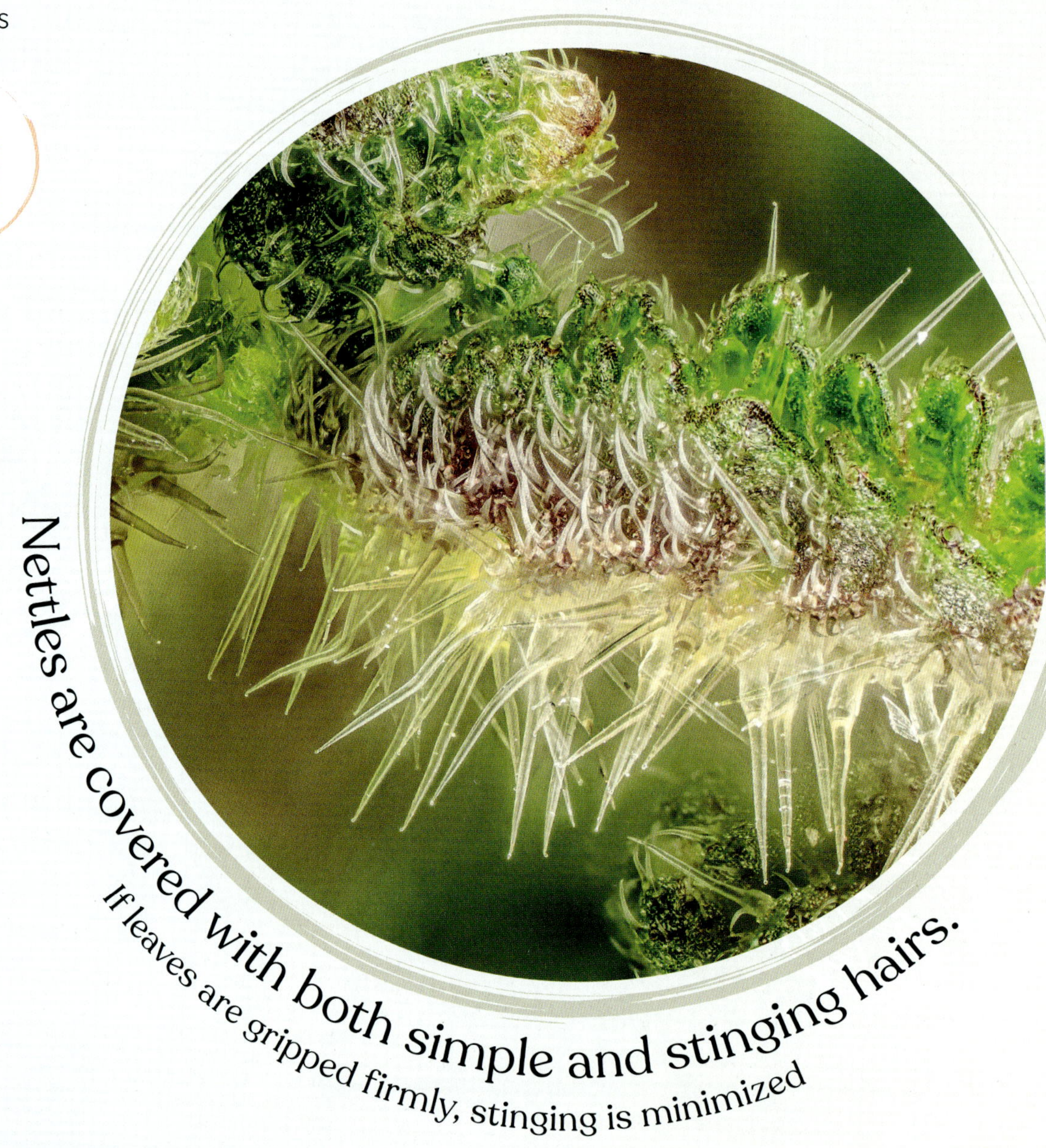

Nettles are covered with both simple and stinging hairs.
If leaves are gripped firmly, stinging is minimized

Stinging Nettle

Urtica dioica

A humble but tenacious herb, stinging nettle is best known for its stinging leaves and stems. However, since ancient times, it has been a popular ingredient in a number of traditional medicines and nutritious recipes, as well as a source of cloth fibres.

The stinging nettle is one of the most common plants in the world. Originally, it grew in moist, fertile soils in woodland, river banks, and fens – in Eurasia and, less commonly, North Africa – but it has long taken advantage of human settlers' tendency to enrich the soil with nitrogen from fertilizer and phosphate from bones and sewage. Today, nettles abound in hedgerows, farmyards, and gardens, and even linger among ruins. They often occur in nettlebeds, with each shoot rising from a rapidly growing network of rhizomes.

Nettle can be used to **activate compost**, or soaked in rainwater to make **"green manure"**

Special sting

The stinging nettle, or common nettle, is dioecious, each individual plant producing only male or female flowers. Some subspecies, however, can be monoecious and have separate clusters of male and female flowers on the same plant. The species name, *dioica*, translates as "two houses", whereas the genus name, *Urtica*, is from the Latin *uro*, meaning "burn", in reference to the burning sensation caused by the plant's stinging hairs.

Most forms of nettle have specialized stinging hairs dispersed among smaller non-stinging ones. The former contain a cocktail of biochemicals. The brittle tips of the stinging hairs break off on contact with the skin, injecting their biochemicals as they do so. The painful, itchy, red rash that appears on the skin is known as urticaria and usually subsides after about half an hour. The age-old remedy of rubbing the affected area with dock leaves (*Rumex obtusifolius*) seems to work, although there is no known reason why it should.

Harming and healing

Although the nettle is commonly associated with its nasty stinging characteristics, the plant can be used to relieve pain. Extracts of nettle have long been used in traditional remedies to treat burns, rashes, and nosebleeds, and it is equally effective against acne or as a treatment for greasy skin. The herb's stinging properties were employed as a counter-irritant to restore circulation or to relieve painful joints. In modern medicine, its roots are used to treat symptoms of benign prostatic hyperplasia.

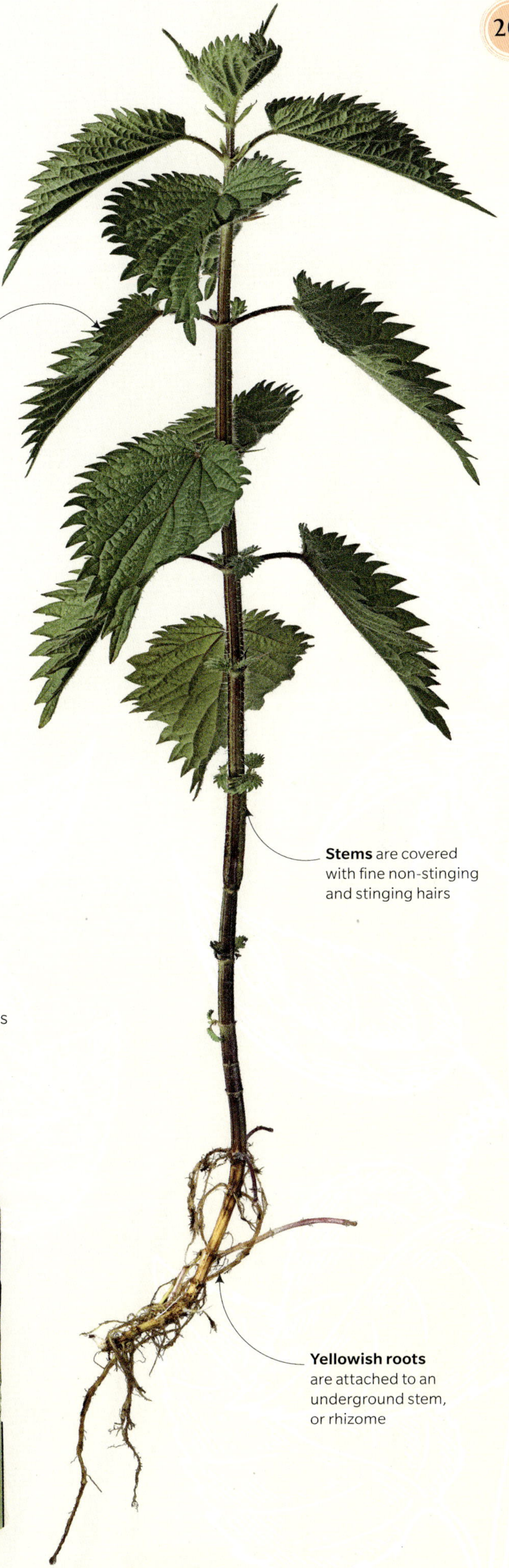

Serrated nettle leaves narrow to a point and are borne in opposite pairs

Stems are covered with fine non-stinging and stinging hairs

Yellowish roots are attached to an underground stem, or rhizome

➤ Nettle plant
This nettle is at pre-flowering stage, having leaves and roots only. Plants vary in height, from less than 1 m (3 ¼ ft) to at least 2 m (6 ½ ft), depending on the substrate.

KNITTING WITH NETTLES

The Wild Swans (1896), a fairy tale by Hans Christian Anderson (illustrated here by Helen Stratton), is the story of Princess Elisa and her 11 brothers, who were turned into swans by their stepmother's curse. In the churchyard, Elisa picks nettles, which she will knit into shirts for her brothers. The nettle shirts will enable them to regain their human shape and release the spell.

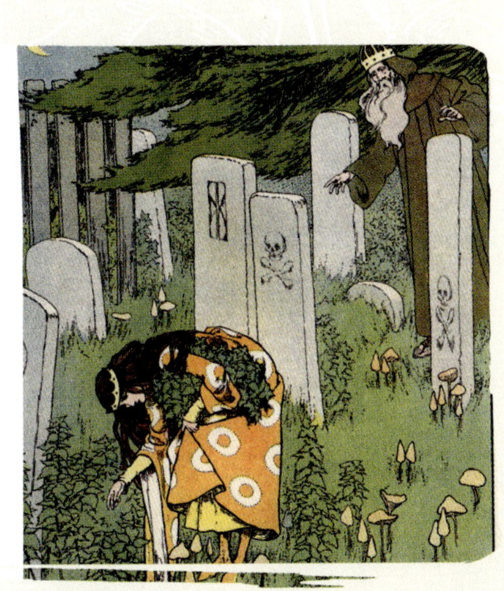

PICKING NETTLES, LITHOGRAPH c.1920

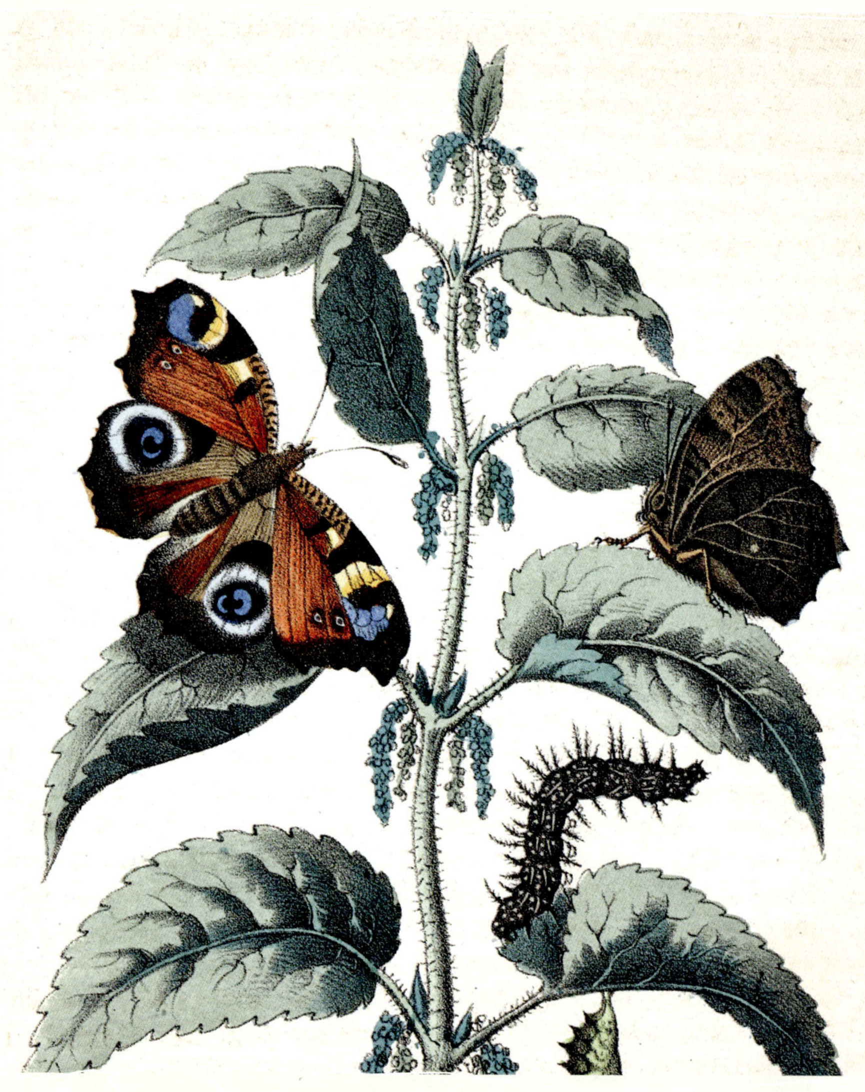

▲ Butterflies and moths
Stinging nettle is the larval foodplant for many butterflies, including the Peacock, and moths, such as the Nettle-tap.

With its contradictory harmful and healing properties, it is not surprising that the stinging nettle has a rich folklore. For example, nettle was seen as a "threshold plant", linking the worlds of the living and the dead. Nettle fibres have been discovered in Bronze Age burial shrouds in Northern Europe, and some folkloric stories describe nettle as growing from or near the dead. This probably also spawned the idea that nettle was associated with fairies.

In Anglo-Saxon times, nettle was one of the nine sacred herbs, used as protection against "elf-shot" – a rheumatic pain in humans or livestock, believed to be caused by invisible arrows fired by elves. In Norse myth, the plant is associated with the thunder god Thor, and it was burnt in fireplaces as a propitiation during storms. The herb is also associated with the trickster god Loki, whose magical fishing net was made of nettle fibres.

Food and fabric

The nettle plant was traditionally harvested in the spring time, when other wild foods are scarce. Used dried, the leaves or flowers make a nutritious tea or they can be brewed to produce nettle beer. Soaking or cooking destroys the sting.

Some of the oldest recipes feature nettle. Examples include nettle pudding, in which chopped nettle leaves and other herbs are cooked with barley grains and salt, and the Scottish "St Columba's broth", in which young shoots are cooked with oatmeal. Today, baby nettle leaves, which have a similar taste to spinach, are often puréed or added to European dishes such as polenta or pasta. In south-east Europe, nettles are sometimes used in place of chard or spinach in the dough filling of *borek* pastries. They are also one of the ingredients in the fillings of savoury *hortopita* pastries in Greece. Frozen first to preserve their freshness, nettle leaves are used as decorative wrapping for Cornish yarg cheese, and also as a flavouring in some varieties of Dutch gouda. Once they are ready to flower, nettles become unpalatable. They develop a gritty texture from calcium carbonate deposits (cystoliths), and this grit remains after cooking.

Nettles have been used in the production of textiles since at least medieval times. The stems contain bast fibres, which can be made into coarse fabric, in the same way as cotton. Using

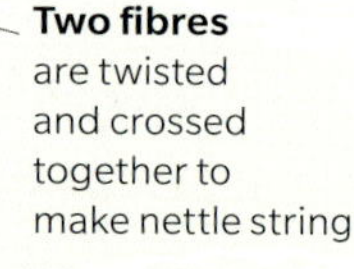

Two fibres are twisted and crossed together to make nettle string

◄ Nettle rope
To make rope fibres, mature nettle stems are stripped and peeled. The pith is removed, and the strings are hung up to dry.

> "Cloth made from the nettle is as good as that made from hemp."
>
> VICTOR HUGO, *Les Misérables*, 1862

nettle fibres to make cloth declined in the late 17th century as the cotton industry expanded, but there was a brief resurgence of demand in Germany during World War I, when embargoes led to a shortage of cotton. Today, there is renewed interest in nettle fibre as a sustainable and biodegradable fabric, and Germany, Austria, and Italy are once again producing nettle-based textiles. The plant can also be used to dye fabric: a yellow dye made from the roots and a yellow-green one from the leaves were used for camouflage netting during World War II.

Stinging nettle is rich in antioxidants, and this property makes it a useful cleansing agent in skincare. It can be applied as facial toner, hand sanitizer, or soap, to cleanse the pores. Nettle-based shampoo is said to strengthen hair and guard against dandruff.

The plant is also exceptionally rich in protein and iron. The leaves contain alpha-linolenic acid, an essential omega-3 fatty acid, and a number of vitamins, including ascorbic acid (vitamin C), riboflavin (vitamin B2), tocopherols (vitamin E), and pantothenic acid (vitamin B5). Although nettle is highly nutritious, livestock are reluctant to graze this fiercely stinging plant. However, dried nettle is useful in animal fodder, and chopped-up nettle leaves have long been fed to chickens as a nutritious treat.

Similar herbs

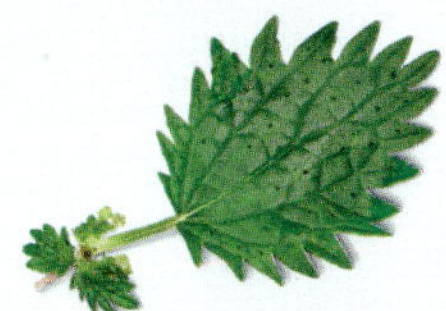

DWARF NETTLE
Urtica urens

Although smaller than the stinging nettle, with more rounded and coarser-toothed leaves, the dwarf nettle still gives a formidable sting.

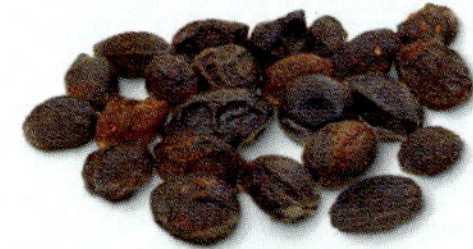

SAW PALMETTO
Serenoa repens

The seeds of this small palm, native to subtropical North America, are used in treatments for benign prostate enlargement.

➤ **Leaf hairs**
Hollow stinging hairs act as needles, piercing the skin and injecting formic acid, histamine, serotonin, and other biochemicals.

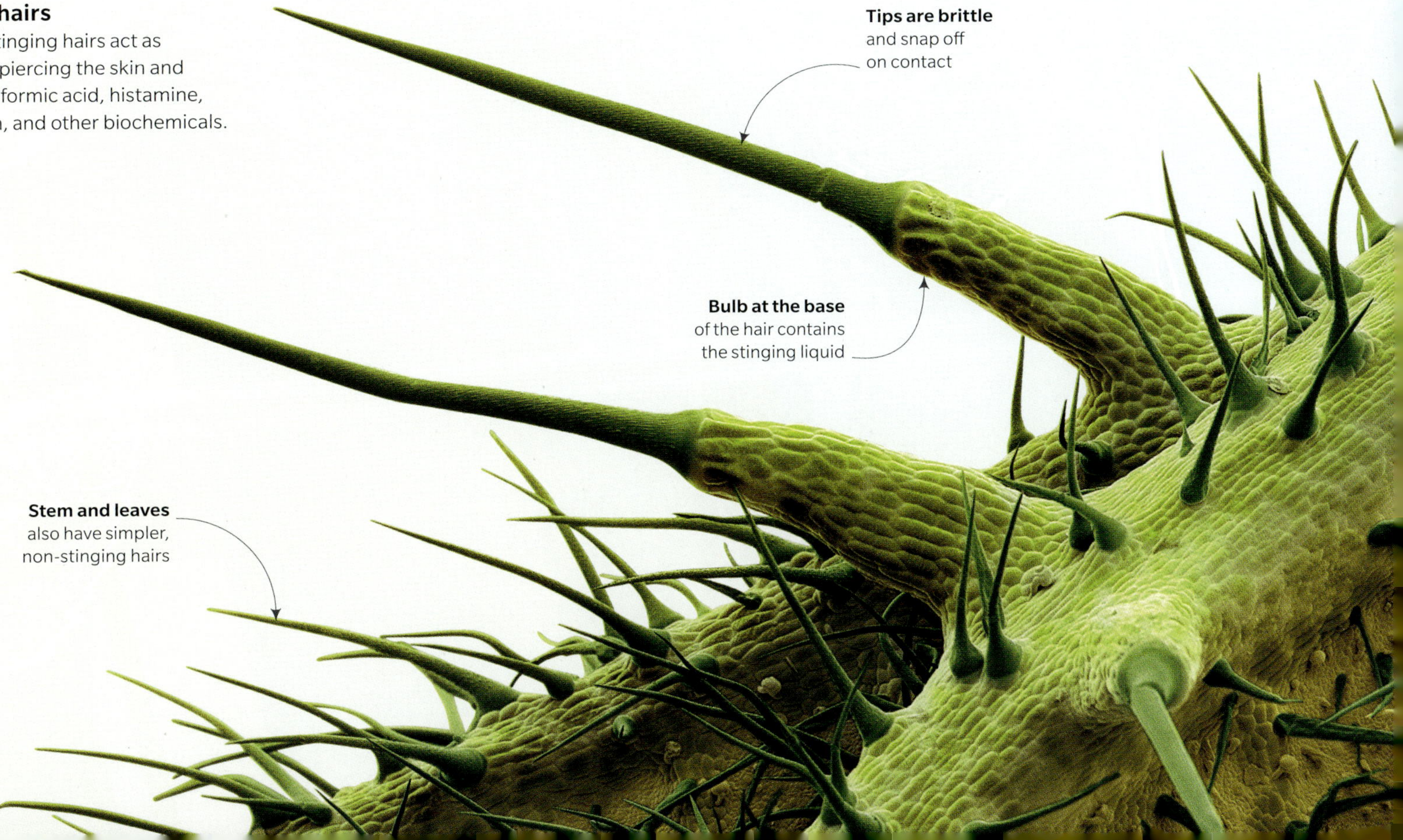

Tips are brittle and snap off on contact

Bulb at the base of the hair contains the stinging liquid

Stem and leaves also have simpler, non-stinging hairs

CHAPTER 4

Annual and Biennial Flowering Herbs

Short-lived plants, annuals germinate, bloom, and die in the space of just one year. Biennials have a slightly longer life cycle of two years, producing leaves in the first year, and flowering in the second.

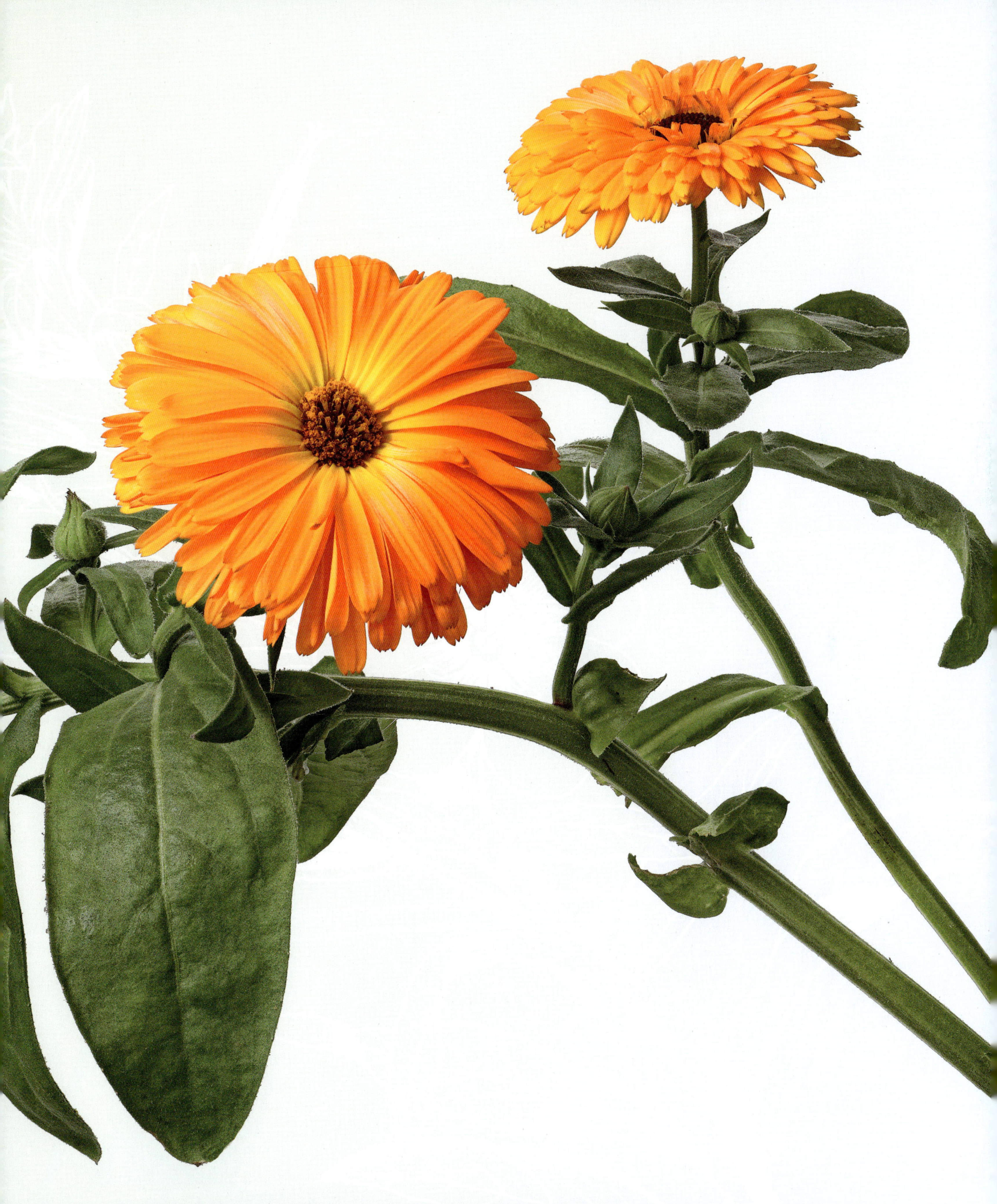

Anise

Pimpinella anisum

Native to Cyprus, Lebanon, Palestine, and Turkey, this flowering plant is similar in taste to liquorice and fennel. It is commonly used to flavour food and drinks, and is well known for its digestive benefits.

Uses Medicines; cooking; perfume

Parts used Fruits (seeds), roots, leaves

Active ingredients Anethole, estragole, pinene, limonene, iron, manganese, calcium

Habitat Mild-temperate regions, on fertile, slightly alkaline soil

The first recorded use of anise seed appears in the Ebers Papyrus (c.1500 BCE), where it is described as a medicine to treat abdominal and dental issues. It also appears in the Bible, alongside mint and cumin, and was documented by Roman scholar Pliny the Elder in *Naturalis Historia* (77–79 CE): "It was generally thought that there is nothing in existence more beneficial to the abdomen and intestine than anise." Pliny also notes the use of anise to dispel vertigo, relieve thirst, act as aphrodisiac, and promote perspiration. The herb continued to be taken to ease digestive complaints, as described by John Gerard in *The Herball, or Generall Historie of Plantes* (1597): "The seede wasteth and consumeth winde, and is goode against upbraidings of the stomache..." Today, anise is known to be a nutrient-rich source of antioxidants, with antimicrobial, carminative, spasmolytic, and expectorant properties. It is also used to balance female hormones.

A sweet treat

Anise is perhaps best known as a warming culinary ingredient, lending its liquorice flavour to a range of Middle Eastern, Italian, Greek, German, Indian, and Mexican recipes, and also to digestif drinks, such as anise tea, anisette, and ouzo. The seed is used as a whole or ground spice – including inside confectionery – or the aromatic leaves and stems can be added as an ingredient or garnish, in a similar way to fennel and tarragon. Anise is not related to the similar tasting star anise (*Illicium verum*), although both herbs contain the compound anethole, which gives them their shared distinctive flavour.

Similar herbs

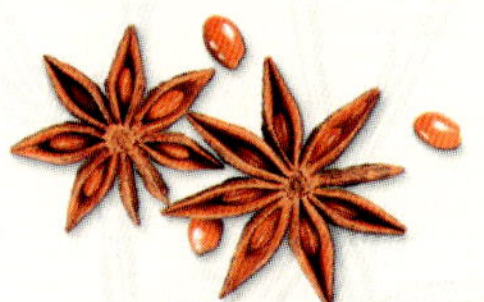

STAR ANISE

Illicium verum

This evergreen tree produces star-shaped fruits that are harvested just before ripening. Fruits, seeds, and oil are used in Asian cooking.

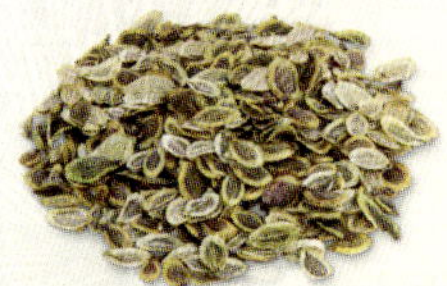

GOLPAR

Heracleum persicum

Native to Iran and Turkey, and now naturalized in Scandinavia, golpar produces anise-like seeds that are often eaten with legumes to aid digestion.

THE SMELL OF DANGER

The *Mallard* train, holder of the official speed record for steam locomotives – 202.59 km/h ($125\frac{9}{10}$ mph) – featured a unique safety device. A "stink bomb" of aniseed oil in the engine would release in the event of overheating, and the smell would alert the crew.

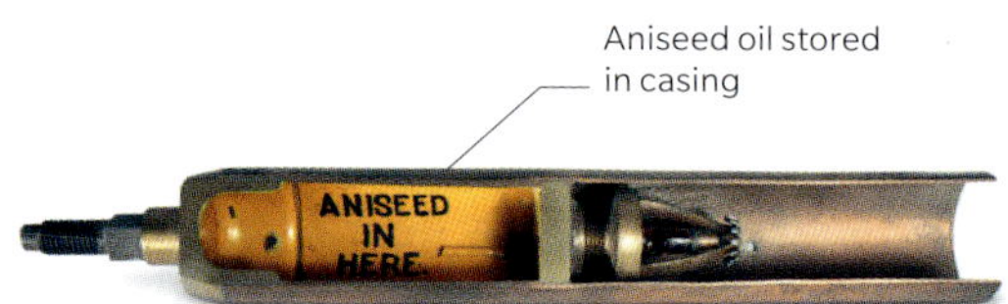

THE *MALLARD*'S "STINK BOMB"

▼ Seed source

Hailing from the same plant family (Apiaceae) as parsley and celery, anise's similarly lacy white flowers produce small, brown fruits that split as they mature.

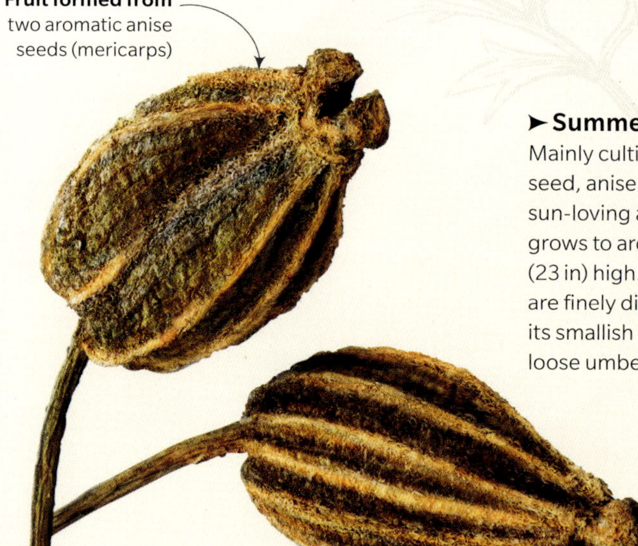

► Summer stalks

Mainly cultivated for its seed, anise is a bushy, sun-loving annual that grows to around 60 cm (23 in) high. Its stem leaves are finely divided, and its smallish flowers form loose umbels.

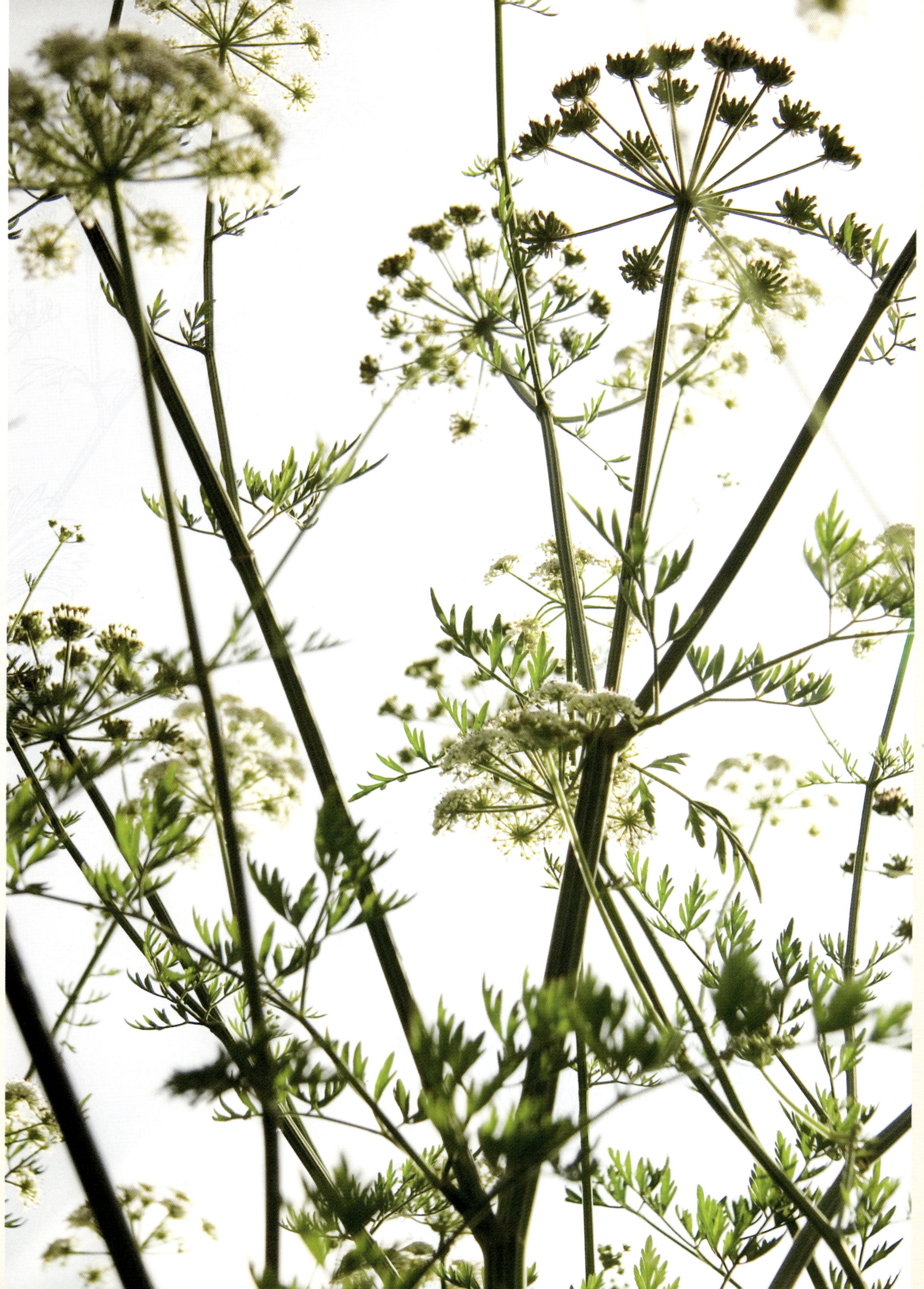

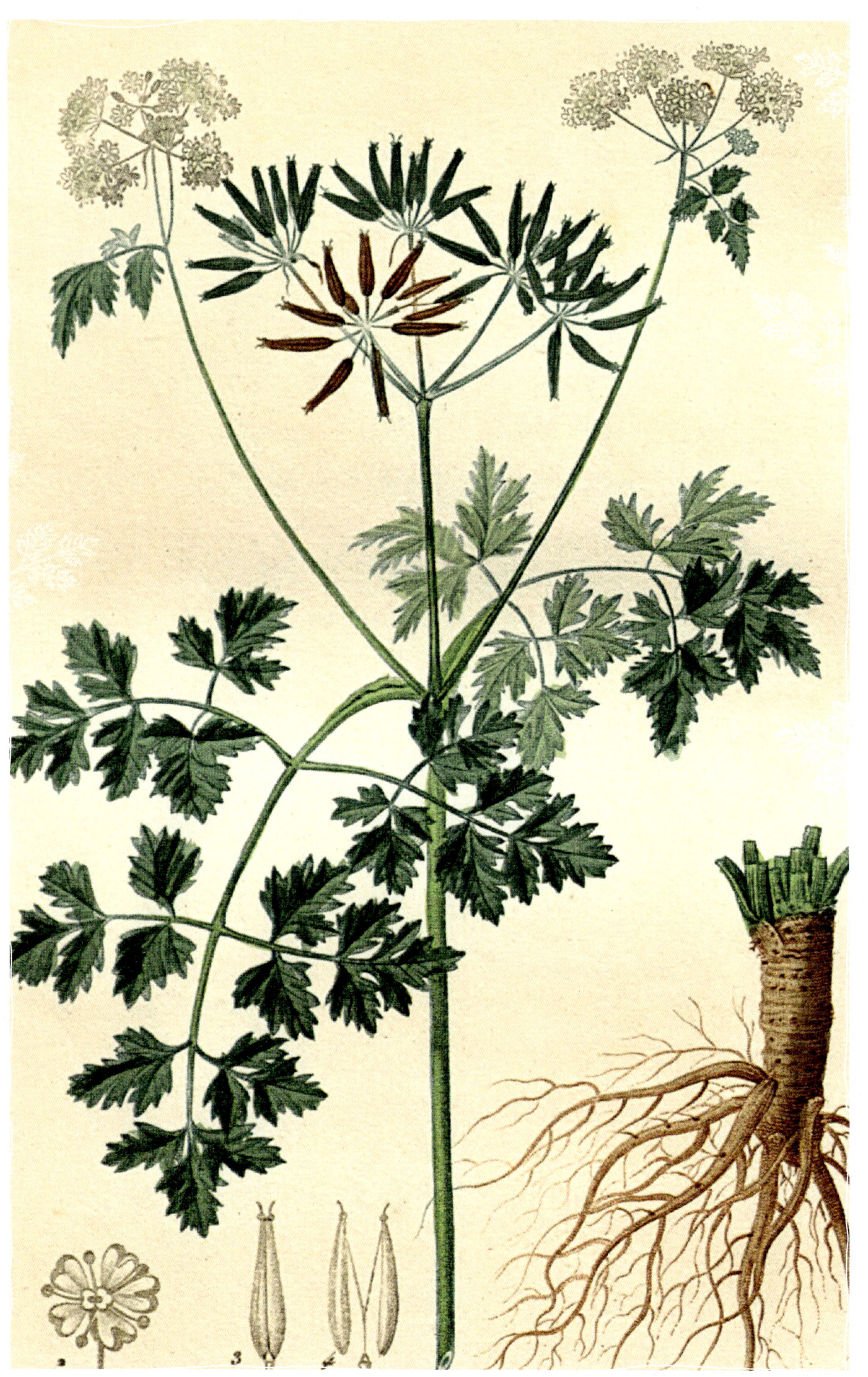

◄ **Edible parts**
This upright biennial is mainly grown as an annual for its parsley-like, mildly anise-tasting leaves, but its lacy white flowers, fine stems and shoots, roots, and fruits are also edible.

> “ [Chervil] rejoiceth and comforteth the heart, and increaseth their lust and strength. ”
>
> JOHN GERARD, *Herball, or Generall Historie of Plantes*, 1597

Uses Various medicines; cooking

Parts used Leaves, stems, flowers, fruits, roots

Active ingredients Bioflavonoids, estragole (methyl chavicol), undecane, iron, calcium, potassium, manganese, vitamin C, dietary fibre

Habitat Cool woodlands and open spaces; sheltered area with dappled shade in summer

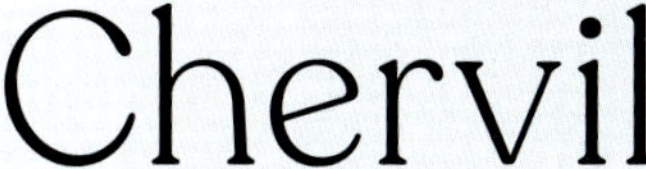

Chervil

Anthriscus cerefolium

This traditional culinary and medicinal herb was thought to bring comfort and joy to those who consumed its parsley–anise tasting leaves, stalks, fruits, or roots.

Chervil is one of the fresh *fines herbes* of French *haute cuisine* – along with parsley (see pp.220–21), chives, and tarragon (see pp.164–65) – used to season chicken, fish, and egg dishes with short cooking times. It can also be used as a substitute for tarragon in a classic Béarnaise (French egg-based sauce). It can be confused with other members of the Apiaceae family such as parsley and cow parsley (see right), as well as toxic relatives such as hemlock (*Conium maculatum*). Chervil can be grown at home, sowing seeds in spring and again at the end of summer. The slightly shiny leaves are harvested about six to eight weeks after sowing, and are best eaten fresh.

A fortifying plant

In his 16th-century *Herball*, British naturalist John Gerard observed “[chervil] seeds eaten as a sallad, whiles they are yet green... exceed all other sallads by many degrees, both in pleasantnesse of taste, sweetnesse of smell, and wholesomnesse for the cold and feeble stomacke”. Chervil root could also be eaten – raw or cooked – and was thought to uplift not just the flavour of a dish but also the spirits of those eating it. Roman naturalist Pliny the Elder is said to have advocated using a chervil-vinegar infusion to cure hiccups.

Traditionally seen as a fully edible, fortifying, and mood-lifting herb, chervil is now known to contain high levels of health-boosting minerals, antioxidants, and dietary fibre. With a flavour combining parsley and sweet cicely, its digestive and diuretic properties are useful for treating gut issues, fluid retention, and high blood pressure.

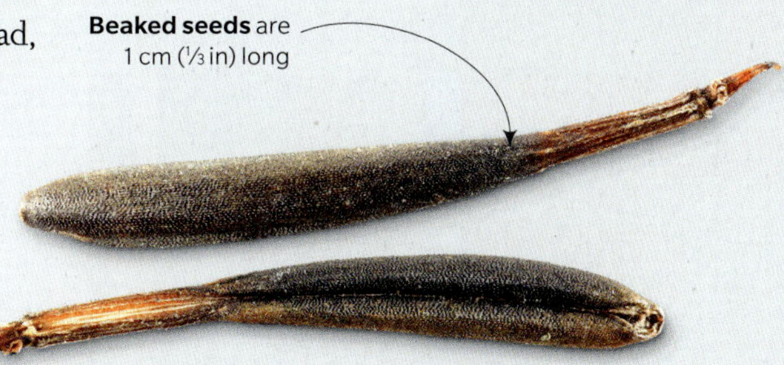

➤ Elongated seeds
Borne in umbels, chervil’s fruits are formed from pairs of oblong-ovoid “seeds” (mericarps), each with a groove running down its length. Fresh seeds are more likely to germinate successfully.

Similar herbs

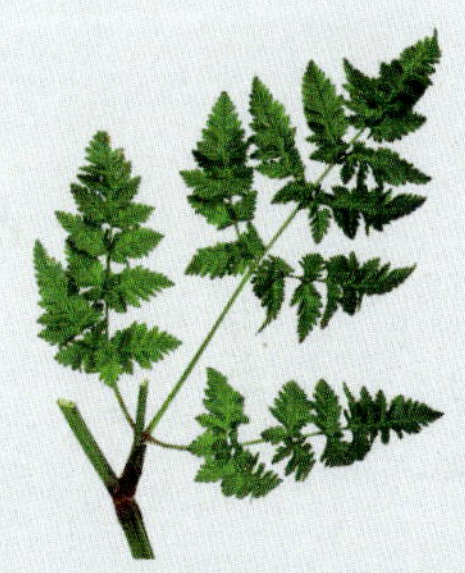

COW PARSLEY
Anthriscus sylvestris
This larger scale version of chervil has a mildly spicy flavour, but can be mistaken with the highly toxic hemlock (*Conium maculatum*).

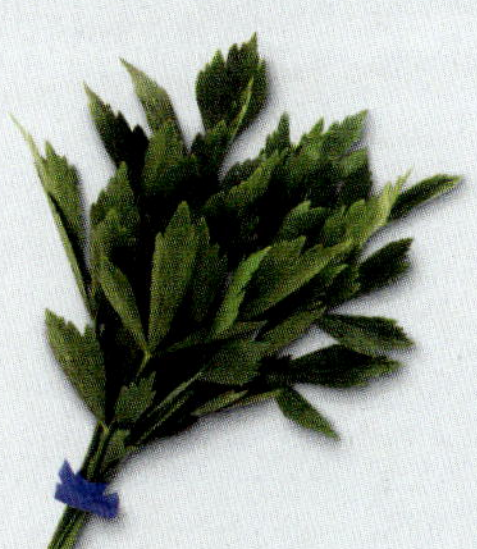

LOVAGE
Levisticum officinale
Lovage’s large, flat leaves are typically used to add a celery–parsley flavour to soups and salads, while the roots can be used as a vegetable.

Uses Medicines, cooking, cosmetics

Parts used Fruits (seeds)

Active ingredients Cuminaldehyde, cymene, terpenoids, petroselinic acid, apigenin, luteolin, vitamin B, vitamin E, iron, magnesium, manganese

Habitat Fertile, well-drained soil

▼ Delicate blossoms
White or pale pink blooms are borne on the ends of the spoked stems of umbels. These mature into tiny green to brown fruits.

Each fruit is a pair of small boat-shaped seeds (mericarps)
Flowers grow amid fine, thread-like, green leaves

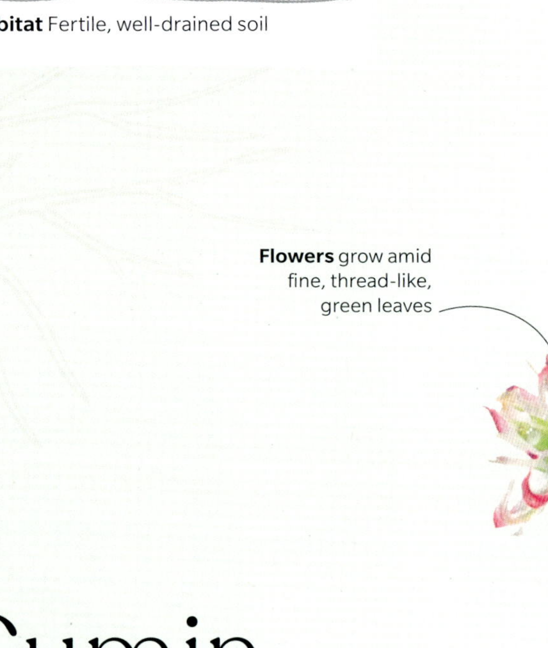

Cumin

Cuminum cyminum

Well known as an ingredient in Indian, North African, Middle Eastern, and Latin American cooking, cumin is also used to treat gut issues and may help to control blood sugar levels.

A characteristic member of the parsley family (Apiaceae), cumin is native to a relatively small part of the Middle East. From at least Sumerian times, its cultivation and use spread to many surrounding countries, continents, and cultures via various overland and then maritime trade routes. The herb can be compared to its close relative caraway (*Carum carvi*) due to its similar shaped seeds and bittersweet undertones. Cumin seeds are, however, slightly larger and have a hotter, more pungent flavour and aroma.

Cumin is thought to be one of the world's most widely used spices

A supportive spice

In India, cumin is an important Ayurvedic ingredient known as *jeera* or *jeeraka*. It is thought to balance all three *doshas* (energies) – *vata* (wind), *pitta* (fire), and *kapha* (water) – and is useful for stomach issues and as a detoxifier. Dry roasted cumin is used to make lassi, an ancient Ayurvedic remedy (and now a popular drink) that combines probiotics and anti-inflammatory agents to support digestion, strengthen

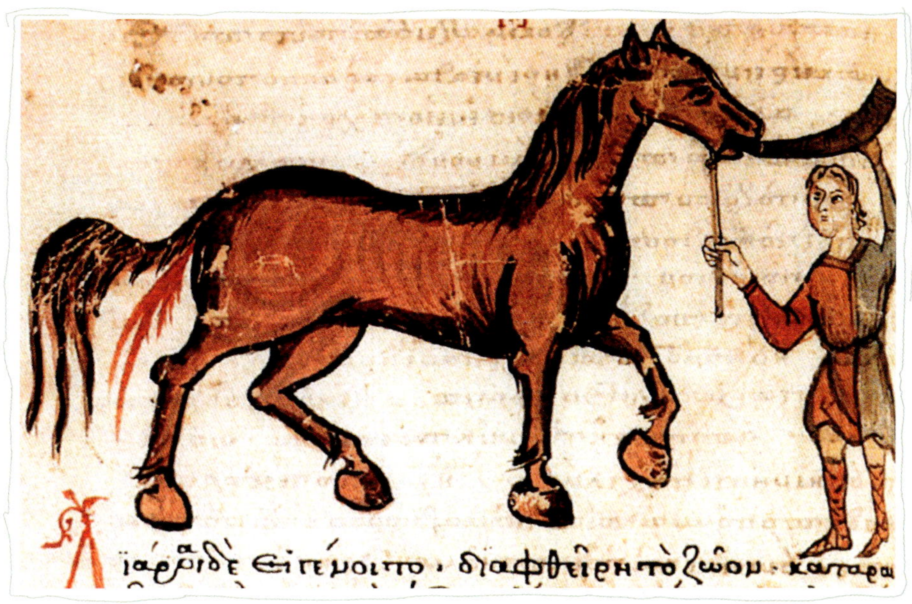

➤ Gut health
Cumin has a long history as a treatment for diarrhoea. Black cumin oil – from unrelated *Nigella sativa* seeds (see below) – was also traditionally used to treat digestive issues in horses, as illustrated in the 14th-century Byzantine manuscript *Hippiatrica*.

> “From Pliny, we learn that the ancients took the ground [cumin] seed medicinally with bread, water or wine.”
>
> MRS M. GRIEVE, *A Modern Herbal*, 1931

the gut, and promote calm. Cumin is also known to have antibacterial, antioxidant, antiseptic, and larvicidal properties. The ancient Egyptians and other ancient civilizations used it to dispel intestinal parasites and may have employed it for embalming. There has also been research into the efficacy of cumin in managing type-2 diabetes and protecting against cancer. Additionally, it may have some potential to boost memory by stimulating the central nervous system. Aside from medicine, it was once believed that cumin kept both chickens and lovers from straying. Today, it is still a popular ingredient of bird seed and is used at weddings as a symbol of loyalty.

Warming touch

The warm, earthy flavour of cumin is harnessed in a range of culinary spice mixtures, including chilli powder blends (such as chilli, garlic, onion, and salt), curry powder (with coriander, cinnamon, cloves, turmeric, and chilli), and garam masala (black pepper, mace, cinnamon, cardamom, cloves, coriander, bay, fennel, and chilli). It also flavours dishes such as falafel and *jeera* rice, as well as various soups, curries, and stews. Whole seeds can be added to hot oil or ghee, or dry roasted to bring out a stronger, more distinctive flavour; dry roasted seeds can also be ground to create a concentrate. Once roasted, seeds can be added to dishes as a final touch as they do not need heat or time to release their flavour.

Canopic jars held key organs, such as the liver, and were put in the tomb with the body

◄ Cumin in ancient Egypt
Ancient Egyptian embalmers may have used cumin as a spice in the mummification process. Cumin is now known to have antibacterial properties, which can aid preservation.

Similar herb

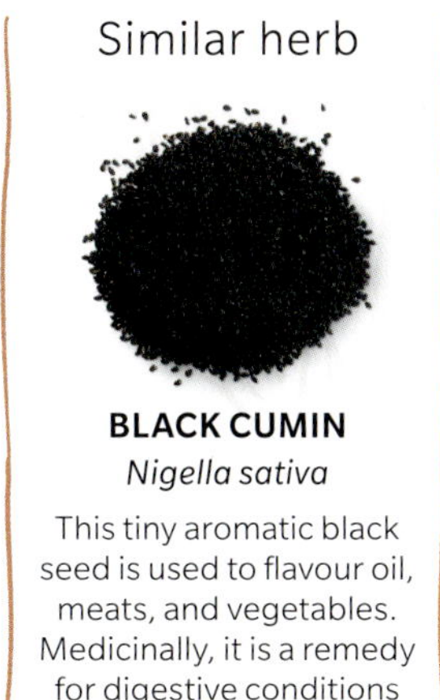

BLACK CUMIN
Nigella sativa
This tiny aromatic black seed is used to flavour oil, meats, and vegetables. Medicinally, it is a remedy for digestive conditions and inflammation.

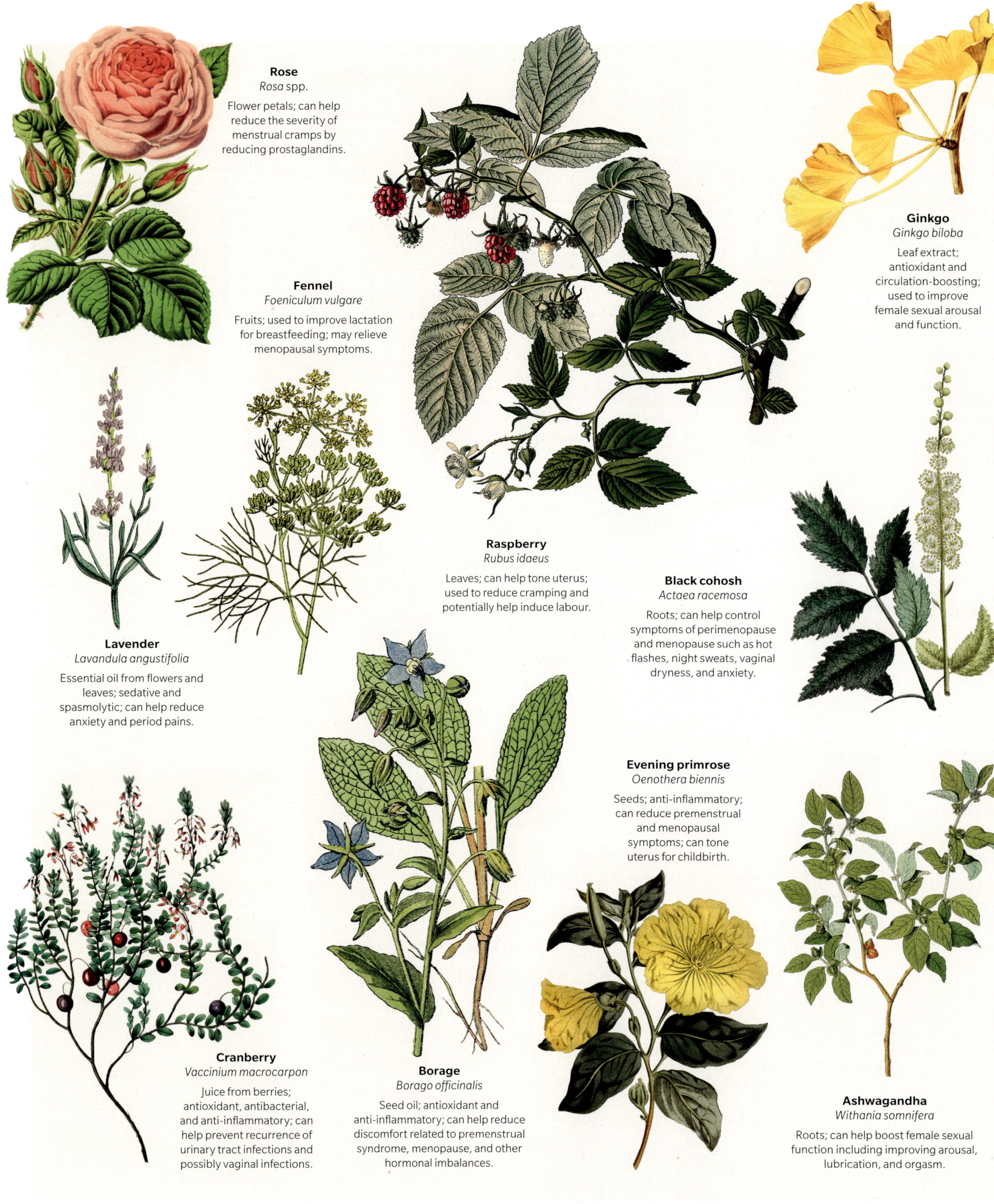

Rose
Rosa spp.
Flower petals; can help reduce the severity of menstrual cramps by reducing prostaglandins.

Ginkgo
Ginkgo biloba
Leaf extract; antioxidant and circulation-boosting; used to improve female sexual arousal and function.

Fennel
Foeniculum vulgare
Fruits; used to improve lactation for breastfeeding; may relieve menopausal symptoms.

Raspberry
Rubus idaeus
Leaves; can help tone uterus; used to reduce cramping and potentially help induce labour.

Black cohosh
Actaea racemosa
Roots; can help control symptoms of perimenopause and menopause such as hot flashes, night sweats, vaginal dryness, and anxiety.

Lavender
Lavandula angustifolia
Essential oil from flowers and leaves; sedative and spasmolytic; can help reduce anxiety and period pains.

Evening primrose
Oenothera biennis
Seeds; anti-inflammatory; can reduce premenstrual and menopausal symptoms; can tone uterus for childbirth.

Cranberry
Vaccinium macrocarpon
Juice from berries; antioxidant, antibacterial, and anti-inflammatory; can help prevent recurrence of urinary tract infections and possibly vaginal infections.

Borage
Borago officinalis
Seed oil; antioxidant and anti-inflammatory; can help reduce discomfort related to premenstrual syndrome, menopause, and other hormonal imbalances.

Ashwagandha
Withania somnifera
Roots; can help boost female sexual function including improving arousal, lubrication, and orgasm.

Supporting Reproductive Health

Herbal remedies have been used for centuries to support the human reproductive system, and to maintain physical and emotional balance through the various stages of life. Herbs can help maintain the general health of reproductive organs as well as hormones.

Rosemary
Salvia rosmarinus
Essential oil in leaves; anti-inflammatory, antioxidant, antimicrobial; can help reduce period pain and boost mood.

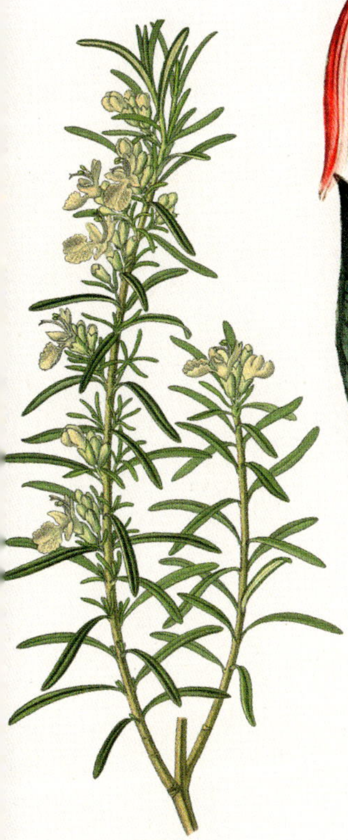

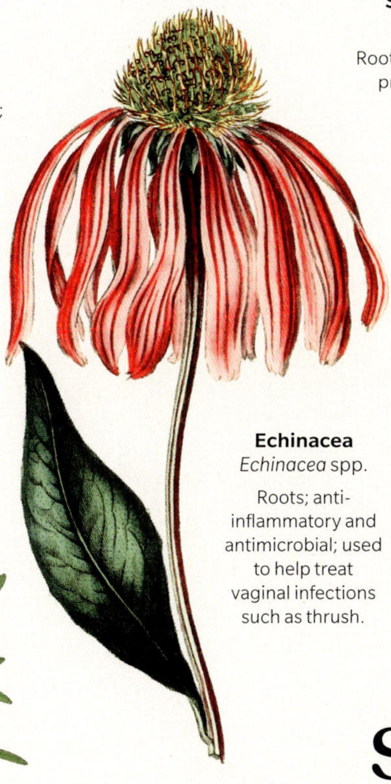

Echinacea
Echinacea spp.
Roots; anti-inflammatory and antimicrobial; used to help treat vaginal infections such as thrush.

Stinging nettle
Urtica dioica
Roots; used for enlarged prostate and heavy menstruation.

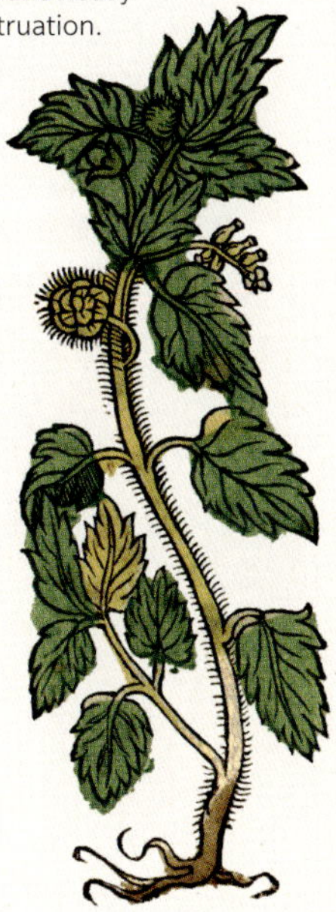

Valerian
Valeriana officinalis
Roots and rhizomes; sedative; can help reduce menopausal hot flashes, anxiety, and insomnia.

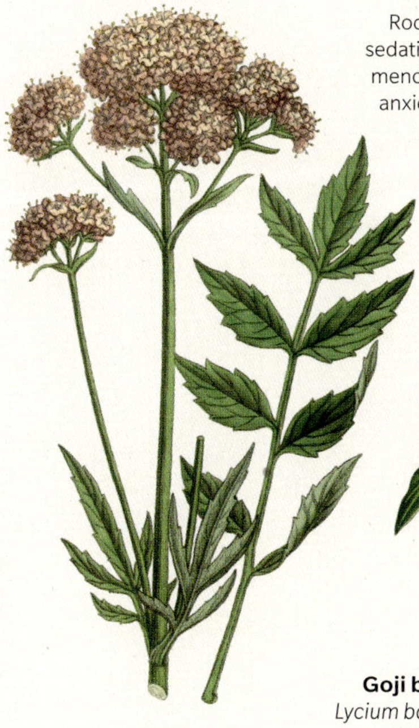

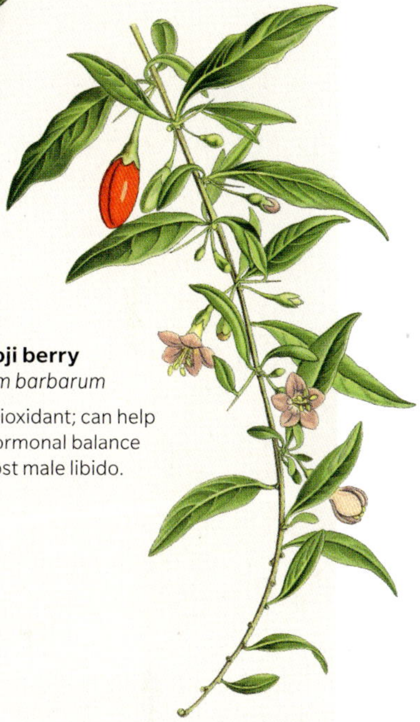

Goji berry
Lycium barbarum
Berries; antioxidant; can help restore hormonal balance and boost male libido.

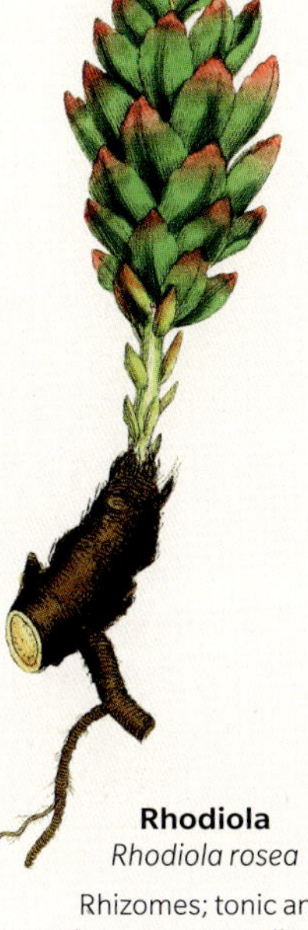

Rhodiola
Rhodiola rosea
Rhizomes; tonic and adaptogen; may alleviate some symptoms of menopause.

St John's wort
Hypericum perforatum
Flowering tops; can help relieve symptoms of premenstrual syndrome including cramps, irritability, mood swings, and lowered mood in menopause.

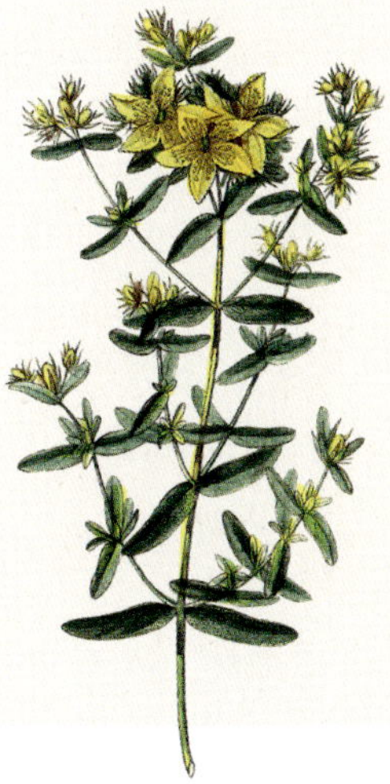

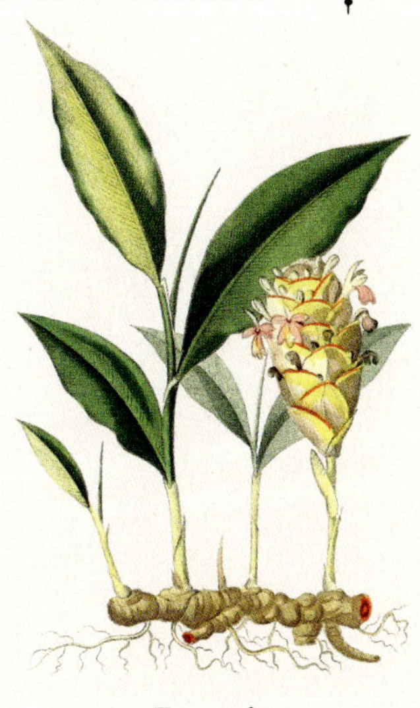

Turmeric
Curcuma longa
Rhizome; anti-inflammatory, and antioxidant; may help polycystic ovary syndrome, uterine fibroids, and endometriosis.

Linden
Tilia spp.
Flowers; antioxidant and anti-inflammatory; can help reduce menopausal anxiety and hot flashes.

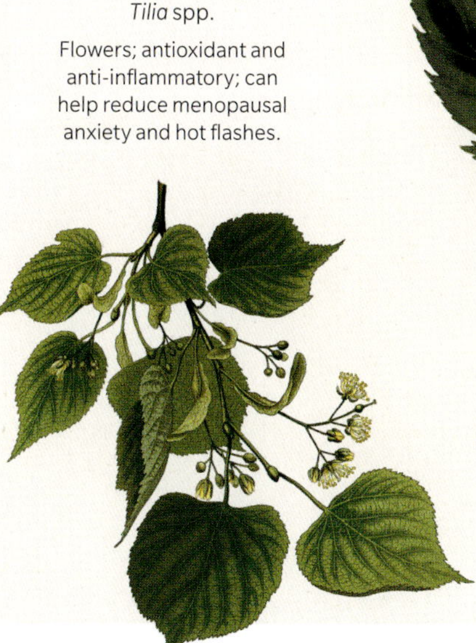

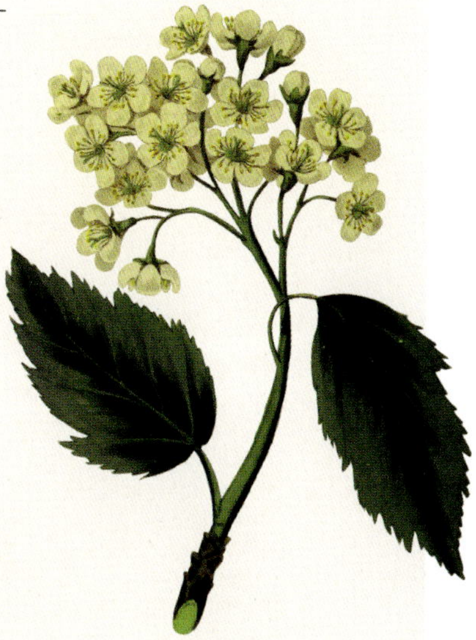

Hawthorn
Crataegus spp.
Berries and flowers; antioxidant and anti-inflammatory; can help strengthen blood vessels and improve circulation; combats anxiety.

Evening Primrose

Oenothera biennis

Uses Medicines, cooking

Parts used Mainly seeds, also leaves, stalks, and buds

Active ingredients Gamma-linolenic acid (GLA), linoleic acid, eicosanoids, flavonoids

Habitat Waste ground, verges, sand dunes

Native to North America, but widely naturalized in Europe and Asia, the evening primrose plant is most prized for the oil derived from its seeds. This oil contains an omega-6 essential fatty acid that can help to reduce inflammation.

As its species name (*Oenothera biennis*) implies, evening primrose is a biennial herb. It has a fleshy rootstock and narrow leaves, and its delicate flowers become fragrant early in the evening to attract night-time pollinators such as moths. Evening primrose is not related to the similarly yellow-flowered common primrose (*Primula vulgaris*), and its closest relatives are willowherbs (*Epilobium* spp.). The plant is native to North America, where its stalks and roots were a staple food of some Indigenous American peoples. It was also valued for its therapeutic properties, and oil was extracted from crushed seeds and used to sooth swellings and pains in joints. From the 17th century, evening primrose was widely grown in physic gardens in Europe, where it became a popular panacea known as "king's cure-all".

Precious oil

The small brown seeds of evening primrose are rich in fibre and protein, but their most valuable commodity is their oil. This is rich in an omega-6 essential fatty acid known as gamma-linolenic acid, or GLA. Although GLA occurs in seeds of other plants, such as blackcurrant and borage, it is most commonly obtained from evening primrose. In animals, GLA is vital for maintaining brain function, skeletal and reproductive health, and general metabolism. It also stimulates hair and skin growth. Evening primrose oil can be used to treat skin disorders, such as eczema, and many women around the world take it to relieve premenstrual symptoms. Other uses of evening primrose oil include the treatment of diabetic nephropathy (kidney disease).

In the kitchen, the roots of evening primrose are generally boiled or fried. They are said to taste like potatoes, whereas the flower buds – pickled or fried – are pleasantly mild and sweet. Young leaves and flowers can be eaten raw in salads. The oily seeds can be roasted and used like sesame seeds. The whole evening primrose plant is edible, although the roots – if eaten raw – may irritate the throat.

▼ Microscopic seeds
Evening primrose plants produce vast quantities of seeds inside clusters of bean-like capsules, which are green when fresh and brown when dry. Each seed measures less than a millimetre.

Irregularly shaped seeds have flattened sides and resemble tiny wood chips

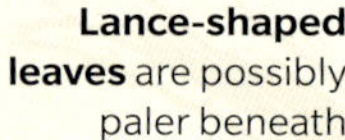

Lance-shaped leaves are possibly paler beneath

"The Evening Primrose opens anew
Its delicate blossoms to the dew."

JOHN CLARE, "Evening Primrose", from *The Rural Muse*, 1835

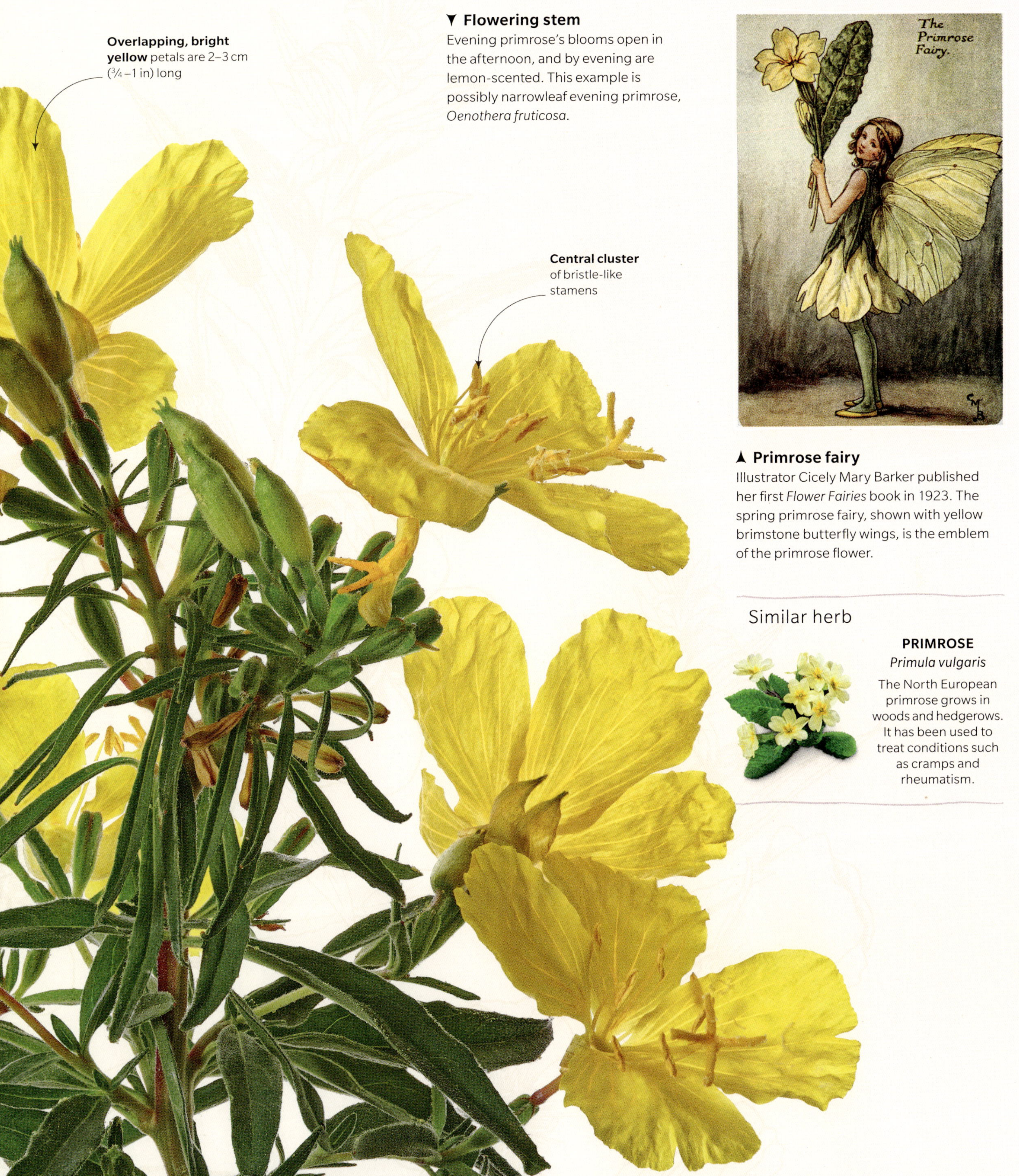

Overlapping, bright yellow petals are 2–3 cm (¾–1 in) long

Central cluster of bristle-like stamens

▼ Flowering stem

Evening primrose's blooms open in the afternoon, and by evening are lemon-scented. This example is possibly narrowleaf evening primrose, *Oenothera fruticosa*.

▲ Primrose fairy

Illustrator Cicely Mary Barker published her first *Flower Fairies* book in 1923. The spring primrose fairy, shown with yellow brimstone butterfly wings, is the emblem of the primrose flower.

Similar herb

PRIMROSE
Primula vulgaris

The North European primrose grows in woods and hedgerows. It has been used to treat conditions such as cramps and rheumatism.

➤ Legume family
Fenugreek is a member of the legume family (Fabaceae) and produces the elongated pods (bottom left) typical of legumes such as beans. The components of the plant are illustrated here in Dr Willibald Artus' *Handbook of All Medical-pharmaceutical Plants* (1876).

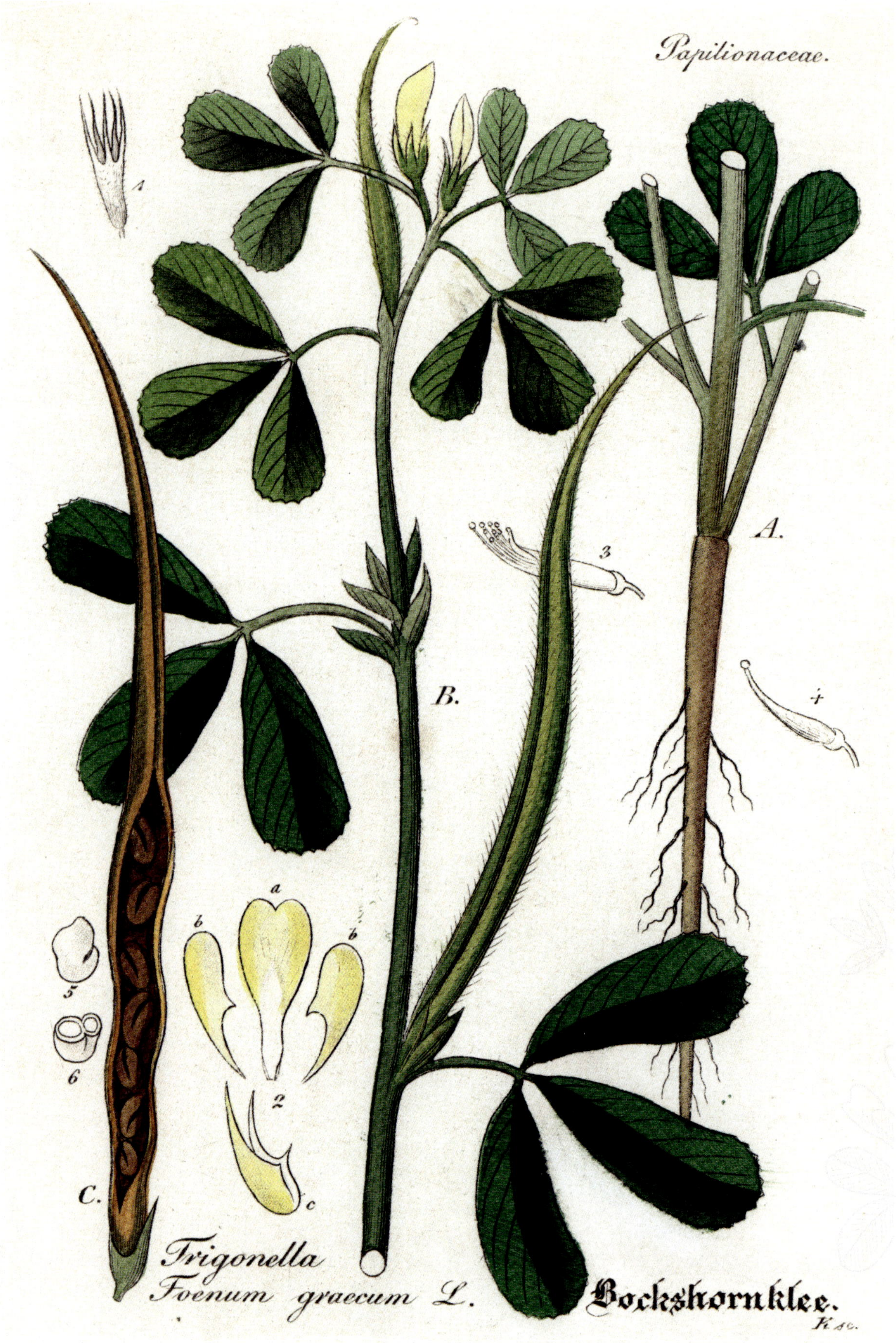

Similar herbs

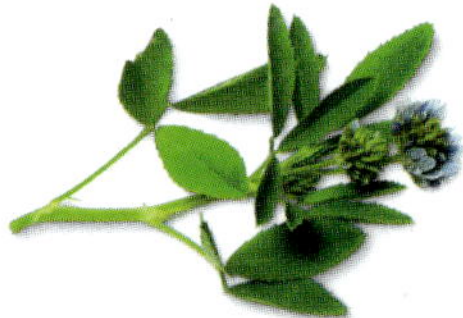

BLUE FENUGREEK
Trigonella caerulea

Possibly originating in the eastern Mediterranean, this species has a milder taste than true fenugreek and is popular in the cuisine of the Caucasian nation of Georgia.

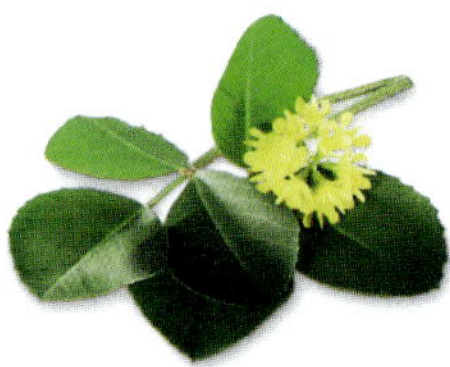

CULTIVATED FENUGREEK
Trigonella balansae

The fresh leaves of this plant (syn. *T. corniculata*) are used as a pot herb, and its dried leaves are ground into a spice. Fruits and leaves are used medicinally in India.

Uses Medicines; cooking

Parts used Leaves, seeds

Active ingredients Diosgenin, coumarins, trigonelline, gentianine, carpaine, fenugreekine, 4-hydroxyisoleucine, sotolon

Habitat Seasonally arid temperate and sub-tropical regions, in field verges, grasslands, and hillsides

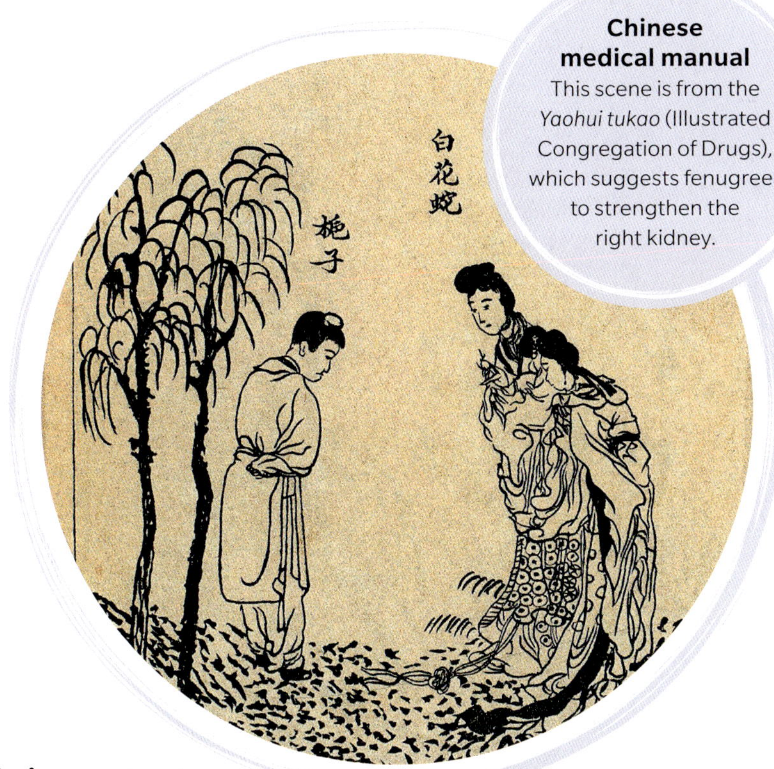

Chinese medical manual
This scene is from the *Yaohui tukao* (Illustrated Congregation of Drugs), which suggests fenugreek to strengthen the right kidney.

Fenugreek

Trigonella foenum-graecum

Cultivated since ancient times, fenugreek is important in the cuisines of many Asian and Mediterranean countries. Although it is used in traditional medicine, it can cause allergic reactions.

Archaeological excavations in the Middle East suggest fenugreek was in use 6,000 years ago. It likely originates in the Middle East – native to a swathe of land from Iraq to Pakistan – but during its long association with humans, it has travelled both east and west and is now an established crop, foodstuff, and medicine in many parts of Africa, Asia, and Europe. The leaves can be harvested as a vegetable, but it is the seeds that are the primary crop.

Seeds, spice, and sotolon

Fenugreek seeds are an important spice and component of spice mixes, such as Indian five spice (*panch phoron*, see right). In Egypt, they are added to bread doughs and used to make a popular herbal tea, while in Yemen they are ground to make *hulbah*, a traditional savoury paste. In India, they are a common ingredient in curries, chutneys, and dhals. The seeds contain the chemical sotolon, which has a curry scent at high concentrations. At low concentrations, it smells of maple syrup and is used in artificial syrups. Medicinally, fenugreek has been used to treat a number of conditions, including type 2 diabetes and inflammation, and is taken as a tea to increase milk production in breastfeeding mothers. However, scientific evidence of its effectiveness is scant. In some people, consuming fenugreek can cause diarrhoea, dyspepsia, and maple-scented sweat. It may also trigger allergic reactions in those with peanut or chickpea allergies.

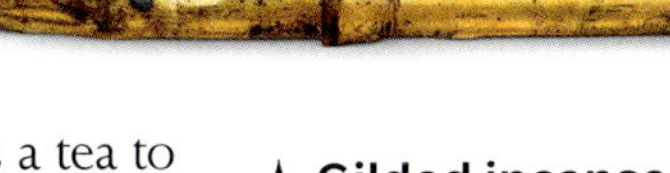

Incense was placed in a cup on the outstretched palm and offered to the deity

▲ Gilded incense burner
Fenugreek may have been used as an ingredient in the seven sacred oils of Egypt, and in incense. This burner is from the Ptolemaic period (330–305 BCE).

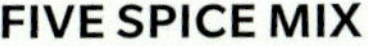

FIVE SPICE MIX

In northern and eastern India, Bangladesh, and Nepal, the spice mix *panch phoron* is a popular cooking ingredient. Made up of five seeds, the mix includes fenugreek, nigella, cumin, black mustard, and fennel in equal portions, although fenugreek can impart a bitter taste and some cooks reduce its share.

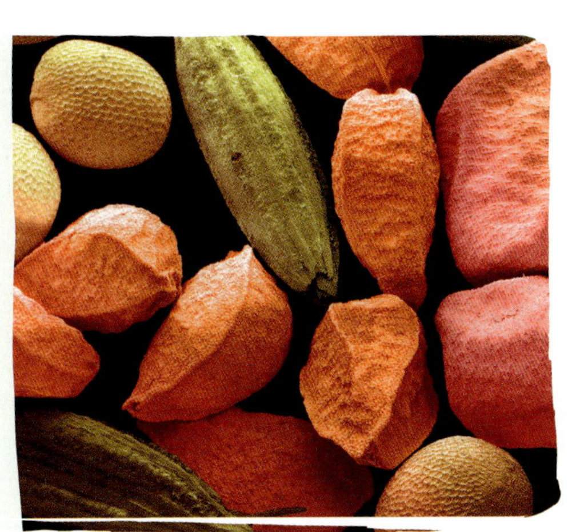

SEEDS USED IN *PANCH PHORON*

Dill fruits are edible and can be used whole or crushed
Fruits are harvested by clipping the entire flower head into a bag
Flavoursome, fibrous stems can be used in pickling, soups, and stocks

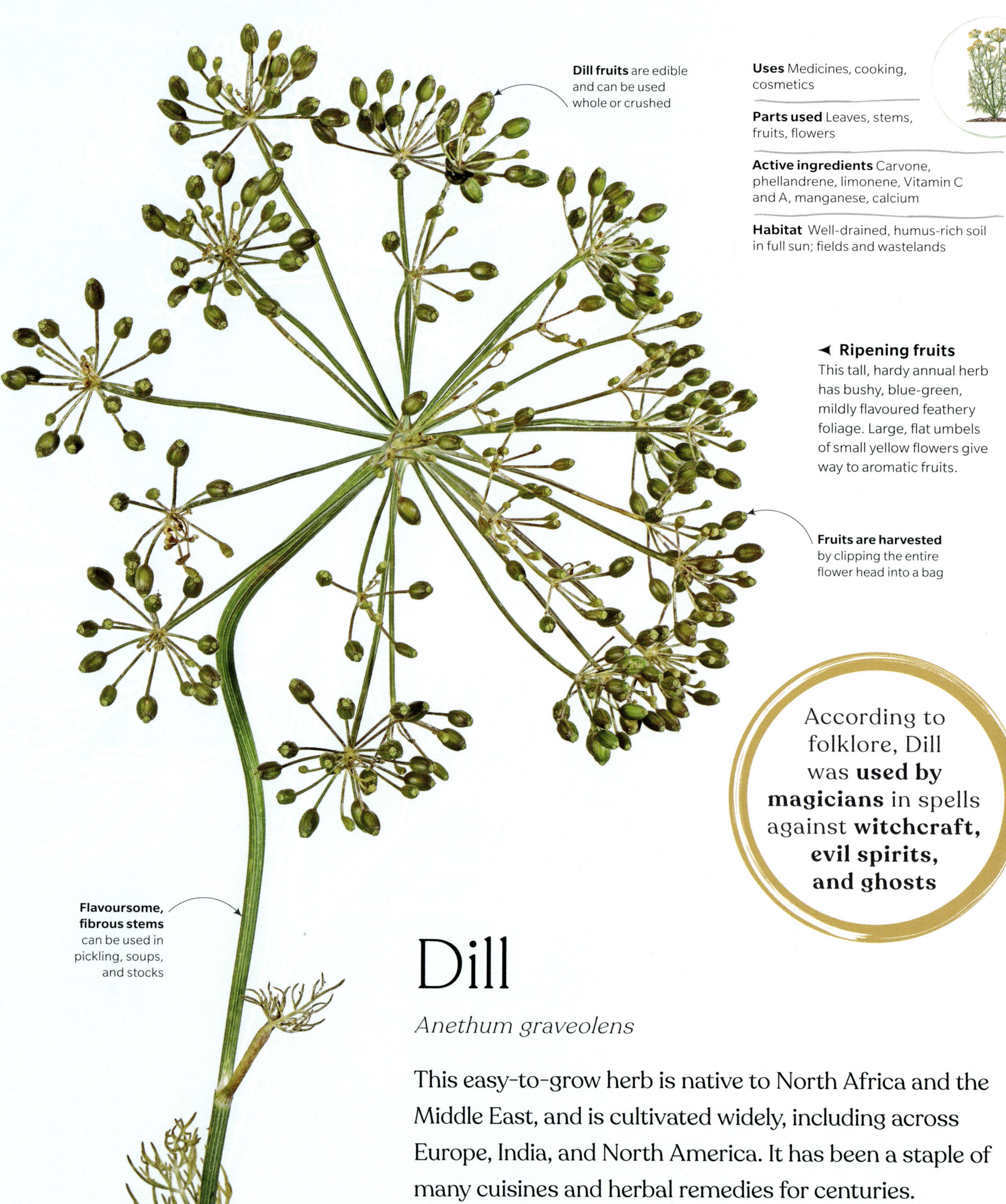

Uses Medicines, cooking, cosmetics

Parts used Leaves, stems, fruits, flowers

Active ingredients Carvone, phellandrene, limonene, Vitamin C and A, manganese, calcium

Habitat Well-drained, humus-rich soil in full sun; fields and wastelands

◄ Ripening fruits
This tall, hardy annual herb has bushy, blue-green, mildly flavoured feathery foliage. Large, flat umbels of small yellow flowers give way to aromatic fruits.

According to folklore, Dill was **used by magicians** in spells against **witchcraft, evil spirits, and ghosts**

Dill

Anethum graveolens

This easy-to-grow herb is native to North Africa and the Middle East, and is cultivated widely, including across Europe, India, and North America. It has been a staple of many cuisines and herbal remedies for centuries.

Recognizable as a member of the carrot family Apiaceae due to its umbel flower heads and physical similarity to relatives such as fennel (see pp.186–87) and anise (see pp.206–207), the popular garden herb dill is fully edible and has a range of medicinal and cosmetic uses. Easy to grow from seed, dill has been widely cultivated and used for thousands of years, with the terms "dill weed" referring to its stems and finely divided leaves. These are largely used for culinary purposes, either fresh or dried, to flavour salads, meats, vegetables, and sauces. The fruits, when dried, appear as flat tan-brown oval seeds, and are used in food, particularly in pickling. Essential oil from the fruits and the leaves is also used in cosmetics to reinforce skin elasticity.

◄ Flavour enhancer
Dill flowers, leaves, and seeds are traditionally used for pickling gherkins (small cucumbers). These June Boy Dill Pickles are made with the addition of garlic.

A herbal soother

As shared by Mrs M. Grieve in *A Modern Herbal* (1931), "the name is derived, according to Prior's *Popular Names of English Plants*, from the old Norse word, *dilla* (to lull), in allusion to the carminative properties of the drug". Dill water (a decoction of dill seeds) was traditionally used by nursing mothers to calm their babies, and is still put in gripe water to combat colic. Dill's volatile compounds make it an effective antibacterial. It is also used to treat hiccups, bad breath, and to support bone health.

Pickles, potatoes, and fish

Dill is particularly popular in Europe, especially in Germany, Poland, the Baltic states, Ukraine, and Russia, where it is used extensively as a garnish, a pickle flavouring, in soups, and mixed with fermented milk. In Scandinavia, the dill umbel is served with crayfish, and snipped foliage is used to flavour potatoes and fish, including gravlax (cured salmon) and herring pickles. It is also used in Asian, Middle Eastern, and Arab cooking, from Vietnamese fish dishes and Lao *mok pa* (steamed fish in banana leaves) to Indian *keema* samosa and Egyptian *mahshi kromb* (stuffed cabbage leaves).

Similar herbs

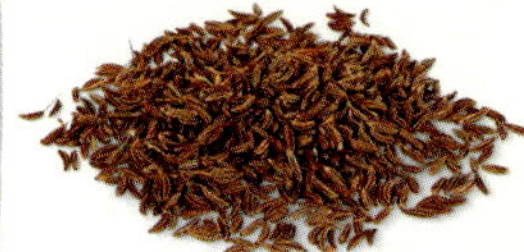

CARAWAY
Carum carvi
Caraway seeds have a pungent anise-like flavour often used to spice breads, cakes, and drinks. The roots can also be eaten as a vegetable.

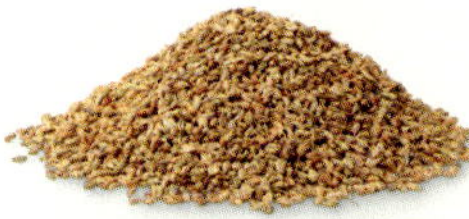

AJOWAN SEEDS
Trachyspermum ammi
Ajowan, or carom, seeds have a bitter and pungent taste with hints of anise, oregano, and thyme. They are used as a spice and in medicine.

Medieval dill recipes for pickling included cucumber and cauliflower

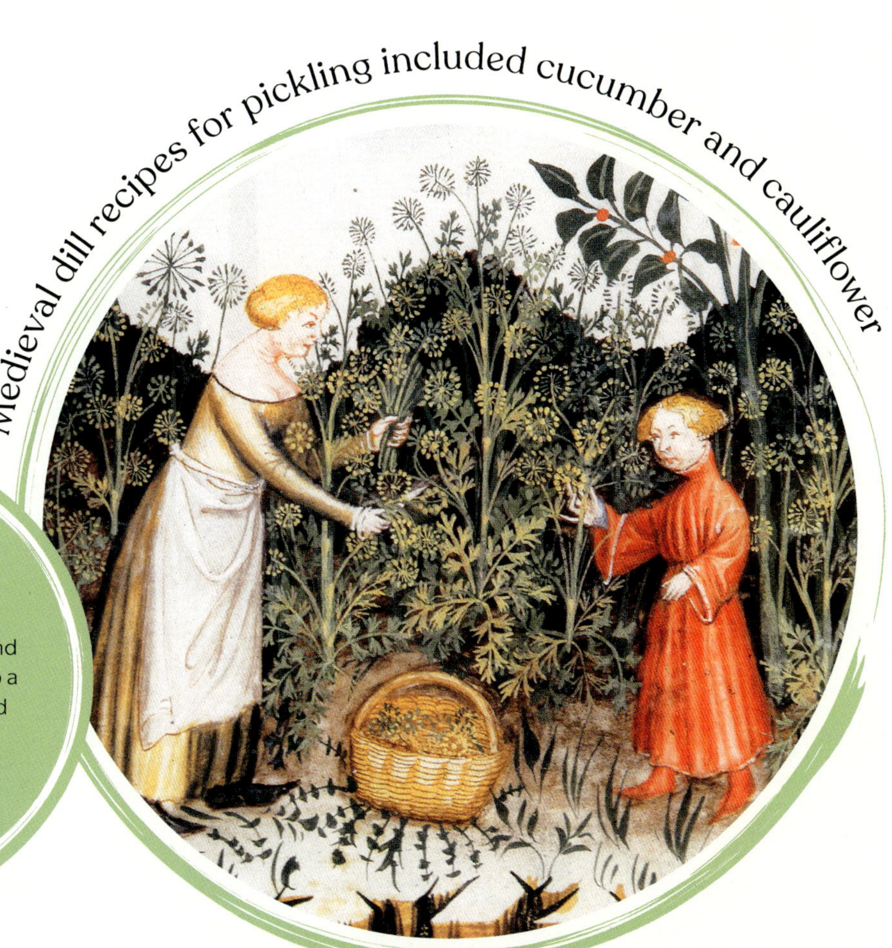

Gainful herb
Dill was a widely cultivated and used garden herb in medieval times. It was commonly used to flavour fish and potatoes but was also baked into a spice cake, alongside cumin and anise, which was eaten to aid digestion after rich foods. Dill cordials were also used to treat hiccups.

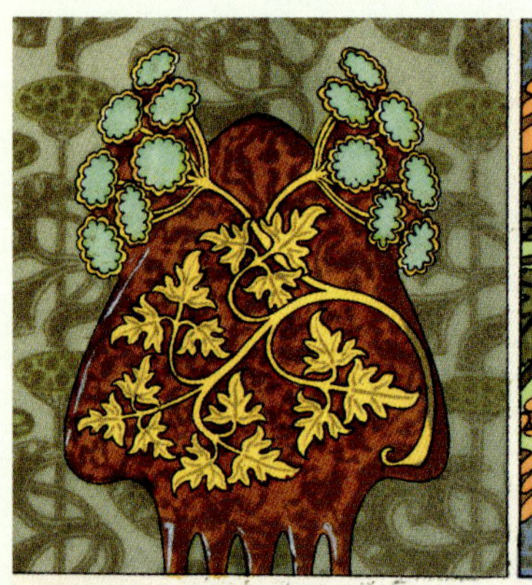

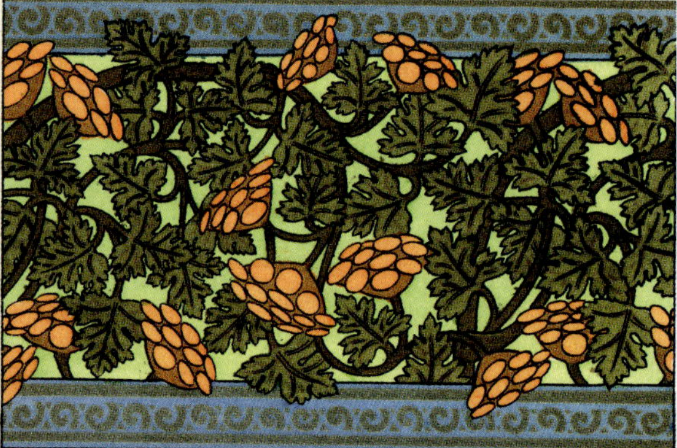

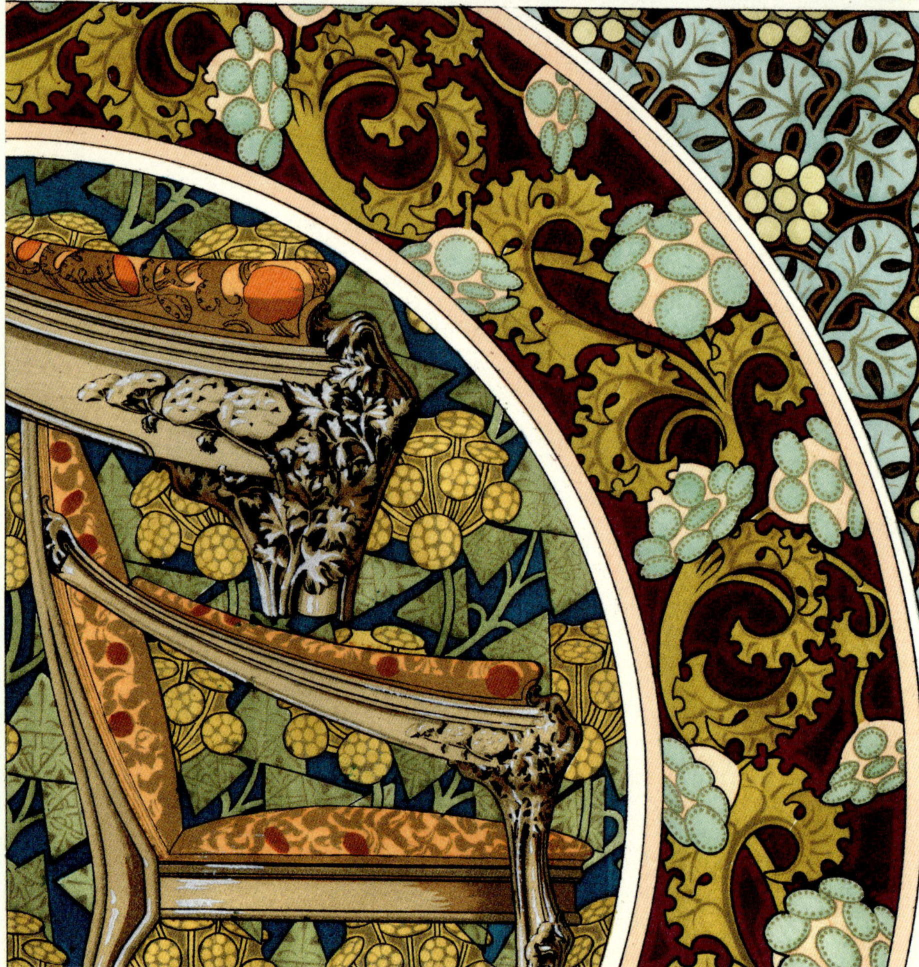

Uses Medicines; cooking; cosmetics

Parts used Leaves, stems, roots, fruits (seeds), flowers

Active ingredients Myristicin, apiole, luteolin, iron, manganese, vitamins A, C, and K

Habitat Mainly in temperate regions; prefers sun, in meadows, fields, or disturbed but well-drained or moist soil

◄ Leafy inspiration
Both the curled and flat leaves of parsley inspired a range of elegant Art Nouveau-style motifs by artist Georges Bourgeot in this illustration for Edward Grasset's *The Plant and its Ornamental Applications* (1896).

Parsley

Petroselinum crispum

A central and eastern Mediterranean native that has spread across the globe, parsley is most well-known as a classic culinary garnish and ingredient. Around its native lands, it has a long history of cultural and medicinal importance.

Verdant leaves grow prolifically in summer and may overwinter in milder regions

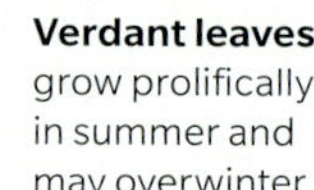

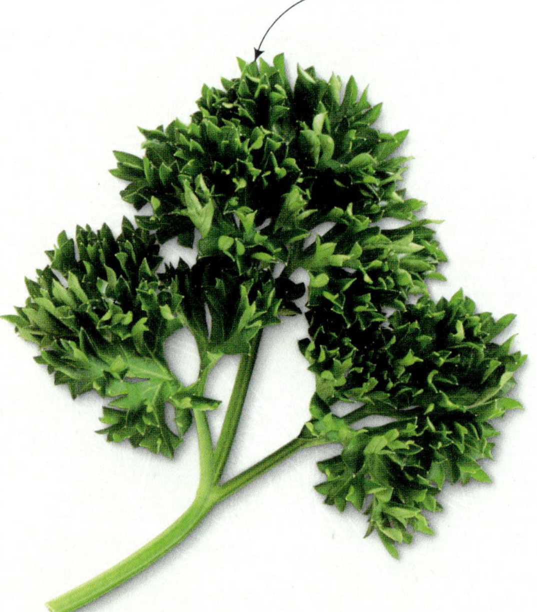

▲ Curled-leaf parsley
The species *Petroselinum crispum* has gently curled edges; *crispum* means "wrinkled" or "finely waved". Varieties such as 'Moss Curled' have leaves with even tighter curls.

This member of the Apiaceae (carrot) family is entirely edible and high in iron and vitamins A and K. The foliage is the main ingredient in various culturally significant dishes including Middle-Eastern *tabbouleh* made with bulgur wheat, lemon, and mint; green sauces such as Argentinian *chimichurri* and Italian *gremolata*, mixing parsley with chilli and garlic or garlic and lemon respectively; the seasoning *persillade*; and in a *bouquet garni* with thyme and bay. In its second year, parsley bears small, pale yellow flowers, which can liven up a salad.

Parsley can be a good companion plant in the garden; its aromatic chemicals help to deter insect pests and even enhance the scent of roses. The slightly grassy aroma is distilled from its seeds (technically its fruits) in an essential oil for use in infusers, blended massage oils, and perfumes.

Lobed leaves with serrated edges are rich in green chlorophyll

▲ Fresh parsley
The leaves and stems of this herb, whether curled- or flat-leaved (shown here), are best used when fresh, but can also be dried.

Medicinal history

As evidenced in the Roman naturalist Pliny the Elder's *Natural History* (77–79 CE), the leaves, seeds, and roots of parsley have a centuries-old history of medicinal use. Traditional applications include as a digestive; as a diuretic, helping to cleanse the kidneys naturally by increasing urine production and flow; as an antioxidant, helping to expel unwanted toxins; to treat eye conditions; and as an anti-inflammatory. Concentrated amounts of parsley may also stimulate menstruation, so the herb is best avoided as a tea, tincture, or juice during pregnancy.

The devil's herb

In the Jewish ritual of Passover, parsley is dipped in salt water as a reminder of slavery in ancient Egypt (see p.30). However, the herb was considered by some ancient cultures to be in league with death or the devil. This reputation arose out of various myths concerning the underworld (see below), its use as a natural deodorizer to mask the stench of death, its slow germination rate, and rumours that only the wicked could grow it or that it grew best where women had more power.

> In Western folklore, the belief that parsley seeds must go to the devil and back nine times before sprouting arose from parsley's very slow germination rate of 4–6 weeks

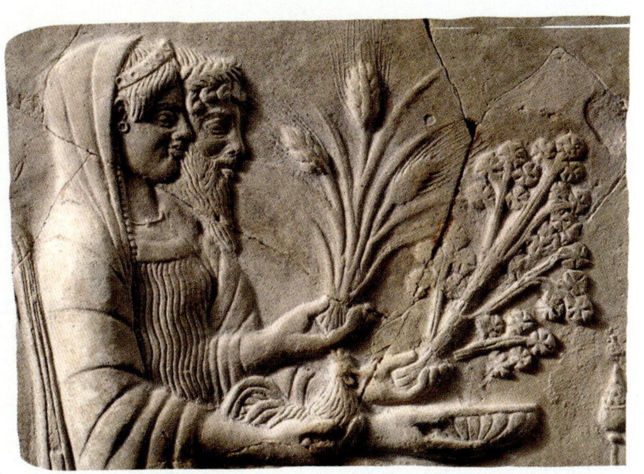

PARSLEY IN GREEK MYTH
This terracotta tablet from the 5th century BCE was found in the shrine of Persephone at Locri in Calabria, Italy. It depicts the daughter of the Greek god Zeus with her abductor husband and king of the underworld, Hades, who is holding a sprig of parsley. The herb symbolized Persephone's associations with nature and the seasons but also death; both Ancient Greeks and Romans included it in their funeral rites.

PERSEPHONE AND HADES

Similar herbs

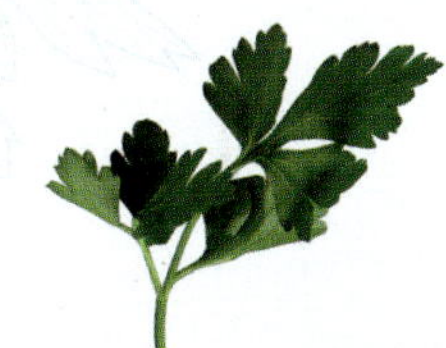

FLAT-LEAVED PARSLEY
Petroselinum crispum var. *neapolitanum*

The leaves of this type of parsley – also known as Italian or plain-leaved parsley – have a stronger aromatic flavour than curled-leaf parsley.

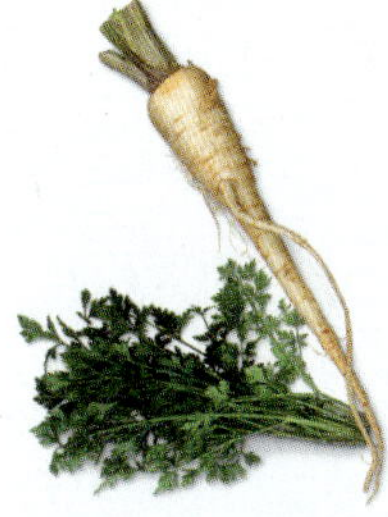

HAMBURG PARSLEY
Petroselinum crispum var. *tuberosum*

Largely cultivated as a vegetable for its parsnip-like roots, this plant offers the bonus of edible parsley leaves and fruits that are valued for medicinal use.

Ruff-like bract expands as the fruit matures
Basal leaves are broadly lobed and aromatic
Leaves on the upper stem are finely divided
CORIANDER LEAF

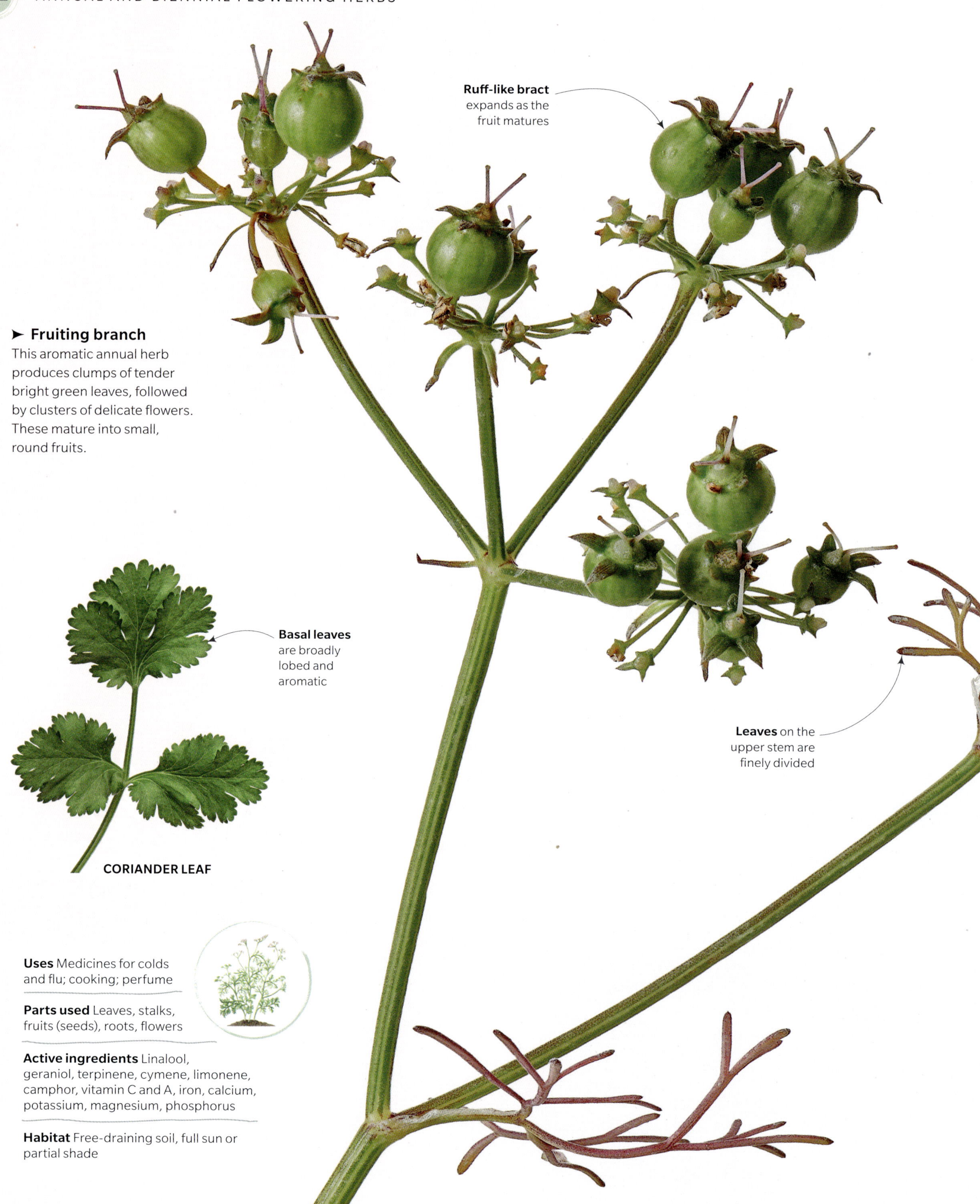

➤ Fruiting branch

This aromatic annual herb produces clumps of tender bright green leaves, followed by clusters of delicate flowers. These mature into small, round fruits.

Uses Medicines for colds and flu; cooking; perfume

Parts used Leaves, stalks, fruits (seeds), roots, flowers

Active ingredients Linalool, geraniol, terpinene, cymene, limonene, camphor, vitamin C and A, iron, calcium, potassium, magnesium, phosphorus

Habitat Free-draining soil, full sun or partial shade

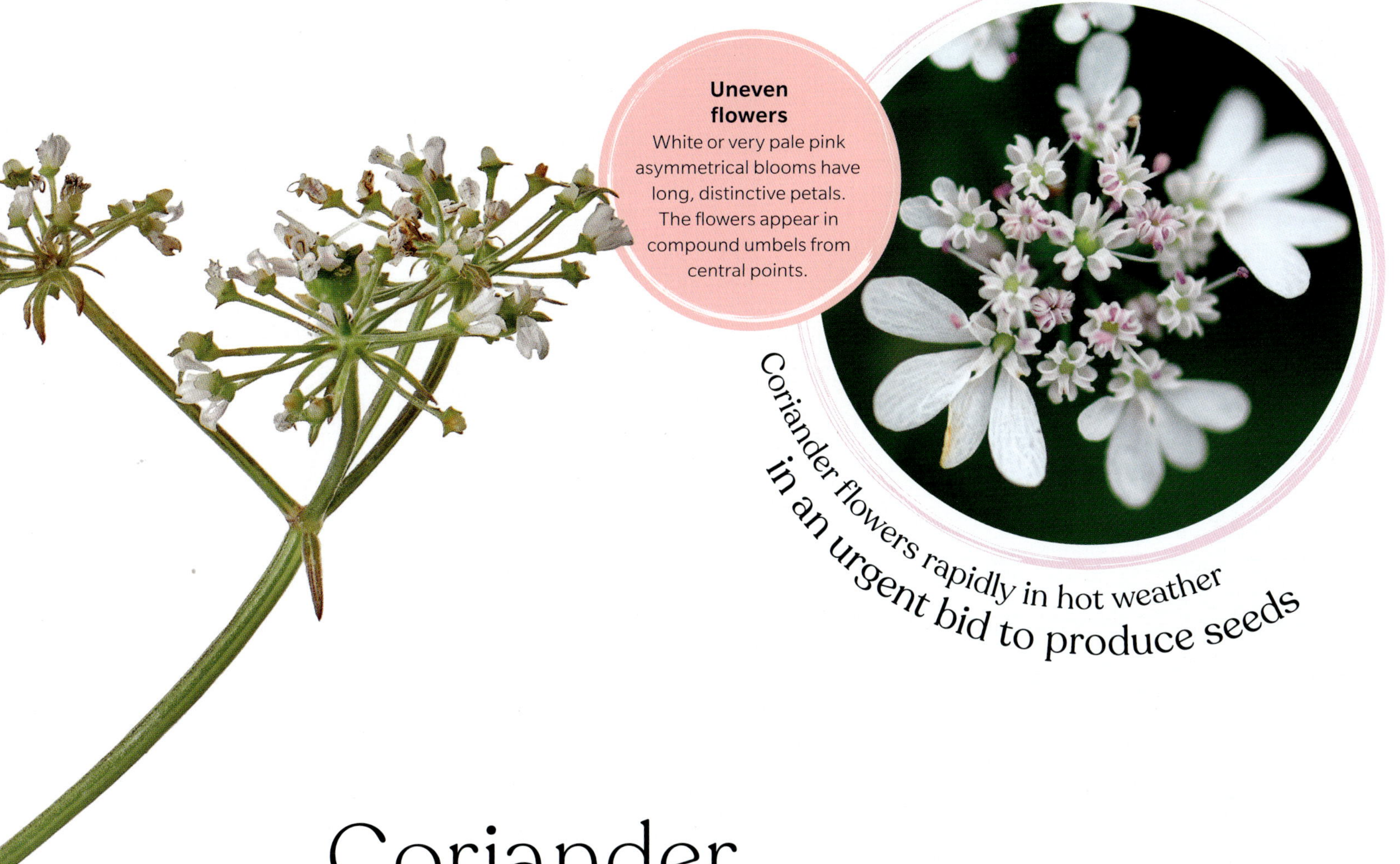

Uneven flowers
White or very pale pink asymmetrical blooms have long, distinctive petals. The flowers appear in compound umbels from central points.

Coriander flowers rapidly in hot weather in an urgent bid to produce seeds

Coriander

Coriandrum sativum

A herbal and culinary classic, coriander's citrus-tasting leaves and spicy, earthy seeds are high in vitamins and minerals, and have digestive, antibacterial, and antiviral properties.

The history of coriander can be traced back to antiquity through the writings of Theophrastus (*Historia Plantarum*, 350–287 BCE), Dioscorides (*De Materia Medica*, 50–70 CE), and Ibn Sina (Avicenna) in *Canon of Medicine*, 1025. Historically referred to as *kopiavvov*, *koriannon*, and *kuzbara*, coriander's genus name *Coriandrum* may stem from the Greek word *koriannon* – relating to the word *koris* meaning "bedbug", likening the strong scent of the herb's unripe fruit to a crushed bug. The Latin word *sativum* means "cultivated" indicating coriander's long standing narrative as a culinary and medicinal herb.

In ancient Egypt, coriander was used to treat fevers and chills, and samples of the seeds were found in King Tutankhamun's tomb as part of the funeral rites that would help take him into the next world. It is also an ancient Ayurvedic herb used for both warming and cooling; a warm and acrid, or pungent, element in Chinese folk medicine; and a staple Roman spice used to treat ailments such as nose bleeds, snake bites, ulcers, and swellings. It is also mentioned in the Jewish Torah and Christian Bible, which compares the substance known as manna with coriander seeds

➤ Regal herb
Coriander may have been included among funerary offerings in the tombs of wealthy ancient Egyptians. The excavation of King Tutankhamun's tomb in 1922 discovered coriander seeds among baskets of food and garlands of flowers.

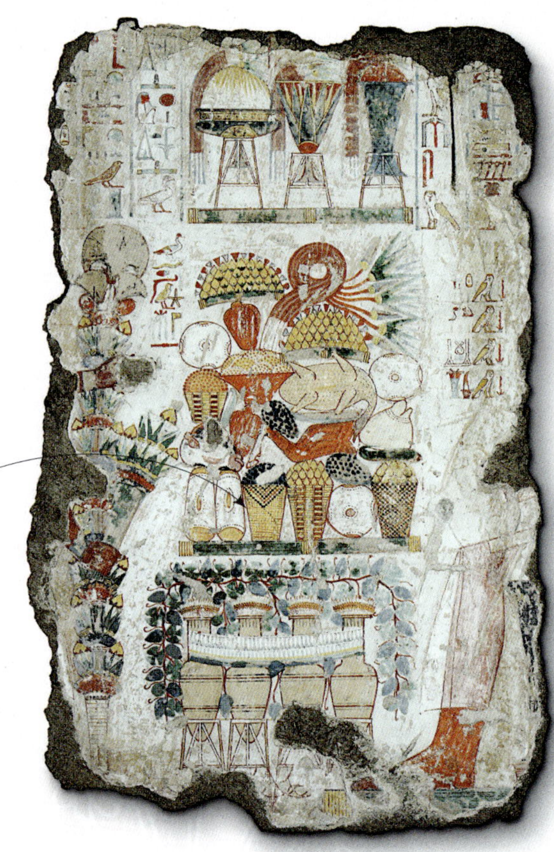

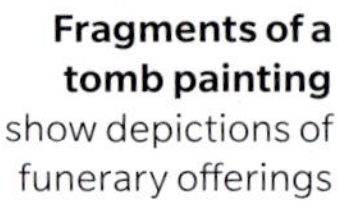

Fragments of a tomb painting show depictions of funerary offerings

Similar herbs

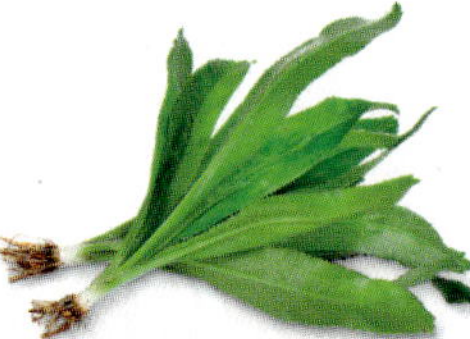

MEXICAN CORIANDER
Eryngium foetidum
Also known as culantro, the long, lance-like leaves of this Central and South American native are used as a coriander alternative and in herbal remedies.

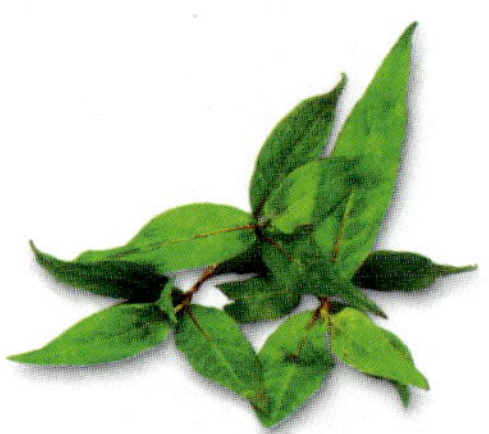

VIETNAMESE CORIANDER
Persicaria odorata
These coriander-flavoured leaves are used in South-East Asian cuisines in salads and noodle soups. It is believed to suppress libido and aid celibacy.

Today, it is known as a highly antioxidant and carminative herb used to help manage gastro-intestinal conditions such as irritable bowel syndrome or constipation, to sooth piles and menstrual issues. Its tender foliage is easy to eat or juice, while the benefits of the seeds are traditionally ingested as a decoction.

Coriander seeds also have antibacterial, antifungal, anti-inflammatory, deodorizing, and uplifting properties, and the essential oil is used to help combat cold and flu, treat aches and pains, aid digestion, soothe nervous tension, address foot infections and odour, reduce blood sugar, and soothe skin complaints. As a perfume, it has a sweet, spicy character with refreshing green notes, while cosmetically it has potential as an anti-ageing ingredient.

Refreshing leaves and earthy seeds

Coriander is best known as a culinary herb. The bright green leaves – also known by the Spanish word cilantro – are similar in appearance to parsley but provide a refreshing, citrus aspect to various cuisines either as an ingredient or as a garnish. However, some people find its taste unpleasantly soapy, which is caused by a genetic sensitivity to the aldehydes (a type of organic compound) present in the plant.

Coriander is popular in Central and South American cuisines, having been introduced by the Europeans in the 17th century. The green sauce *mojo de cilantro*, hailing from the Spanish island of Tenerife, is made with coriander leaves and is traditionally served with *papas arrugadas* (salt-crusted potatoes) and chilli. Many Asian cuisines use the tangy stems and peppery roots in sauces, broths, curries, and soups, while the traditional Indo-Chinese lemon coriander soup, uses chopped leaves for a particularly immune-boosting combination. The more earthy coriander seeds are commonly used in Indian cuisine, as well as featuring in Middle Eastern, and Mediterranean sweet and savoury dishes.

Small, creamy-brown fruits are often toasted and ground into a powder

◄ Ripened fruits
The dried, round fruits of the coriander plant splits into two seed-like mericarps when ripe. They lend a warm, aromatic flavour to dishes and contain a medicinal oil.

> “ It is sweet in taste... and possesses hot potency... and helps to pacify all three doshas. ”
>
> BHAVAMISHRA
> *Bhavaprakasha Nighantu* (Ayurvedic text), 16th century

Celery

Apium graveolens

Celery is commonly cultivated for its highly nutritious, fibrous leaf stalks, known as celery sticks, and its leaves and seeds. It is also used medicinally for its antioxidant, anti-inflammatory, carminative, nervine, and diuretic properties.

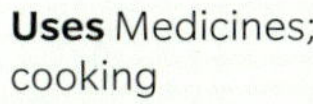

Uses Medicines; cooking

Parts used Leaf stalks, stems (celeriac)

Active ingredients Limonene, apiole, sedanolide, butylphthalide, luteolin

Habitat Open, damp locations, often coastal, in temperate regions

The ancient Greeks named this herb *selinon*, from *heleioselinon* (from the marshes). The name *petroselinon* (rock selinon) was given to its relative parsley (see pp.220–21), which is indicative of celery's preference for moist, nutrient rich soil. Native to a wide area of the Mediterranean, it is thought to have been used and cultivated for thousands of years as a vegetable, flavouring, and medicinal herb.

Fibrous ingredient

As described by Mrs M. Grieve in *A Modern Herbal* (1931) celery is useful for "promoting restfulness and sleep, and diffusing through the system a mild sustaining influence". It is now known to include high levels of dietary fibre, vitamins, and minerals, and it can be used for supporting brain and heart health. The leaf stalks are a popular addition to the tomato-based Bloody Mary cocktail; they also combine well with onions and carrots in the French base *mirepoix*, or with onions and peppers in Cajun cuisine. The seeds can be ground down into a powder, and used to make flavourful celery salt, as can the extract of root, or the dried leaves.

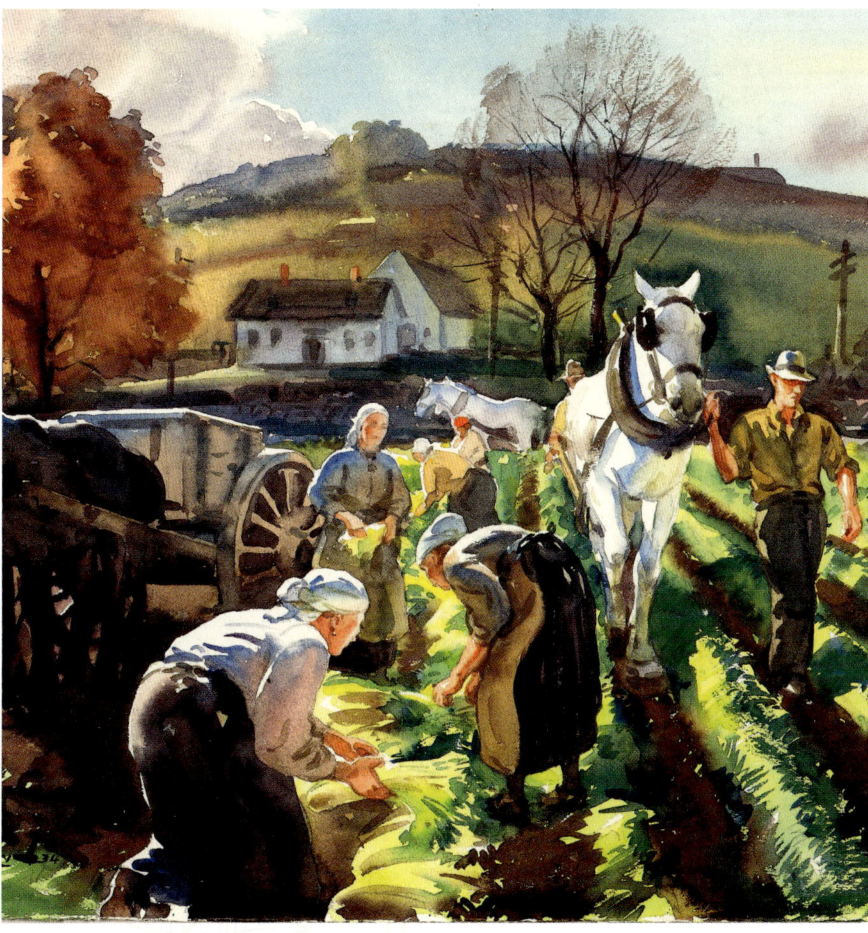

▲ Celery garden
Cultivation of celery in the US, as depicted in *Celery Garden, Lexington* by Aiden Lassell Ripley (1896–1969), was pioneered by Dutch immigrants in the late 1800s.

► Nutritious tops
Celery is typically grown as an annual for its thick, crunchy edible leaf stalks, but the leafy tops are also edible and highly nutritious. The leaves are useful in salads, stir fries, and soups.

Twice-pinnate leaves are divided into toothed leaflets

The ancient Greeks used wild celery to crown the winners of their Panhellenic games

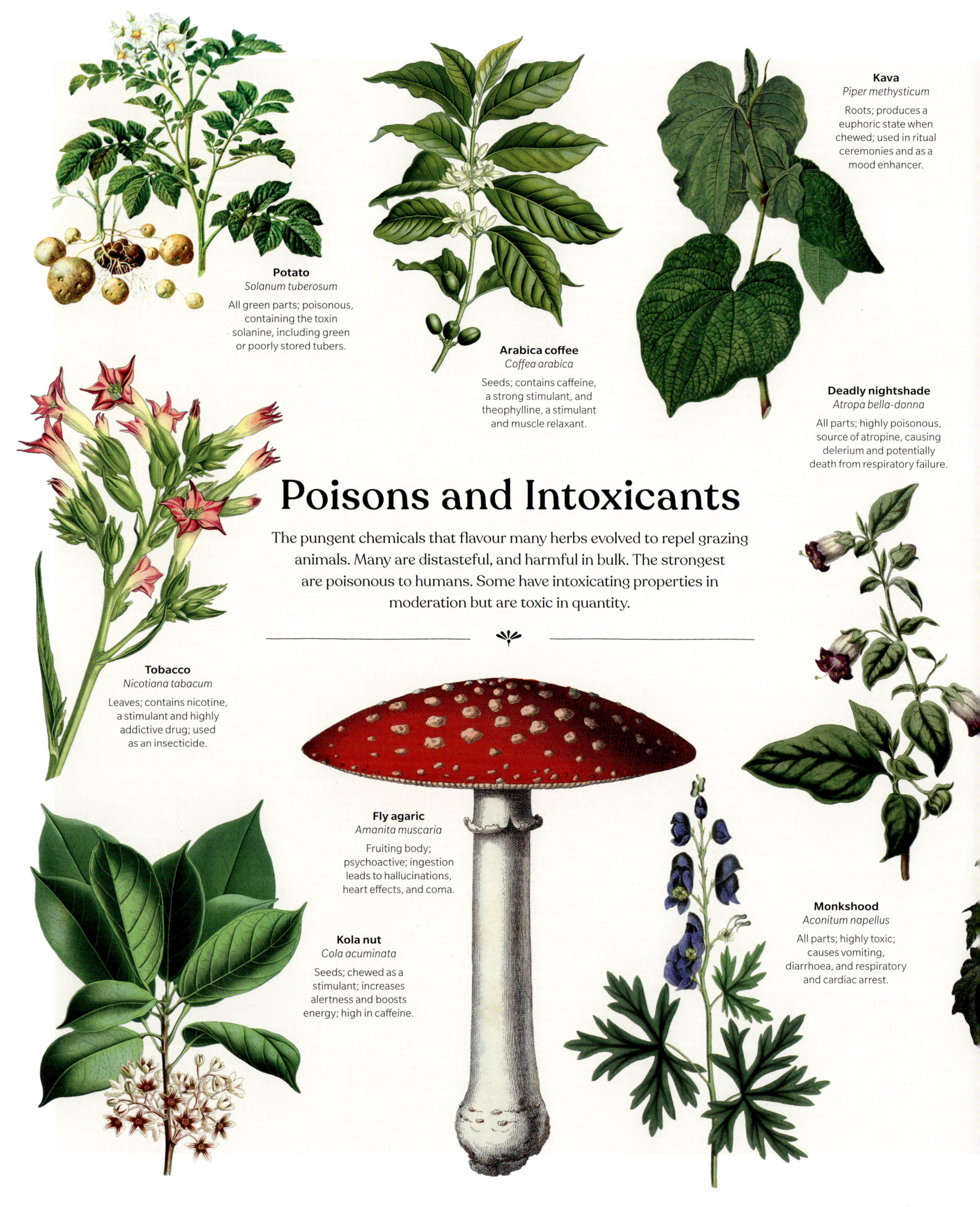

Poisons and Intoxicants

The pungent chemicals that flavour many herbs evolved to repel grazing animals. Many are distasteful, and harmful in bulk. The strongest are poisonous to humans. Some have intoxicating properties in moderation but are toxic in quantity.

Potato
Solanum tuberosum
All green parts; poisonous, containing the toxin solanine, including green or poorly stored tubers.

Arabica coffee
Coffea arabica
Seeds; contains caffeine, a strong stimulant, and theophylline, a stimulant and muscle relaxant.

Kava
Piper methysticum
Roots; produces a euphoric state when chewed; used in ritual ceremonies and as a mood enhancer.

Deadly nightshade
Atropa bella-donna
All parts; highly poisonous, source of atropine, causing delerium and potentially death from respiratory failure.

Tobacco
Nicotiana tabacum
Leaves; contains nicotine, a stimulant and highly addictive drug; used as an insecticide.

Fly agaric
Amanita muscaria
Fruiting body; psychoactive; ingestion leads to hallucinations, heart effects, and coma.

Kola nut
Cola acuminata
Seeds; chewed as a stimulant; increases alertness and boosts energy; high in caffeine.

Monkshood
Aconitum napellus
All parts; highly toxic; causes vomiting, diarrhoea, and respiratory and cardiac arrest.

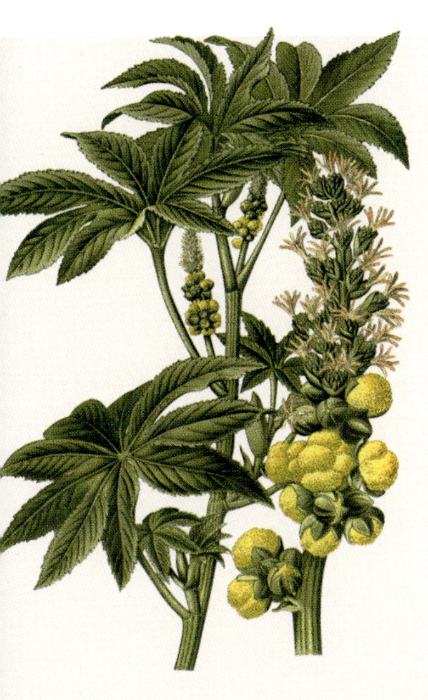

Castor oil plant
Ricinus communis

Seeds; very poisonous; contains toxic protein ricin; the toxin-free oil is used as a strong laxative.

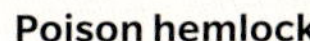

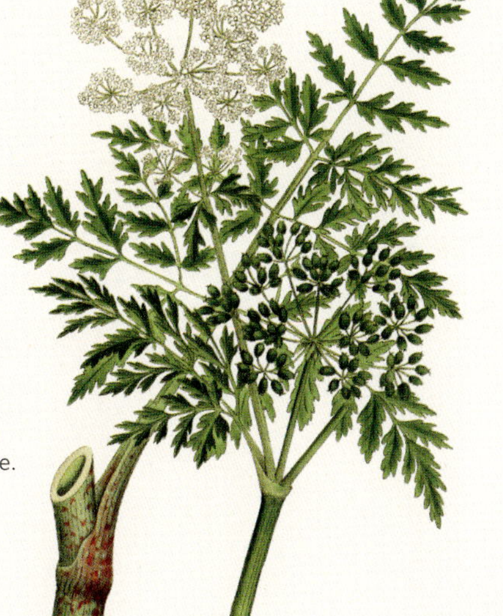

Poison hemlock
Conium maculatum

All parts; highly poisonous; causes paralysis, and death from respiratory failure.

Mandrake
Mandragora officinarum

All parts; poisonous; alkaloids hyoscine and hyoscyamine historically used to relieve pain in surgery.

Marijuana
Cannabis sativa

Resin and leaves; contains cannabinoids; consumed for psychoactive effects; can be addictive.

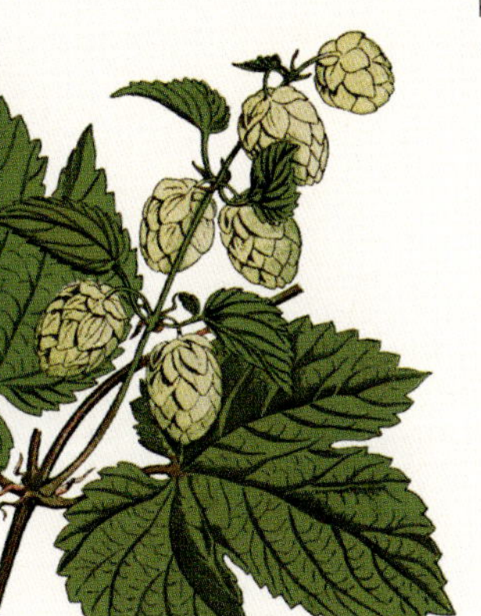

Hop
Humulus lupulus

Resin; inhibits the central nervous system; strongly sedative, used to treat insomnia.

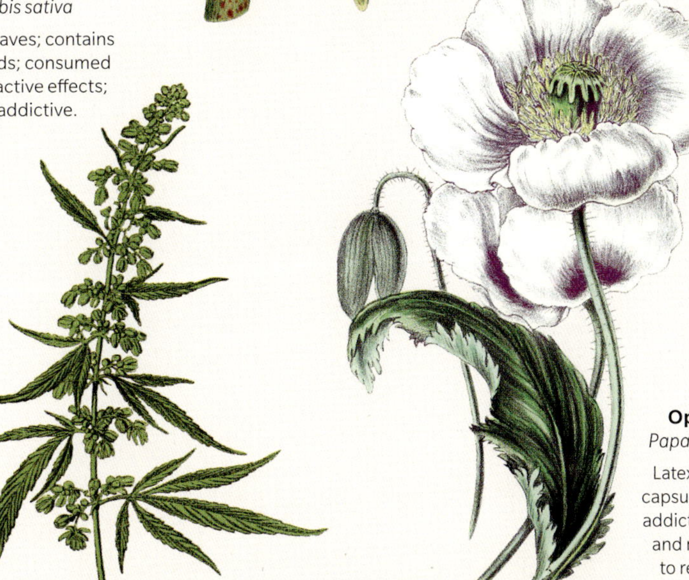

Opium poppy
Papaver somniferum

Latex of unripe seed capsules; source of the addictive drugs opium and morphine, used to relieve pain and induce sleep.

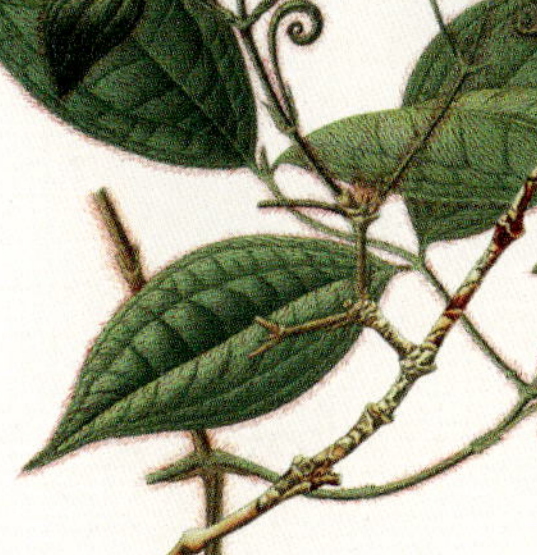

Curare
Chondrodendron tomentosum

Bark; poisonous; pounded and mixed with other plants to make a paralyzing poison (curare) to put on arrows.

Coca
Erythroxylum coca

Leaves; chewed as a stimulant and to combat altitude sickness; source of the drug cocaine, used medically and as an addictive narcotic.

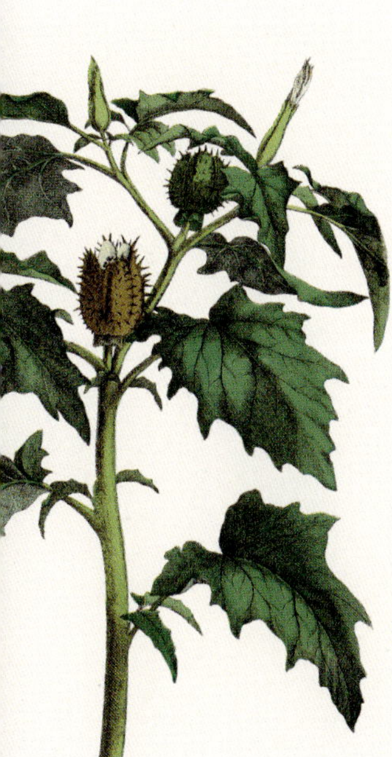

Jimsonweed
Datura stramonium

All parts; poisonous and potentially deadly; lower doses cause hallucinations.

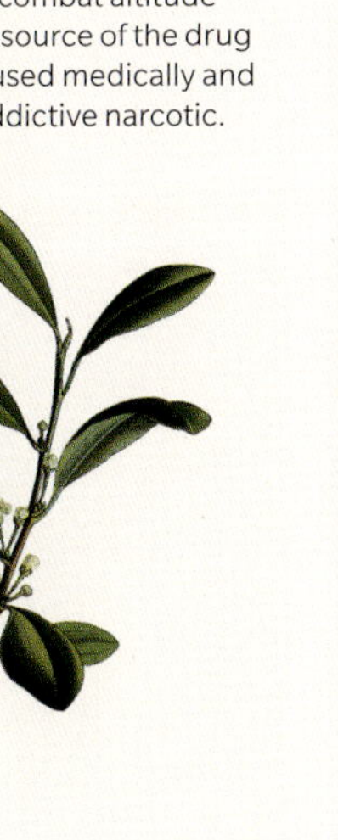

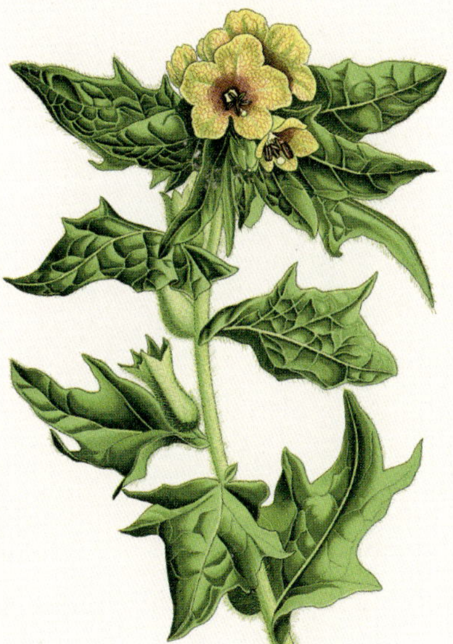

Henbane
Hyoscyamus niger

Leaves and seeds; poisonous; causes hallucinations, seizures, and potentially death; used as herbal sedative and painkiller.

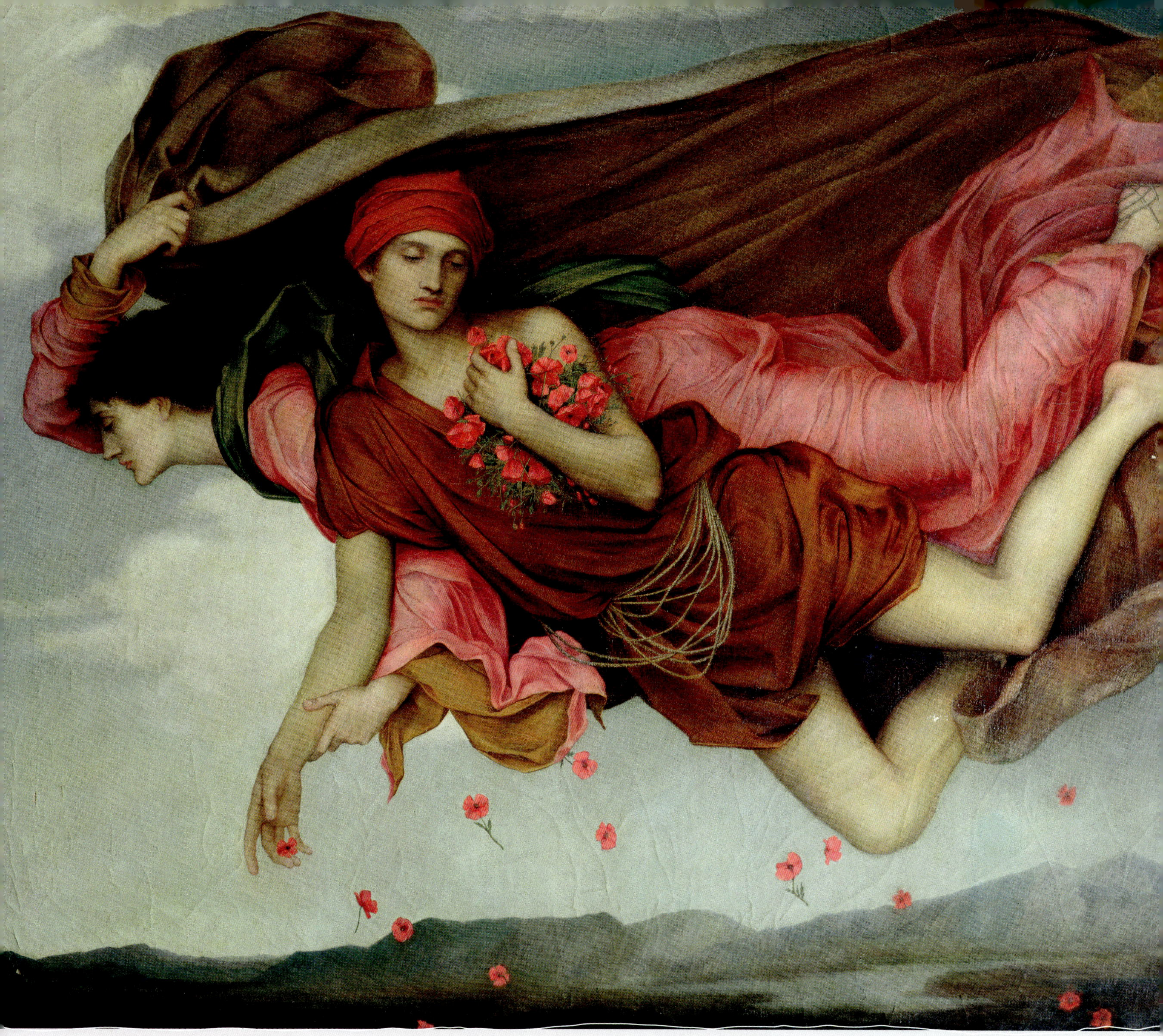

Opium Poppy

Papaver somniferum

The fleeting beauty of this herb belies its potency: its produce is one of the oldest and most powerful medicines for pain and insomnia, but is also a narcotic that has generated misery and even led to wars.

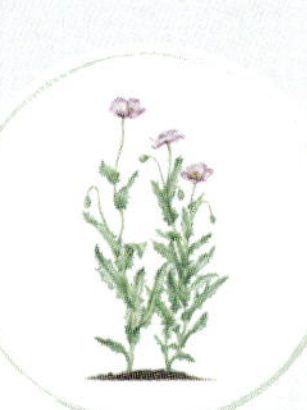

Uses Medicines; cooking; horticulture; narcotic

Parts used Latex, fruits, seeds

Active ingredients Opium, which contains morphine, codeine, papaverine, and other alkaloids

Habitat Sunny, well-drained soil on arable field margins, waysides, and open land, mainly in temperate climates

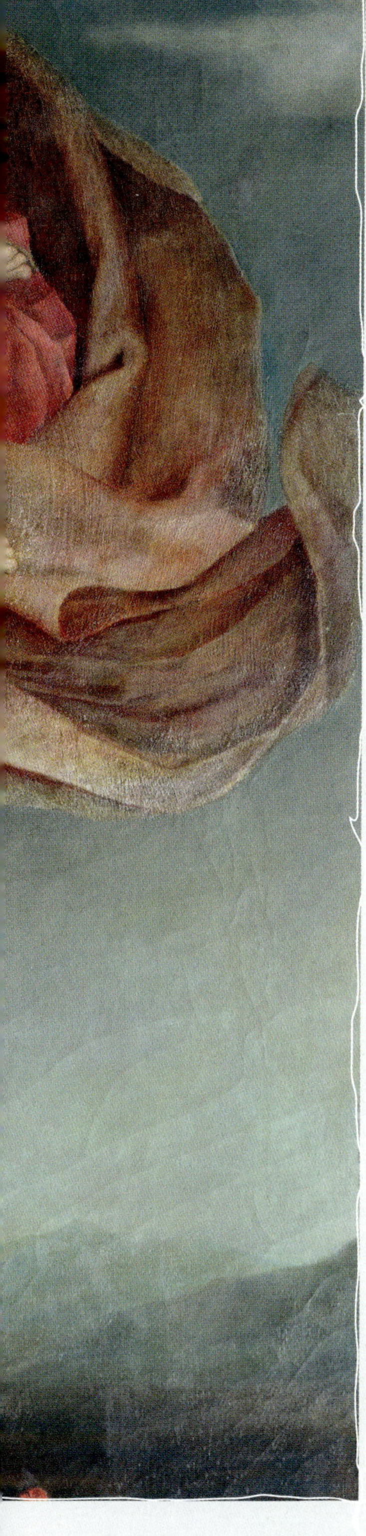

Opium is concentrated in a sticky latex found in the walls of the opium poppy's seed capsule. It is obtained by scoring the ripened capsule with a sharp blade and scraping off the exuding white latex, or poppy tears, as it dries into a brownish gum. Opium was known as a pain reliever and inducer of relaxation in Ancient Greece, Rome, and Persia. It was probably the *hul gil* or "joy plant" described in Ancient Sumerian texts from 3,400 BCE. In Ancient Egypt, opium was said to be a gift from the ibis-headed god, Thoth. The Ancient Greek father of medicine, Hippocrates, recommended drinking poppy juice mixed with nettle seeds to treat pain. It was the most powerful of stupefying drugs, equally effective for bowel disorders, toothache, and battle wounds.

In China, opium was administered to patients before surgery by doctor Hua To in the 2nd century CE. It was also thought to aid masculinity by strengthening sperm and general vigour. In traditional Ayurvedic medicine, opium was used for pain, diarrhoea, and dysentery; it is still prescribed in herbal pills and pastes, which can be addictive, to relieve ailments such as pain, impotence, coughs, and colds.

In 16th-century Europe, powdered opium was sold in herbal mixtures. One called Fracastorius's diascordium was used for easing childbirth pains, malignant (serious, infectious) fevers and plague, and was praised by English herbalist Nicholas Culpeper in 1653 as "a well-composed Electuary" (medicinal remedy sweetened with honey).

> " The whyte Popy is colde and moyste and it is good to cause one to slepe. "
>
> ANON, *Banckes's Herbal*, 1525

Large flowers, to 10 cm (4 in) wide, have four overlapping petals
Grey-green leaves have wavy margins; upper leaves clasp the stem
Stout stem is slightly hairy and 1–1.5 m (3–5 ft) tall
Seed capsule is ready to yield opium when fully swollen and green

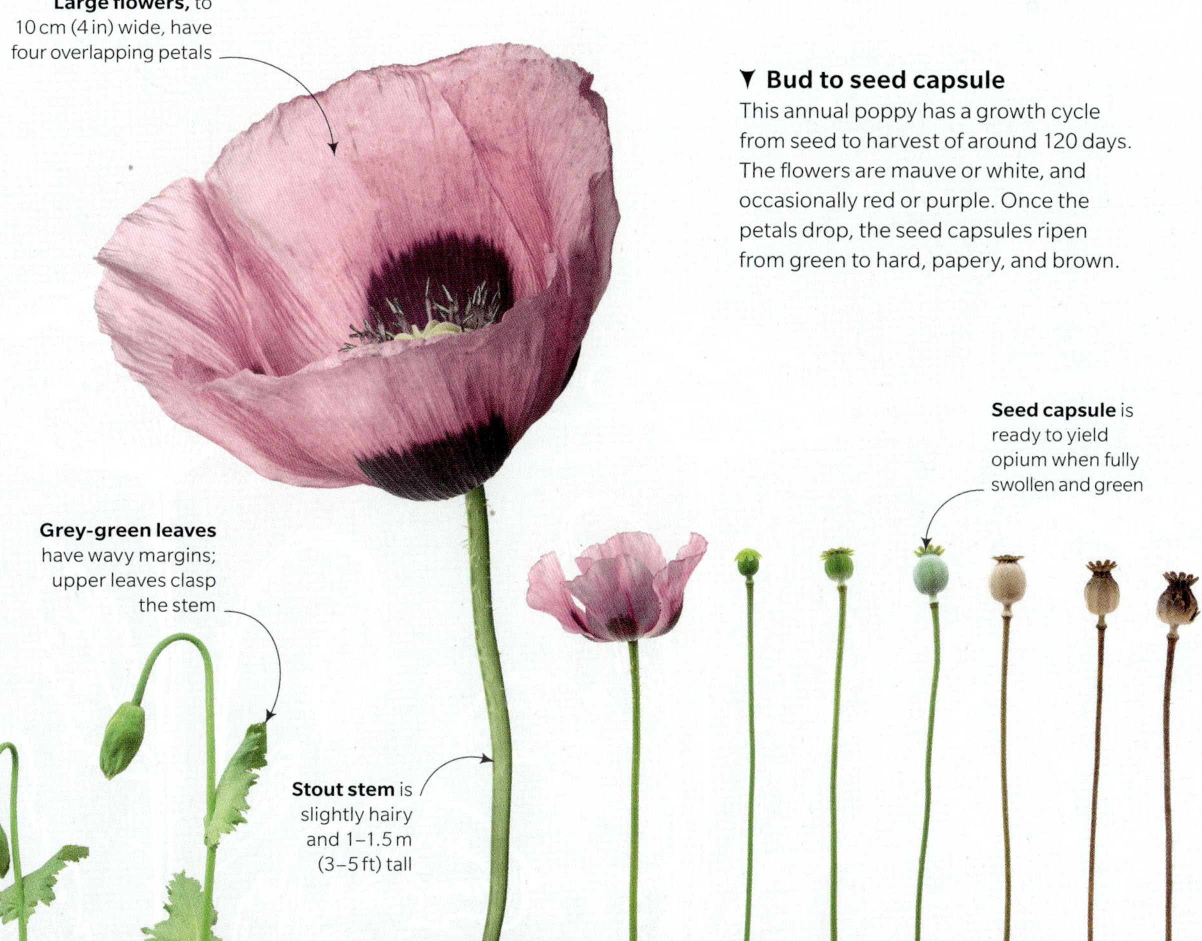

▼ Bud to seed capsule
This annual poppy has a growth cycle from seed to harvest of around 120 days. The flowers are mauve or white, and occasionally red or purple. Once the petals drop, the seed capsules ripen from green to hard, papery, and brown.

▲ Night and Sleep
Evelyn de Morgan's 1878 painting was inspired by Nyx, the Greek goddess of night, and her son Hypnos, god of sleep. Hypnos was always shown with opium poppies; here, Nyx carries Hypnos as he scatters poppies to the earth below.

➤ Soldier's morphine
Tins with morphine syrettes (single doses of morphine with a needle) were issued to individual soldiers and the British Royal Army Medical Corps in World War II.

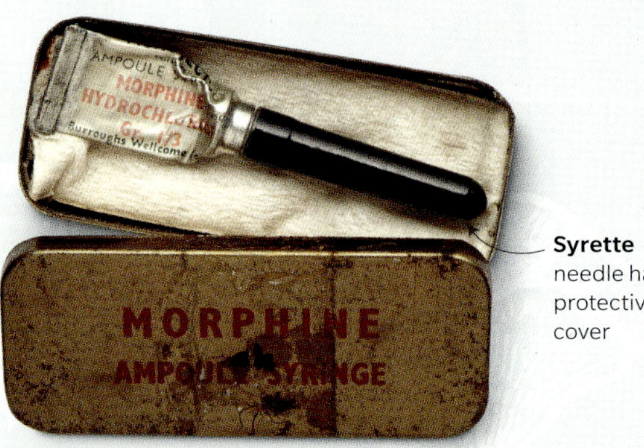

Syrette needle has protective cover

The opium trade

By the 1830s, India was the largest exporter of opium, under control of the British government. Most was exported to China, where its use, often smoked in pipes, was illegal. The profits funded British trade in Chinese tea and other goods. China tried to ban the trade in 1839, because of widespread opium addiction, seizing opium stocks from British warehouses. This led to two opium wars (in 1840–43 and 1856–60), the outcome of which was to preserve the trade for much of the 19th century. Opium dens sprung up in cities in the West as well as Asia. Clients were supplied with pipes and lamps to heat the opium, and couches to lie on as the drug took effect, as described in Charles Dickens' last novel, *The Mystery of Edwin Drood*. The opium dens were eventually outlawed.

Laudanum and heroin

Made from opium dissolved in alcohol, laudanum was a popular 19th-century drug, available at drug stores and pharmacists. Reddish-brown and very bitter, it relieved pain, diarrhoea, stress, and sleeplessness and was widely used as a sleeping draught. It was also addictive; laudanum addiction became widespread in Europe and the US. It is now banned from sale, but is still used in drugs such as dropizol, a treatment for diarrhoea.

▼ Poppy field
Contrary to belief, walking in poppy fields does not make you drowsy. Opium poppies are grown legally in some nations, here in Germany, for the pharmaceutical industry. The world's largest illegal grower of opium is Afghanistan.

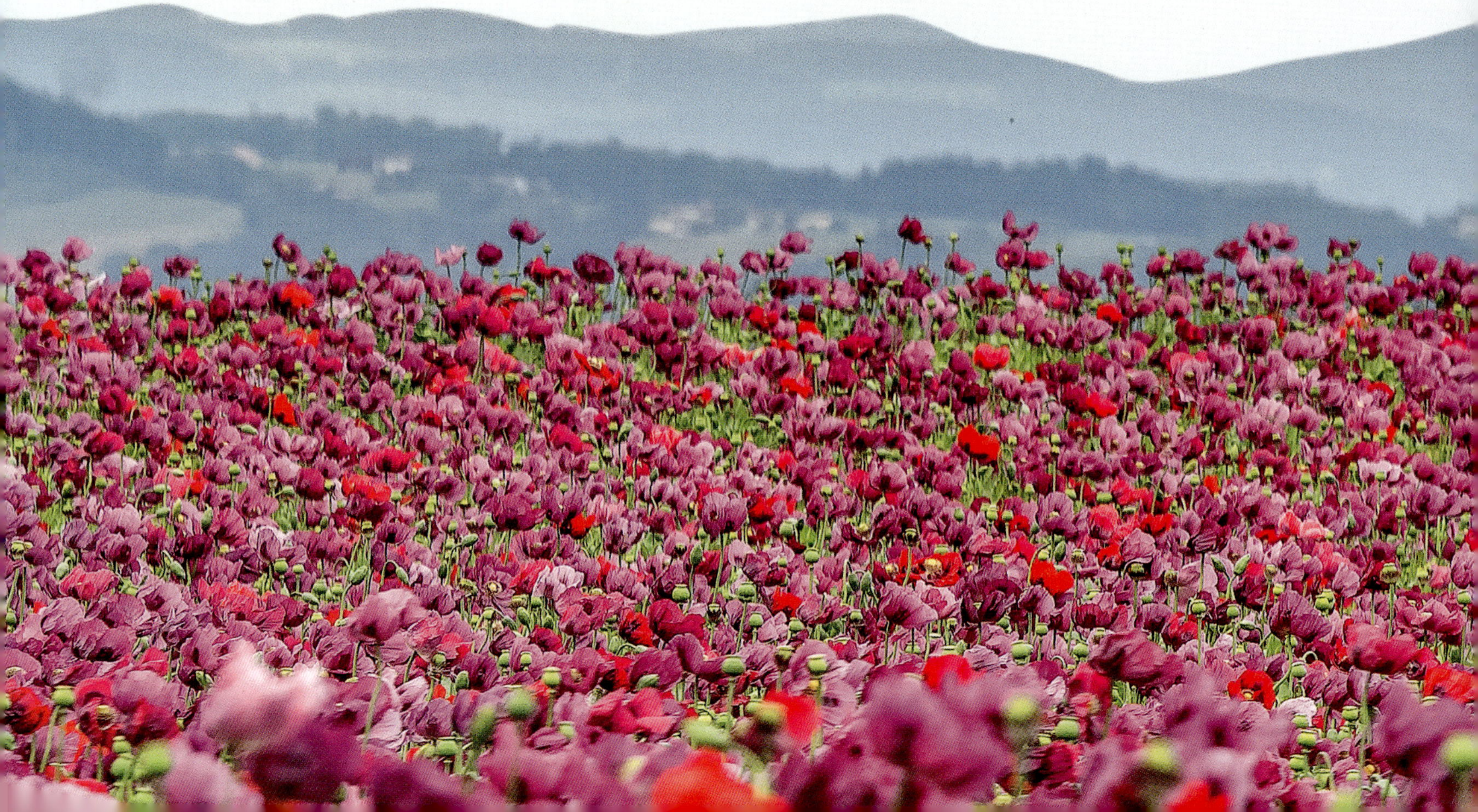

The main ingredient in opium is an alkaloid first isolated in 1803 by German pharmacist Friedrich Sertürner, and named morphium (now morphine), after Morpheus, Greek god of dreams and son of Hypnos (see p.228). Other alkaloids to be isolated from opium were codeine in 1832 and papaverine in 1848; today both have medical uses in their pure, synthesized forms.

The narcotic heroin was first synthesized from morphine in 1874 and was believed to be non-addictive and less dangerous than morphine, even being added to children's cough medicine. It is still used in pain relief and palliative care as diamorphine. In its pure form, heroin is highly addictive, especially if smoked or injected.

By 2015, an estimated 17 million people worldwide regularly used illegal opiates, of which heroin is the most common. As other clinical

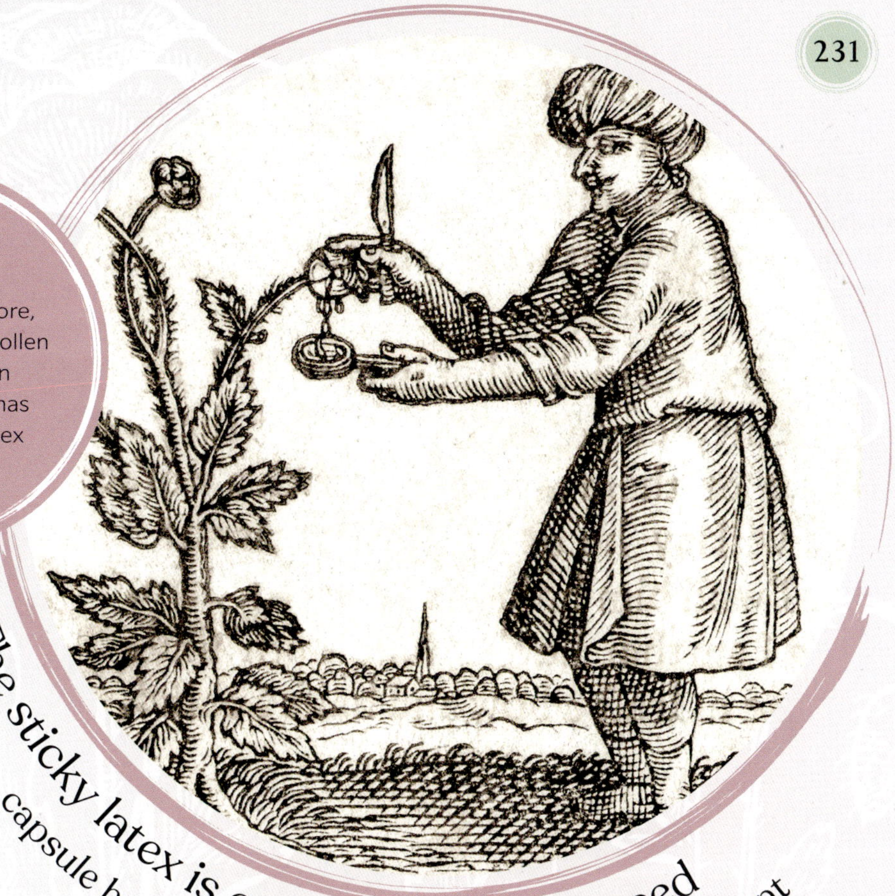

Harvesting raw opium
For 5,000 years or more, scoring the walls of swollen seed capsules, as in this 1614 woodcut, has yielded the milky latex called opium.

The sticky latex is collected once the seed capsule has hardened and while it is still on the plant

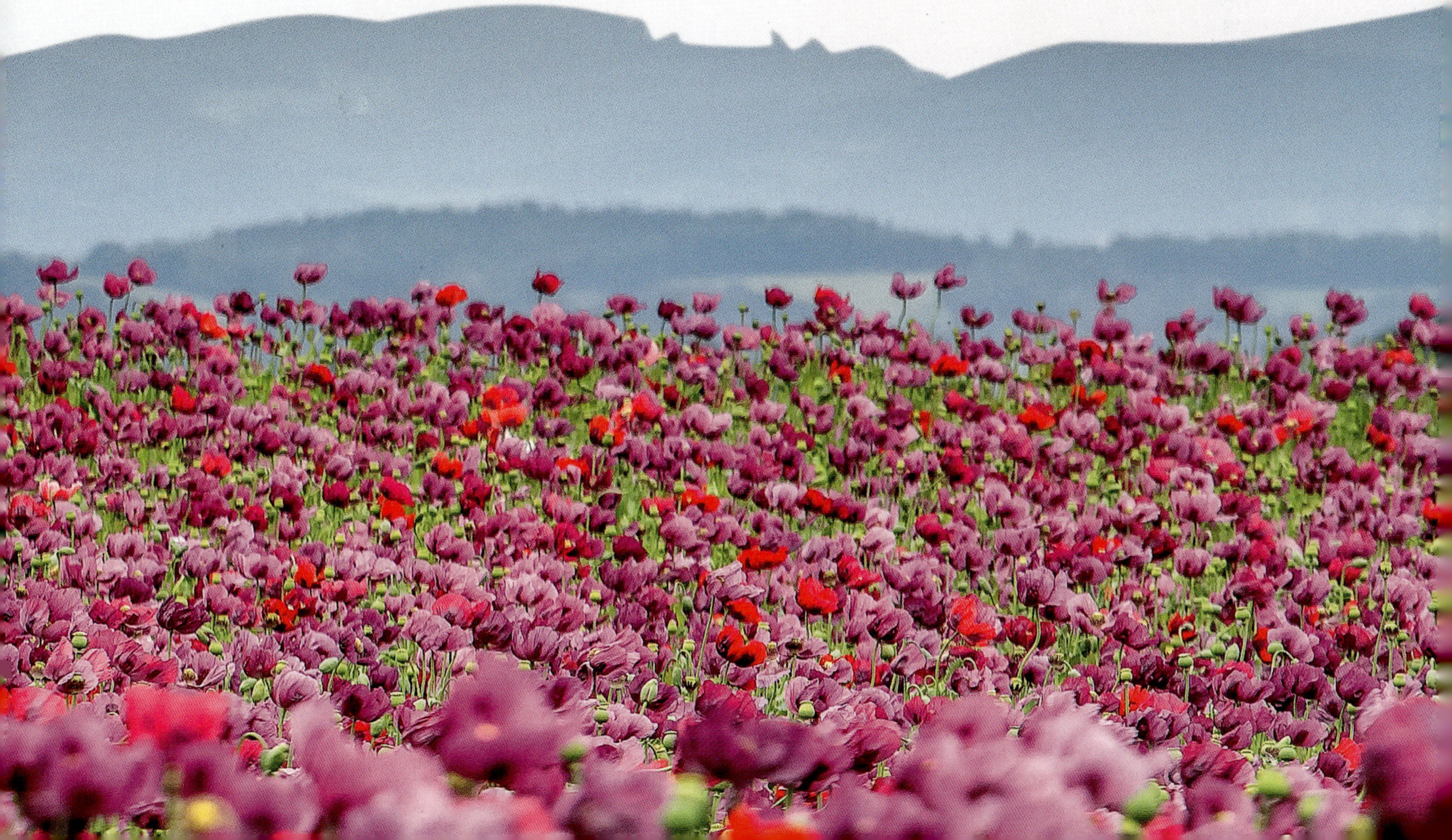

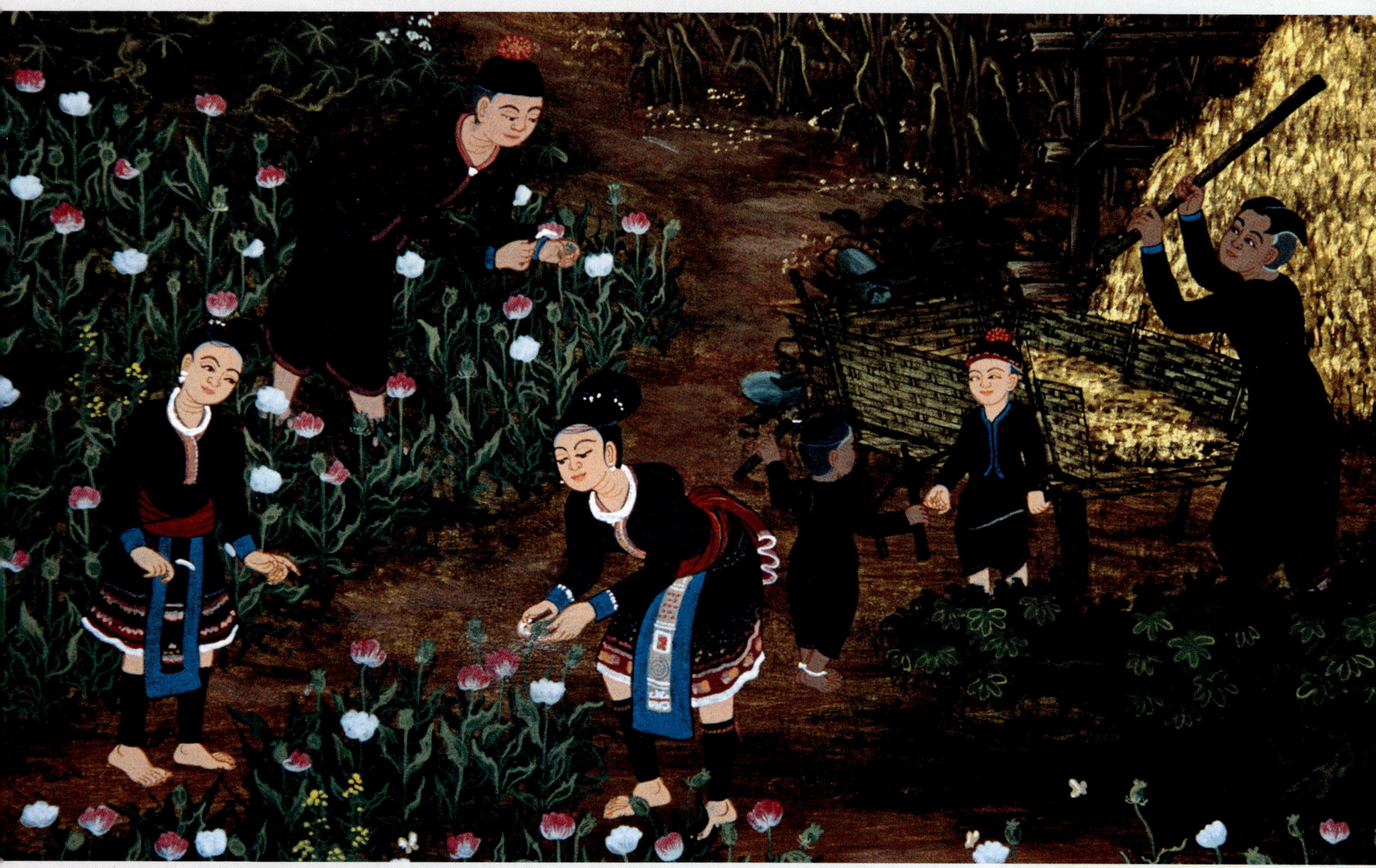

▲ **Harvesting poppies, Thai miniature**
Here, hill farmers in northern Thailand harvest opium in the cool season, between December and February. The most concentrated illegal opium cultivation is in the "Golden Triangle" of Laos, Myanmar, and Thailand.

HOW DO ANALGESIC HERBS WORK?

Analgesic herbs relieve pain by modulating, or temporarily inhibiting, the pain receptors in the brain. Some also decrease inflammation by inhibiting the release of inflammatory compounds. The principal clinically-used analgesics for moderate to acute pain are opiates, derived from the opium poppy and used in the treatment of a post-operative pain, trauma, and cancer pain. Other analgesic herbs include feverfew (see pp.156–57), ginger (see pp.170–73), and white willow (see pp.40–41), the source of compounds related to aspirin.

drugs became available and the harmful effects of addiction more widely known, an international commission was set up to control and reduce the production and trade of opium. It is now called the International Narcotics Control Board (INCB).

Opium poppy as a crop

While it originated in the Mediterranean region, this herb has been grown as a medicinal crop and for its edible seeds for centuries, especially in China, Southeast Asia, and the Middle East. Today, it is cultivated under government control, mainly in India, Turkey, and Tasmania, but is grown illegally worldwide, especially in the Middle East, Southeast Asia, and South America.

The disease-resistant plant tolerates a range of soils and arid conditions. Hardy even in northern climates, it readily spreads into the wild. Once the seed capsules have been "tapped" for opium or emptied of seeds, the poppy straw (dried plants) is burned for ash as a soil fertilizer. Dried seed capsules can be processed to extract more morphine. Poppies are a break crop; they restore soil fertility after years of cereal growing.

Edible seeds

Poppy seeds lack narcotic alkaloids so can be sold legally for culinary use. The seeds are rich in oil, dietary fibre, vitamins, and minerals such as iron, calcium, and magnesium. With its nutty taste, the seed is widely used for baked goods – sprinkled over loaves, buns, and pastries. Ground seeds make a sweet paste, as in Poland where the paste fills a rolled cake, called *makowiec*. The pressed seeds produce a straw-coloured, odourless oil with a pleasant taste of almonds. In Indian cooking, poppy seed, or *khus khus*, is an important food ingredient, said to improve digestion, boost fertility, and even improve libido; *khus khus* also appears in Ayurvedic skincare products. The principal exporters of poppy seed are the Czech Republic, Turkey, and Spain.

Opium poppies are hardy and are popular garden plants because of their large, showy flowers, and "pepperpot" seed capsules that suit dried flower arrangements. Cultivated varieties have colours and forms rarely found in nature.

IN FLANDERS FIELDS

In Europe, the field, or corn, poppy (*Papaver rhoeas*) has become a symbol, exploited by many poets, to commemorate those fallen in battle. The soil churned up by battles in World War I in Flanders, Belgium, threw poppy seeds to the surface. In the spring, swathes of blood-red poppies covered the fields of war.

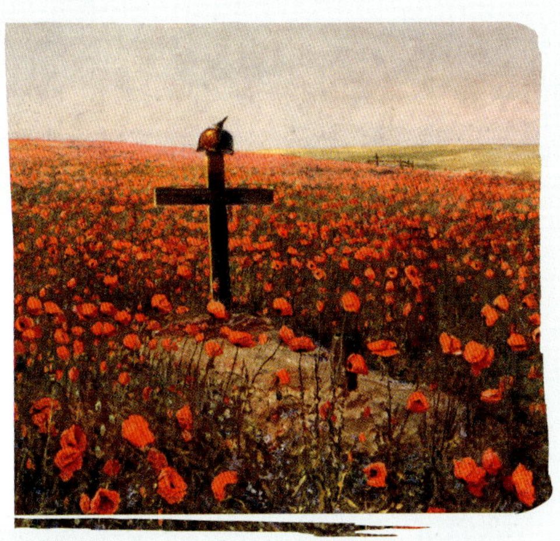

WAR GRAVE AMONG POPPIES

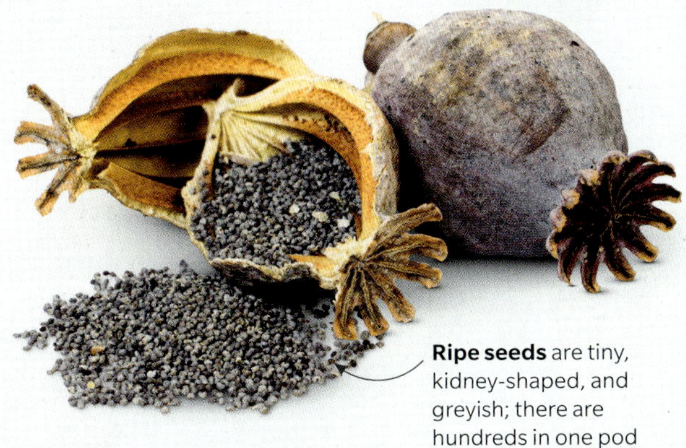

Ripe seeds are tiny, kidney-shaped, and greyish; there are hundreds in one pod

▲ **Seed capsules**
Seeds are harvested when the round to urn-shaped capsules are brown and dry. Below the crown, formed from stigmas, are pores that release the seeds when the wind shakes the capsule.

> " I have struggled against this fascinating enthralment, and... untwisted... the accursed chain which fettered me. "
>
> THOMAS DE QUINCEY, *Confessions of an English Opium-Eater*, 1821

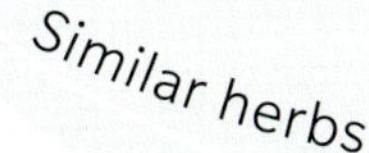

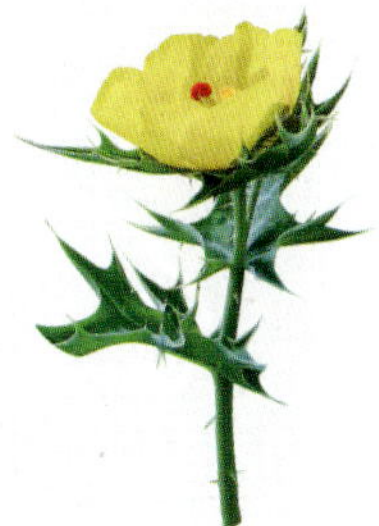

MEXICAN POPPY
Argemone mexicana
A perennial poppy that exudes a toxic, yellow latex. It has many uses in traditional medicine, including as a pain reliever, skin treatment, and laxative. Its toxic seed oil is used in soap.

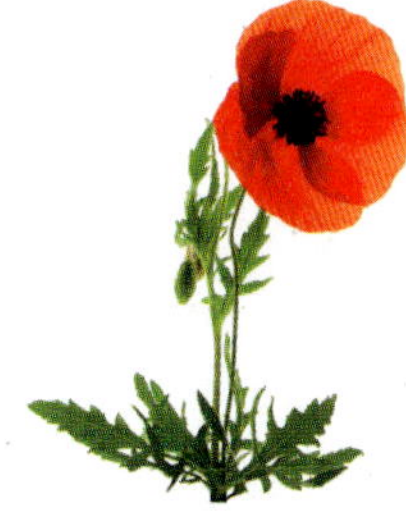

FIELD POPPY
Papaver rhoeas
A well-known, annual weed of arable fields in temperate areas across the world. Its edible, black, oily seeds are used in baking, and the red petals to colour wine and as a herbal tea.

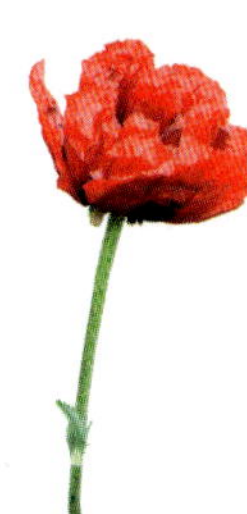

IRANIAN POPPY
Papaver bracteatum
This perennial from Iran and Russia is 1 m (3 ft) tall. It is cultivated as a source of thebaine, which can be converted into codeine and synthetic opiates, but it lacks any morphine.

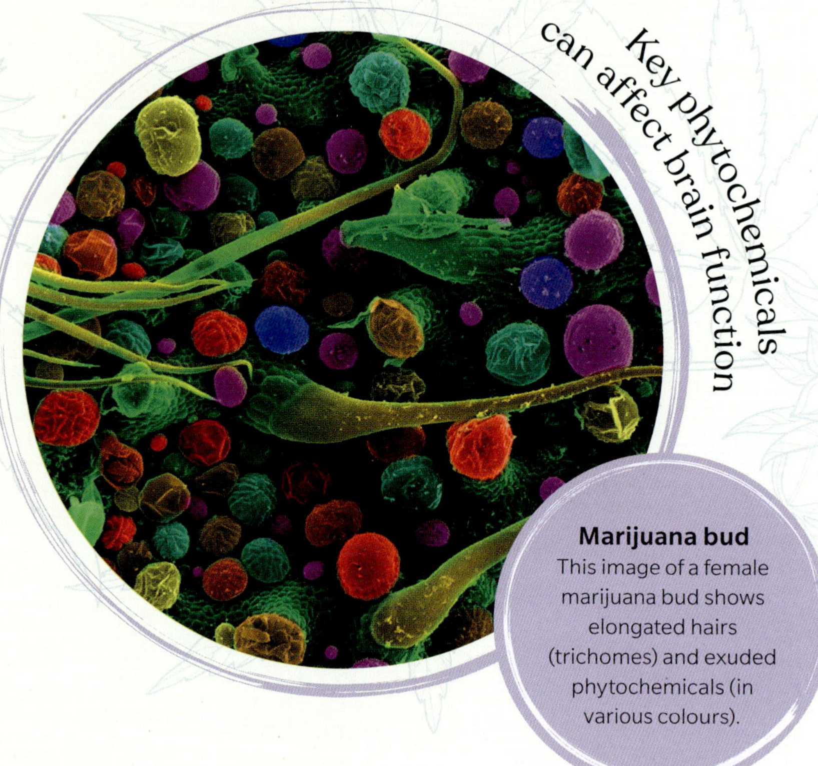

Marijuana bud
This image of a female marijuana bud shows elongated hairs (trichomes) and exuded phytochemicals (in various colours).

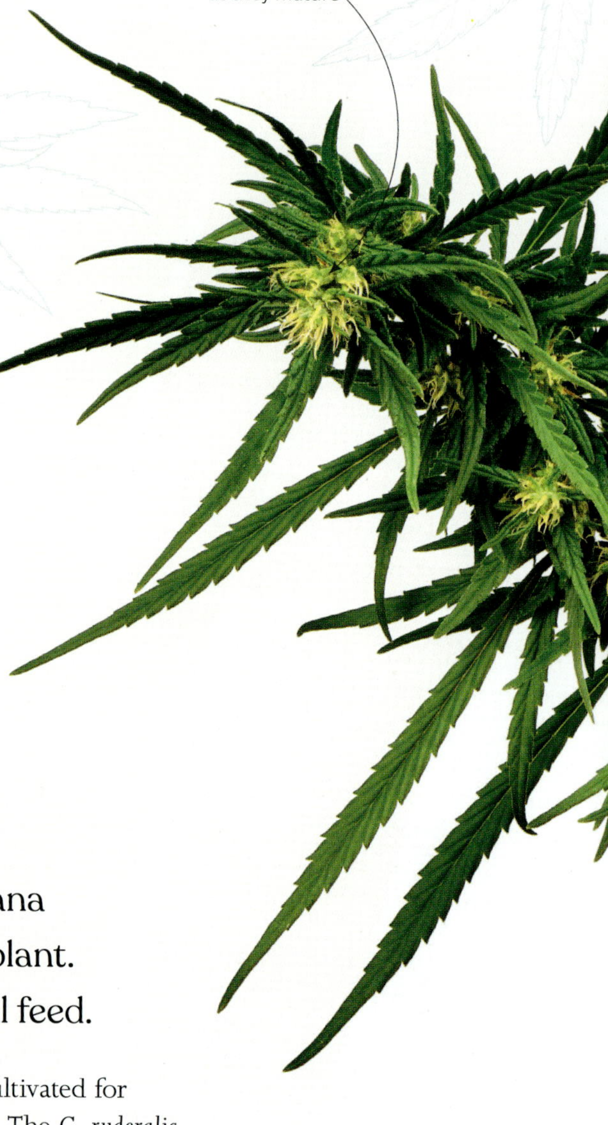

Marijuana

Cannabis sativa

First domesticated in China around 12,000 years ago, marijuana has one of the longest histories of human association of any plant. Its many uses include medicine, clothing, edible oil, and animal feed.

Marijuana is native to central Asia and is closely related to brewer's hops (*Humulus lupulus*, see pp.148–49). The term "marijuana" can refer to the whole plant, or to the most basic preparation – herbal cannabis – comprising dried flowers, buds, and leaves. A powdered form is known as "kief", while "hashish" refers to a concentrated resin. Scientists and others disagree on whether there is a single variable species (*Cannabis sativa*) or three separate species – the others being *C. indica* and *C. ruderalis* (see p.237). The three names are often used to indicate different characteristics. *C. sativa* is tall and is used for fibre and seed production (widely known as hemp), while *C. indica* is shorter and cultivated for medicinal and recreational use. The *C. ruderalis* form is the shortest and is used for breeding only.

Cannabis culture

Using cannabis as a recreational drug remains controversial. Its cultivation and possession are controlled by

Harvested bud includes flowers and leaves

➤ Cannabis bud
At the tip of the female plant, clusters of flowers (colas) develop. These are the most sought-after parts for drug manufacture.

"The Scythians take the seed of this hemp and... throw it on the red-hot stones... no Greek vapor-bath could surpass it."

HERODOTUS,
History, c.425 BCE

Uses Medicines; cooking; fibre

Parts used Flower buds and resin, leaves, stems

Active ingredients
Tetrahydrocannabinol (THC), cannabidiol (CBD), other cannabinoids, terpenes such as sesquiterpenes

Habitat Temperate and subtropical climates

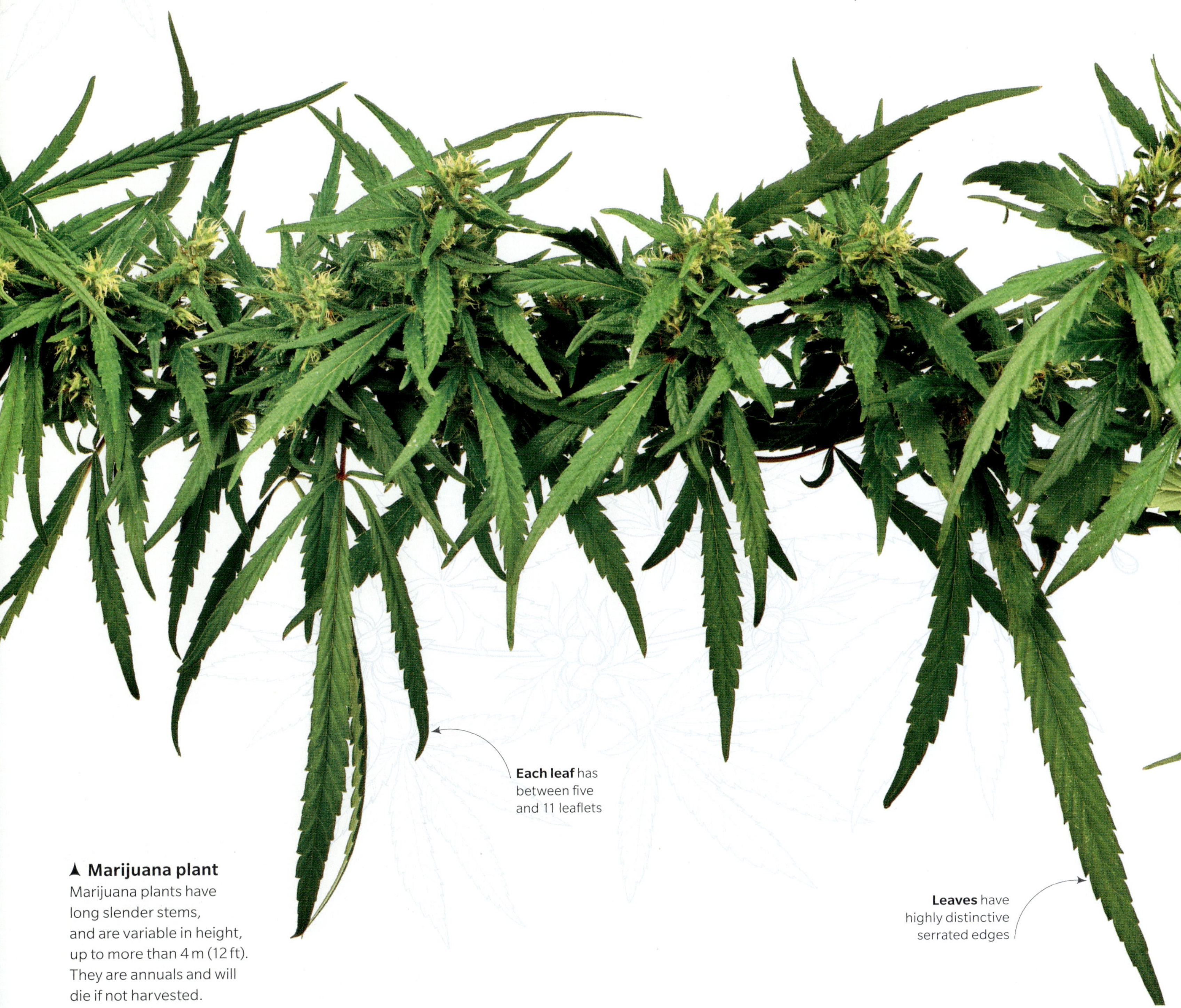

Each leaf has between five and 11 leaflets

Leaves have highly distinctive serrated edges

▲ Marijuana plant
Marijuana plants have long slender stems, and are variable in height, up to more than 4 m (12 ft). They are annuals and will die if not harvested.

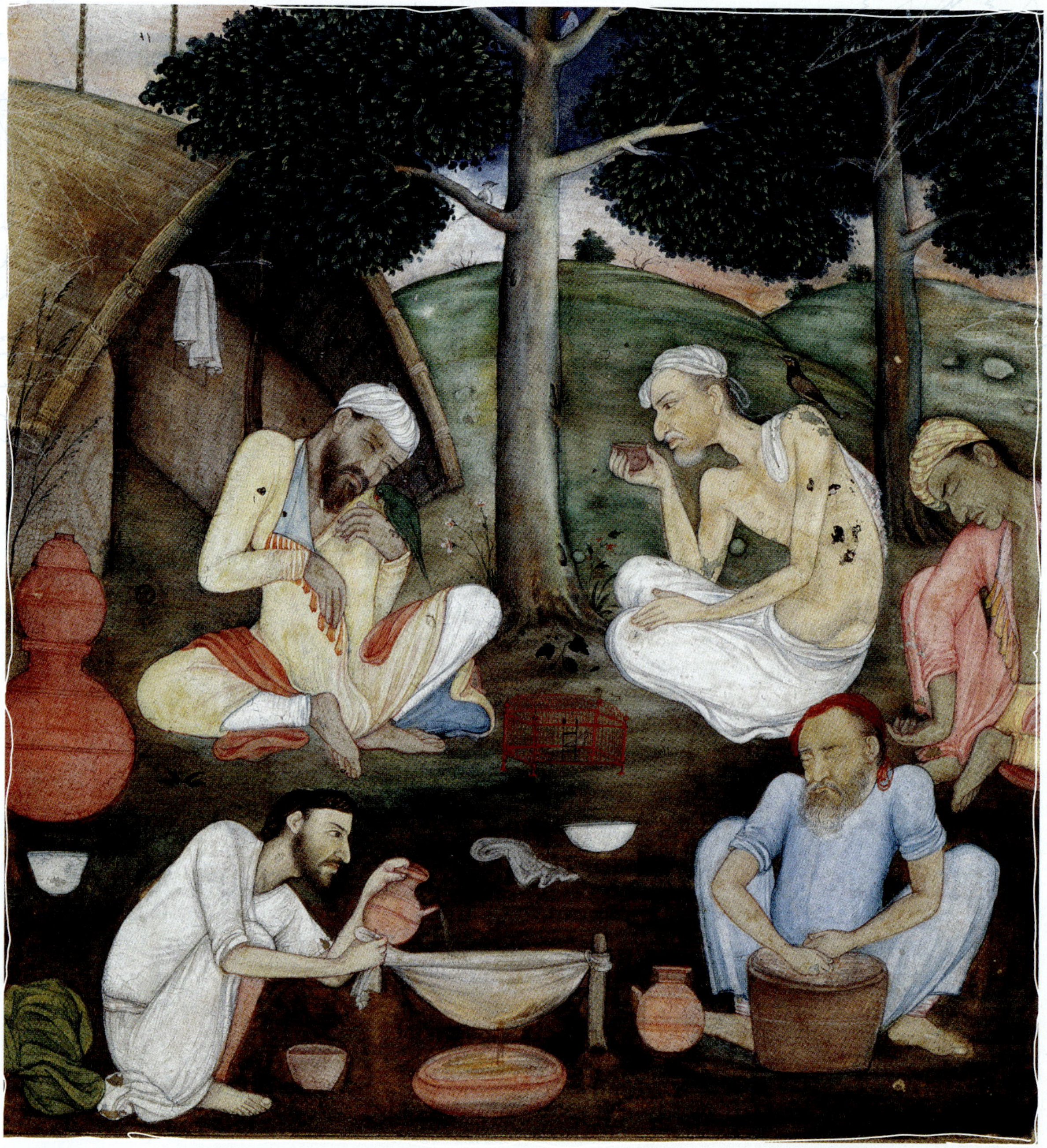

◄ **Bhang users**
In this painting from northern India, created around 1600, addicts consume bhang, an edible preparation of marijuana leaves used in religious festivals such as Holi.

Marijuana is among the **6 per cent** of flowering plants to be **dioecious,** having separate male and female plants

CULTURAL IMPORTANCE

Among adherents of the Rastafari religion, cannabis, or ganja, is a sacred herb and is often smoked during ceremonial "groundings". In many countries with significant Rastafari communities, including Jamaica (pictured), smoking cannabis represents an act of defiance, although it is also considered to have healing properties.

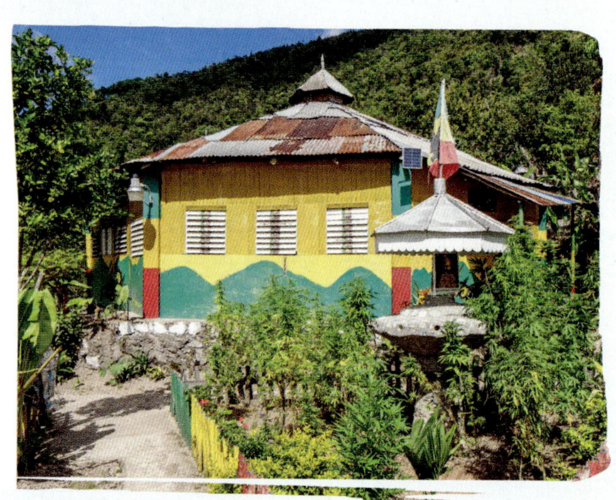

MARIJUANA GARDEN AND TEMPLE

law in many countries, although legalization for medicinal or recreational purposes is increasingly common. Aside from smoking, it can be taken in a variety of ways, including in food.

The active ingredient of marijuana that is responsible for most of the herb's psychoactive properties – causing euphoria, introspection, anxiety, and paranoia, for example – is the phytochemical tetrahydrocannabinol (THC). THC has also been used to treat multiple sclerosis and neurodegenerative diseases such as Parkinson's and Alzheimer's. Another phytochemical in cannabis is cannabidiol (CBD), which is also psychoactive but does not produce the same "high" as THC. CBD has been used to treat epilepsy, and research continues into its use for other medical conditions. A lucrative industry has developed utilizing CBD in herbal, medical, veterinary, and cosmetic applications. As a result, forms of cannabis with low THC levels are widely grown in some countries to supply CBD.

Hemp for ropes, clothes, and oil

Forms of marijuana with low levels of THC are commonly cultivated for their seeds and fibre. Hemp seeds can be eaten raw or sprouted, converted into hemp milk, or pressed to produce edible oil. They are a component of wild bird foods, and the oil has numerous industrial uses, including in wood varnish, cosmetics, and plastics. Hemp fibre is used in cloth production and an increasing number of construction items, including insulation and wood alternatives. Historically, the fibre was significant in the production of rope and canvas to outfit naval ships from the late 15th to mid-19th century, and countries needed to ensure a ready supply of such materials to enable their defence.

WHAT ARE CANNABINOIDS AND TERPENES?

The better-known phytochemicals in cannabis, such as THC and CBD, are members of a group called cannabinoids. In humans, cannabinoid receptors are found primarily in the brain and immune system. The other major group of cannabis compounds are terpenes, which produce the plant's distinctive fragrance. Terpenes are also found in many other plants, and provide the fragrance of herbs such as rosemary, sage, and basil, for example.

> " Hemp flourishes even to rankness, so that we need not want cordage. "
>
> THOMAS PAINE, *Common Sense*, pamphlet advocating for independence for the American colonies, 1776

Similar herbs

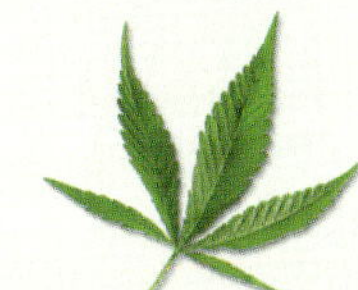

DWARF CANNABIS
Cannabis ruderalis
This name is often applied to early flowering plants, used in crossbreeding for faster harvests.

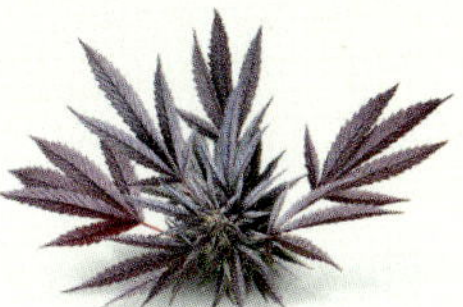

PURPLE KUSH
Cannabis sativa 'Purple Kush'
Bred in California, US, this purple-leaved form has high levels of THC.

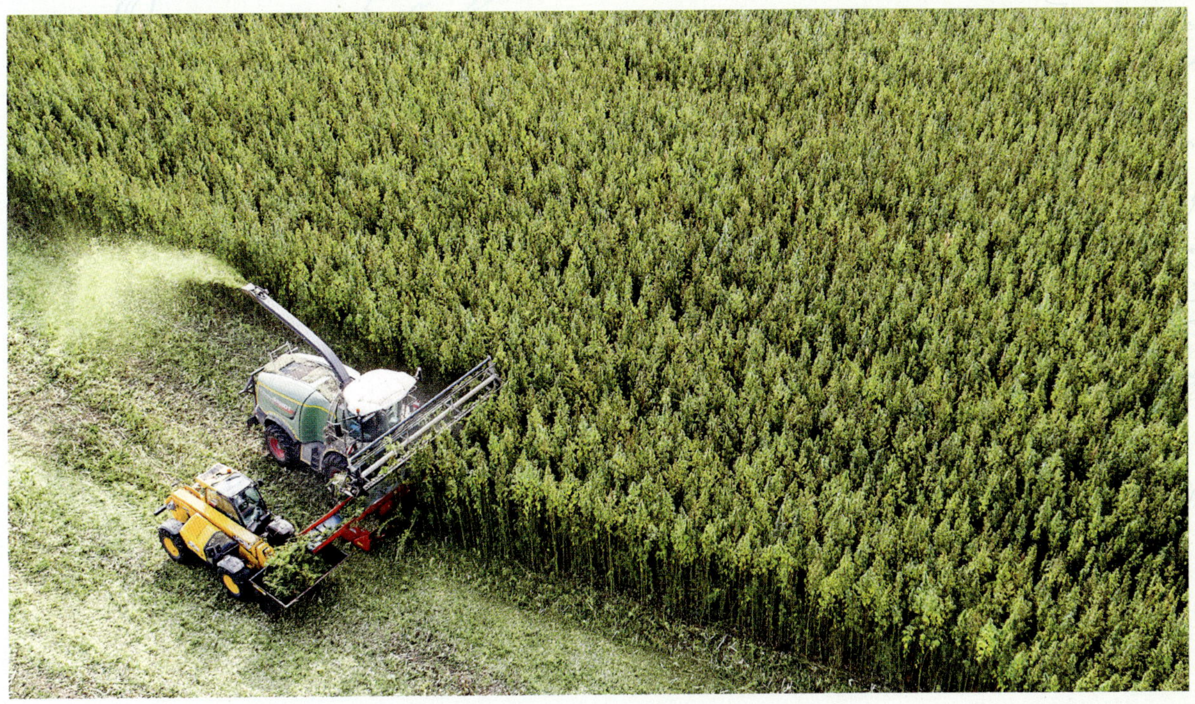

◄ Field of cannabis
A farmer harvests marijuana in Germany using modified machinery. Cannabidiol is extracted from the buds for medicinal purposes.

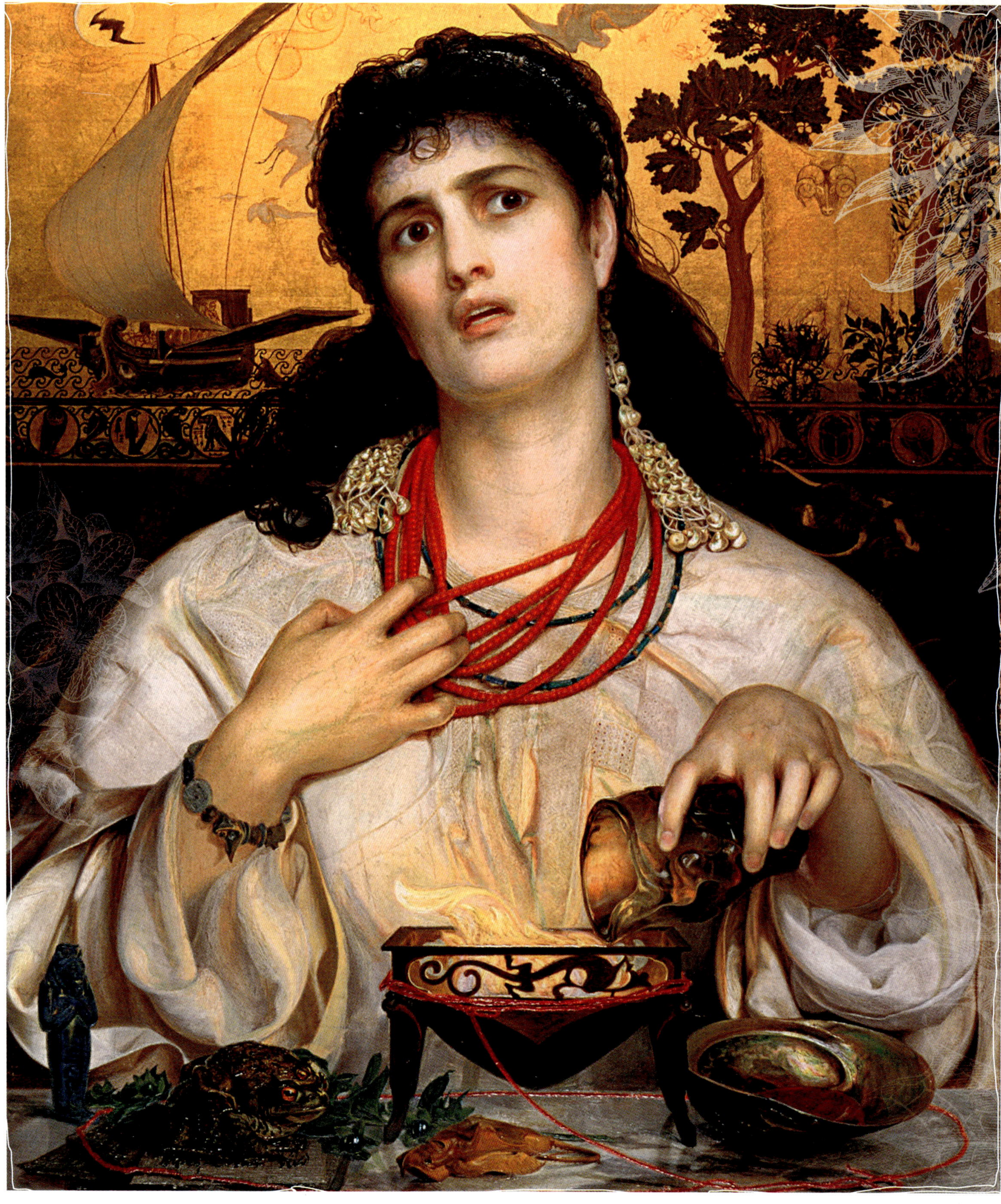

Uses Medicines for travel sickness and to dry up secretions; sedative and muscle relaxant

Parts used Leaves, roots

Active ingredients Hyoscine (scopolamine), hyoscyamine

Habitat Usually lime-rich soils; often near the sea; abandoned areas; roadsides

Flowers are parchment coloured, with purple veins and a dark purple centre
Ragged leaves are sticky and with a musty, unpleasant smell

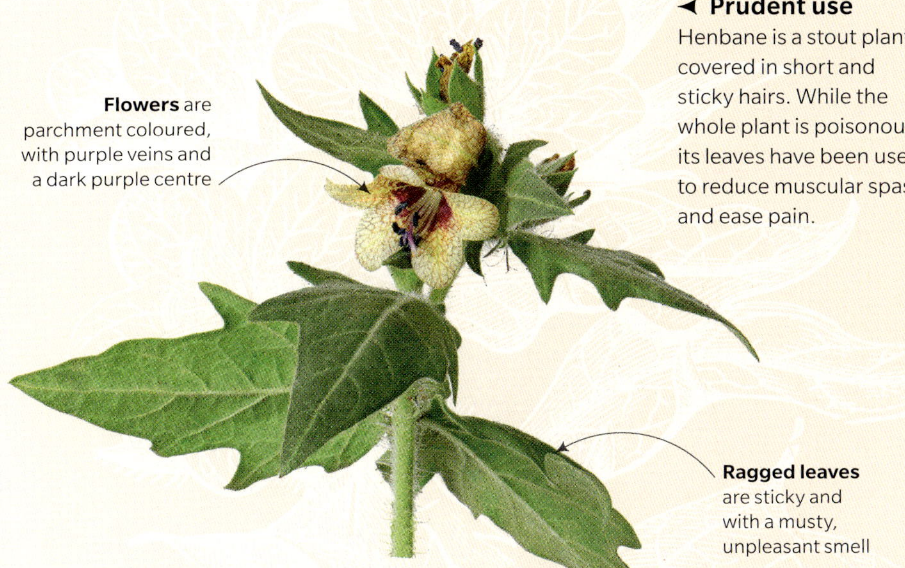

◄ Prudent use
Henbane is a stout plant, covered in short and sticky hairs. While the whole plant is poisonous, its leaves have been used to reduce muscular spasm and ease pain.

Henbane

Hyoscyamus niger

An ancient herb associated with witchcraft and prophecy, henbane was a part of many traditional medicines. It is also known for its narcotic, psychoactive, and poisonous properties.

Henbane is a 1 m-(3 ft-) tall plant with ragged, greyish green leaves and purple-veined flowers, which are replaced later by rows of capsules. These capsules, held in the clasp of stiff sepals, contain numerous black seeds. Henbane is native to temperate Eurasia and northwest Africa, and is frequently called black henbane. Its other names include: hog's-bean, Jupiter's bean, poison tobacco, and stinking nightshade.

Henbane through history

Historically cultivated for medicinal and ritualistic purposes, henbane now persists in abandoned farms, waste lands, and ruins – something that perpetuates its association with the occult. It is a narcotic as well as poisonous, and causes symptoms including dizziness and altered states of consciousness. As a result, the plant was used in religious rituals, witchcraft, and sorcery. It also has a history of being used as a poison.

In parts of Europe, henbane was used as a bitter-tasting additive to beer. Its leaves were dried and smoked as a treatment for asthma. It served as a painkiller in primitive dentistry and was also used as a hallucinogenic or recreational drug. In Chinese medicine, henbane seeds were used as a body strengthener, consumed after being soaked in milk or vinegar to reduce their toxicity.

◄ A famous poison
Painter Frederick Sandys portrays the Greek mythical sorceress Medea preparing a fatal brew to poison her husband's mistress. Deadly nightshade (*Atropa bella-donna*) can be seen on the table, and it would possibly have also included henbane, which was widely used in Greece in antiquity.

Sedative and healing

Henbane is a member of the Solanaceae family, which includes deadly nightshade (see pp.154–55). Like deadly nightshade, it contains tropane alkaloids, including hyoscine and hyoscyamine, named after its genus *Hyoscyamus*. These alkaloids affect the nervous system and in measured doses can be used medically as a sedative or muscle relaxant. An oil-based extract of henbane is still used for skin treatments such as scar healing.

Similar herbs

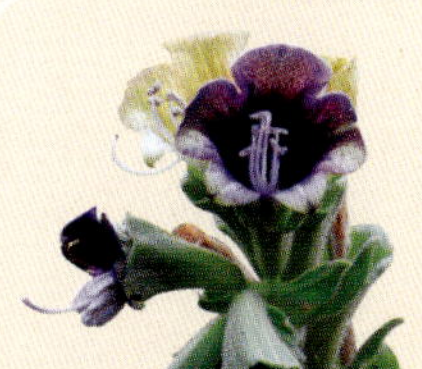

EGYPTIAN HENBANE
Hyoscyamus muticus
Found in North Africa and east to India, it is used locally as a painkiller and recreational drug. It has a higher alkaloid content.

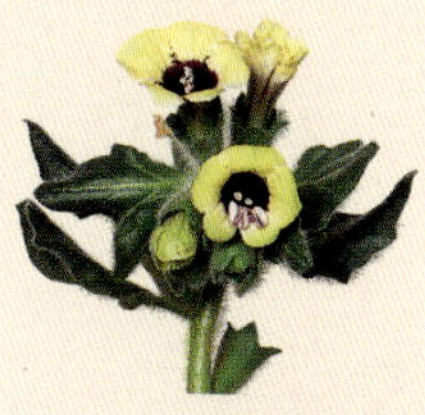

WHITE HENBANE
Hyoscyamus albus
This Mediterranean plant was considered sacred in ancient Greek rituals. While poisonous, it is a source of medicinal drugs.

Uses Medicines for heart conditions

Parts used Leaves

Active ingredients Digoxin, digitoxin, digoxigenin

Habitat Rough ground, river banks, rocky slopes, heaths and open woodland; in acidic soil; on land that has been disturbed or burnt

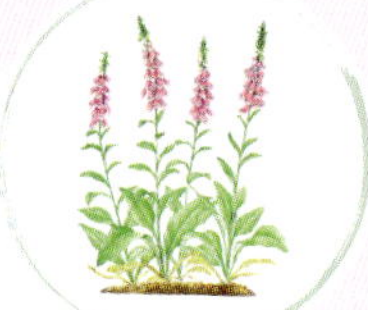

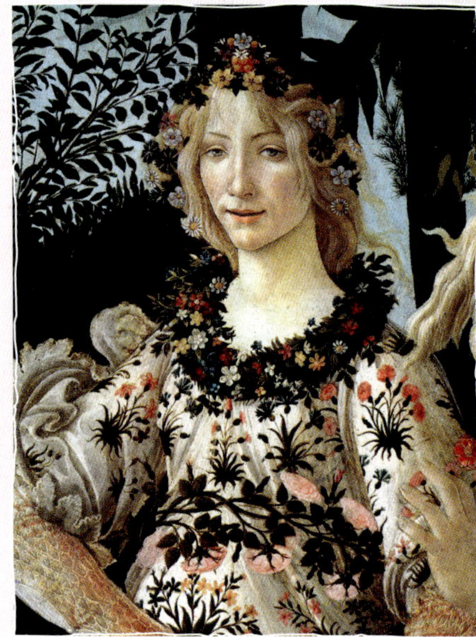

➤ Flora
This detail from Italian painter Sandro Botticelli's *La Primavera* (c.1478) depicts Flora – the Roman goddess of flowers and springtime. According to some interpretations of Roman mythology, Flora held foxglove to be sacred.

Common Foxglove

Digitalis purpurea

With its bell-shaped blossoms held in statuesque racemes, foxglove is well known in both medicine and folklore. When administered in measured doses, this highly toxic plant can heal.

Over time, foxglove has earned a number of names – from fairy thimbles to goblin gloves – reflecting the whimsy and fear this plant can inspire. Its tubular flowers are reminiscent of "gloves", each the width of a human finger. The common foxglove is widespread in temperate parts of Eurasia, and has been naturalized in North America and elsewhere. It is a biennial, forming a rosette of leaves in the first year, flowering in the second, and then dying. A popular ornamental plant, foxglove has a variety of cultivars.

Kill or cure

All parts of foxglove, including its flowers and seeds, are poisonous, and an overdose of this herb can lead to cardiac arrest. However, it also has proven medicinal uses.

Long used in folk medicine, common foxglove came to the attention of the pharmaceutical industry in the late 18th century, when English physician William Withering discovered that it acted on the human heart and was a good diuretic (causing increased urination). Foxglove extracts regulate an irregular heartbeat, slowing it down and increasing the strength of the contractions so the heart fills and empties properly. This reduces fluid accumulation in the extremities. Foxglove's active ingredients digoxin and digitoxin are still used in precisely measured doses as pharmaceutical heart medicines. Another ingredient, digoxigenin, is used in genetic research as a molecular probe – to detect and study molecules.

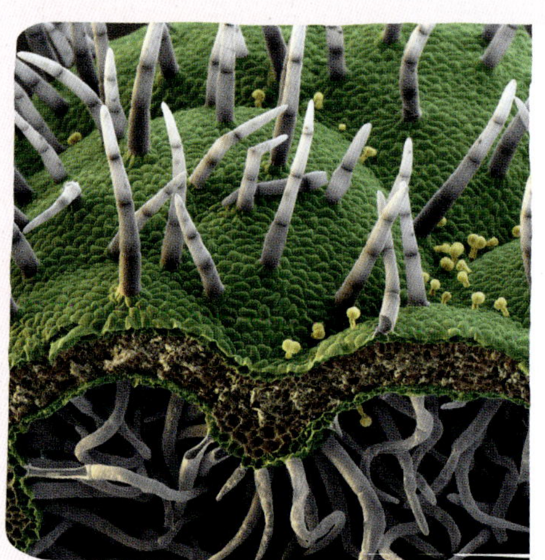

DEFENCE MECHANISMS
Foxglove leaves are covered on both sides with two different kinds of hairs. One is long and downy, and may protect the plant from water loss and solar radiation. The other kind is glandular, and releases a toxin when disturbed. This gives the leaf an unpleasant taste, and is thought to deter any animal tempted to eat it.

MAGNIFIED VIEW OF LEAF SECTION

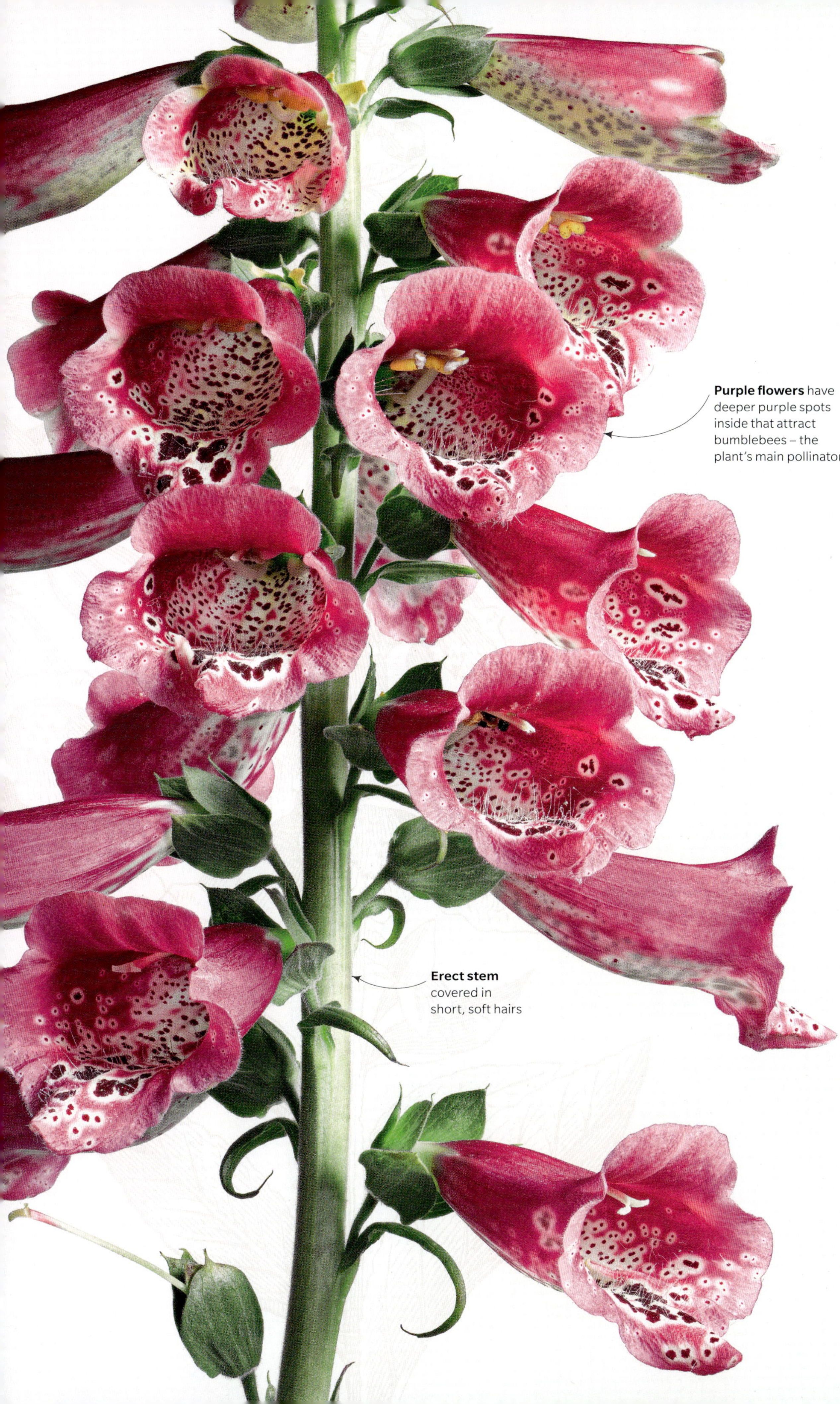

Purple flowers have deeper purple spots inside that attract bumblebees – the plant's main pollinator

Erect stem covered in short, soft hairs

Similar herb

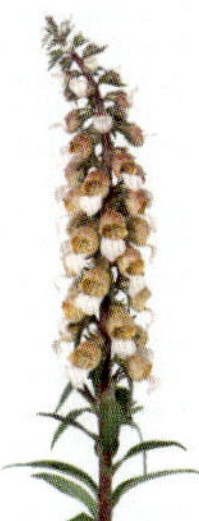

GRECIAN FOXGLOVE
Digitalis lanata
This Mediterranean foxglove has a coating of shaggy hairs and white-lipped, ochre coloured flowers. It is the main source of digoxin today.

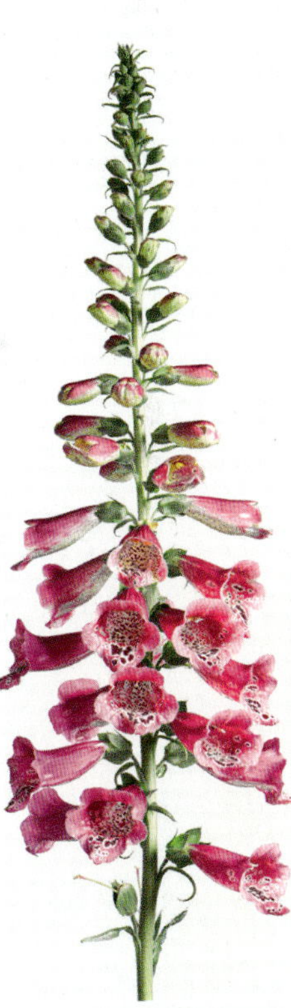

FOXGLOVE RACEME

◄ Standing tall
Foxglove flowers are spirally arranged on a long raceme, with the flowers at the bottom opening first. In the wild form, the flower stalks bend so the flowers face the same direction.

Stem leaves are smaller with wrinkled edges; grey-green and downy below
Flower heads (capitula) appear in late summer; drying out to form burs when the seeds mature
Pale yellow-brown taproot is around 2 cm (¾ in) across
Heart-shaped lower leaves are up to 50 cm (20 in) long; green above, grey-green and softly hairy below; borne on long stalks
BURS, LEAVES, AND ROOTS

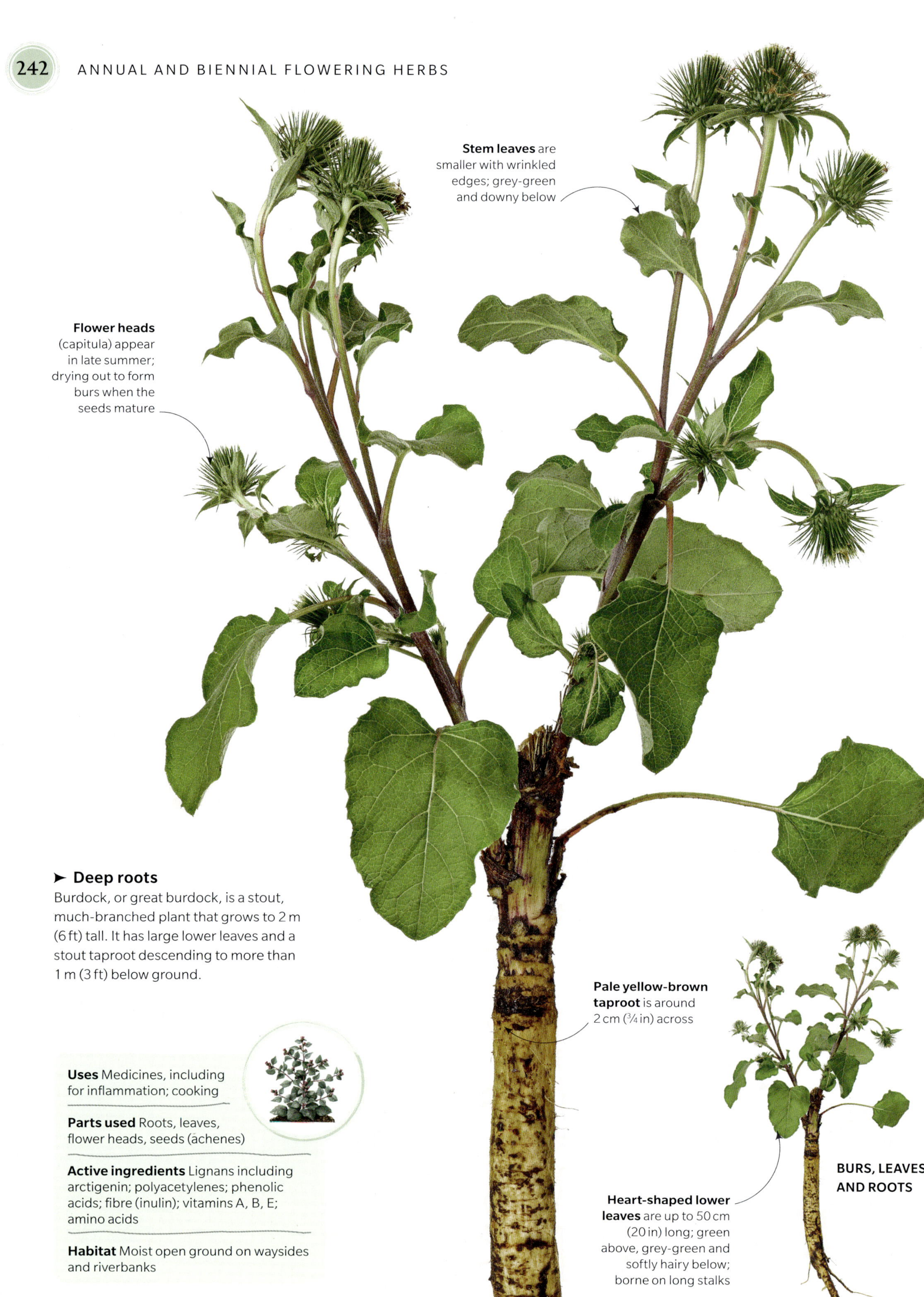

➤ Deep roots

Burdock, or great burdock, is a stout, much-branched plant that grows to 2 m (6 ft) tall. It has large lower leaves and a stout taproot descending to more than 1 m (3 ft) below ground.

Uses Medicines, including for inflammation; cooking

Parts used Roots, leaves, flower heads, seeds (achenes)

Active ingredients Lignans including arctigenin; polyacetylenes; phenolic acids; fibre (inulin); vitamins A, B, E; amino acids

Habitat Moist open ground on waysides and riverbanks

Burdock

Arctium lappa

This imposing plant has downy leaves and attractive, reddish-purple flowers clustered within large burs. Its fleshy root has various uses in food and medicine.

Burdock is a biennial or short-lived perennial. It produces a rosette of leaves in its first year, then flowers in its second year when enough reserves have accumulated in the plant's deep and fleshy taproot. The rough texture of the fruit heads, known as burs or burrs, is referenced in its genus name, *Arctium*, meaning "bear", a name coined by Roman naturalist Pliny.

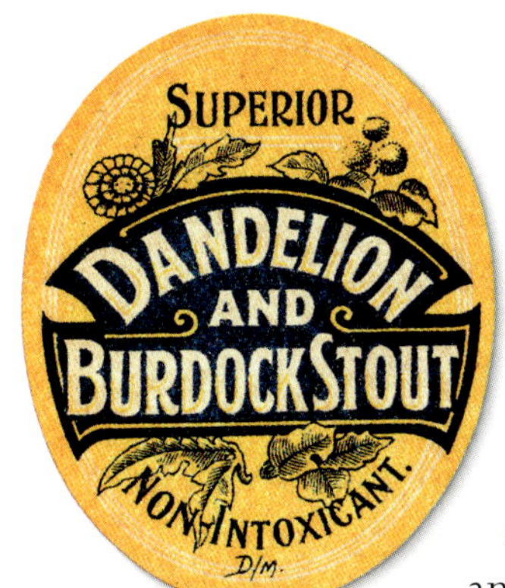

◄ **Dandelion and burdock stout**
A popular, beer-like soft drink, dandelion and burdock stout was thought to be good for health.

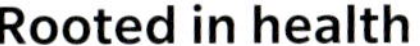

Rooted in health

Burdock roots have a mild, earthy flavour and are popular in East Asian cuisine. They are referred to as *niubang* in China and *tong-u-eong* or "whole burdock" in Korea. In Japan, the shredded roots, called *gobo*, are often braised or stir-fried with carrots and onions, and seasoned with soy sauce and *sake*. Roots are dug up in spring, when they are relatively tender, and can be soaked in water for some hours to reduce any harsh, muddy taste. Its tender leaves are also sometimes eaten, as are the peeled flower stalks and immature flower heads, which taste like artichoke.

Dandelion-and-burdock stout – a fizzy, non-alcoholic drink first produced in Scotland in 1871 – is a popular drink in Europe. The roots of these plants are peeled, roasted, and then simmered in water to form a dark-coloured syrup. Sweetened, diluted, and mixed with spices such as ginger and anise, the resulting drink tastes like liquorice, and is marketed in bottles and cans.

Burdock roots, leaves, and seeds have been used worldwide in traditional medicine. It is mildly diuretic, and functions as an appetite stimulant and blood purifier. It is used to stimulate organs such as the liver and pancreas. An anti-inflammatory, it can also be taken as an infusion to treat rheumatic complaints. Since burdock is a healthy, low-calorie vegetable rich in fibre, calcium, and potassium, its potential as part of a macrobiotic diet is being explored.

Similar herbs

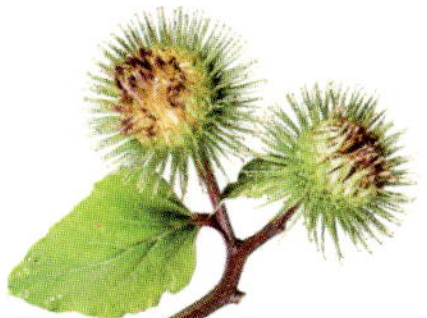

LESSER BURDOCK
Arctium minus
With smaller burs than *A. lappa*, this European native also has edible roots, though it is not harvested as much.

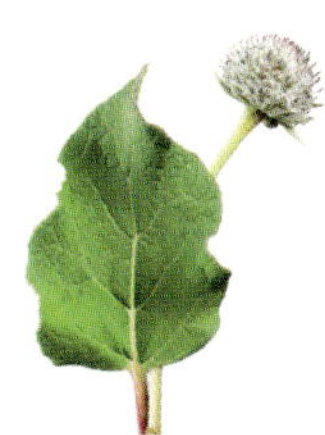

WOOLLY BURDOCK
Arctium tomentosum
With similar herbal uses as *A. lappa*, this Eurasian plant has woolly flower heads and has been naturalized in North America.

▼ **Fresh burdock roots**
Burdock roots are brittle and best harvested when they are tender, from young plants before the flowering stalks develop.

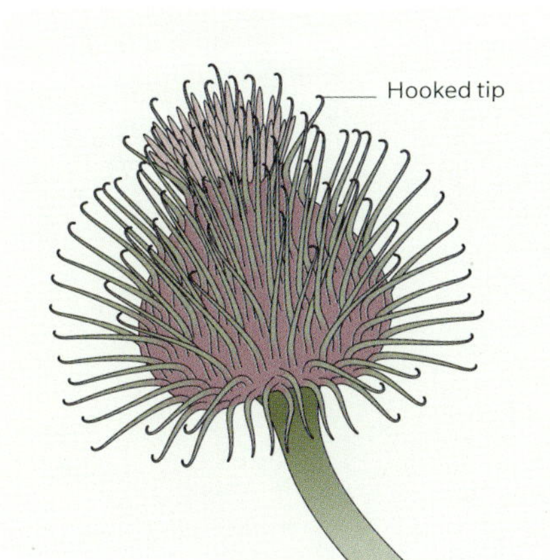

NATURAL MECHANISM

Burdock's burs are covered in long, fine hooks. Not only do these sharp, protective bracts deter potential predators, they latch on to fur or clothing to enable the seeds within to be transported far and wide. These burs were the inspiration for the mechanism of the hook-and-loop-fastener.

BURDOCK BUR

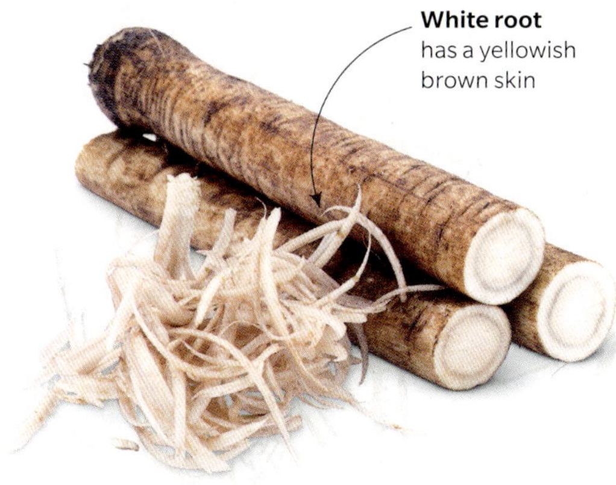

German Chamomile

Matricaria chamomilla

German chamomile has long been cultivated across many parts of the world for its healing powers. The herb is commonly used to soothe inflammation and fevers, and to calm the nervous and digestive systems.

Uses Medicines, cosmetics, perfume, home scents, cooking

Parts used Flower heads

Active ingredients Terpenoids including bisabolol, chamazulene, and matricin; flavonoids including apigenin, quercetin, and kaempferol

Habitat Cultivated and waste ground; well-drained, light, sandy soil

Native to disturbed ground in Europe, North Africa, Eurasia, and Asia but now widespread, German chamomile is often referred to simply as chamomile – from the ancient Greek word *chamaimelon*, *chamai* meaning "on the ground" and *melon* meaning "apple". It is often confused with the similar but botanically distinct Roman chamomile (*Chamaemelum nobile*).

A tale of two chamomiles

Both these plants have a tradition of medicinal use – to treat skin complaints, flush out infections, relieve pain, and relax the mind. However, they are slightly different and have unique chemical constituents.

German chamomile is a hairless, branching, upright annual. It produces a few small, white-"petalled" flower heads, of which the yellow centre is raised in a cone shape. The plant is propagated by seed in spring and blooms throughout the summer, smelling like sweet straw. It is best to wait until two-thirds of the flower heads have opened before harvesting. Importantly, German chamomile contains chamazulene, which gives its oil (produced by steam-distilling the dried flower heads) its characteristic deep blue colour. The compound also gives the herb its alternative common name, blue chamomile. German chamomile is especially good for maintaining and healing

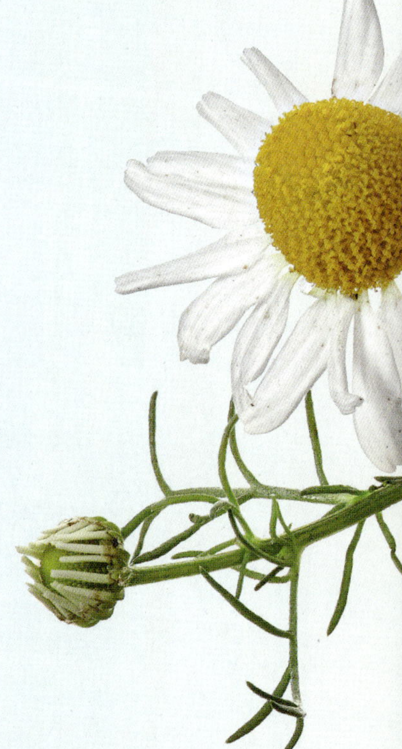

➤ Flowering stem
German chamomile has long, tender stems with feathery foliage, on top of which bloom its yellow and white flower heads. The whole plant can grow to around 0.5 m (1½ ft) tall.

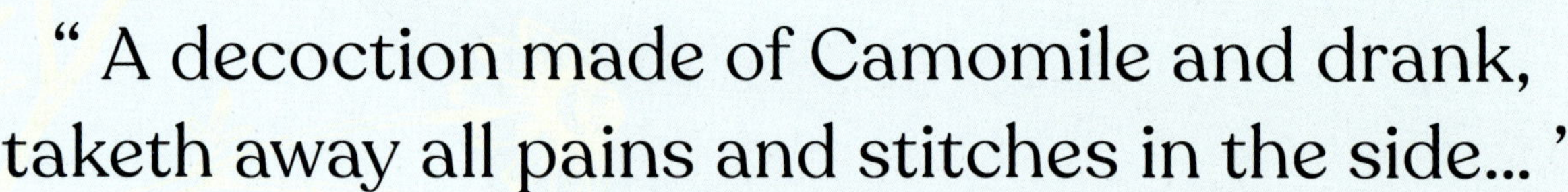

" A decoction made of Camomile and drank, taketh away all pains and stitches in the side... "

NICHOLAS CULPEPER, *Complete Herbal*, 1653

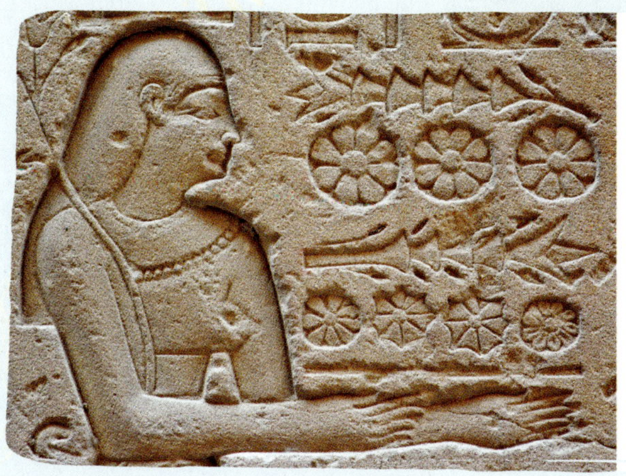

A SACRED EGYPTIAN HERB

Chamomile had myriad uses in ancient Egypt, from honouring the gods – especially the sun god Ra – and embalming the dead to curing disease, warding off colds, and treating skin problems caused by a dry, harsh climate. Depictions of daisy-like flower heads, thought to be chamomile, have been found on many Egyptian hieroglyphs. Here, a young woman is shown in profile holding out an offering of flower heads and stems.

ANCIENT EGYPTIAN BAS-RELIEF

White ray florets encircling yellow disc florets

Tender leaves are light green. Technically, they are edible if they are free from pesticides

Immature flower heads open to be about 1–2.5 cm (½–1 in) in diameter

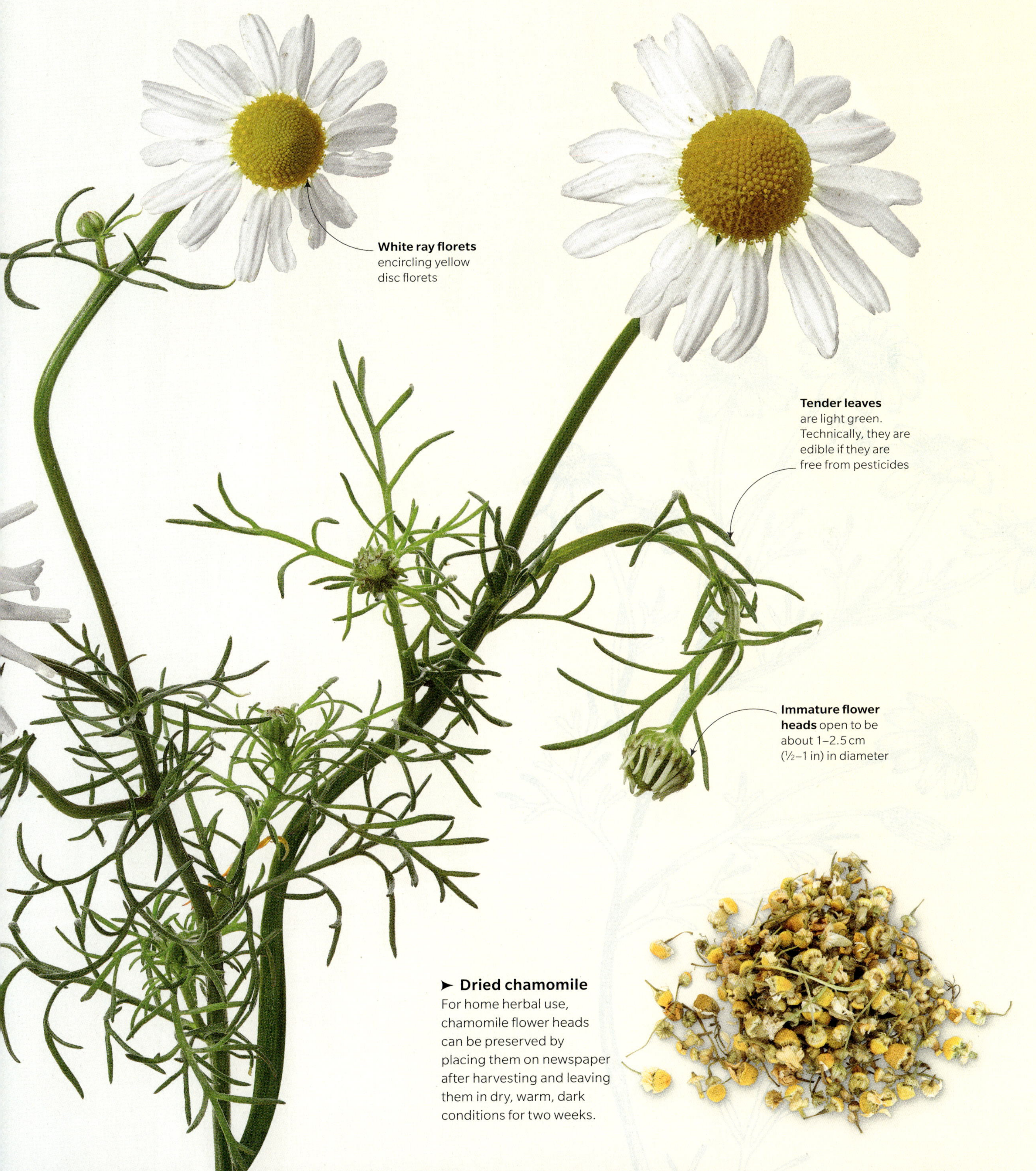

➤ Dried chamomile
For home herbal use, chamomile flower heads can be preserved by placing them on newspaper after harvesting and leaving them in dry, warm, dark conditions for two weeks.

Trimming German chamomile **encourages** new growth and **flower production**

skin – from a dry, flaky, or irritated complexion to conditions such as eczema, psoriasis, or dermatitis. It can stimulate the liver, kidneys, and gall bladder to help improve digestion, remove toxins, and treat gastrointestinal problems. It is also used to ease anxiety, including during menstruation and menopause.

The "other" chamomile – Roman chamomile – is a much lower-growing perennial herb. It has finely divided leaves on hairy stems and slightly larger flower heads, with a flatter yellow centre. Sometimes, the plant is grown as ground cover (the non-flowering, mat-forming cultivar 'Treneague' is used for chamomile lawns), propagated by division. Roman chamomile has a light apple fragrance and contains high levels of esters of angelic, butyric, and tiglic acids. The essential oil is yellow with a blue tint and has anti-spasmodic, antimicrobial, and sedative properties. Consequently, it is used to help promote sleep and to provide pain relief from sore muscles, joints, or headaches. It is thought to be effective in reducing anxiety or balancing emotions, including in children.

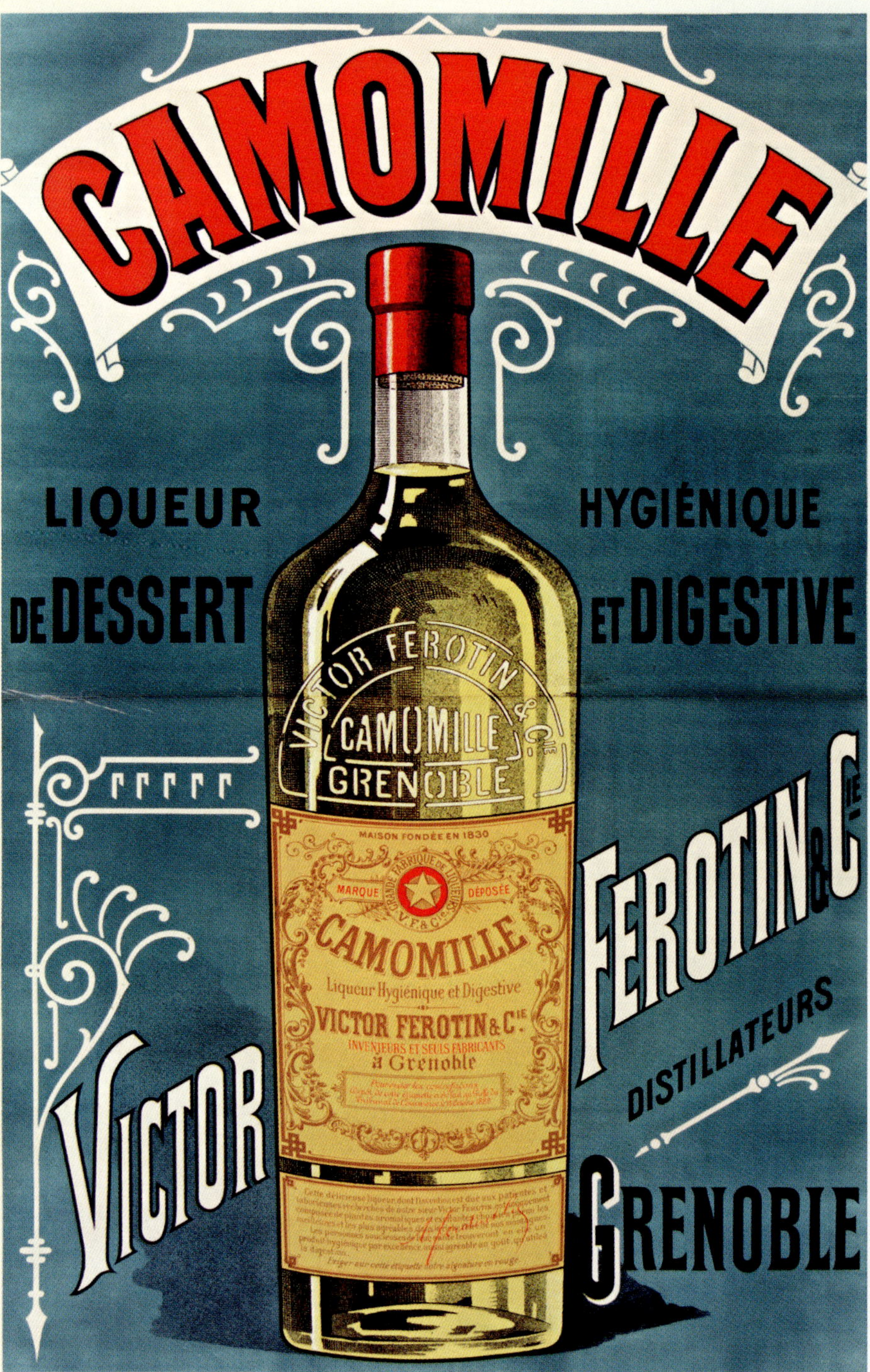

▲ Sweet digestif
Chamomile dessert liqueur, such as this French one produced by Victor Ferotin, was a popular late 19th-century digestif. The drink was made by infusing alcohol with dried chamomile flowers.

Traditionally speaking

Although Roman chamomile is thought to have the more ancient history in both name and within the canon of historical herbals (it is known as "true chamomile"), the native spread and cultivation of both herbs mean it is difficult to prove which species was used for which application. Today, German chamomile is cultivated across the globe for medicinal use. It is available as dried flower heads and also as a tea, extract, essential oil, powder, or ointment. The genus name *Matricaria* is thought to stem from the Latin word *matrix*, referring to the womb. This is based on the herb's historical use to treat menstrual cramps and female sleep problems.

Roman scholar Pliny the Elder, working in the 1st century, identified three species of chamomile, one of which may relate to German chamomile. The herb is also thought to have been used by Germanic tribes long before documentation began and was likely grown in monastic gardens under the medieval emperor Charlemagne. German chamomile is mentioned in Mrs M. Grieve's comprehensive book *A Modern Herbal* (1931) as "wild chamomile", being frequently found in cornfields at the time. (This is the chamomile commonly used in wildflower seed mixes.) The plant's popularity has since risen, with shared knowledge of cultivation and high-yield varieties.

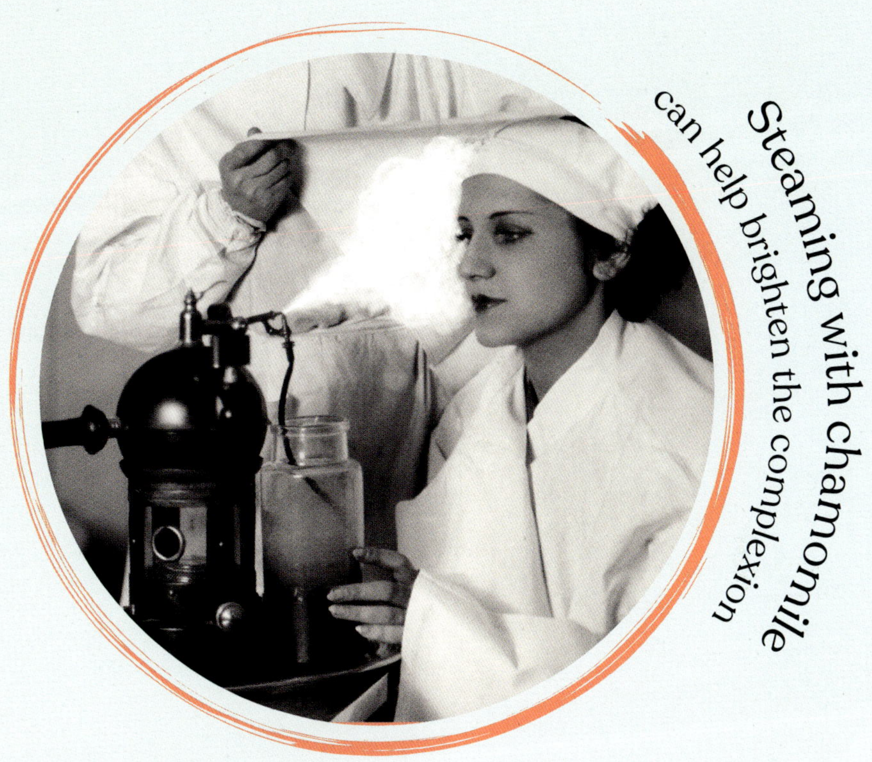

Steaming with chamomile can help brighten the complexion

More than tea

The most common way to take German chamomile is as a tea, by steeping fresh or dried flower heads in just-boiled water. Any preparation should be covered to stop the steam escaping. This will prevent the beneficial properties – including antioxidants, anti-inflammatory flavonoids, and nerve-calming phytochemicals – being lost before infusion completes. German chamomile tea is known for delivering a sweet and soothing taste and aroma via its volatile oils. A cup is recommended an hour before bed to encourage more restorative sleep, or at breakfast to help instil calm before a busy day. A few drops of the essential oil on a pillowcase or handkerchief can have the same effect. Cooled chamomile tea can also be used to bathe puffy or tired eyes, as a rinse to lighten hair or to combat dandruff (harnessing its antimicrobial properties), to heal and beautify the skin, or as a flavouring for food, including jams and dressings.

Chamomile is an ingredient in cosmetics and perfumes and introduces herbal, sweet, fresh notes. German chamomile is sweetly smoky with a hint of apple, which works well as a base note, while Roman chamomile has a similar earthy apple aroma, but is sweeter and headier.

▲ Chamomile steam bath
Inhaling steam infused with dried chamomile flower heads or with a few drops of chamomile essential oil can help combat symptoms of the common cold, such as a blocked nose or congested sinuses.

"For though the camomile, the more it is trodden on, the faster it grows, yet youth, the more it is wasted, the sooner it wears."

WILLIAM SHAKESPEARE, *Henry IV, Part I*, 1597

Similar herbs

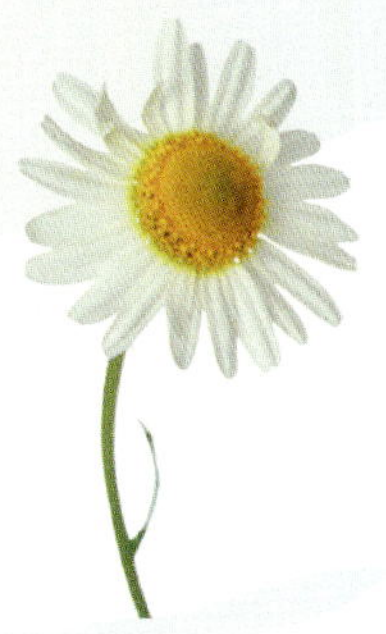

ROMAN CHAMOMILE
Chamaemelum nobile
This ancient herb has similar properties to German chamomile. However, although the two are related, Roman chamomile is from a different genus.

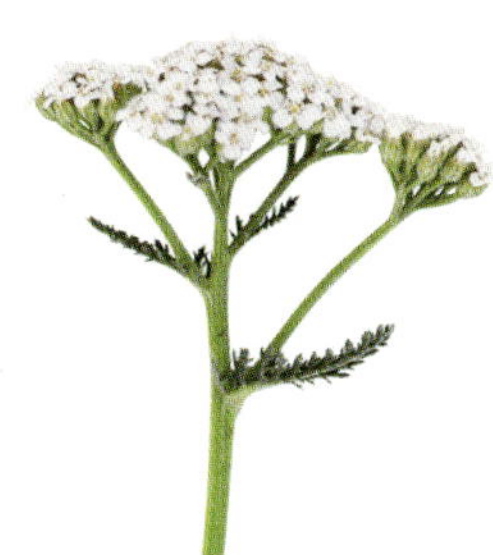

YARROW
Achillea millefolium
Yarrow, like German chamomile, hails from the daisy (Asteraceae) family. It is used to treat cold symptoms and reduce fever and pain.

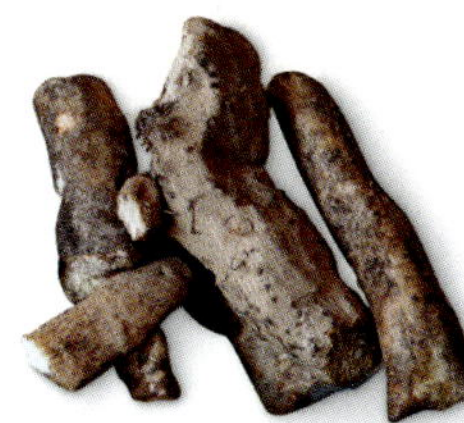

WILD YAM
Dioscorea villosa
Like chamomile, wild yam contains phytoestrogens. It is traditionally used to help treat menstrual cramps and female reproductive health issues.

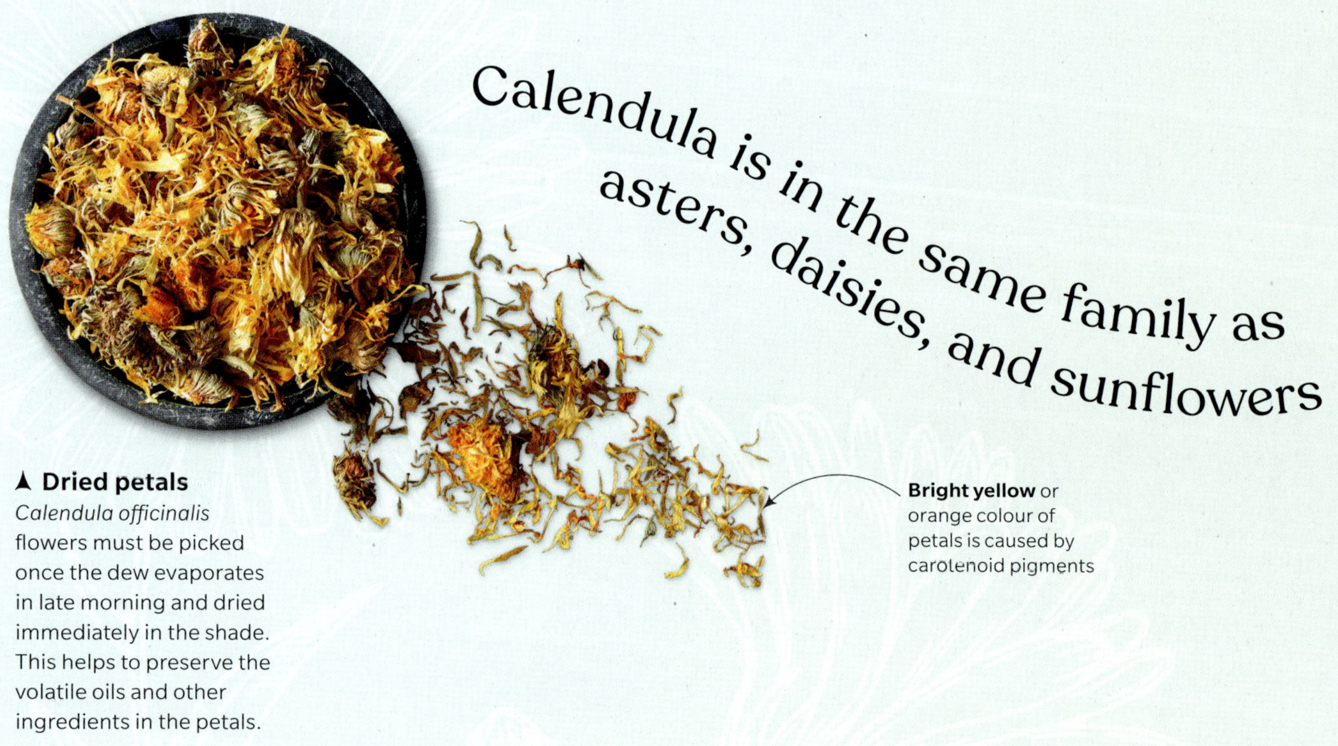

Calendula is in the same family as asters, daisies, and sunflowers

▲ Dried petals
Calendula officinalis flowers must be picked once the dew evaporates in late morning and dried immediately in the shade. This helps to preserve the volatile oils and other ingredients in the petals.

Bright yellow or orange colour of petals is caused by carotenoid pigments

Pot Marigold

Calendula officinalis

Uses Medicines; cooking; cosmetics

Parts used Flowers, leaves

Active ingredients Triterpene glycosides (saponins); carotenoids; flavonoids including quercetin;

Habitat Well-drained soil and full sun in fields and open spaces; temperate zones

The vibrant flowers of this easy-to-grow herb have been used for thousands of years to flavour food, gently heal skin, soothe senses, and aid digestion.

The European name of pot marigold harks back to Renaissance times, when the herb bloomed during various Christian festivals of the Virgin Mary – "mari" stood for Mary, "gold" for the yellow-orange glow of its flowers. The herb was also added to the pot for feasts. As described by Nicholas Culpeper in his 1653 *Complete Herbal*, the flowers were "much used in possets, broths, and drink, as a comforter of the heart and spirits".

Originally native to Spain and its surrounds, but now introduced across the globe, pot marigold is related to several other plants known as marigolds in the daisy family, Asteraceae. The other species hail from the *Tagetes* genus. Although they typically share the same carotenoid-rich, sunset-hued petals, any edible or medicinal uses are plant specific and should be checked; some *Tagetes* species can cause gastrointestinal issues.

Edible petals and leaves

Pot marigold has featured in cooking since ancient times. The fresh, slightly peppery petals season and give a golden hue to cheeses, rice dishes, and butter. They can also garnish or be added sparingly to salads, salsas, and summer rolls, to scrambled eggs, quiches, and frittatas. Referred to as "poor man's saffron", the petals provide a cheap alternative to real saffron (see pp.122–23) and also

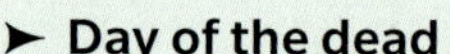

➤ Day of the dead
The calendula's relative, *Tagetes erecta*,shown in Saturnino Herrán's 1913 painting *The Offering*, is also called the Mexican, Aztec, French, or African marigold. In Mexico, its vivid colour and scent is said to attract the dead.

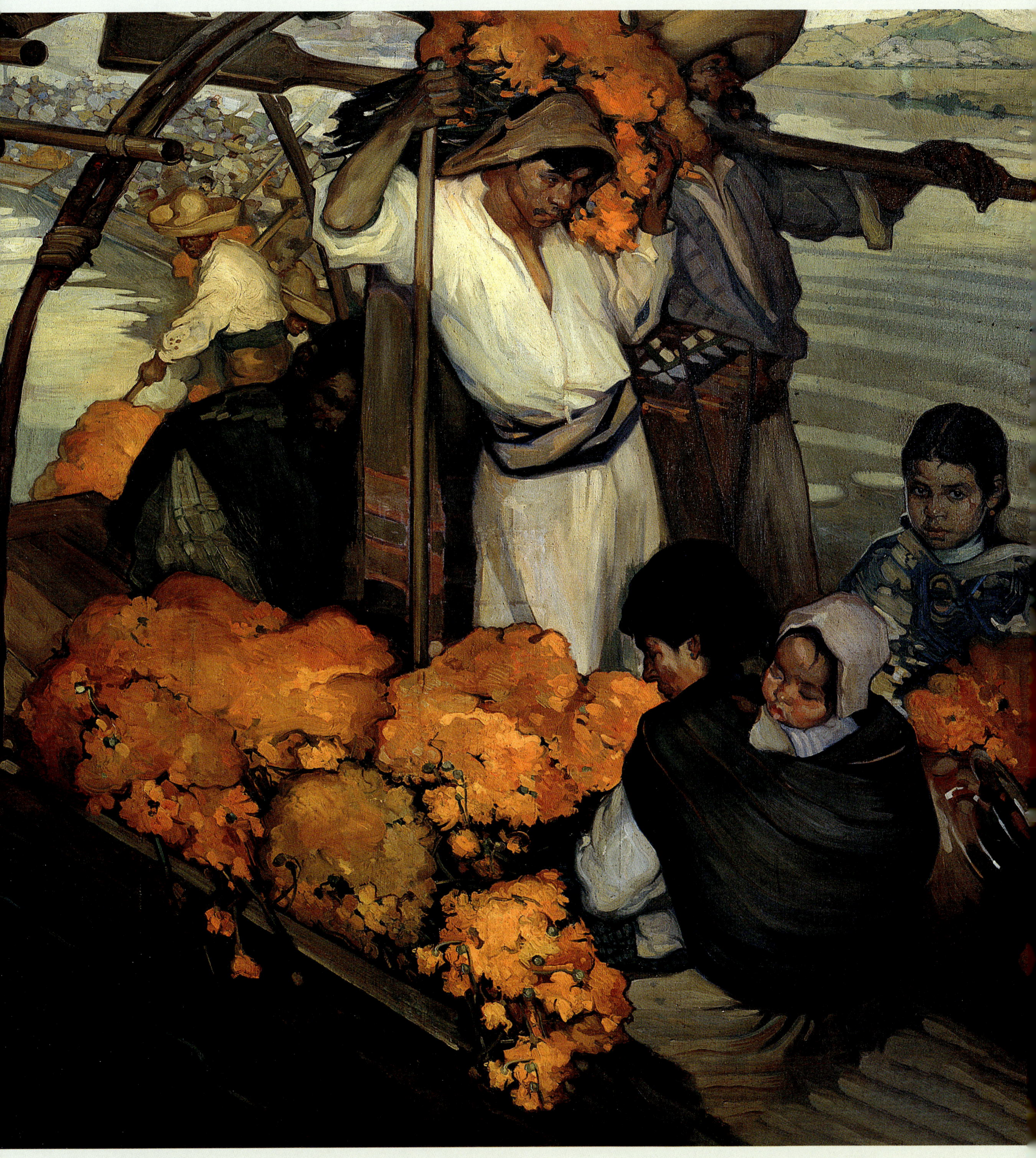

Similar herbs

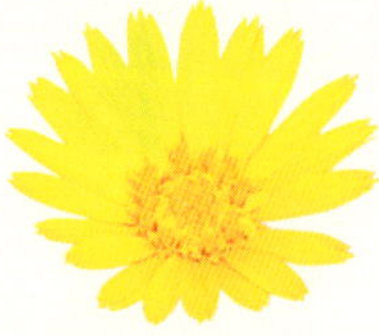

FIELD MARIGOLD
Calendula arvensis

A native of Europe, parts of Asia, and North Africa, this annual has yellow or orange blooms, which are used for skin problems.

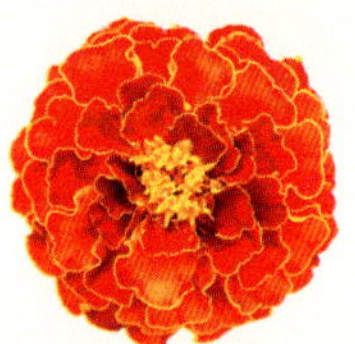

FRENCH MARIGOLD
Tagetes erecta

This annual is sometimes used for digestive ailments. It is known as the "flower of the dead" in Mexico.

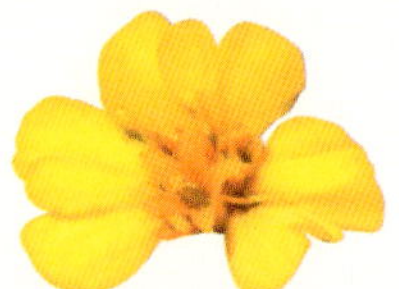

SWEET MARIGOLD
Tagetes lucida

Also known as sweet mace, this perennial has glossy, long leaves that are used as a tarragon substitute in Mexican cooking.

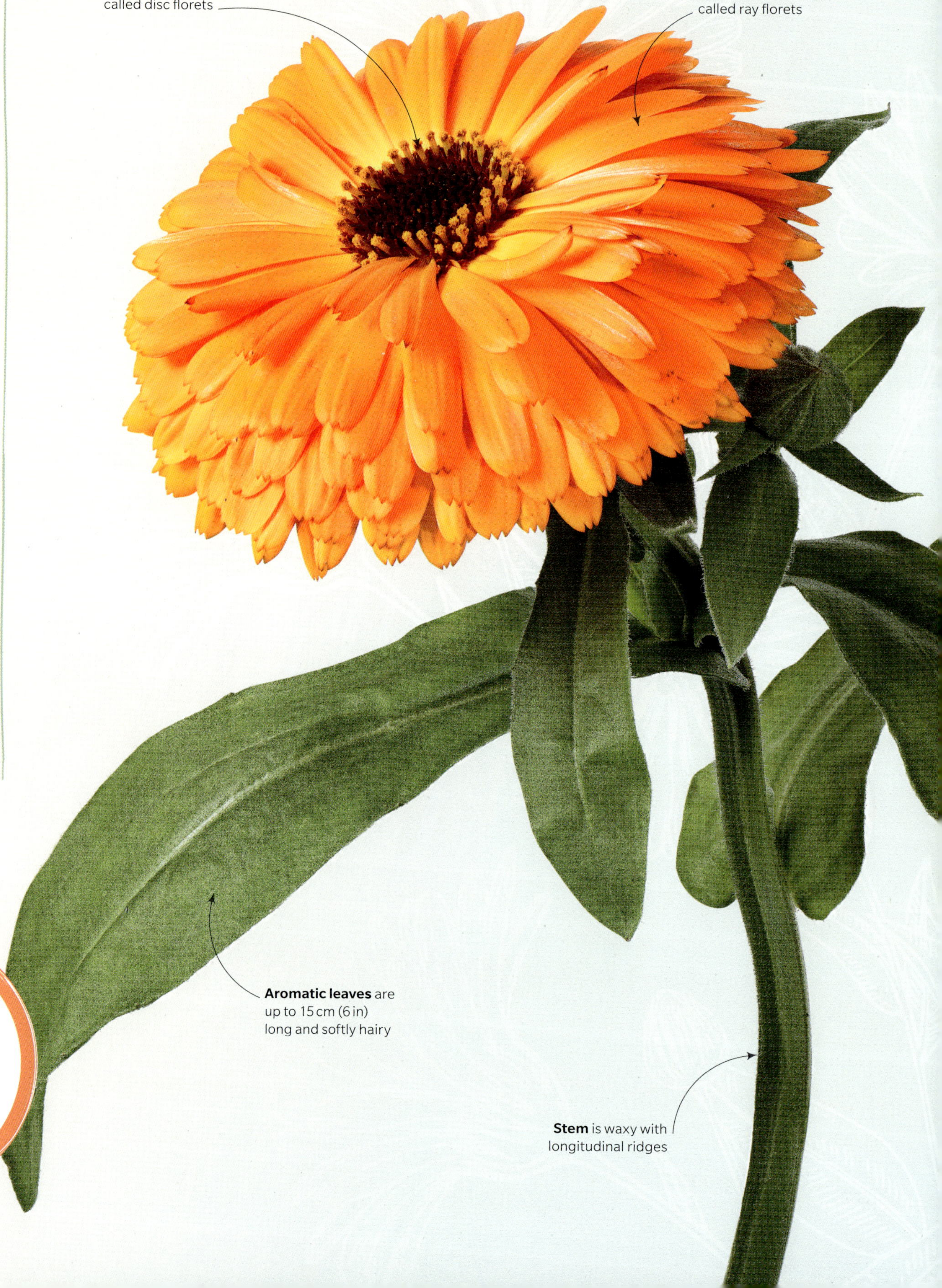

Central disc of flowerhead made of short, fertile flowers, called disc florets
Flower head "petals" are sterile, strap-shaped flowers, called ray florets
Aromatic leaves are up to 15 cm (6 in) long and softly hairy
Stem is waxy with longitudinal ridges

Calendula comes from the Latin **calendae**, meaning **"first of the month"**

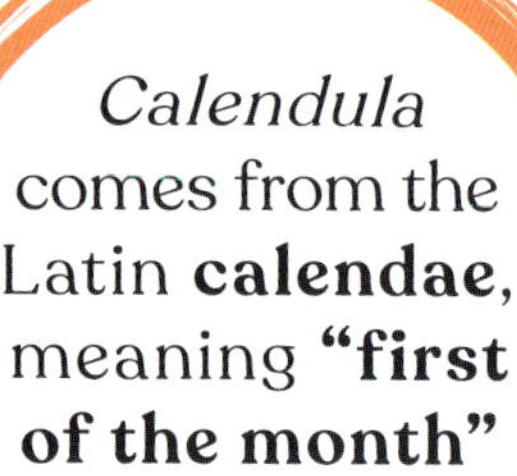

MARIGOLDS IN ART

Marigold flowers are a popular motif in the history of art, variously symbolizing grief, pain, joy, and youth, all possible readings of this Pre-Raphaelite painting of model and muse Fanny Cornforth by Dante Gabriel Rossetti. The painting's title alludes to an Italian proverb: "The mouth that has been kissed does not lose its good fortune, rather, it renews itself just as the moon does".

***BOCCA BACIATA* (1859)**

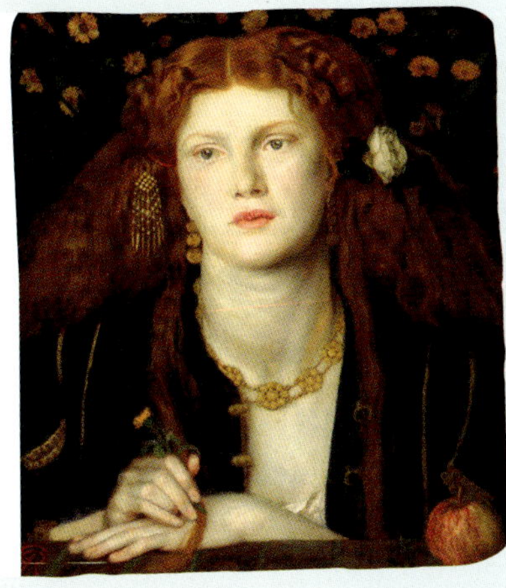

reducing redness and supporting skin healing without exposing infants to harsh chemicals. These benefits are delivered through the topical application of an ointment or salve or in a bath soak, all of which are fairly easy to make at home. Anti-inflammatory flavonoids and saponins in the flowers are best accessed by infusing the petals in oil. Pot marigold's high levels of saponins made it useful for making soap.

Historically, the herb was also used as a hair dye and to soothe stomach cramps, toothache, and the hot swellings of smallpox and measles. Some people are allergic to Asteraceae plants; pot marigold also should not be taken in pregnancy.

◄ Bright blooms
Calendula officinalis is a fast-growing annual or biennial, up to 50cm (20in) tall. It blooms readily and successively through the summer and autumn, but will not survive frosts.

are served in a soothing tea. The leaves are relatively bitter, but also work well in salads and soups. Pot marigolds are rich in vitamins and minerals, and easy to grow in beds or containers for a continuous summer and autumn harvest.

A soothing remedy

Pot marigold is a popular ingredient in skincare products. The active ingredients, extracted from the petals, have antioxidant, antibacterial, antifungal, and anti-inflammatory properties. It is utilized for a variety of skin problems, including inflammation, wounds, burns, scalds, scars, lip chaffing, and eczema. It is said to soothe nappy rash,

Ritual flower

Pot marigold's brilliantly hued flowers have been used by various peoples throughout history as ceremonial decorations, along with other, native marigolds. The tradition crosses many civilizations, cultures, and religions, from the Ancient Greeks and Romans, to Perisans, Hindus, and Aztecs. Today, ritual garlands of marigolds are still worn in countries such as India, Bali, and Saudi Arabia.

▼ Harvesting marigold blooms
Entire, fully open flowerheads are picked before they go to seed and are laid out to dry on screens, so no excess moisture remains. Picking also prompts new flowers to grow.

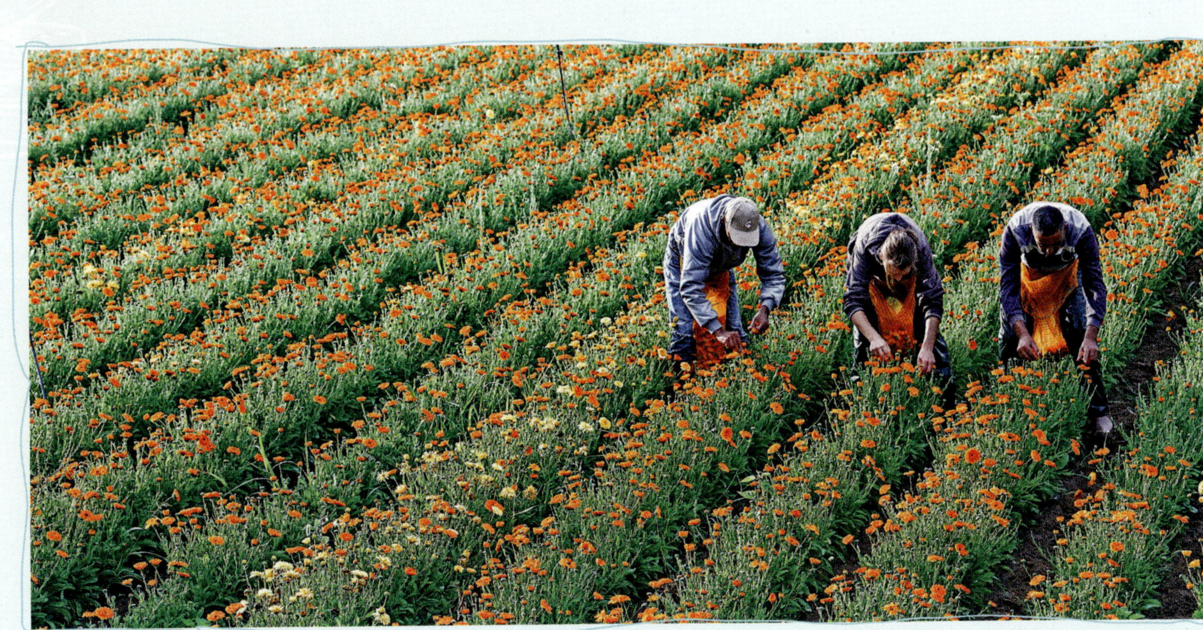

Traditions and Customs

Many traditional cultural practices around the world use herbs as tokens and talismans, from bringing good luck to deterring witches. Others have more prosaic yet customary uses around the home, including as pest control, as fertilizer, and as decoration.

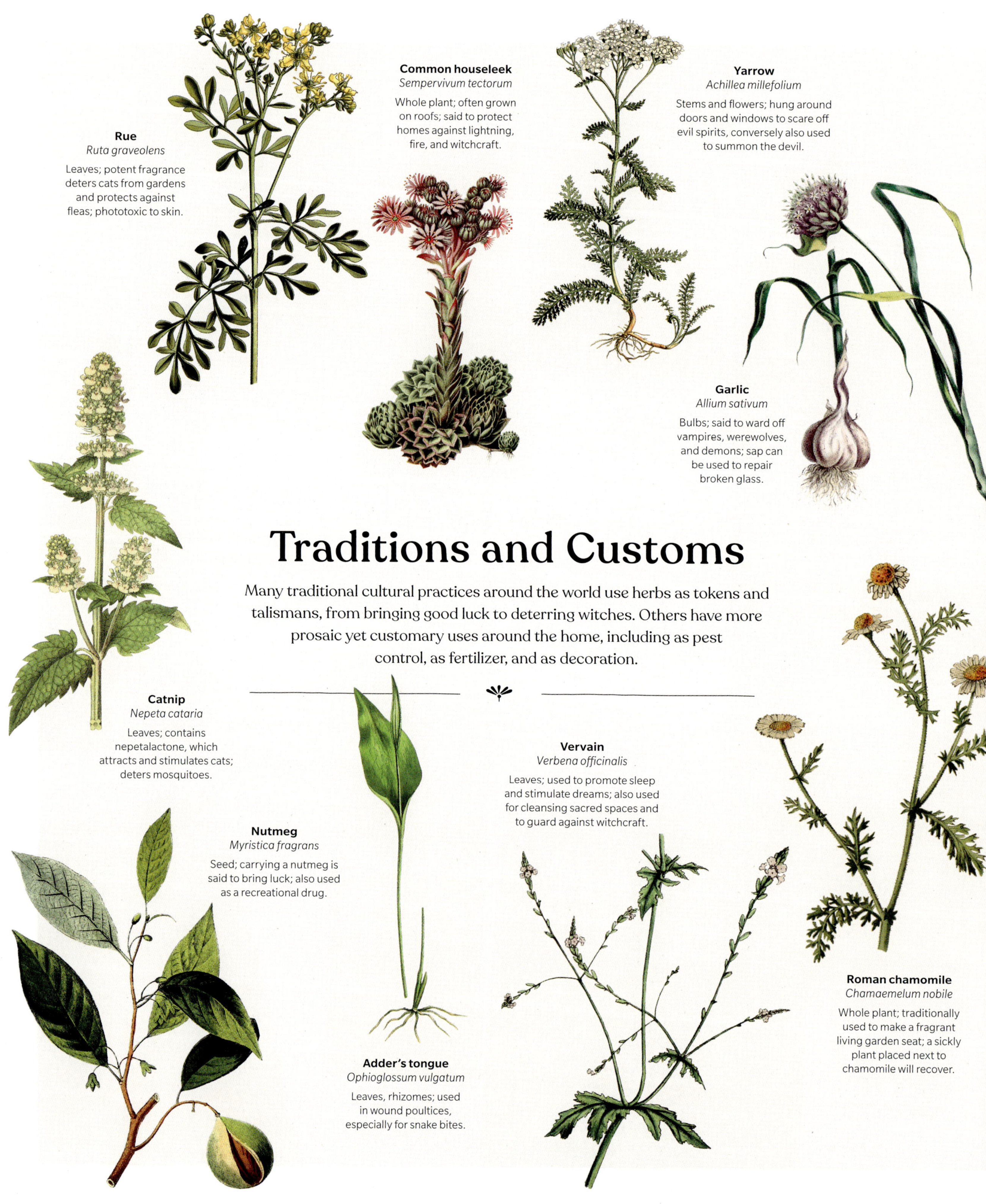

Rue
Ruta graveolens
Leaves; potent fragrance deters cats from gardens and protects against fleas; phototoxic to skin.

Common houseleek
Sempervivum tectorum
Whole plant; often grown on roofs; said to protect homes against lightning, fire, and witchcraft.

Yarrow
Achillea millefolium
Stems and flowers; hung around doors and windows to scare off evil spirits, conversely also used to summon the devil.

Garlic
Allium sativum
Bulbs; said to ward off vampires, werewolves, and demons; sap can be used to repair broken glass.

Catnip
Nepeta cataria
Leaves; contains nepetalactone, which attracts and stimulates cats; deters mosquitoes.

Vervain
Verbena officinalis
Leaves; used to promote sleep and stimulate dreams; also used for cleansing sacred spaces and to guard against witchcraft.

Nutmeg
Myristica fragrans
Seed; carrying a nutmeg is said to bring luck; also used as a recreational drug.

Roman chamomile
Chamaemelum nobile
Whole plant; traditionally used to make a fragrant living garden seat; a sickly plant placed next to chamomile will recover.

Adder's tongue
Ophioglossum vulgatum
Leaves, rhizomes; used in wound poultices, especially for snake bites.

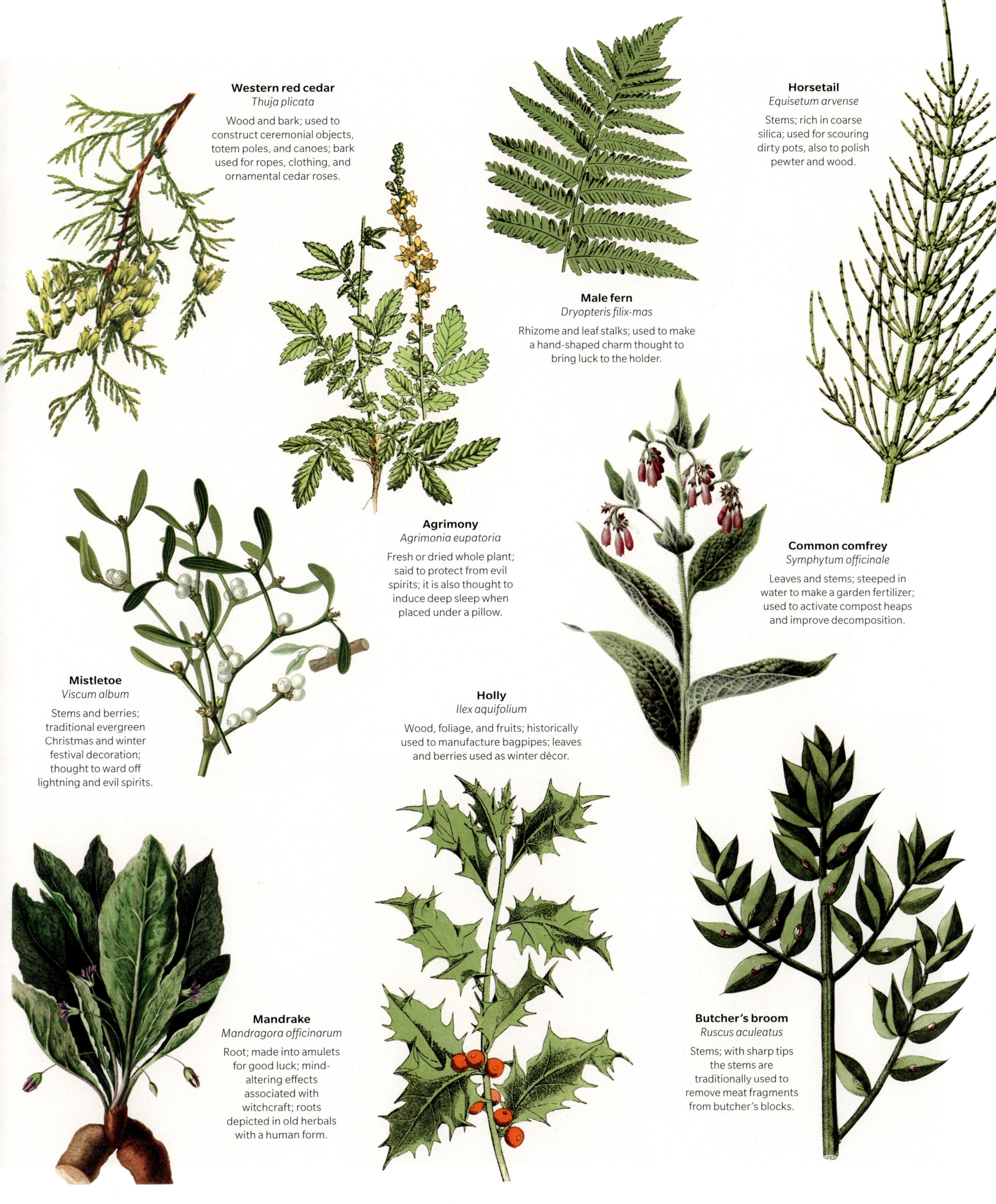

Western red cedar
Thuja plicata
Wood and bark; used to construct ceremonial objects, totem poles, and canoes; bark used for ropes, clothing, and ornamental cedar roses.

Agrimony
Agrimonia eupatoria
Fresh or dried whole plant; said to protect from evil spirits; it is also thought to induce deep sleep when placed under a pillow.

Male fern
Dryopteris filix-mas
Rhizome and leaf stalks; used to make a hand-shaped charm thought to bring luck to the holder.

Horsetail
Equisetum arvense
Stems; rich in coarse silica; used for scouring dirty pots, also to polish pewter and wood.

Mistletoe
Viscum album
Stems and berries; traditional evergreen Christmas and winter festival decoration; thought to ward off lightning and evil spirits.

Common comfrey
Symphytum officinale
Leaves and stems; steeped in water to make a garden fertilizer; used to activate compost heaps and improve decomposition.

Holly
Ilex aquifolium
Wood, foliage, and fruits; historically used to manufacture bagpipes; leaves and berries used as winter décor.

Mandrake
Mandragora officinarum
Root; made into amulets for good luck; mind-altering effects associated with witchcraft; roots depicted in old herbals with a human form.

Butcher's broom
Ruscus aculeatus
Stems; with sharp tips the stems are traditionally used to remove meat fragments from butcher's blocks.

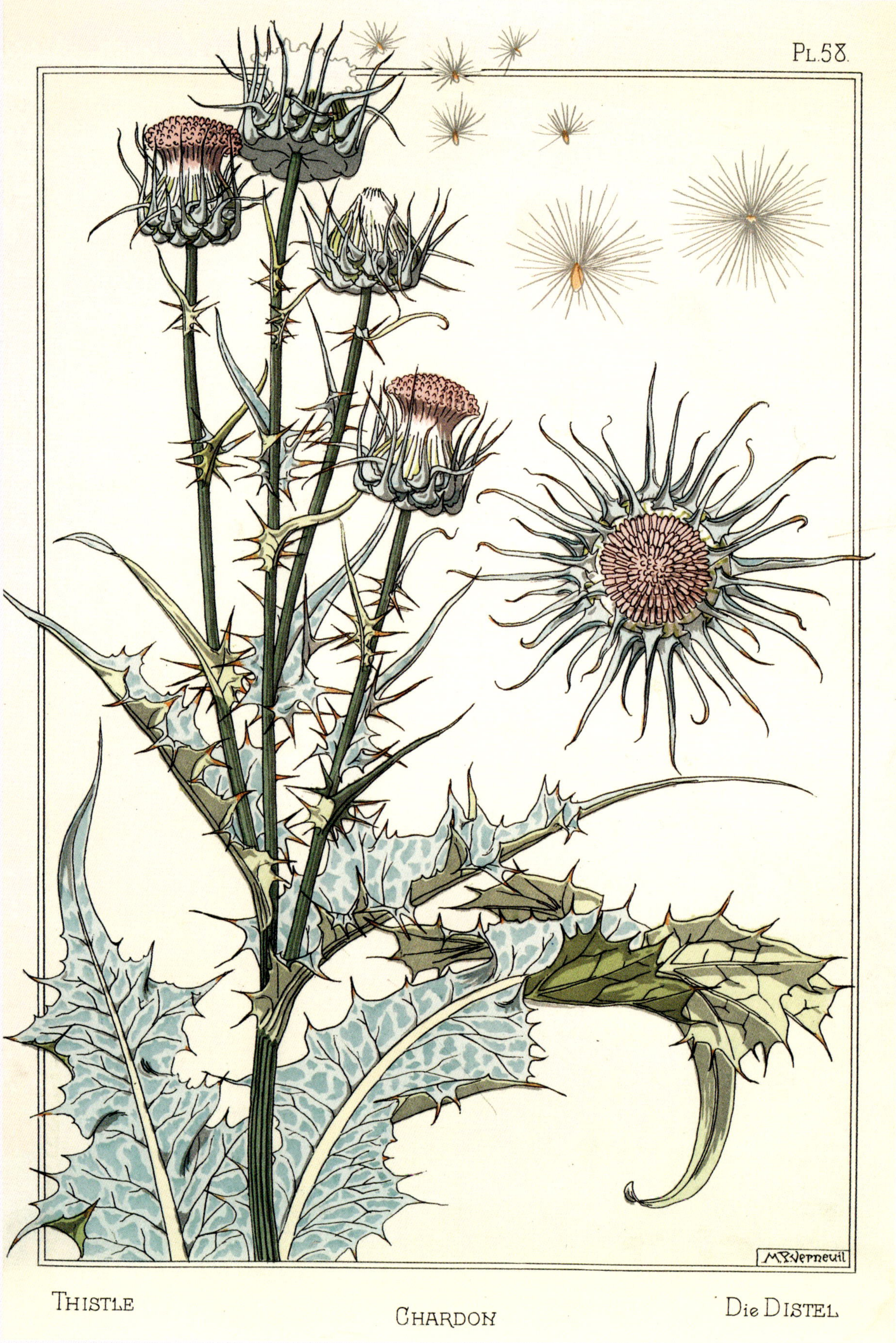

PL. 58.

M.P. Verneuil

THISTLE CHARDON Die DISTEL

◄ Fabled foliage
According to folklore, when the Virgin Mary was nursing baby Jesus, a drop of breast milk fell on the leaves of a nearby thistle plant, leading to its white-mottled colouration. This connection is alluded to in the plant's species name *marianum*.

Similar herbs

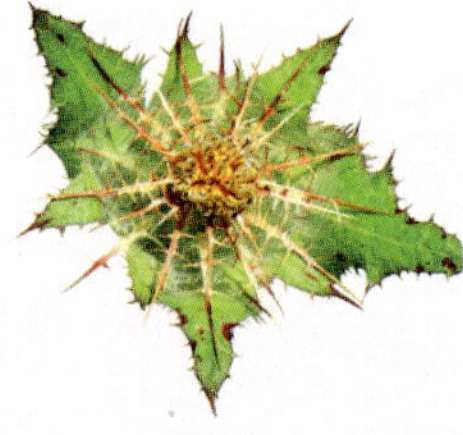

HOLY THISTLE
Centaurea benedicta
Native from Spain east to Central Asia, and widely introduced elsewhere, this non-edible thistle is used to promote lactation in mothers and to treat wounds, digestive ailments, and plague.

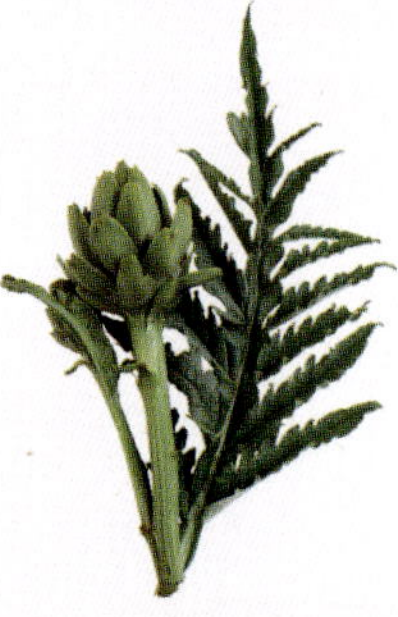

GLOBE ARTICHOKE
Cynara cardunculus
This large Mediterranean thistle has a long history as an edible crop, especially leaf stalks (cardoon) and flower heads (artichokes). Domesticated forms are less spiny than wild plants.

Milk Thistle

Silybum marianum

Uses Medicines for liver conditions; cooking

Parts used Seeds; occasionally roots, leaves, flowers

Active ingredients Silymarin (a mixture of silibinin, silidianin, and silicristin)

Habitat Disturbed or waste ground in temperate and subtropical regions, including fields and roadsides

Despite its ferocious, prickly appearance, almost every part of milk thistle is edible, and the seeds contain an important medicinal compound traditionally used in the treatment of liver disease.

Milk thistle gets its name from the milky white mottling splashed across its leaves. The herb has been used as a galactagogue – a booster of milk supply in lactating mothers – although clinical evidence supporting its effectiveness is sparse. Silymarin, the active ingredient extracted from the seeds, is used to treat a variety of medical conditions and as a food supplement.

Perhaps the most common application for silymarin is in treating conditions of the liver, including alcoholic hepatitis and cirrhosis, and viral hepatitis (or hepatitis C). Scientific studies of its efficacy showed mixed results. Milk thistle extract may counteract the effects of consuming poisonous amatoxin-containing mushrooms by reducing the degree of liver damage caused.

Wonder weed

Native to the Mediterranean Basin and east to India, milk thistle is now found as a weed on every continent except Antarctica, with laws prohibiting its cultivation in some regions. Its leaves can be used in a similar way to spinach and its roasted seeds can be a coffee substitute. Almost every part of the plant is edible, though spines must be removed before consumption.

" [Milk thistle] can... recreate your liver from a memory of health. "

AURORA LEVINS MORALES, *Remedios: Stories of Earth and Iron from the History of Puertorriqueñas*, 2001

Each seed is carried away by a silky parachute formed from the calyx
Outermost florets open first and the innermost last, extending the blooming season
Prickly protective bracts known as phyllaries surround the flower head
Each flower head produces numerous seeds (achenes), one from each pollinated floret

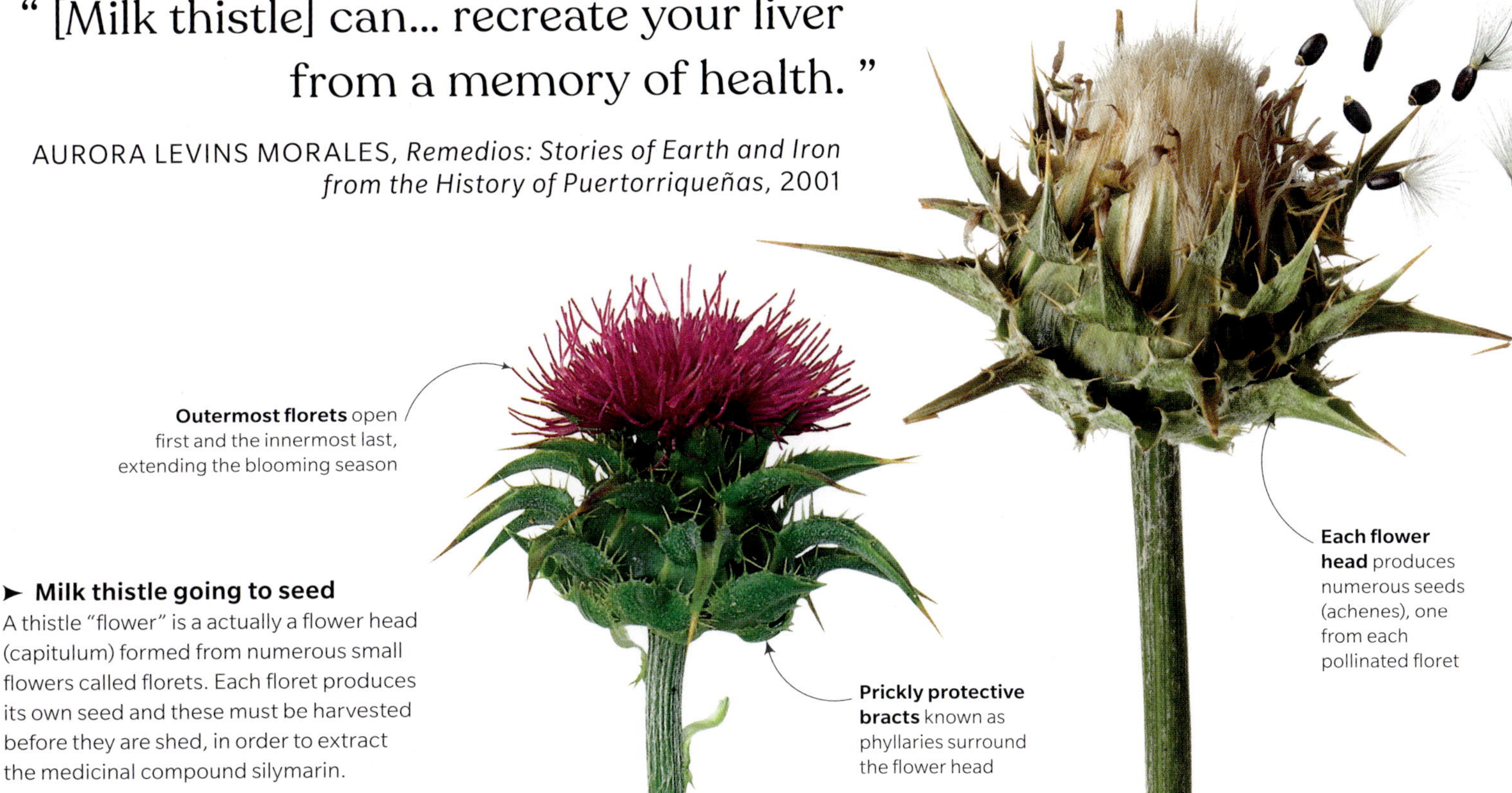

➤ **Milk thistle going to seed**
A thistle "flower" is a actually a flower head (capitulum) formed from numerous small flowers called florets. Each floret produces its own seed and these must be harvested before they are shed, in order to extract the medicinal compound silymarin.

Holy Basil

Ocimum tenuiflorum

Uses Medicines; religious symbol; insect repellent, tea

Parts used Leaves, flowers, stems, seeds

Active ingredients Eugenol, elemene, caryophyllene, germacrene-D, ursolic acid, rosmarinic acid, oleanolic acid

Habitat Tropical and subtropical regions in a variety of sunny habitats, often in agricultural areas and as a weed

The culinary properties of sweet basil (*Ocimum basilicum*) have long been enjoyed by many cultures, but few medicinal herbs attract such veneration as does holy basil among the many adherents of Hinduism.

Holy basil, also known as tulsi or tulasī, is close kin to sweet basil, the famed culinary herb. Both originate from the Indian subcontinent and east to Southeast Asia and northern Australia. Holy basil is cultivated widely around the world, especially in tropical and subtropical climates. *Ocimum tenuiflorum* has several forms; the most commonly cultivated is a green-leaved form known as Rama tulsi, which has a sweet flavour. Purple-leaved Krishna tulsi is rarer and has a more peppery flavour, the dark leaves supposedly recalling the Hindu deity Krishna's dark skin.

Less common in cultivation but widely available as a wild plant, Vana tulsi has a spicy, clove fragrance due to high levels of eugenol in its essential oil. This wild tulsi is a different species (*O. gratissimum*) and occurs naturally in both Africa and Asia. While there are notable differences between *tulsi* species and forms, products containing tulsi do not always specify which is included; forms of tulsi are also used interchangeably in cultural practices.

The venerated herb

The Hindu religion respects nature; many plants and animals are subjects of worship. Holy basil is considered the most sacred of all plants and a gateway between heaven and earth. In many Hindu homes, a holy basil plant is cultivated in the central courtyard, with its every need catered for by residents. It is grown on a raised plinth, called the *Tulsi Vrindavan* in Hindi or *Tulasī Chaura* in Odia. Various customs dictate how and when to care for the plant. Holy basil is positioned only on the north or northeast sides of the house – never the south side – and away from kitchens and bathrooms. Plants are worshipped during the *tulsi puja*, where a lamp

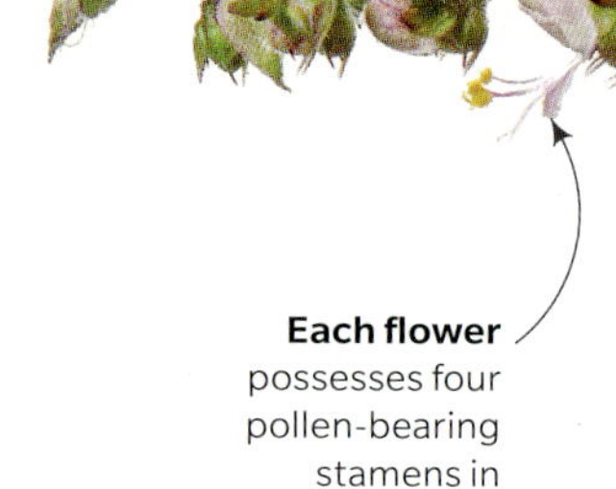

Each flower possesses four pollen-bearing stamens in two pairs

Holy basil is considered an earthly manifestation of the Hindu goddess Tulsi

◄ Tulsi malas
Made from the roots and woody stems of holy basil, a tulsi mala is a set of Hindu prayer beads, worn around the neck or held in the hand like a rosary in order to connect the wearer with the Great Lord Vishnu.

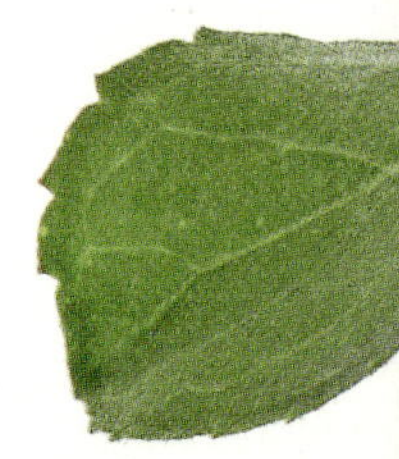

Whorls of flowers, called verticillasters, each made up of six small, pink flowers
Uppermost flowers open last; each is enclosed within a tubular calyx
Holy basil leaves have serrated edges, and are smooth or have fine hairs

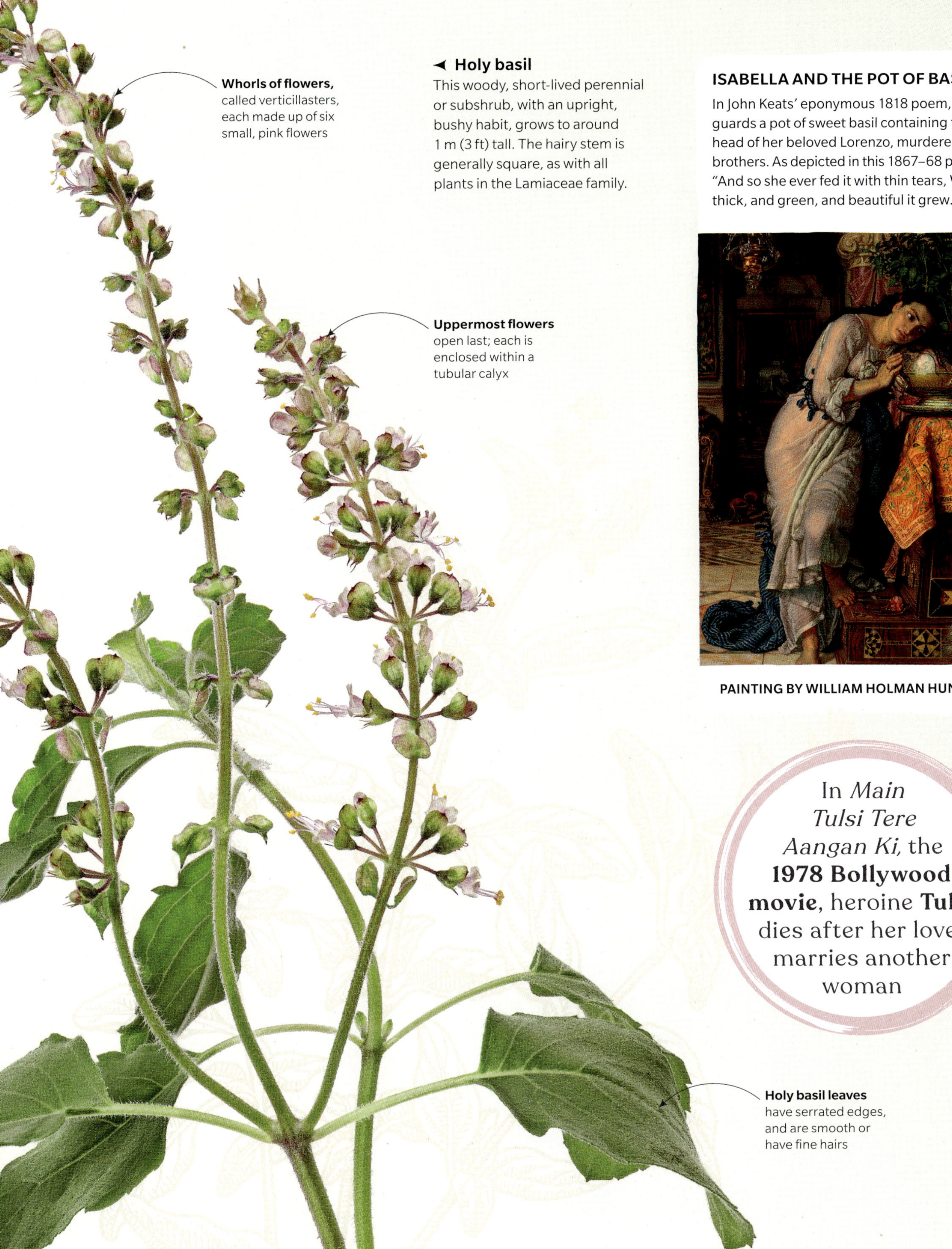

◄ Holy basil
This woody, short-lived perennial or subshrub, with an upright, bushy habit, grows to around 1 m (3 ft) tall. The hairy stem is generally square, as with all plants in the Lamiaceae family.

ISABELLA AND THE POT OF BASIL

In John Keats' eponymous 1818 poem, Isabella guards a pot of sweet basil containing the head of her beloved Lorenzo, murdered by her brothers. As depicted in this 1867–68 painting, "And so she ever fed it with thin tears, Whence thick, and green, and beautiful it grew."

PAINTING BY WILLIAM HOLMAN HUNT

In *Main Tulsi Tere Aangan Ki,* the **1978 Bollywood movie,** heroine **Tulsi** dies after her lover marries another woman

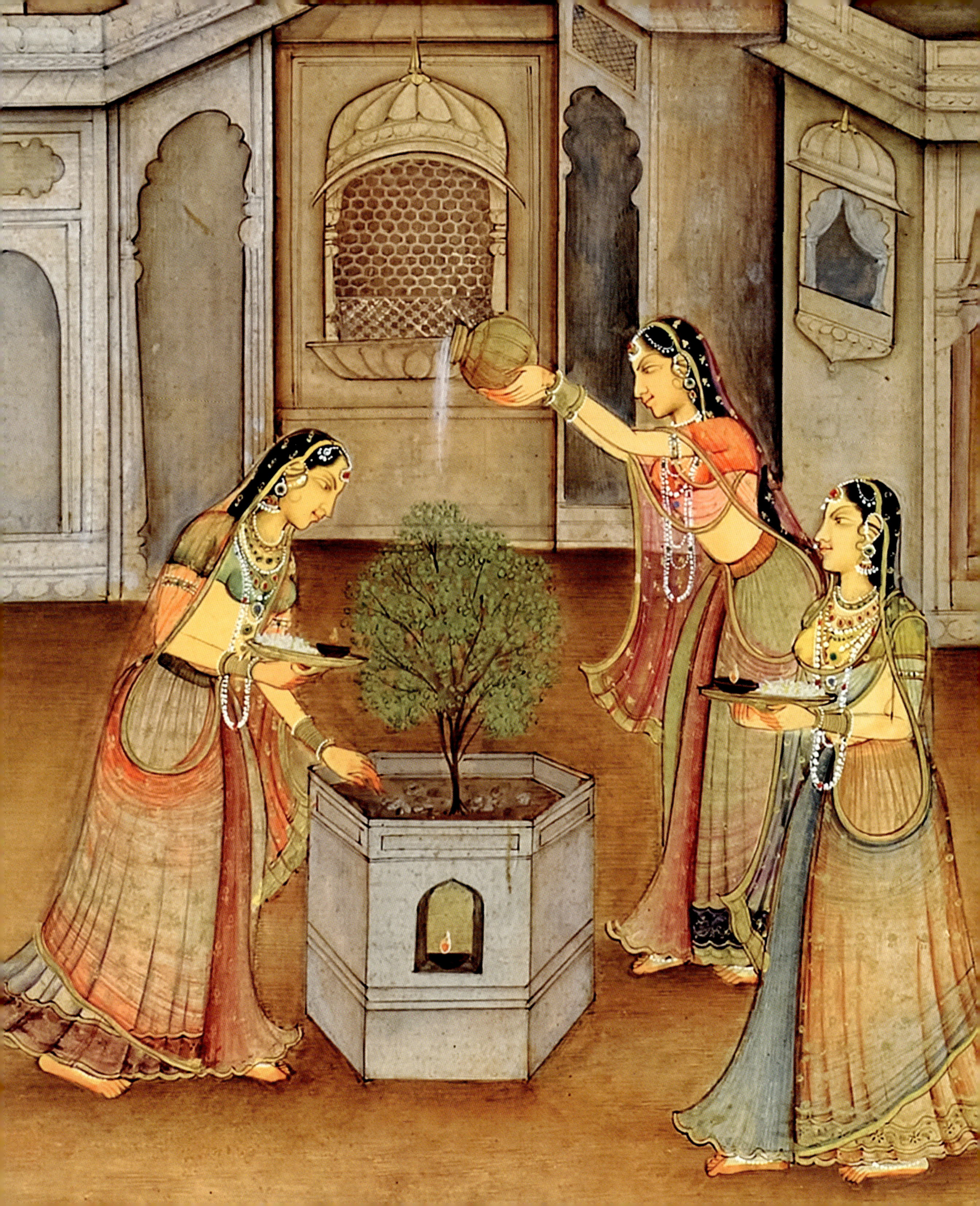

Similar herbs

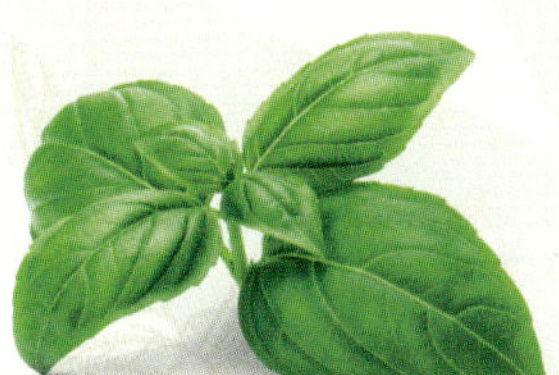

GENOVESE BASIL
Ocimum basilicum 'Genovese'
This Italian form of culinary or sweet basil, with glossy leaves and a strong aroma, is grown worldwide. It is often used in tomato-based dishes.

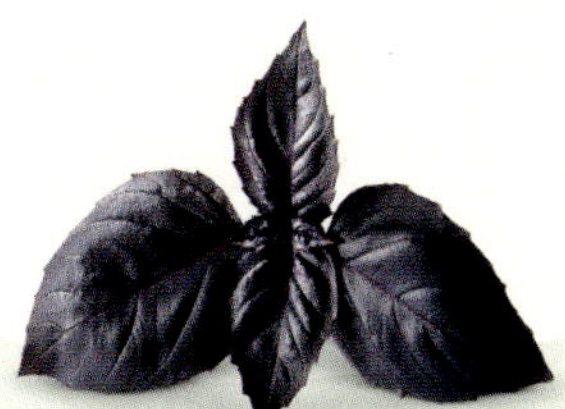

PURPLE BASIL
Ocimum basilicum. var. *purpurascens*
Its spicy, purple leaves make this sweet basil a popular ornamental; it is used in salads and rice dishes.

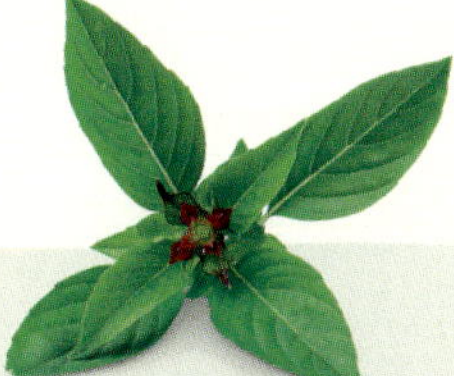

THAI BASIL
Ocimum basilicum 'Horapha Nanum'
Favoured in Thai and Vietnamese cuisines for its potent liquorice taste, this form has tough leaves that take cooking better than Genovese basil.

of ghee (clarified butter) is lit and water is offered after circling the plant three times. The water is never given on a Sunday and milk can be offered to ward off bad luck. Offerings of flowers, cow dung, incense, and Ganges water may be made to the holy basil plant while chanting mantras.

Most of the devotional activities regarding tulsi are tendered by women and it is often considered a women's deity. A tulsi leaf may be placed on the forehead of a dying person to ease their passage, and tulsi water may help their soul reach heaven.

Divine origins

In Hinduism, it is not uncommon for deities to be reincarnated in human or animal forms known as avatars. The goddess Tulsi (or Tulasī) is an avatar of Lakshmi, the consort of the god Vishnu. His two best known avatars are Krishna and Rama, after which are named the two common forms of this herb. Holy basil derives its mythological significance from the connection between the plant and Vishnu.

The *Tulsi Vivah* is a *puja* that marks the end of the monsoon and the start of the Hindu wedding season; the details of the ceremony vary across India. *Tulsi Vivah* takes the form of a marriage between a holy basil plant representing the goddess Tulsi and a symbol of Vishnu, such as a *shaligrama* stone (a black fossil from the Kali Gandaki River in Nepal) or a branch of an Indian gooseberry tree (*Phyllanthus emblica*). The ritual is conducted in homes or temples; the holy basil plant is adorned with a sari, jewellery, and even a paper image of Tulsi's face and the basil "bride" and groom are linked with a cotton thread.

Childless couples may take on the ceremonial role of "parents" to the tulsi plant, sometimes providing bridal offerings, such as bangles, which are then donated to an unmarried girl or to a priest. This is said to bring upon the couple the blessing of a child.

◄ Tulsi puja
Holy basil plants adorn many Indian homes and may be worshipped daily in a ceremony called the *tulsi puja*: the plant is watered and offered gifts such as flowers and an oil lamp is later lit nearby.

> " Where there is a Tulasī, there is no poverty... no fear, and no disease. "
>
> *Padma Purana*,6: 23: 28–33, 4–15th century CE

Sacred role in Assam

Tulsi also plays a role in the Kati Bihu ceremony in Assam, which coincides with the period during which young rice plants are transplanted into the fields. Grain supplies are beginning to wain and the harvest has yet to come, so prayers are said around the household tulsi plant to encourage a robust harvest. A lamp is lit in front of the plant; other lamps are lit in the fields to attract insect pests, which die when drawn into the flames.

▼ Fresh tulsi leaves
In the past, holy basil's role as a culinary herb has been limited to some Thai dishes. Some Western recipes now substitute sweet basil with holy basil, for its more pungent, aniseed flavour and its health benefits.

Fresh leaves of holy basil can be mashed with oil into a spicy pesto

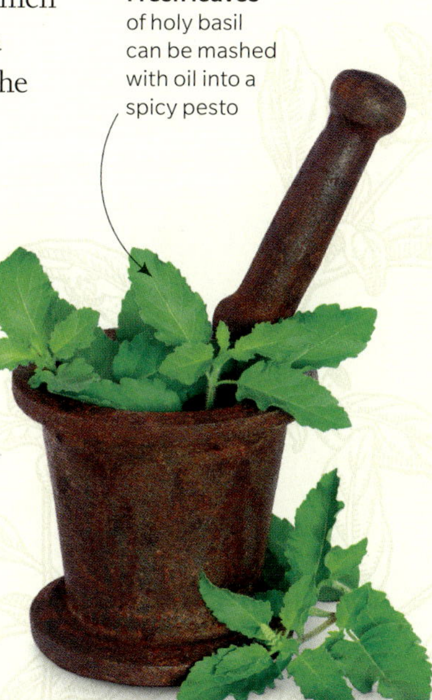

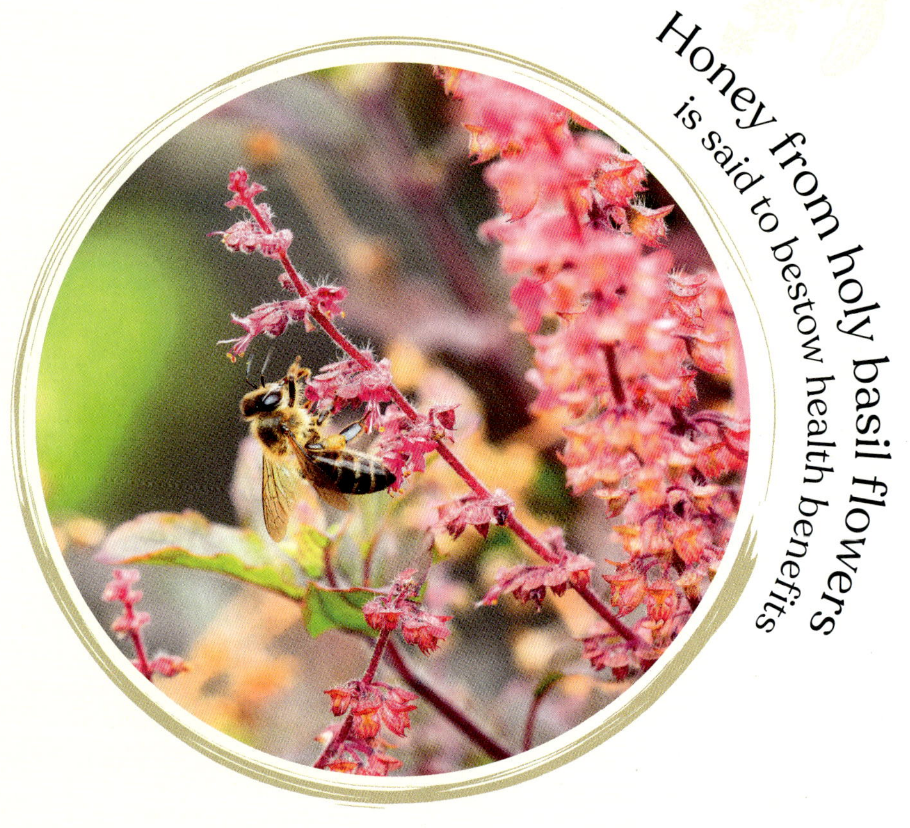

Honey from holy basil flowers is said to bestow health benefits

▲ Holy basil flowers
Tulsi flowers are harvested for use in herbal teas and ointments. They can also be left to be pollinated, usually by bees, in order to harvest the seeds for culinary or medicinal use.

Holy basil and Ayurveda

Considering its great cultural significance, it is no surprise that tulsi is very important in traditional medicines – especially of the Ayurveda system of India, in which it is a principal herb. Holy basil is typically utilized as a hot-water infusion of fresh leaves, stems, and flowers. It has been used to treat a wide range of ailments, from abdominal conditions, arthritis, and eye diseases to coughs and colds, leprosy, and lumbago. It is considered an adaptogen (a plant extract that helps the body to resist stress and improves well-being). Few scientific studies demonstrate clear benefits of using holy basil medicinally, but it may improve breathing function in asthma sufferers and help patients with type 2 diabetes to better control their blood-sugar levels. Its antioxidants may reduce the neural damage that causes Alzheimer's disease, and it has been used externally to treat a range of skin conditions, including ringworm.

Tea and Thai food

Beyond its medicinal uses, holy basil is most often consumed as a tea, which can have a flavour reminiscent of cloves, liquorice, mint, or pepper, depending on the form of tulsi used. It can taste bitter, so is also blended with other herbs and spices; tulsi tea is free of caffeine. While fresh basil leaves are preferable, the leaves can be dried and ground to make a long-lasting powder for use as a tea.

Although sweet basil (*Ocimum basilicum* and its cultivars) has long been an important culinary herb in Mediterranean and Southeast Asian cuisines, tulsi is seldom used in food preparation in India. In Thailand, it is the key herb in *pad kra pao*, a dish of pork, chicken, beef, or seafood stir-fried with holy basil, chilli, and garlic. Holy basil in Thai dishes should not be confused with Thai basil (see p.259), which is a form of sweet basil. If soaked in water, holy basil seeds become mucilaginous and can be used as a substitute for the seeds of its relative, chia (*Salvia hispanica*); they also impart a slight basil flavour.

Both holy basil species can be used in companion planting schemes to deter insect pests. Tulsi may also be effective as a mosquito repellent and organic pest control.

Tulsi is often combined in a tea with ginger, lemon, and honey
Dried flowers and leaves can be stored for brewing in a tea

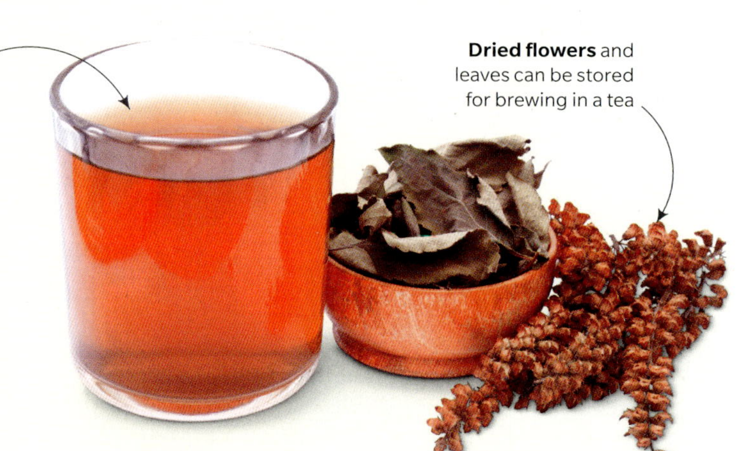

► Herbal tea
One of the most common methods of consuming holy basil is as a tea, made from the leaves or flowers. Tulsi tea is rich in antioxidants and has adaptogenic properties, reducing stress and boosting immunity to respiratory conditions.

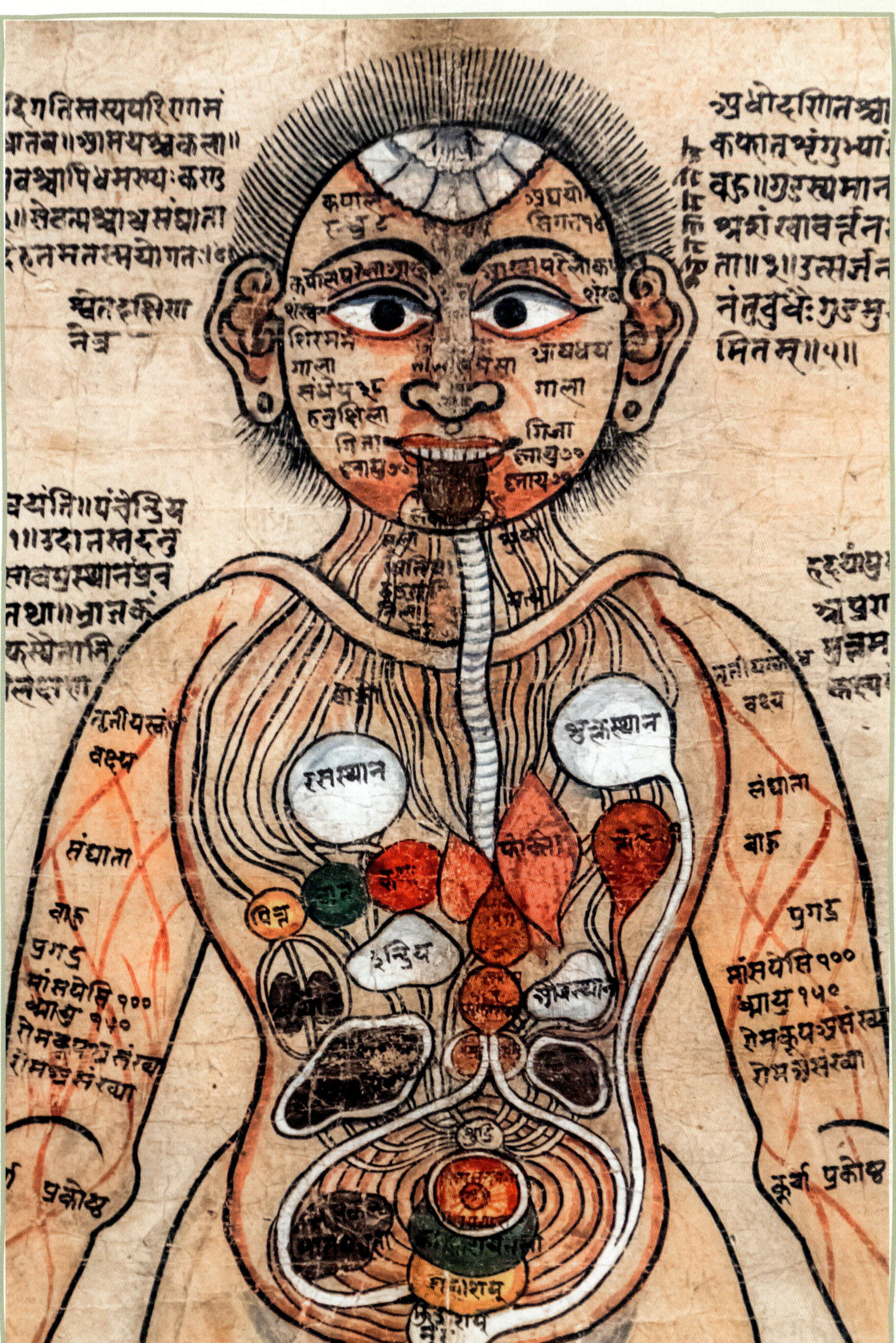

◄ Ayurvedic man
This 18th-century diagram from Nepal depicts the human body as seen by practitioners of Ayurvedic medicine. The Sanskrit text describes anatomical details and Ayurveda theory.

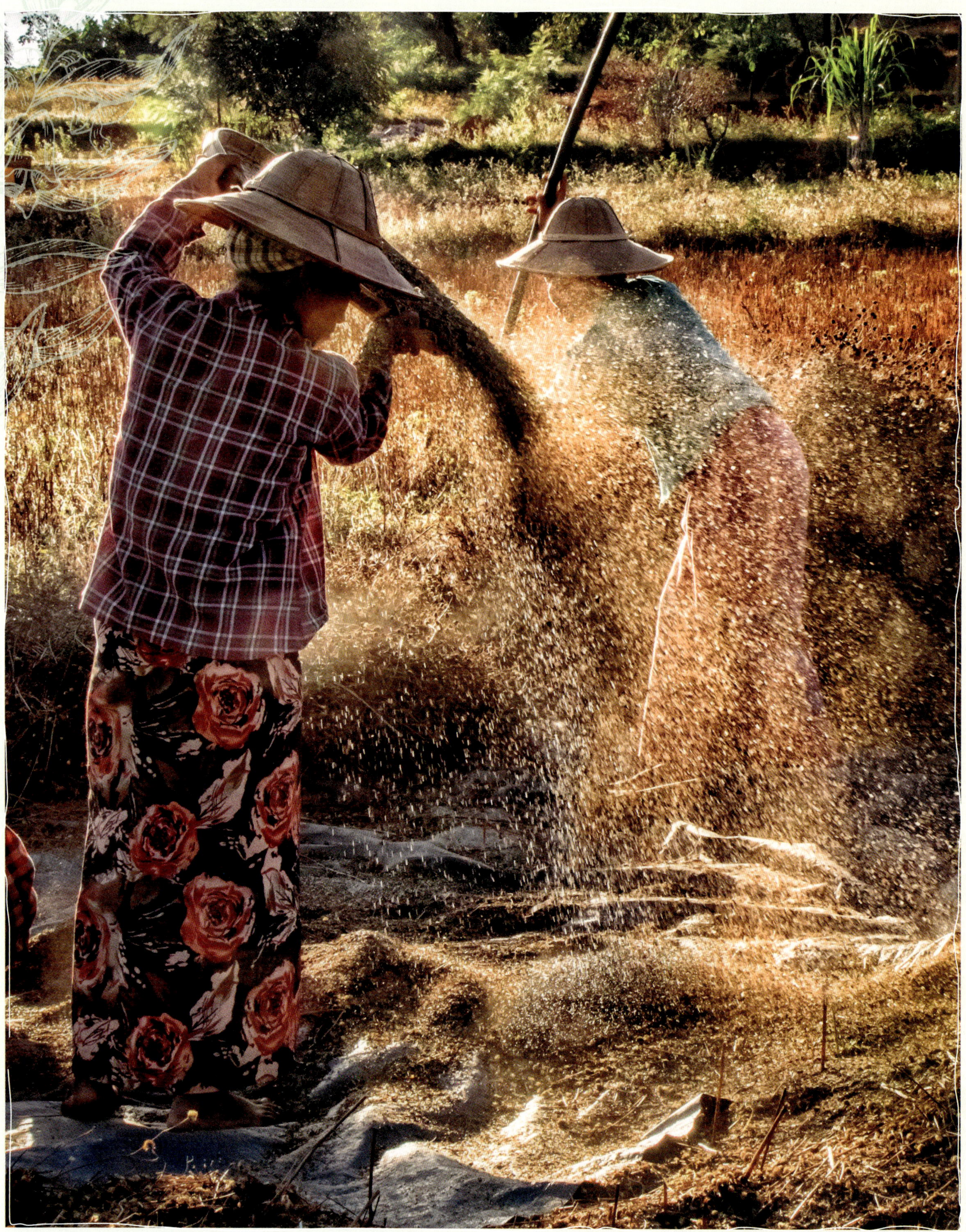

Sesame

Sesamum indicum

From flavouring baked goods to making biofuel, sesame has a multitude of uses. This versatile plant is also extremely tolerant to droughts, making it a crucial crop in arid parts of the world.

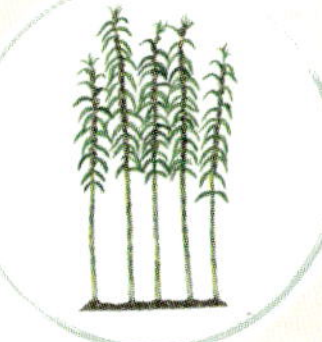

Uses Medicines for diabetes, hypertension; cooking; biofuel

Parts used Seeds

Active ingredients Sesamin, sesamolin, linoleic acid, oleic acid, palmitic acid, fibre, protein

Habitat Unknown in the wild; tropical and sub-tropical regions; drought tolerant

Sesame is not a grass, like so many other popular grains, but a colourful flowering plant and a significant commercial crop in countries with a seasonally dry climate. Probably originating in the Indian subcontinent, sesame cultivation dates back at least 5,000 years. It is thought to be the oldest oilseed known to humans. While sesame is easy to grow and drought-tolerant, traditional varieties have fruits that spontaneously split open, or shatter, when ripe, losing the valuable seeds into the soil, and these varieties are not suited to mechanical harvesting. In the 20th century, plant breeders developed varieties with capsules that do not split open when mature, but research continues to look for a sesame variety that can be efficiently harvested by machine.

◄ Green sesame pods
Sesame's seed pod is an oblong, ridged capsule containing 50 to 100 oil-rich seeds. These may vary in colour from creamy white to black.

Flattened, oval seeds are covered in an edible husk

A primary use of the seeds is to yield sesame oil, which is widely used in cooking, especially in South and eastern Asia. Beyond its culinary significance, sesame oil is attracting attention as a biofuel. It is also used in cosmetics, as a solvent for intravenous drugs, and in products such as lubricants.

Similar herb

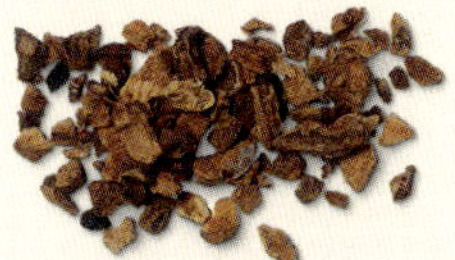

DEVIL'S CLAW
Harpagophytum procumbens

The roots and tubers of this sesame relative are used to treat back pain, heartburn, and inflammation including arthritis. It is native to southern Africa.

Seeds, oil, and paste

Sesame seeds are used in a variety of foods including benne wafers in South Carolina, US, sesame snaps in Poland, sesame balls (*jian dui*) in China, and *goma dofu*, a sesame tofu in Japan. They are sprinkled on baked goods such as breads, bagels, and buns to add texture and flavour. In the Middle East, the seeds are ground to make tahini, a topping for falafel, or a component of some hummus and halvah recipes.

► Source of seeds
Sesame is an annual plant grown each year from seed. Flowers may be white, pink, or purple, and each produces a seed capsule.

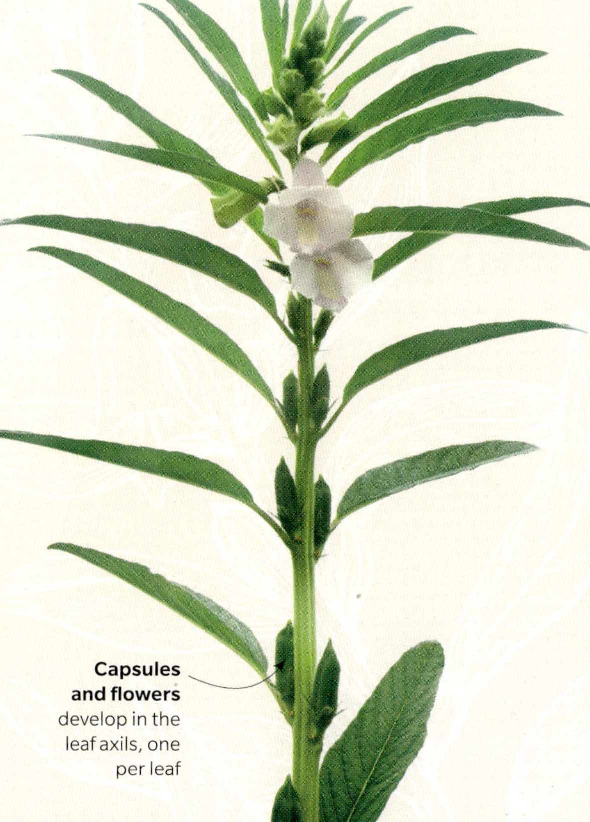

Capsules and flowers develop in the leaf axils, one per leaf

Sesame can cause **allergic reactions** such as anaphylaxis

◄ Winnowing sesame
Sesame capsules must be harvested once dry, but before they split open. Seeds are separated from the capsules manually, then hulled to remove the outer coat.

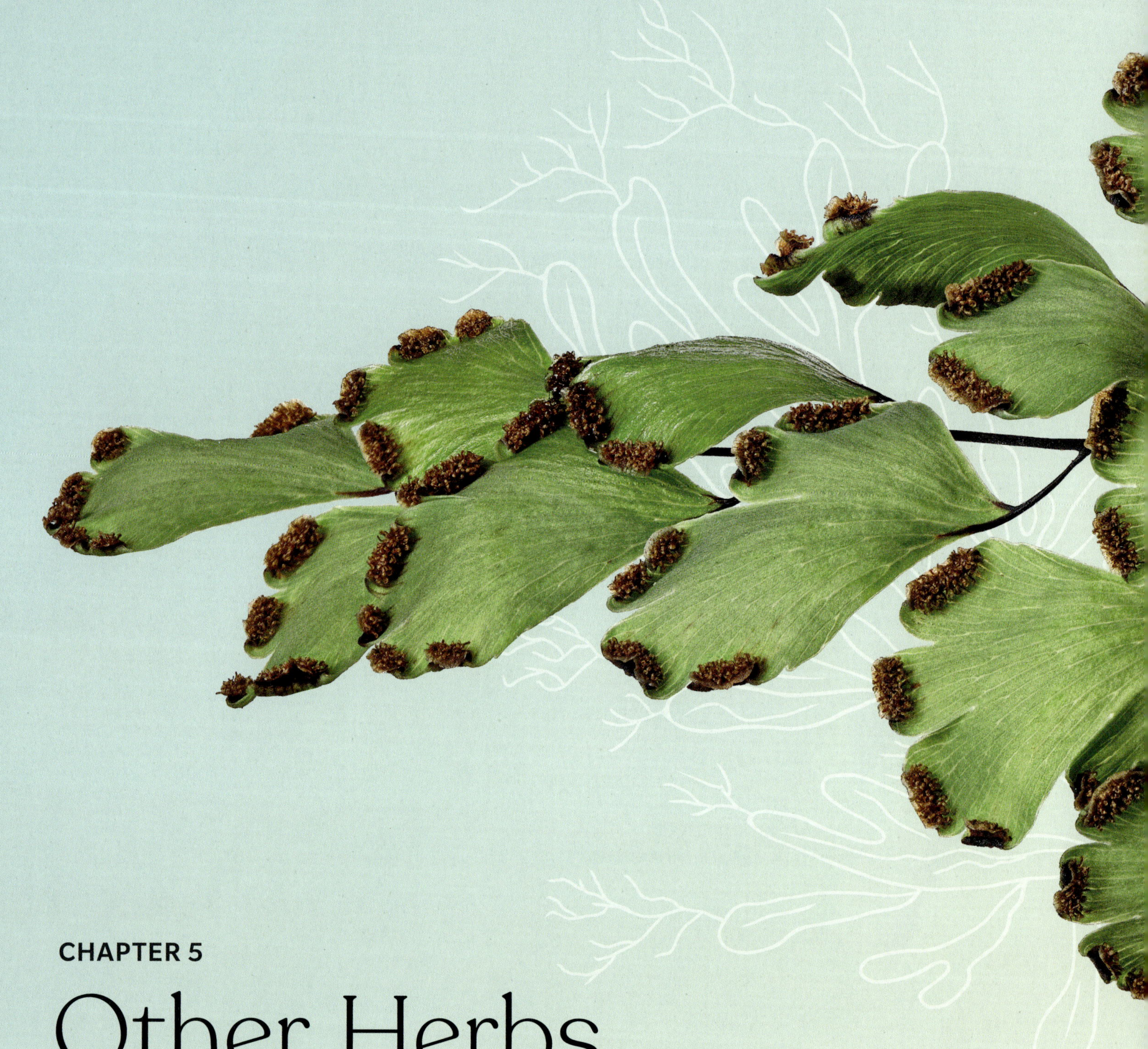

CHAPTER 5

Other Herbs

Herbs span the entire breadth of the plant kingdom, including non-flowering plants like ferns. Some non-plant organisms – fungi and algae – also have herbal uses.

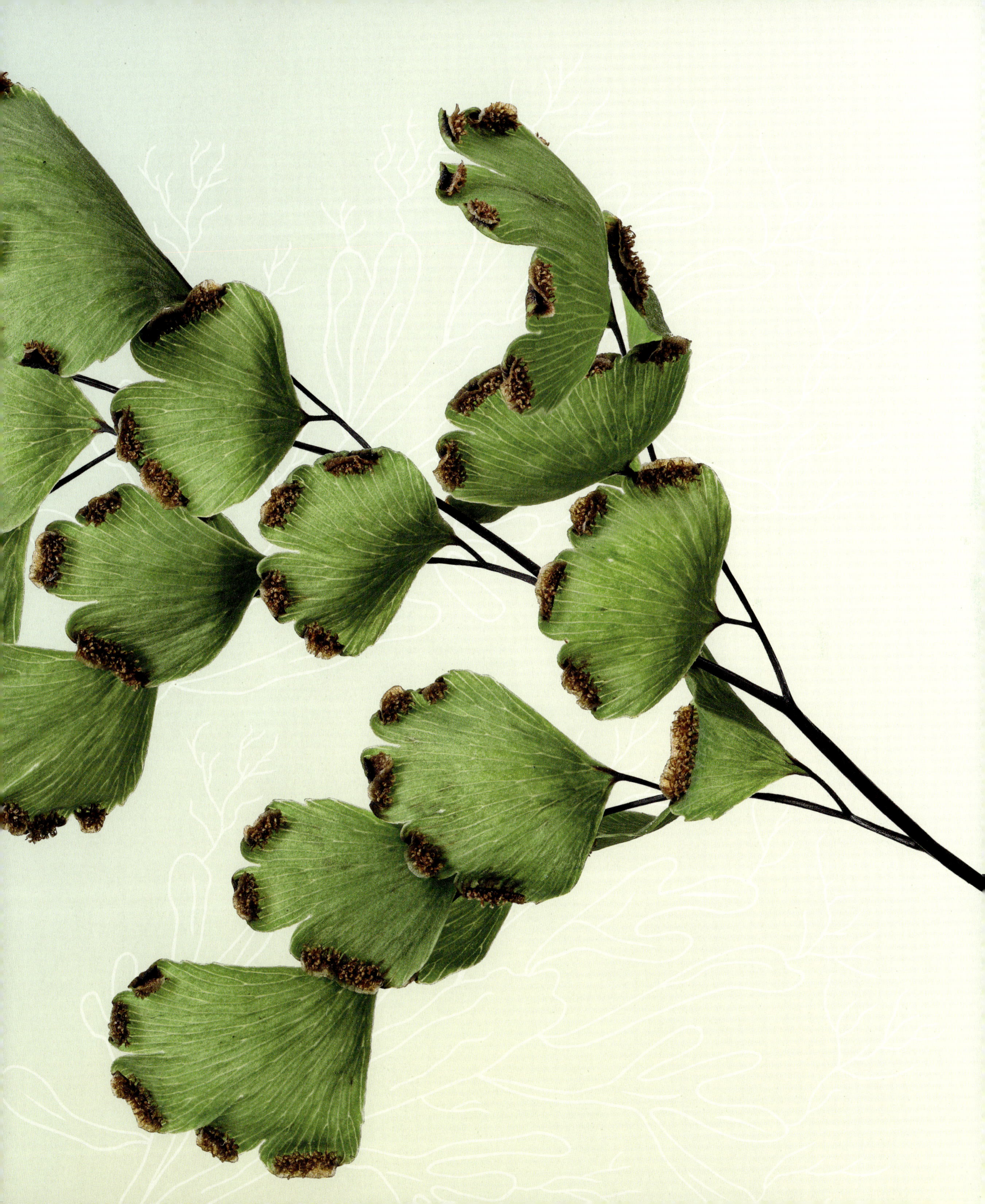

Royal Fern

Osmunda regalis

Royal fern, found in wet soils in temperate regions of the northern hemisphere, has been used as a growing medium and medicinal remedy, and is still valued as a garden plant and a culinary delicacy.

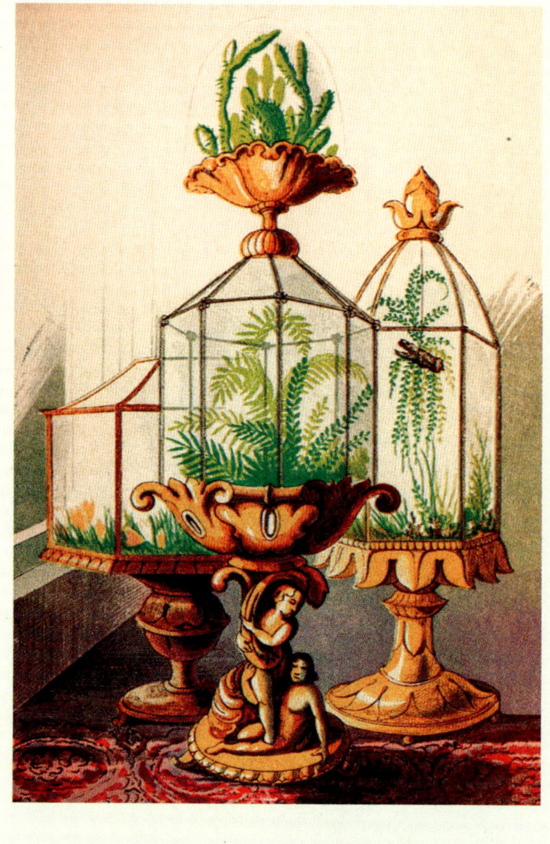

▲ **Wardian cases**
These glazed containers, perfect for growing delicate ferns, were invented by Nathaniel Bagshaw Ward in 1829. They sparked off a craze, called pteridomania, for general fern cultivation in Britain, Australia, and elsewhere.

Royal fern originates from Europe, east as far as Iran, and from northwest Africa. It is a large, handsome, architectural plant, often grown in water gardens and damp woodland plantings. The fern's spores are borne on fertile fronds. Their modified frond tips are smothered in spore-bearing structures (sporangia) that make the tips look like rusty-brown tassels and led to the plant's other name of flowering fern. The beauty of the royal fern led to mass pillaging of plants from the wild, but it is now legally protected in many countries.

Exploiting the plant

In the 19th and early-20th centuries, the fern was also collected for its root fibre. Osmunda fibre is water- and air-retentive, fine-textured, and long-lasting – a perfect medium for growing orchids. Luckily, the trade has largely ceased since more sustainable and less costly growing media became available.

In the past, royal fern was gathered for medical use. In Europe, rickets was widely treated with extracts from the rhizome. The rhizome has astringent and diuretic properties, and was used as a remedy for jaundice and "obstructions of the viscera" (the internal organs).

A starchy mash made from the crushed rhizome of royal fern was made into a poultice and applied to burns and bruises or as a rub for sciatica and painful joints. In Spain, the pounded rhizomes provided a mucilaginous drink called *antojil* wine, taken as a treatment for muscular-skeletal disorders, bruises, and sprains. The mucilage contained in royal fern has also made it a useful ingredient for natural skincare products, as well as shampoo.

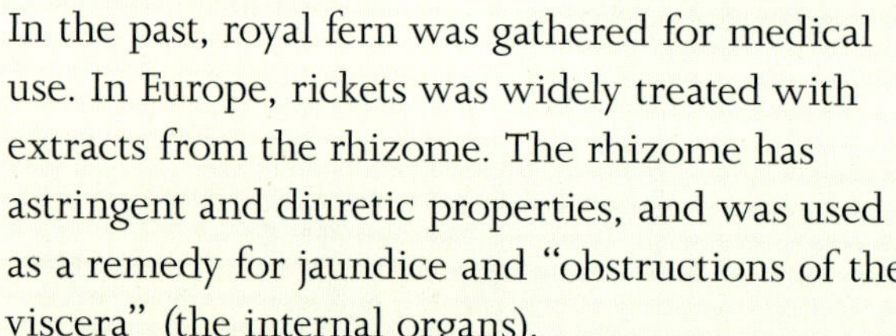

◄ **Royal fern shoots**
Tightly furled, new shoots emerge each spring. They are known as croziers, because of their similarity to bishops' crooks, or fiddleheads, alluding to the scrolls of violins.

Similar herbs

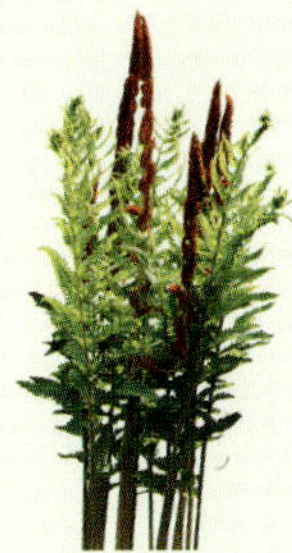

CINNAMON FERN
Osmundastrum cinnamomeum
In the Americas, this fern was harvested by Indigenous peoples for food and medicines. Like royal fern, it is one of the world's oldest plants.

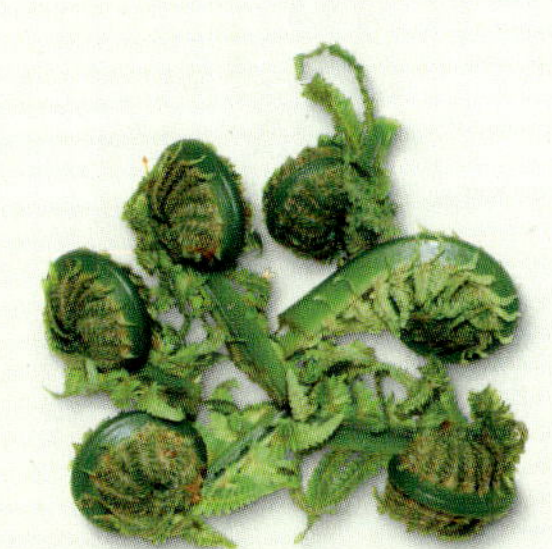

OSTRICH FERN
Onoclea struthiopteris
The fronds of this large fern resemble ostrich plumes. It spreads by creeping stems in damp woods, and is a popular garden plant. In Japan, its fiddleheads are eaten as *kogomi*.

Royal fern is a "living fossil": it has changed little since the Cretaceous – the last age of the dinosaurs – 80 million years ago

Large fronds form a clump up to 2.5 m (8 ft) tall

➤ Fern frond
Most of the broad, upright fronds of royal fern are sterile. In cool-temperate climates, they are deciduous, turning red-brown in autumn, but are evergreen in warmer areas.

Uses Medicines, cooking, horticulture, cosmetics

Parts used Stems, rhizome

Active ingredients Terpenes, phenols,flavonoids, starch

Habitat Bogs, water margins, and damp woodlands in temperate areas

Pinnule, or second-level leaflet, is oval to oblong and has a short stalk

➤ Young frond

Bracken stems, or stipes, are attached to underground horizontal structures called rhizomes. Technically, a rhizome is not a root but a creeping stem.

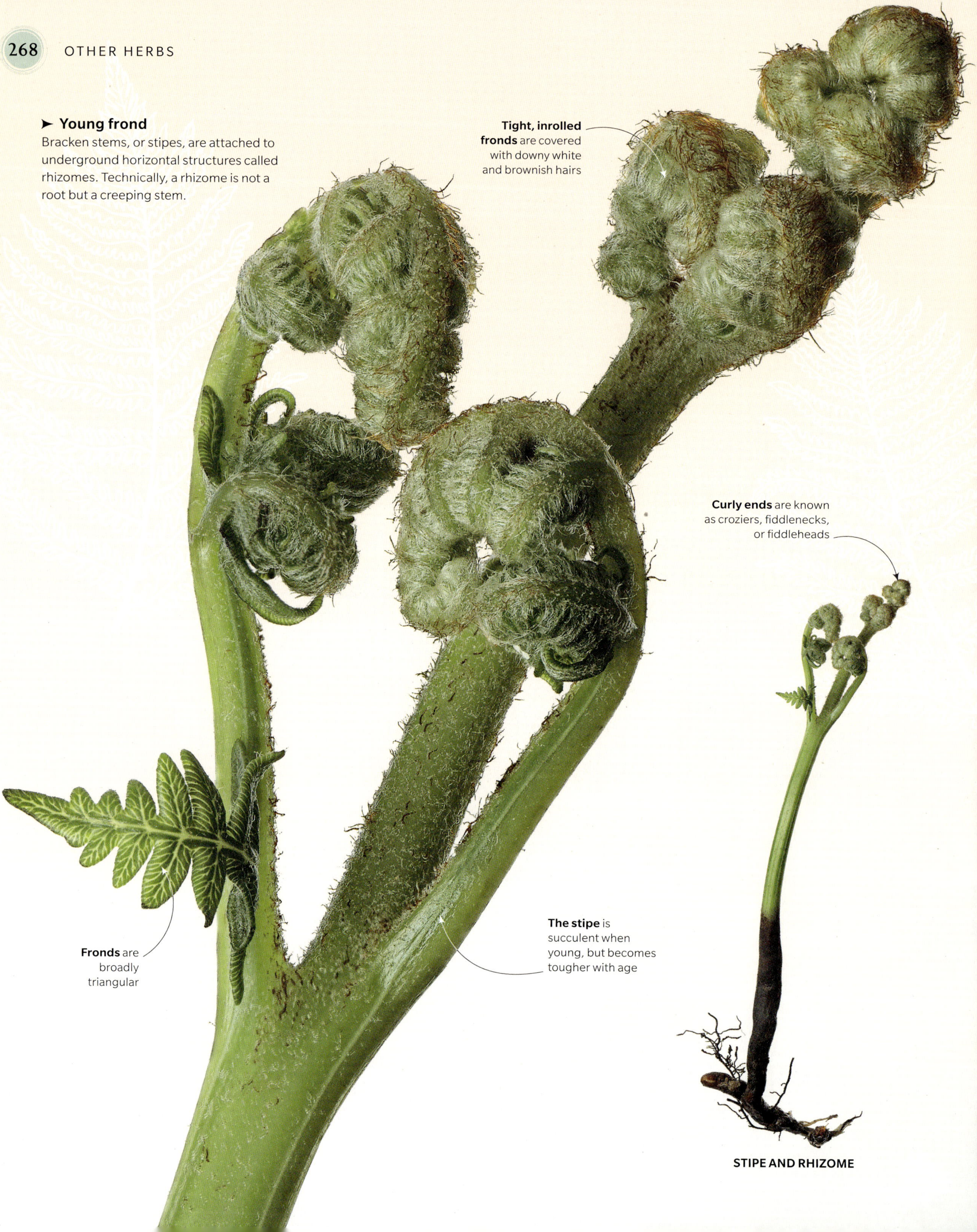

Tight, inrolled fronds are covered with downy white and brownish hairs

Curly ends are known as croziers, fiddlenecks, or fiddleheads

Fronds are broadly triangular

The stipe is succulent when young, but becomes tougher with age

STIPE AND RHIZOME

Uses Medicines, cooking, fuel, animal bedding, fertilizer, garden mulch

Parts used Young shoots, fronds, rhizomes

Active ingredients Ptaquiloside, thiaminase, prunasin

Habitat Woodland, heaths, and grassland on acidic soils

In Japan, bracken shoots are deep fried as tempura

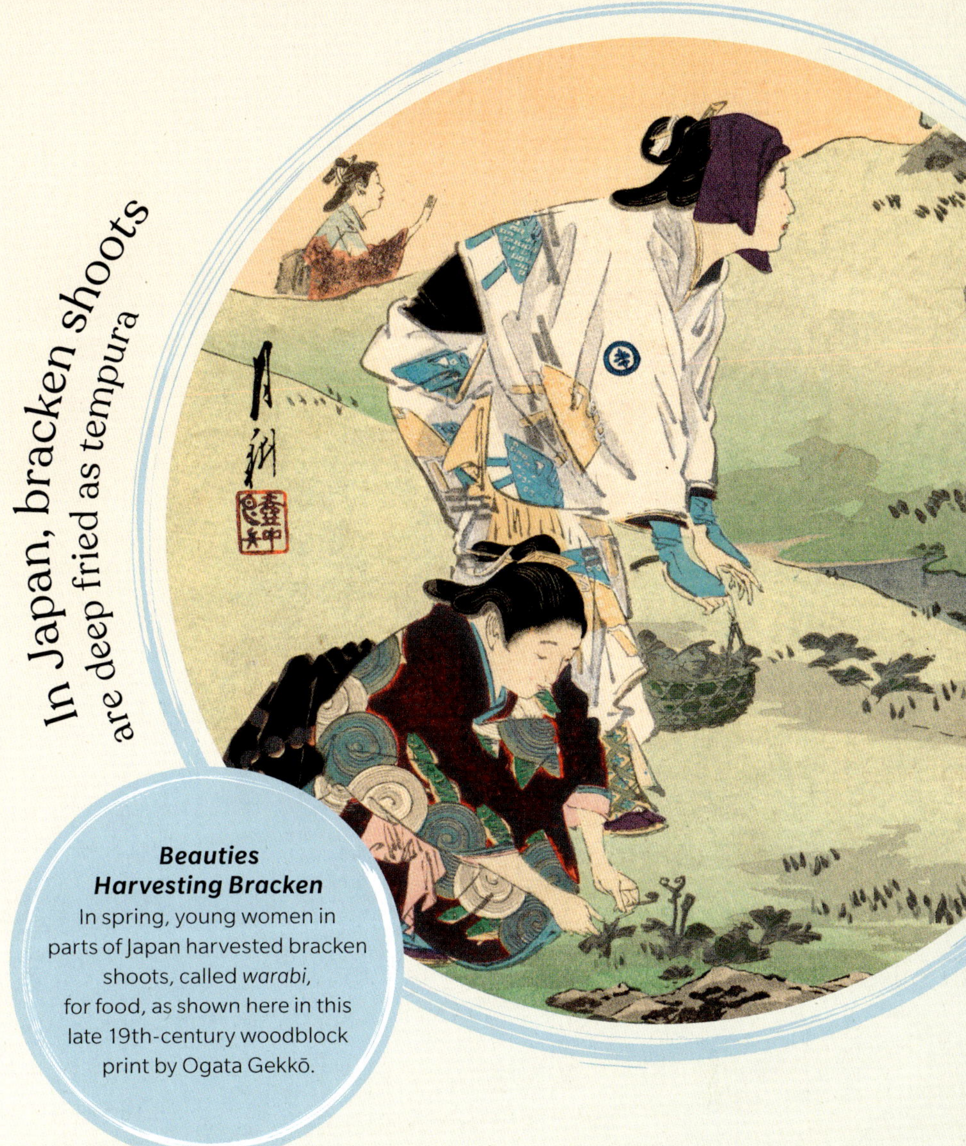

Beauties Harvesting Bracken
In spring, young women in parts of Japan harvested bracken shoots, called *warabi*, for food, as shown here in this late 19th-century woodblock print by Ogata Gekkō.

Bracken

Pteridium aquilinum

Bracken is an aggressive fern that can colonize hillsides and invade grazing land. Nonetheless, it has many uses, including medicine and animal bedding, and it is a traditional food source in East Asia.

In growing terms, bracken – also known as brake, bracken fern, eagle fern, hog brake, and turkey-foot bracken – is the world's most successful fern. It inhabits every continent except Antarctica, and every habitat apart from polar regions and deserts. The fast-growing plant is also one of the world's largest ferns, standing up to 2.5 m (8¼ ft) tall. Its secret is its rhizome, the thick, rootlike, underground stem that puts up shoots at regular intervals and enables the plant to spread rapidly when conditions are right. The thick mat of leaf litter that forms beneath the fern's fronds and the grass-suppressing biochemicals (allelochemicals) released into the soil by the plant allow bracken to invade grassland and dominate whole hillsides.

Fiddleheads should be fully dehydrated and then stored in an airtight container

▲ **Dried bracken**
Bunches of dried bracken are widely sold in Korea, Japan, and parts of China. The herb grows as a wild vegetable and is popular among foragers.

Commonly, ferns are associated with damp growing conditions, but unlike most fern species, bracken is tough enough to tolerate drying winds on open hillsides. However, it is sensitive to frost and so cold springs will delay its growth.

The plant has branched fronds, with each branch (pinna) a triangular shape and further divided into pinnules and pinnulets. As the season advances, these fronds become leathery and resistant to water loss. On well-drained hillsides on acidic soil, bracken forms dense stands. They are pale green in spring, become darker later on, and finally die back to a russet brown in autumn.

Spore capsules release spores, which are carried by wind currents

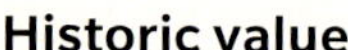

Historic value

Today, bracken is often regarded as a pernicious weed, but in the Middle Ages it was valued enough to be used as currency in rent disputes. The fern was gathered to make thatch for roofing, and it was also used as a packing material. Multiple layers of fronds made a cool lining for baskets of fruit or fish. In the past, bracken was a source of fuel and was especially useful where a hot flame was needed, for example in brewing and baking. Potash collected from burnt bracken was used in the glass-making and soap-making industries until the late 19th century, and it was also an ingredient in bleach. A yellow dye was extracted from bracken rhizomes and used to tan leather and dye wool.

Historically, the fern's fronds were packed together to make bedding for livestock, and the plant is still used for this purpose in parts of Wales. However, bracken is known to be poisonous to cattle, sheep, horses, and pigs if consumed in quantity. Despite this, bracken mulch – made from silage or by mixing the chopped-up fronds with poultry manure – is still sometimes used as fertilizer. One of its traditional uses was to feed and cover potato beds.

◄ Mature frond
Spore capsules form on the folded-over edges of the underside of each segment (pinnule) of the bracken frond. A single frond may produce 300 million spores annually.

Folklore and traditional medicine

According to folklore, sleeping on a bed of fresh bracken helps to cure rickets. It also deters insects and is said to be as effective as a mosquito net. Bracken also has applications within traditional medicine. Some claim that a steam bath made with the fronds can help ease arthritis. A tea made from the rhizomes has been used to treat diarrhoea and stomach cramps, and also to expel intestinal worms. Smoke from smouldering

> "I love to see the old heaths withered brake
> Mingle its crimpled leaves with furze and ling..."
>
> JOHN CLARE, "Emmonsails Heath in Winter", early 19th century

Similar herbs

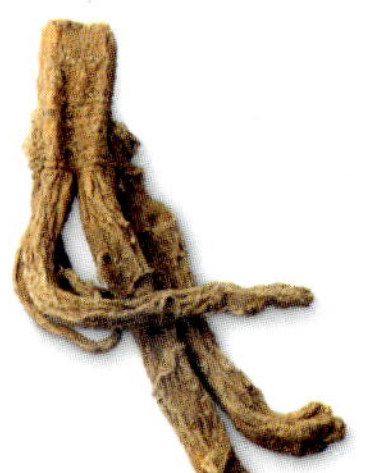

GENTIAN
Gentiana lutea
The dried roots of gentian taste extremely bitter. Root extract has long been used as a remedy for digestive complaints and also to calm irritated skin.

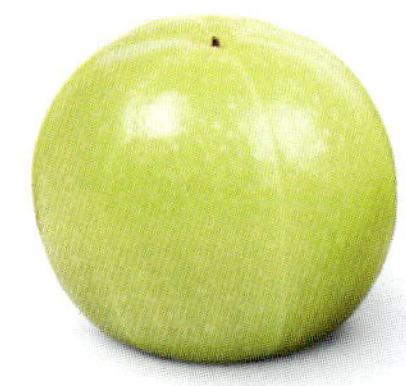

AMLA
Phyllanthus emblica
Also known as Indian gooseberry, amla is used in traditional medicine to relieve a number of conditions, including diarrhoea and abdominal pain.

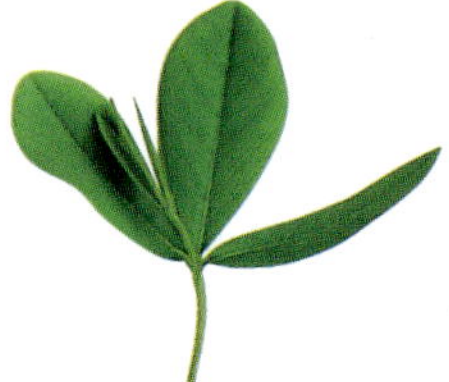

FALSE INDIGO
Baptisia australis
This attractive but bitter-tasting, blue-flowered plant is used in traditional North American medicine as a cold or fever remedy, purgative, or mouthwash.

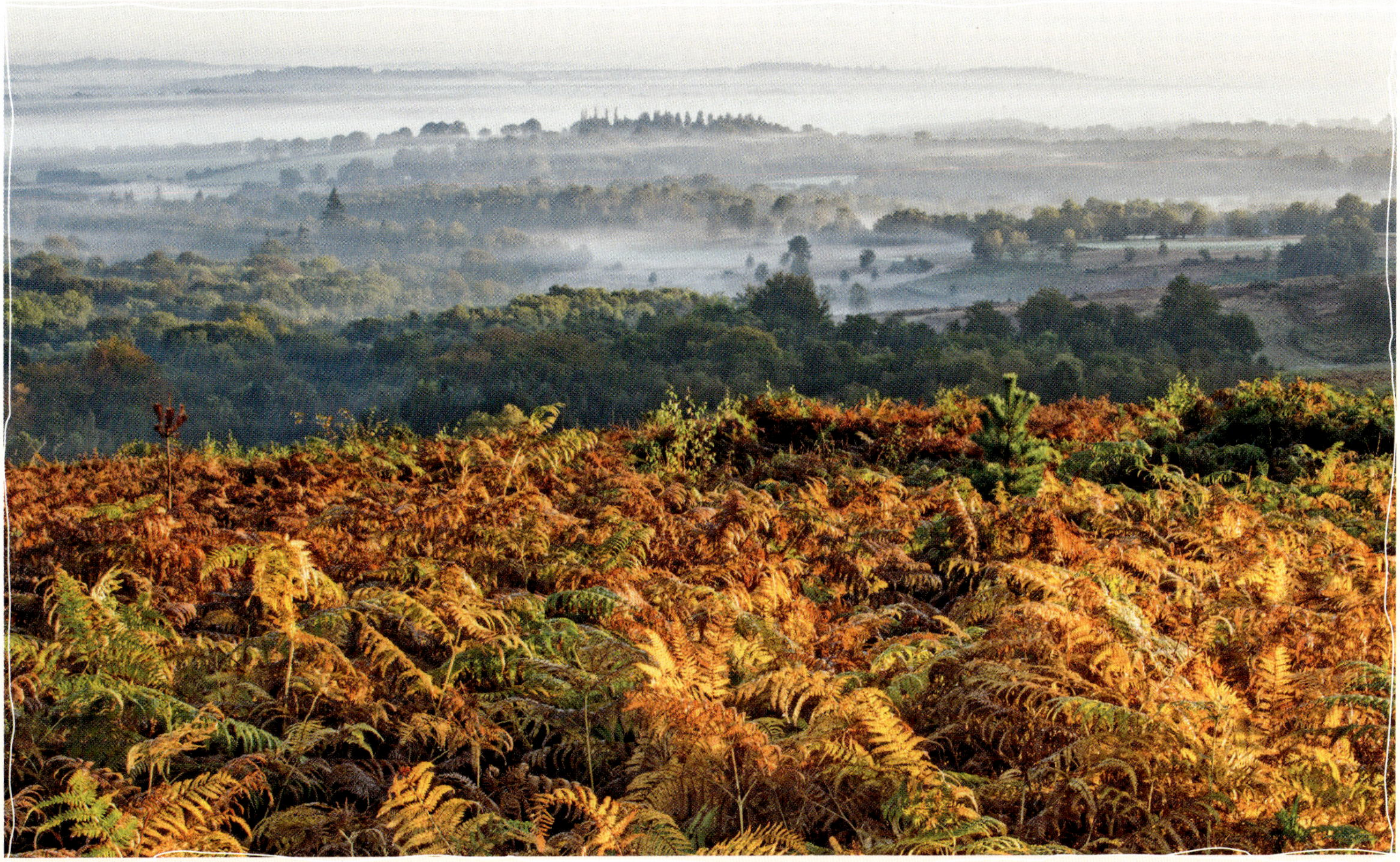

bracken may ease an aching head, and a poultice made from the rhizomes is said to provide relief from burns and sores.

Culinary uses

Bracken is a key ingredient in some East Asian cuisines. Although all bracken fronds are carcinogenic when raw, levels of the chemical responsible – ptaquiloside – are reduced by boiling or drying. Harvested before the fronds expand, bracken shoots are relatively tender and have a texture similar to asparagus. In mountain areas in Japan, the young shoots are collected in baskets, and then steamed or boiled. Fiddleheads, or *warabi*, can also be preserved in salt or miso, a seasoning made from fermented soya beans. Another bracken product is *warabimochi*, a sweet confection made from bracken starch and covered in toasted soya bean flour. In South Korea, bracken shoots, known as *gosari* or fernbrake, are a popular ingredient in the vegetable rice dish called *bibimbap*. Dried fiddleheads are sold in grocery stores in tight bundles; seasoned with soya sauce or minced garlic, they are used to make soups or side dishes.

A related species of bracken (*Pteridium esculentum*), used by the Māori people in New Zealand, was planted as a crop. The edible part is the rhizome, known as *aruhe*. It is first dried, and then heated and pounded to separate the starch-rich flesh from the fibres. The resulting paste, which can be sweetened with fruit juice, is regarded as an important source of carbohydrate.

▲ **Bracken landscape**
In autumn, bracken turns a rich reddish brown (bracken brown) colour, marking out whole hillsides and heaths. It often quickly collapses afterwards.

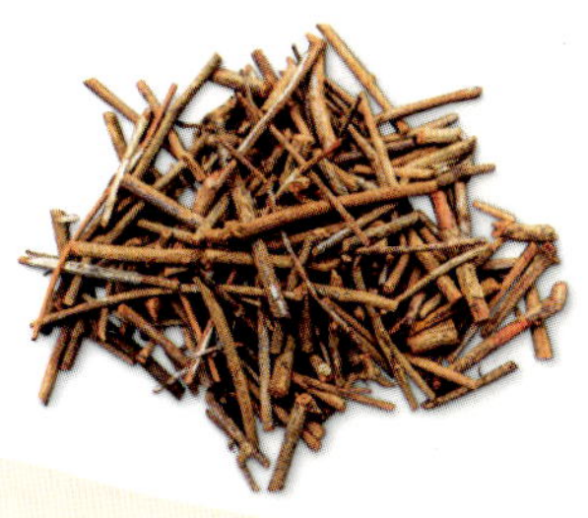

MANJISTHA
Rubia cordifolia
This coffee relative is used in traditional Indian (Ayurvedic) medicine as a blood purifier. It can also be applied as a poultice to treat wounds and skin disorders, such as acne.

Bracken has a **fossil record** dating back **55 million years**

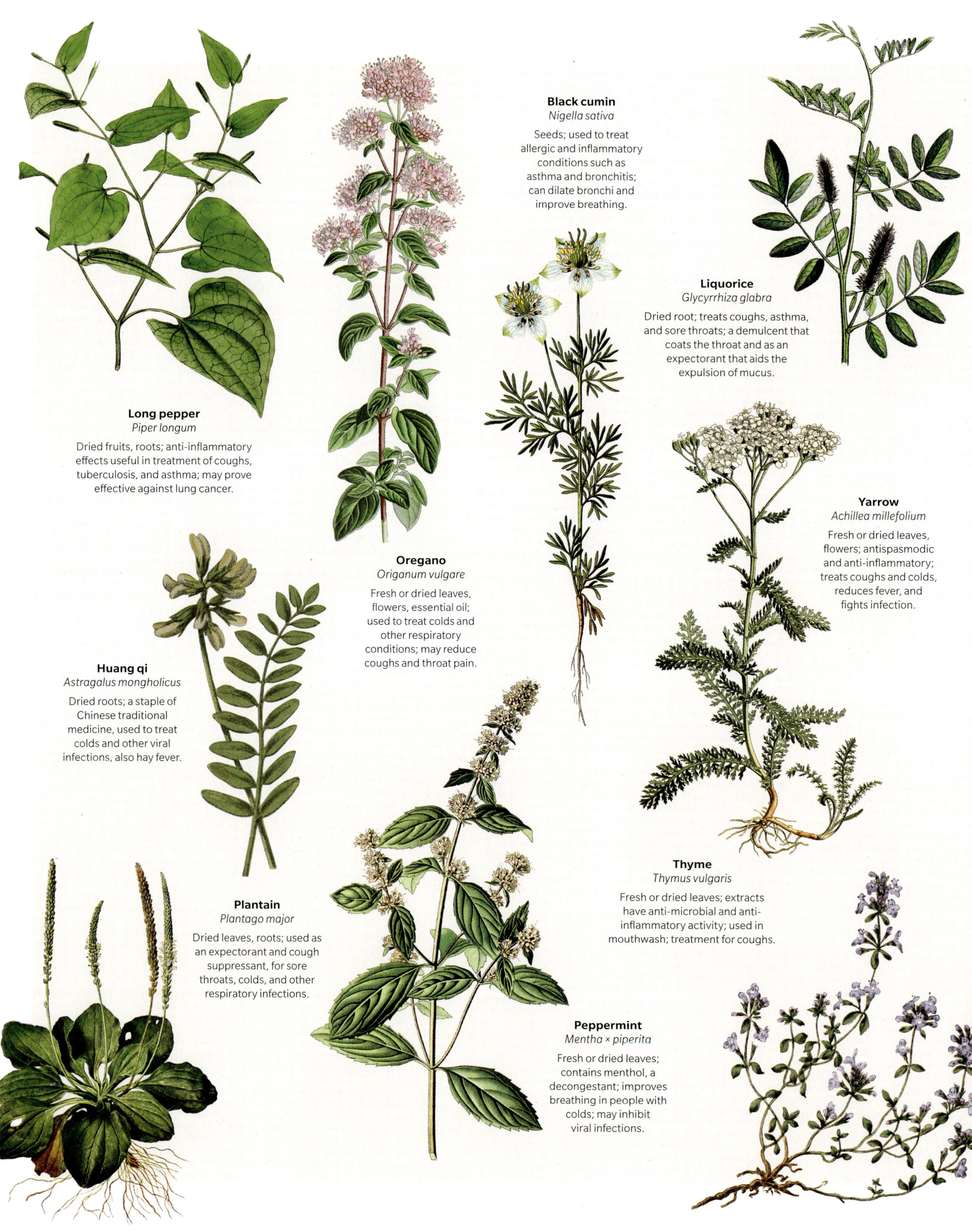

Black cumin
Nigella sativa
Seeds; used to treat allergic and inflammatory conditions such as asthma and bronchitis; can dilate bronchi and improve breathing.

Liquorice
Glycyrrhiza glabra
Dried root; treats coughs, asthma, and sore throats; a demulcent that coats the throat and as an expectorant that aids the expulsion of mucus.

Long pepper
Piper longum
Dried fruits, roots; anti-inflammatory effects useful in treatment of coughs, tuberculosis, and asthma; may prove effective against lung cancer.

Yarrow
Achillea millefolium
Fresh or dried leaves, flowers; antispasmodic and anti-inflammatory; treats coughs and colds, reduces fever, and fights infection.

Oregano
Origanum vulgare
Fresh or dried leaves, flowers, essential oil; used to treat colds and other respiratory conditions; may reduce coughs and throat pain.

Huang qi
Astragalus mongholicus
Dried roots; a staple of Chinese traditional medicine, used to treat colds and other viral infections, also hay fever.

Thyme
Thymus vulgaris
Fresh or dried leaves; extracts have anti-microbial and anti-inflammatory activity; used in mouthwash; treatment for coughs.

Plantain
Plantago major
Dried leaves, roots; used as an expectorant and cough suppressant, for sore throats, colds, and other respiratory infections.

Peppermint
Mentha × piperita
Fresh or dried leaves; contains menthol, a decongestant; improves breathing in people with colds; may inhibit viral infections.

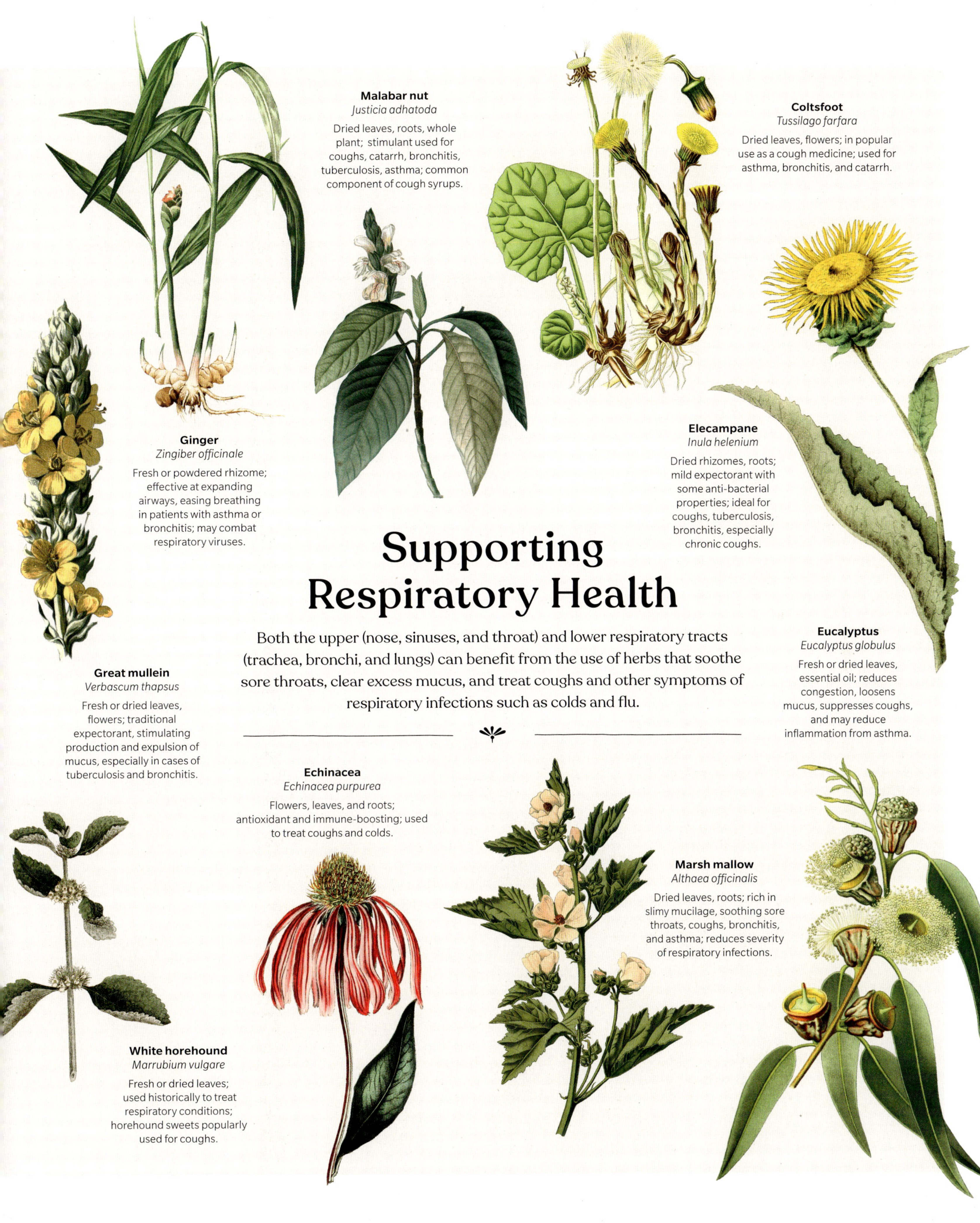

Supporting Respiratory Health

Both the upper (nose, sinuses, and throat) and lower respiratory tracts (trachea, bronchi, and lungs) can benefit from the use of herbs that soothe sore throats, clear excess mucus, and treat coughs and other symptoms of respiratory infections such as colds and flu.

Ginger
Zingiber officinale
Fresh or powdered rhizome; effective at expanding airways, easing breathing in patients with asthma or bronchitis; may combat respiratory viruses.

Malabar nut
Justicia adhatoda
Dried leaves, roots, whole plant; stimulant used for coughs, catarrh, bronchitis, tuberculosis, asthma; common component of cough syrups.

Coltsfoot
Tussilago farfara
Dried leaves, flowers; in popular use as a cough medicine; used for asthma, bronchitis, and catarrh.

Elecampane
Inula helenium
Dried rhizomes, roots; mild expectorant with some anti-bacterial properties; ideal for coughs, tuberculosis, bronchitis, especially chronic coughs.

Great mullein
Verbascum thapsus
Fresh or dried leaves, flowers; traditional expectorant, stimulating production and expulsion of mucus, especially in cases of tuberculosis and bronchitis.

Eucalyptus
Eucalyptus globulus
Fresh or dried leaves, essential oil; reduces congestion, loosens mucus, suppresses coughs, and may reduce inflammation from asthma.

Echinacea
Echinacea purpurea
Flowers, leaves, and roots; antioxidant and immune-boosting; used to treat coughs and colds.

Marsh mallow
Althaea officinalis
Dried leaves, roots; rich in slimy mucilage, soothing sore throats, coughs, bronchitis, and asthma; reduces severity of respiratory infections.

White horehound
Marrubium vulgare
Fresh or dried leaves; used historically to treat respiratory conditions; horehound sweets popularly used for coughs.

Uses Medicines; cooking; horticulture

Parts used Fronds, rhizome

Active ingredients Triterpenoids

Habitat Caves and shaded, damp crevices on cliffs and rocks, or in walls; in moist soil or on rocks in woodlands; grows worldwide, mainly in warm-temperate, but also in tropical climates

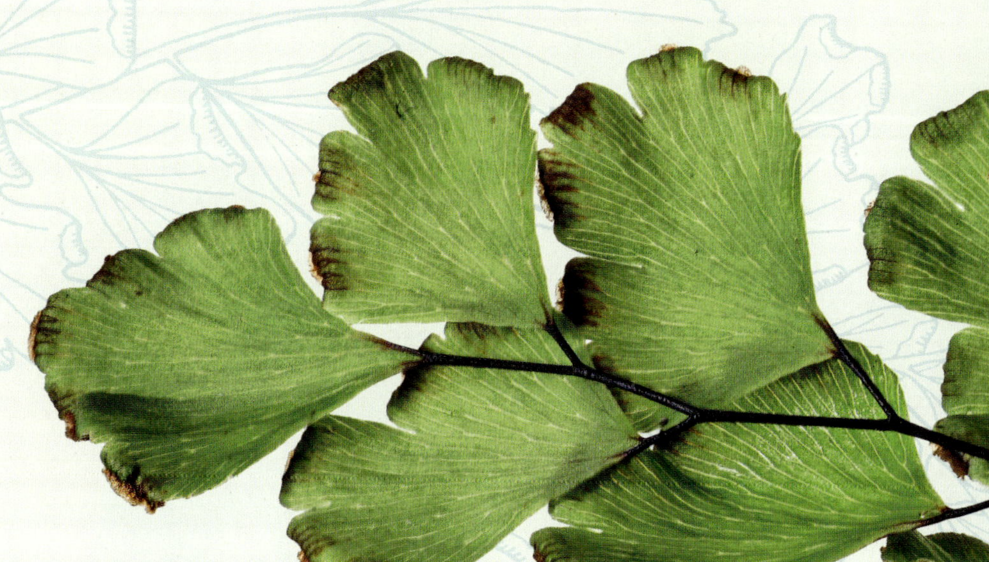

➤ **Maidenhair fern frond**
The 35 cm- (14 in-) long fronds arise from a short, creeping rhizome. Like all ferns, the plant produces spores, not seeds, on fertile frond segments.

Curled-back lobe edges protect spore-producing parts

Maidenhair Fern

Adiantum capillus-veneris

This dainty fern is a popular ornamental plant for its fan-shaped frond segments, which are unusual in ferns. However, it is its resemblance to hair that has inspired its use as a hair-loss remedy since antiquity.

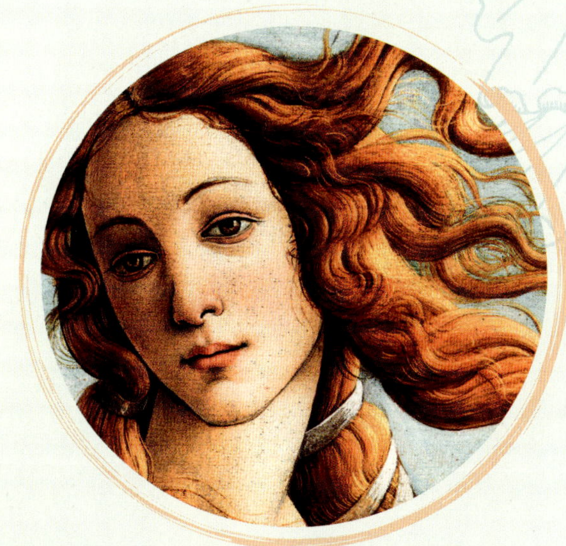

▲ ***The Birth of Venus***
As in this detail from Sandro Botticelli's painting, c.1485, the Roman goddess Venus arose from the waves with her hair magically unwetted by the water, like the leaves of the maidenhair fern.

Maidenhair fern requires a fairly high humidity, so occurs on sheltered, permanently wet rocks and seepages, or in moist woodland. The waxy fronds have a silvery sheen under water. This semi-evergreen fern is sensitive to frosts; in cool areas, it dies back in autumn and pink-tinged crosiers (young fronds) emerge again in spring. It is instantly recognizable and often grown as an indoor plant where, apart from looking good, it acts as an air freshener. It quickly dies back in dry conditions, but regrows once watered again.

The generic name *Adiantum*, means "unwetted", recalling maidenhair fern's ability to grow under trickling water without getting soaked. The species name, *capillus-veneris*, means "hair of Venus" and the fern is also called the Venus hair fern or Venus maidenhair fern. By the Middle Ages, the plant had become associated with the Roman goddess, who is usually depicted with long, flowing locks that were miraculously dry when she emerged from the sea. Whether it was due to the massed, water-repellant fronds that

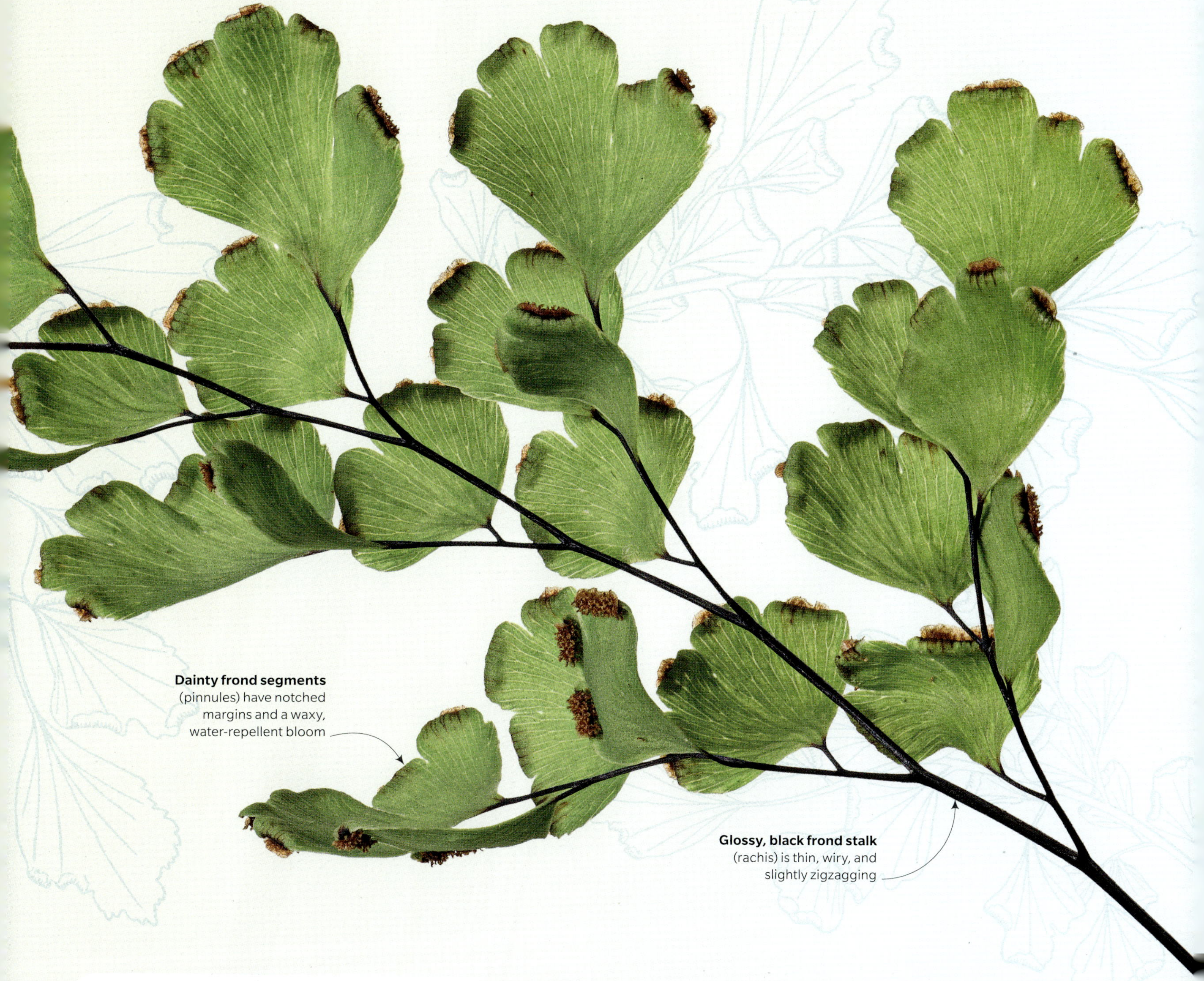

Dainty frond segments (pinnules) have notched margins and a waxy, water-repellent bloom

Glossy, black frond stalk (rachis) is thin, wiry, and slightly zigzagging

ANTITUSSIVE AND EXPECTORANT HERBS

Antitussive herbs are used to suppress or relieve a cough by inhibiting the cough reflex in the brain or the respiratory passages. They are particularly useful for dry, hacking coughs that interfere with rest and sleep. Examples include maidenhair fern, thyme (see pp.100–103), and the roots of angelica (see pp.188–89) and liquorice (see pp.192–94). Expectorant herbs such as maidenhair fern, garlic (see pp.118–21), and fenugreek (see pp.216–17) help to thin and loosen mucus in the respiratory passages, making coughing more effective.

> " The ruffled leaves
> of vapory green
> Fringe mimic branches,
> fine as thread. "

EDGAR FAWCETT, "Maidenhair", 1880

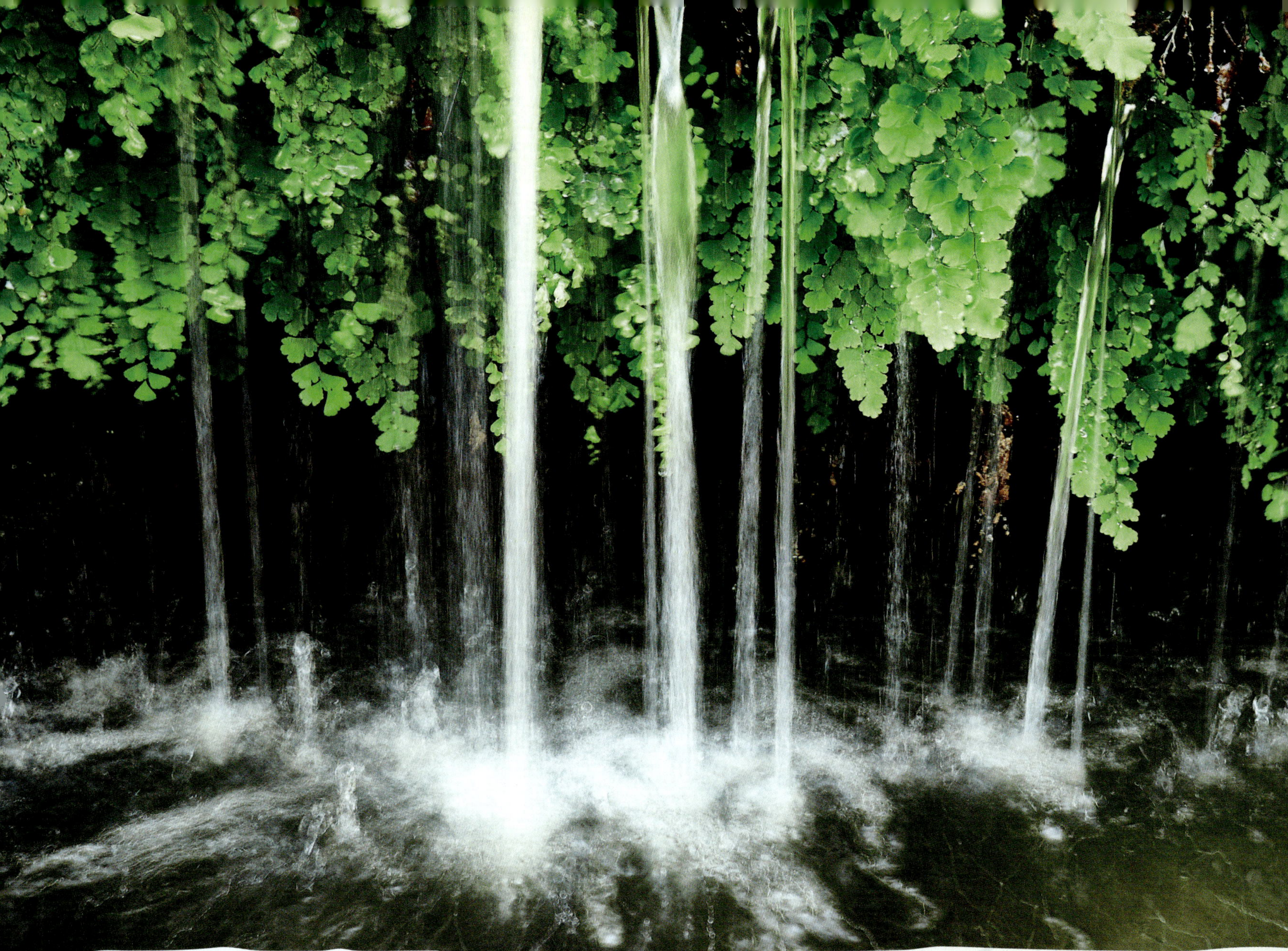

look a little like curly, luxuriant locks, or the black, wiry, hair-like stems, maidenhair fern's appearance led to its reputation as a herb that would prevent baldness.

The Ancient Roman writer Pliny the Elder referred to its Greek name of *callitrichos* ("fine" or "beautiful hair"). He also noted that the fronds were simmered with parsley or celery seeds in wine and oil. This made a tonic to stop hair loss that also promoted lush hair growth. A decoction of the bitter-tasting fronds was produced as an antidote to snake and spider venom; it was also used to break and expel bladder stones, for asthma, and for liver complaints.

Traditional medicines

Maidenhair fern's beneficial properties were discovered independently around the world. The Diné (Navajo people) in North America made it into a decoction, for bee stings and centipede bites. They also smoked the fronds and used the fern to treat mental illness. In Peru, the rhizome and fronds treated ailments such as hydrophobia, gallstones, and jaundice. In Mexico, it was said to purify the blood and purge the body of toxins.

Adiantum capillus-veneris and several related species featured in Chinese folk medicine. The fern was seen as a "cool" herb capable of clearing heat and detoxifying; it was used to treat ailments such as feverish colds and coughs, as well as kidney and bladder conditions.

Maidenhair fern was an important herb in the Unani system of traditional Iranian medicine, in which the plant was known as *parsiawashan*. An infusion of the fronds, administered singly or in combination with other herbs, was used to treat respiratory-tract diseases, menstrual problems, scrofula, and jaundice, and to assist childbirth.

▲ Watery habitat
Maidenhair fern grows best where water trickles over rocks. Its wiry, flexible frond stalks and water-repellent pinnules shrug off the water, while its rhizome is kept constantly moist.

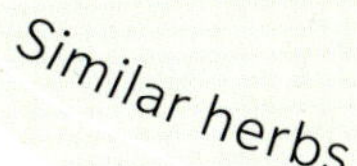

Similar herbs

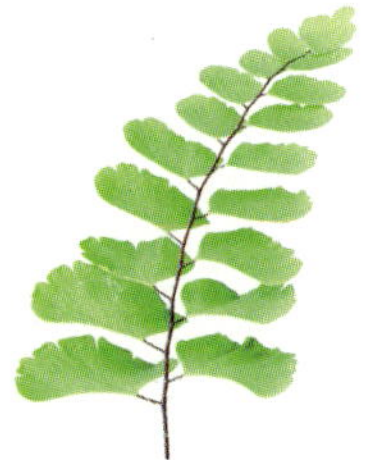

FIVE-FINGERED MAIDENHAIR FERN
Adiantum pedatum
This deciduous fern grows in moist, acidic soils, mainly in temperate areas, in North America, the Himalayas, and Central and Far East Asia. It is used medicinally in the same way as maidenhair fern.

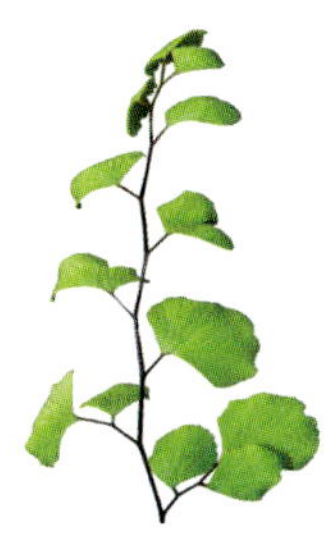

COMMON MAIDENHAIR FERN
Adiantum aethiopicum
A widely planted native of Australasia and southern Africa, this evergreen, clumping fern has been used medicinally in cough syrups and by First Australians for bronchial complaints.

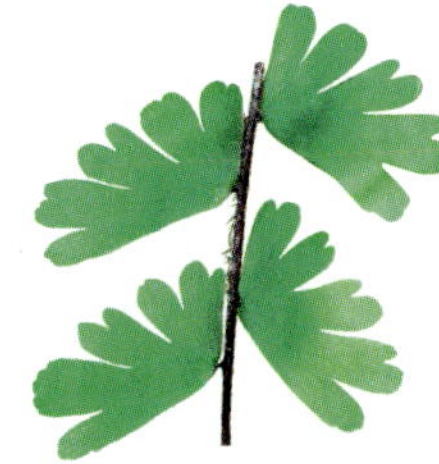

WALKING MAIDENHAIR FERN
Adiantum caudatum
This evergreen native of southeast Asia "walks" by rooting new plantlets where the tips of its 60 cm (2 ft), ladder-like fronds touch soil. It has been used to treat skin complaints.

In Ayurvedic medicine, maidenhair fern and its allies were used to treat many disorders, such as coughs, diarrhoea, urination pain, infected insect bites, and hoarseness of voice. Dried fronds from India are available today under names such as *hansraj* and *pershosha* as the basis for a health tonic.

In Europe and the US, the fern was used in some skin creams, and occasionally as a sudorific (herb that induces sweating). It was also utilized to reduce inflammation and prevent bleeding.

Pharmaceutical studies have affirmed many maidenhair fern attributes, but it has rarely found its way into modern clinical medicine. There is no scientific foundation for the fern's age-old use as a cure for baldness.

Tonic drink

The best-attested medical use of maidenhair fern in modern times is as a remedy for catarrh and congestion. One such 17th-century, French remedy, *sirop de capillaire* (syrup of maidenhair), was a herbal cough syrup produced by infusing dried or fresh, chopped fronds in boiled water for 45 minutes. The resulting mucilaginous, earthy-tasting liquid was then sweetened with sugar and orange water. *Sirop de capillaire* became extremely popular in 19th-century France as a drink flavouring – alcoholic spirits were added to it or it was made into a hot drink with eggs and milk.

Hair loss herb
This illustration of maidenhair fern appeared under the name of *capelvenere* in Pietro Andrea Mattioli's 16th-century translation of *De Re Medica*. In this herbal, Dioscorides echoes the long-held belief that the fern prevented male baldness and promoted lush hair growth in women.

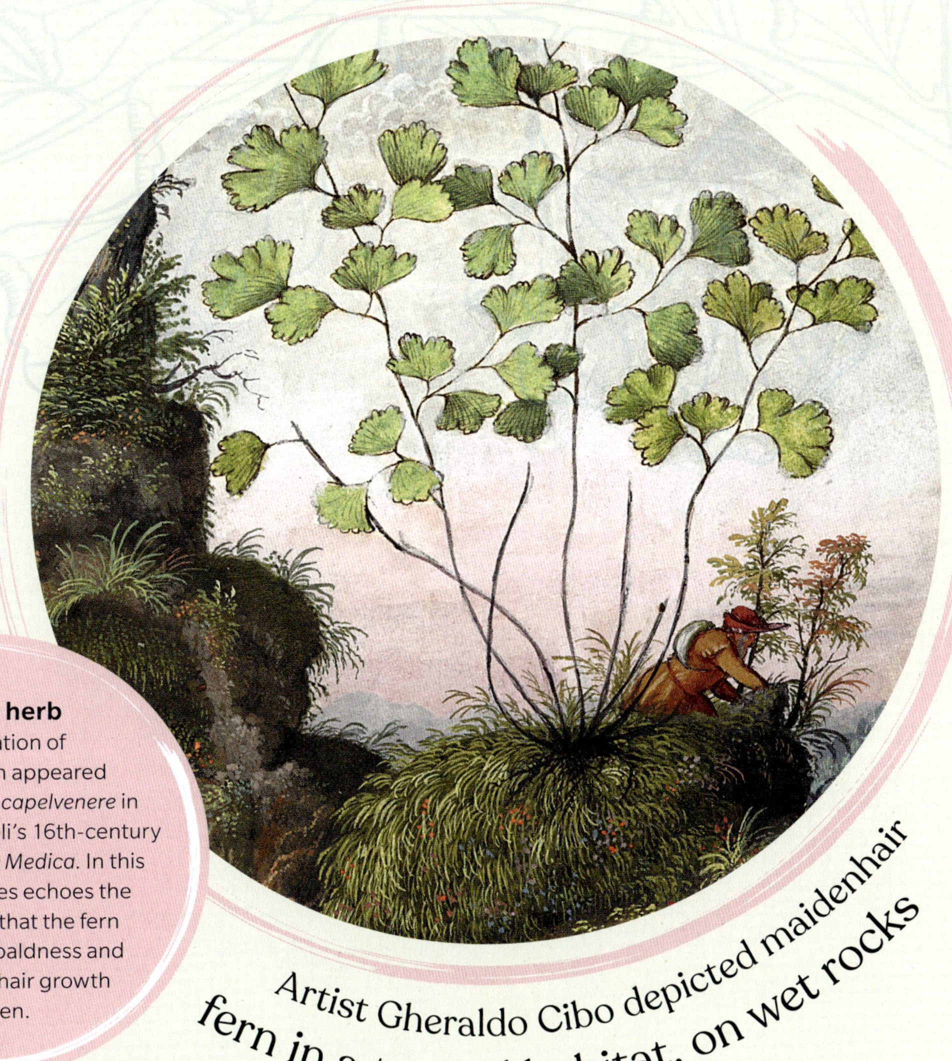

Artist Gheraldo Cibo depicted maidenhair fern in a typical habitat, on wet rocks

Hai Zao

Sargassum fusiforme

Hai zao is a marine algae species that is popularly harvested for use as a fibre- and mineral-rich, low-fat food product. It is also known for its healing properties.

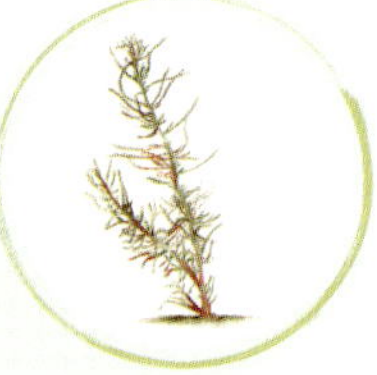

Uses Medicines to treat goitres, cysts, and swellings; cooking

Parts used All

Active ingredients Alginic acid, fucoidan, laminarin

Habitat Temperate coastal regions, along the shore

Seaweeds are macroalgae, alluding to their large size. Macroalgae are divided into three groups: red, green, and brown. *Hai zao* in China, known as *hijiki* in Japan, is a brown seaweed that occurs along the Pacific coasts of China, Korea, and Japan. In the Sargasso Sea – an area of the Atlantic Ocean hemmed in by currents called the North Atlantic Gyre – *Sargassum* seaweeds form broad, floating mats.

Several seaweeds are harvested as sea vegetables, and *hijiki* is especially popular in Japan and Korea. Brown when harvested, it turns black once dried and processed, providing the natural food colouring used in Japanese *konnyaku*. This "cake", made from the powdered tuber of the arum or calla lily family (Araceae) member konjac (*Amorphophallus konjac*),

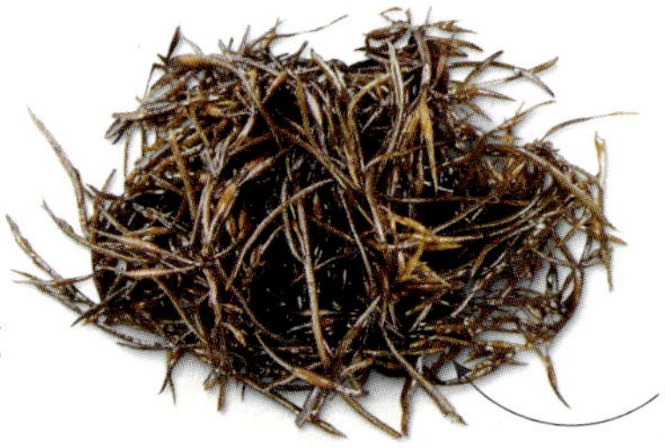

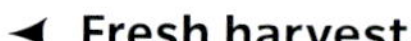

Fresh harvest
Hijiki can be eaten raw (as here) or cooked and is often dried for long-term storage. It is rich in fibre and minerals like iron

Stipes (equivalent of stems) and needle-like blades are harvested for consumption

Food from the sea
Hai zao is harvested by hand using a sickle. It is air-dried, washed, and steamed, or boiled to remove bitterness.

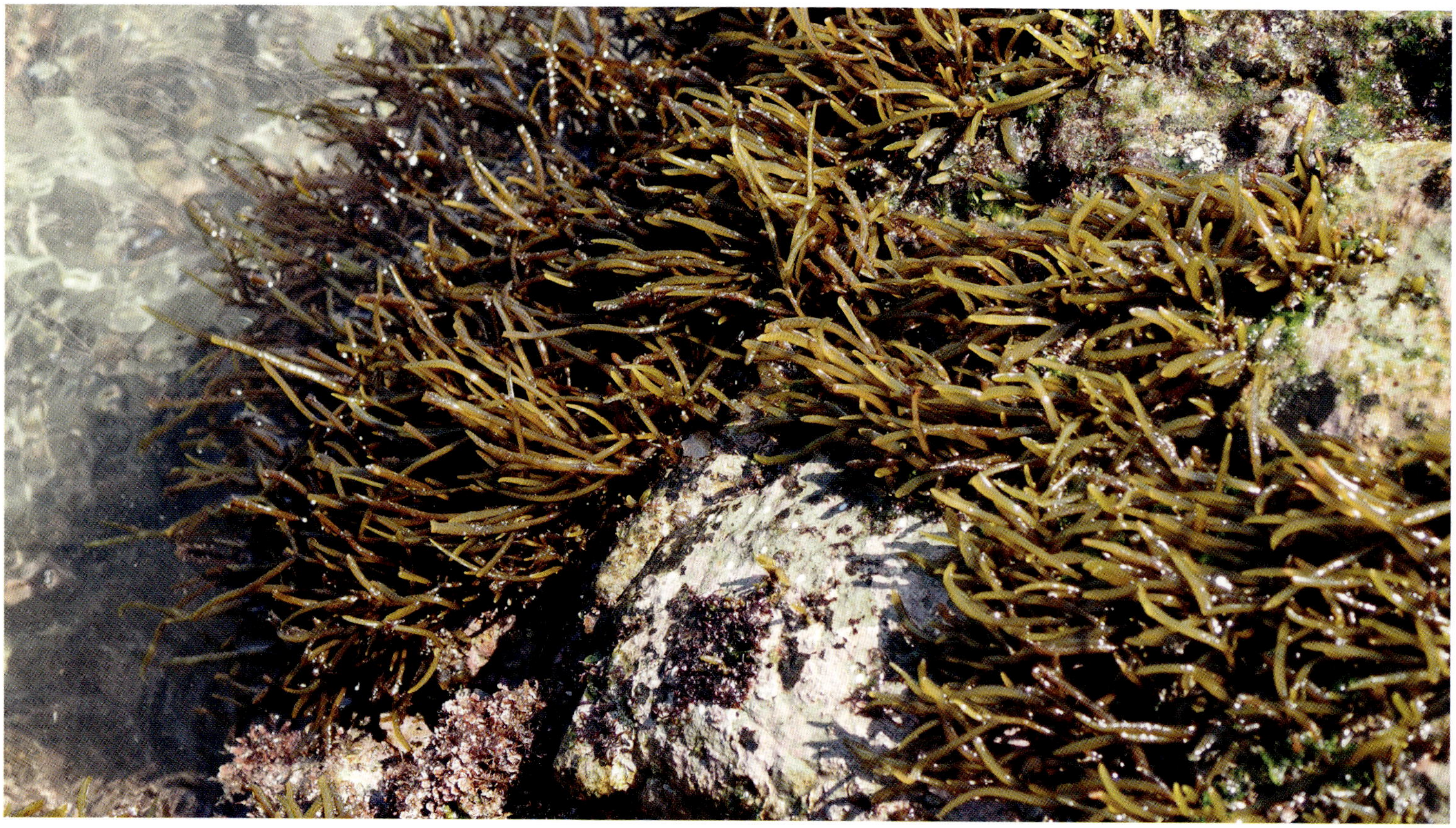

➤ Study of seaweed
The Japanese have a long history of harvesting wild seaweed for consumption. This image of *S. fusiforme* is from a 1913 study of Japanese native seaweeds and shows the long narrow fusiform blades.

has a gelatinous, rubbery texture and is used as a low-calorie meat substitute, or in stews and stir fries. *Hijiki* is also a common ingredient in Japanese cuisine, as a vegetable side, mixed with rice, or in soups and sushi. In Korea, where it is known as *tot*, it is a common side dish, mixed with rice (*tot-bap*), tofu, or beansprouts.

Medicines and macronutrients

Like many other edible seaweeds, *hai zao* is a popular component of macrobiotic diets, which stress the importance of locally grown foods and a diet rich in plant material. While it is unclear whether a macrobiotic regime is good for health, *hai zao* is rich in dietary fibre, a macronutrient often lacking in modern processed foods. It is also a useful source of iron, calcium, magnesium, and potassium. In traditional Chinese medicine, *hai zao* is used to treat a variety of swellings including goitres, cysts, and lipomas. It may also prove effective in treating some cancers, arthritis, and viruses. Food and health authorities in some countries advise against consumption of *hai zao* due to its high levels of inorganic arsenic compared with other seaweeds. Others maintain that the small quantities consumed by most citizens are insufficient to cause serious health concerns.

The Sargasso Sea is the only region where **European eels** (*Anguilla anguilla*) **breed**

SARGASSO WEED

This lithograph by Scottish illustrator Edward S. Hodgson takes its name from a line in English poet Samuel T. Coleridge's poem *The Rime of the Ancient Mariner* (1798). It shows ships stranded in the Sargasso Sea, where seaweed was thought to catch the rudders and keels of ships, holding them in place. Calm seas and a lack of wind were a more likely cause.

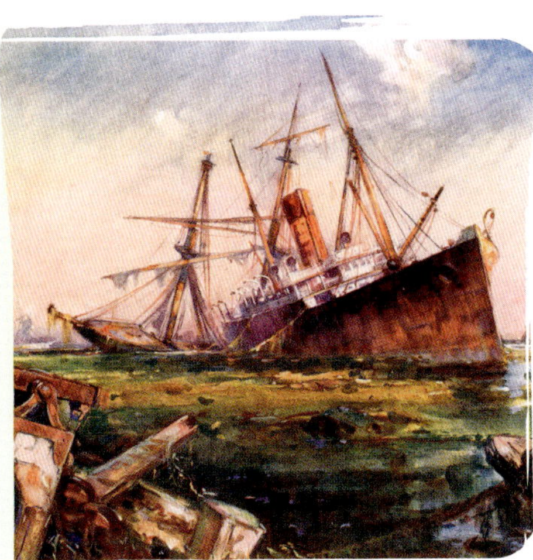

***THE VERY DEEP DID ROT*, 1915**

Similar herbs

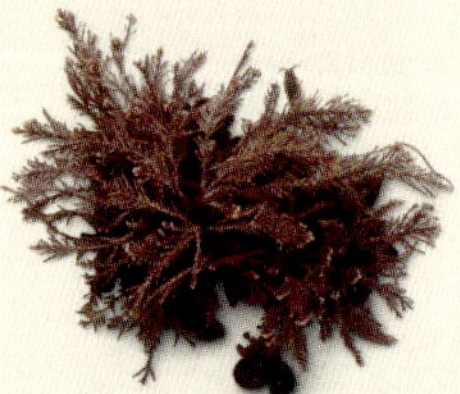

CORAL WEED
Corallina officinalis

This seaweed stores lime (calcium carbonate) in its cell walls and can be used as a bone-forming material, in the cosmetics industry, and as an emulsifier.

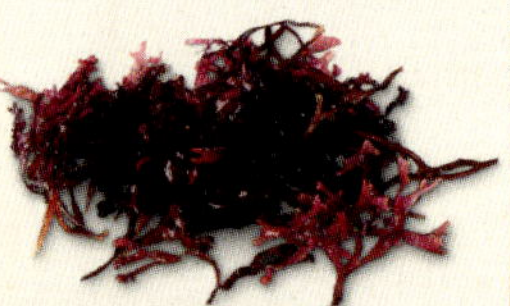

FALSE IRISH MOSS
Mastocarpus stellatus

This red seaweed is gathered and sold dried as food and as a gelling agent. It has also been used in remedies for coughs and sore throats.

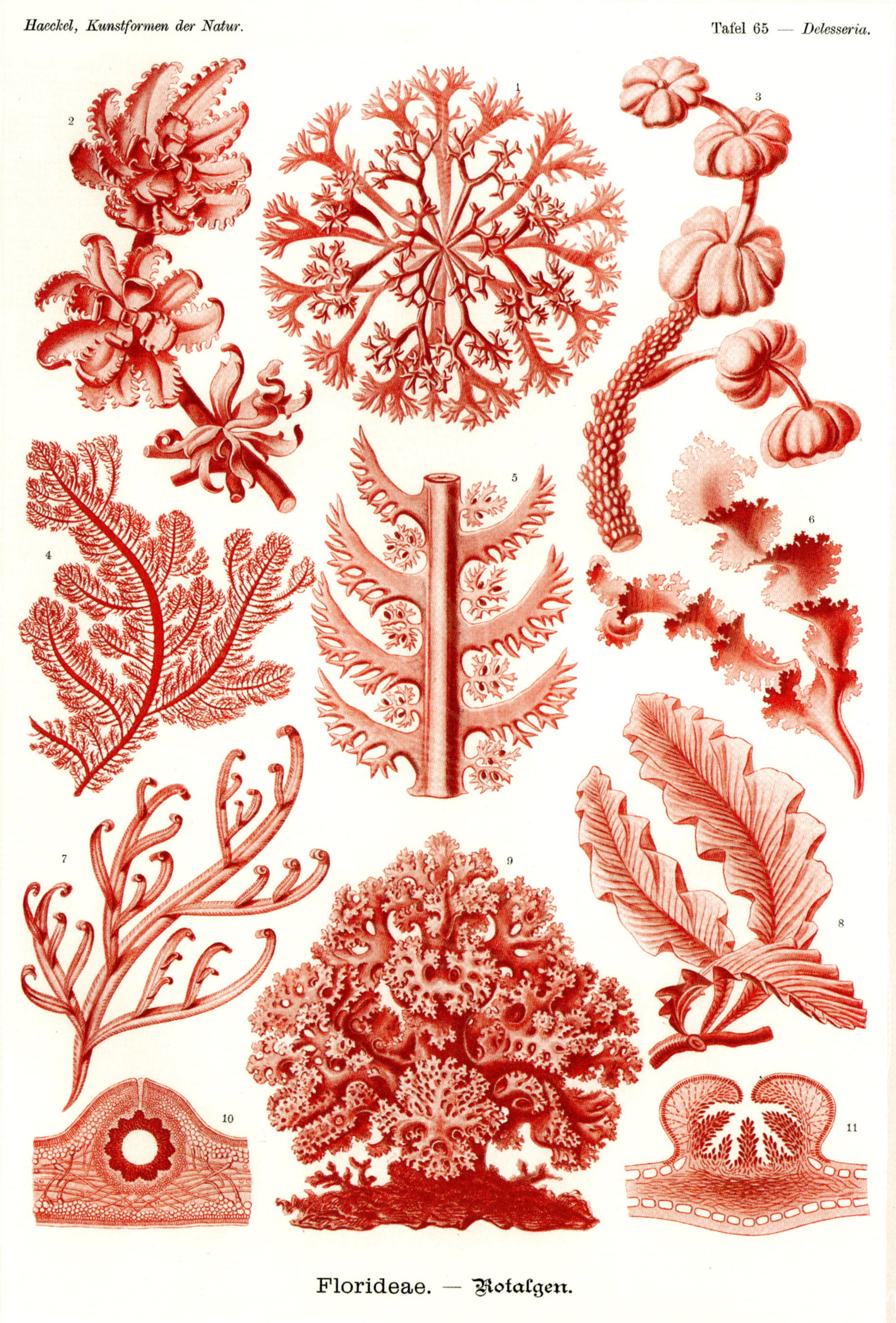

Haeckel, Kunstformen der Natur. Tafel 65 — *Delesseria.*

Florideae. — Rotalgen.

➤ Red seaweeds
This illustration of red seaweeds from German zoologist Ernst Haeckel's 1904 book *Kunstformen der Natur* (Art Forms in Nature) depicts carragheen at the top centre.

Carragheen

Chondrus crispus

Uses Medicines, food additive and stabilizer; beer fining; fabric printing, paper marbling

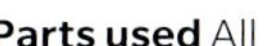

Parts used All

Active ingredients Carrageenan, proteins, sulphur, potassium

Habitat Rocky coasts, intertidal pools

Carragheen is one of a large and varied group of primitive seawater algae distinguished by their reddish pigments. This edible seaweed is commonly used as a gelling agent.

Carragheen (spellings of its name vary) is a small, fan-shaped seaweed with flat, branching fronds and measuring around 10–20 cm (4–8 in) in length. It grows along rocky coasts on both shores of the North Atlantic and gets its name from the Irish word for "little rock". Despite being a seaweed, it is often called Irish moss, since it is found in abundance on the west coast of Ireland.

Bounty of the sea

The seaweed is rich in proteins and minerals, especially iodine, potassium, and sulphur. When softened in water, it smells of the sea and when boiled, it forms a glutinous jelly containing 20–100 times its own weight in water. Both the seaweed and its jelly are edible, with a strong flavour of the sea, and the main use of carragheen is in food processing. More than half its dry weight is made up of a polysaccharide called carrageenan, which is used as a thickening agent in a wide variety of products, including toothpaste, cottage cheese, milkshakes and smoothies, jellies and puddings, and processed food in general. In Europe, the presence of carrageenan is indicated by E-numbers E407 and E407a. Used as a thickener in fabric printing and paper marbling, it is also used for fining, or clarifying, beer.

While its medical attributes are somewhat controversial, carragheen has long been used to treat coughs and colds, as a stomach settler, and even as a hangover cure. It is naturally rich in vitamins B, C, and protein. However, questions are currently being raised over the safety of using this herb in large doses.

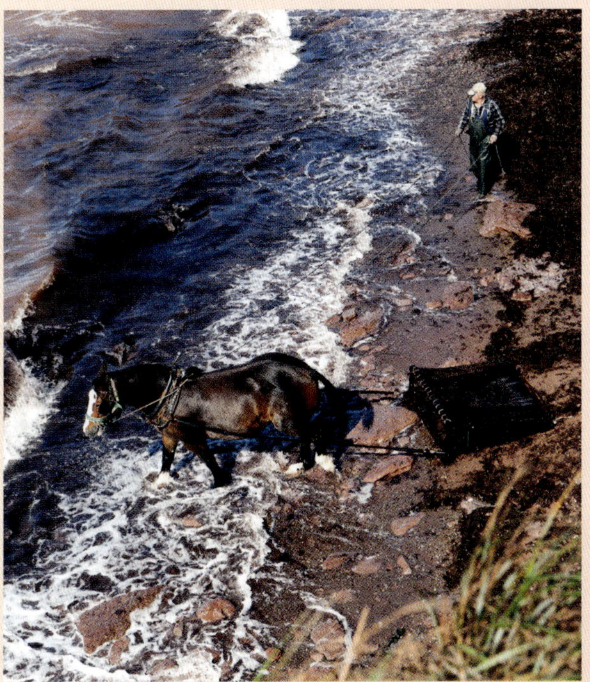

◄ Commercial harvesting
Some seaweed harvesters, as seen here on Prince Edward Island, Canada, still employ draft horses to work in heavy surf. These powerfully built horses drag large rakes through the water at low tide to gather seaweed.

SEAWEED FARMING

Seaweed farms, like those on Palawan Island, Philippines, are among the main producers of carrageenan. *Kappaphycus* and *Eucheuma* seedlings (propagules) are planted on staked rope lines. When the seaweed is fully grown, a harvester spools the lines in, onto a boat, which automatically cuts and separates the weed. It is then dried and can be sold as food, fertilizer, or an emulsifying agent.

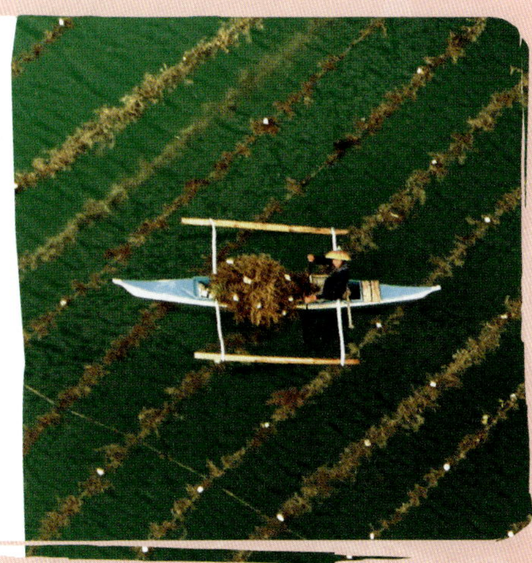

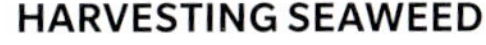

HARVESTING SEAWEED

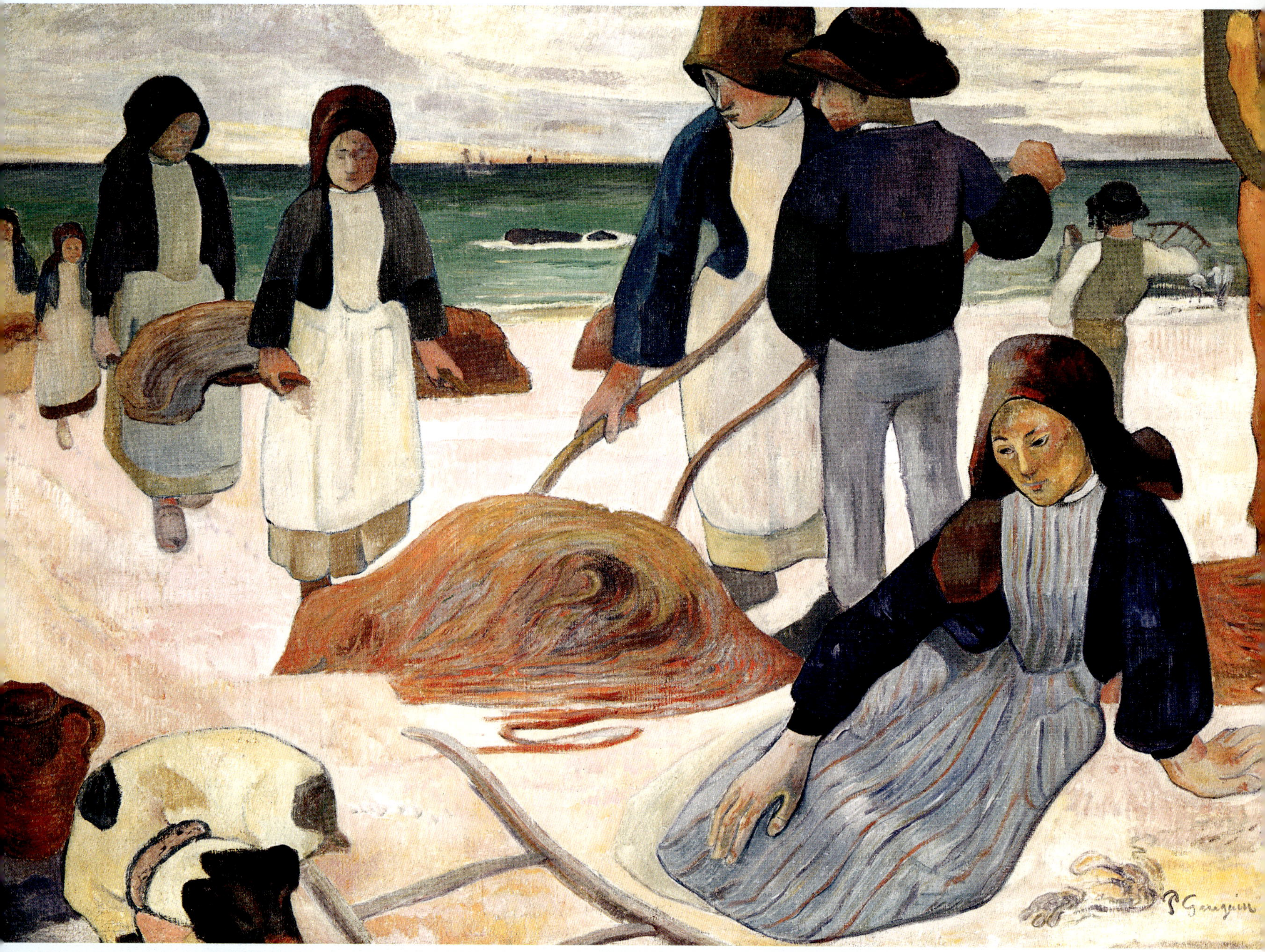

Dulse

Palmaria palmata

Dulse is a species of red alga that is common along the colder shores of Europe and North America. In addition to its nutritional value and medical benefits, this seaweed is now being used in skincare products.

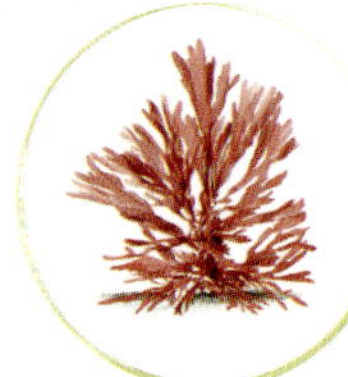

Uses Medicines to treat goitre, improve blood circulation; food, flavouring; cosmetics

Parts used All

Active ingredients Rich in fibre, protein, and iodine; lutein, zeaxanthin, Vitamin A (as carotene)

Habitat Rocky shores on either side of the Atlantic

◄ Gathering seaweed
Seaweeds including dulse are harvested on the Brittany coast, as depicted by French painter Paul Gauguin's *Seaweed Gatherers* (1889). It is traditionally dried in the sun, turning once or twice

Dulse is found in the intertidal zone and in shallow seas along the northern coasts of the Atlantic and Pacific oceans (the Pacific alga may be a different, closely related species). It has a number of flat blades, or fronds, radiating from a short, stem-like stipe. A single holdfast – an organ for attaching algae to another surface – affixes it to rocks or larger seaweeds such as kelp (see p.284). Dulse is rich in protein, fibre, and minerals, especially iodine and potassium, and has been gathered as a health food and for medical purposes for at least 1,500 years.

Colour coded
In dulse, phycoerythrin (a protein-pigment complex) reflects red light, making the seaweed appear red. It absorbs blue-green light, which has greatest penetration into the water. The captured light energy is passed on to chlorophyll, facilitating the photosynthesis of this underwater plant.

Dulse is one of more than 7,300 species of red algae

Savour flavour

Dulse is hand-gathered at low tide from June to September when it is fully grown. It is popular in Iceland, Ireland, and France's northwestern region of Brittany, as well as across the Atlantic on the east coast of Canada and northeast US. Although it can be eaten raw, as a snack, dulse is usually cooked in butter or oil. In Iceland, where it is known as *söl*, it is either eaten straight from the packet as a snack, or ground into flakes or powder as a topping for soups, sandwiches, or pizza. In the past, dulse gathered from the shore was even traded for meat.

Ireland, too, has a long tradition of gathering dulse. Also called *dillisk*, the cleaned weed can be smoked over beech, oak, or apple wood to impart a smoky bacon-like flavour to it, and is often used as "vegan bacon". Dulse is also the key ingredient of white soda bread, made by mixing rehydrated sun-dried flakes into the dough before baking it. It is said that there are as many recipes of this bread as there are families, some of which involve adding beer or buttermilk, or both, to the dough. Devoid of yeast, soda bread has a biscuity taste with a mild tang of the ocean. Dulse pairs well with cottage cheese and can be mixed with butter to spread on breads.

The west coast of Scotland has a similar dulse-gathering tradition, dating back to the Dark Ages (500–1000 CE). Known in Gaelic as *creathnach*, it was often combined with oatmeal. It was also simply roasted in the embers of a fire, turning from red to green in the process, and served with vinegar.

The world's best dulse is said to come from the Grand Manan Island in Canada's Bay of Fundy. Gathered from rocks below the cliffs in the island's Dark Harbour, this dulse is darker,

Dulse flakes are red if the seaweed used to make them is dried at a low heat

◄ Dried and ground
Dulse flakes can be sprinkled on any dish, from curries to smoothies. Not only do they impart a strong flavour, they are high in mineral, protein, and fibre content and low in calories.

Fresh
DULSE
Dulse IS A SEA VEGETABLE GROWN AT LOW TIDE AND TAKES

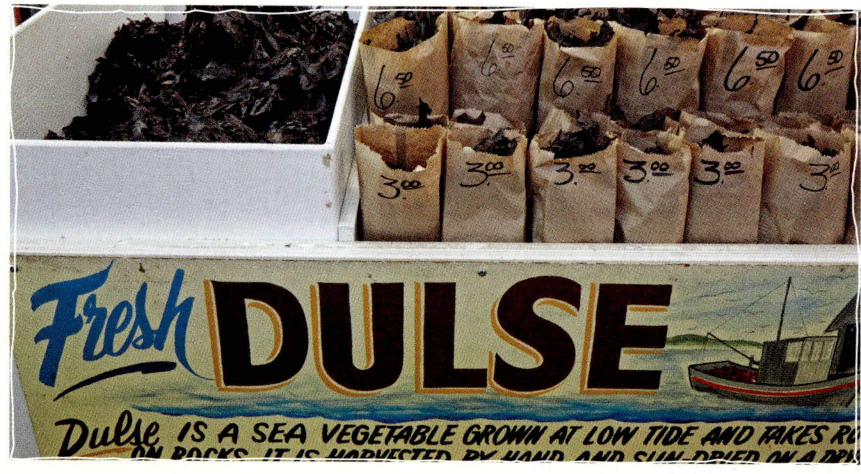

➤ **Fresh dulse**
Seen here on sale at a seafood market in St John, New Brunswick, Canada, dried fresh dulse can be eaten as a snack.

thicker, and more flavoursome. It is spread on nets over salty, sun-baked rocks to dry, and sold as smoked "whole leaf", flakes, granules, or powder in stores and fish markets. There is a dulse-gathering industry in Maine, US, centred in Hancock County.

Health food

Dulse has earned a reputation as a health food and pick-me-up. It is known to be an important source of dietary fibre, rich in vitamins and iron. There was a saying in Orkney, Scotland, that when drunk with water from the Well o' Kildingie, dulse would guard against all maladies bar one – the Black Death, or the bubonic plague. It was a well-known treatment for goitre, a thyroid condition caused by iodine deficiency. It was also used to treat scurvy and to relieve constipation. A tradition reported from the Outer Hebrides in Scotland was to lay fresh dulse on the belly of a woman who had just given birth to help expel the afterbirth – the placenta and fetal membranes left in the uterus after childbirth. It is said to improve blood circulation and lower blood pressure.

Commercial cultivation

There has been a renewed interest in dulse both as a health food and as a cosmetic. In North America, it is marketed as a luxury skincare ingredient, used in soaps, shampoo bars, and face oils. With the depletion of the wild dulse populations, owing perhaps to a combination of overharvesting and habitat degradation, research is underway into the possibility of commercial cultivation to meet the growing demand for this seaweed. One potential method is attaching its seedlings (young tetrasporophytes) to ropes under salmon farms, where the weed would also soak up nutrients from salmon feed.

➤ **Dulse seaweed**
Dulse is divided into blades, or fronds, that vary in shape but broaden outwards and branch out at the tips. Its colour varies from rose-pink to reddish purple or brown.

Claimed health benefits of dulse include **strong bones, improved digestion**, and **sharper sight**

Similar herbs

SEA KELP
Laminaria spp.
Kelp occurs in dense beds along the cold rocky shores of the world's oceans. An important resource and habitat for marine life, it is gathered for food and for medicinal use as well.

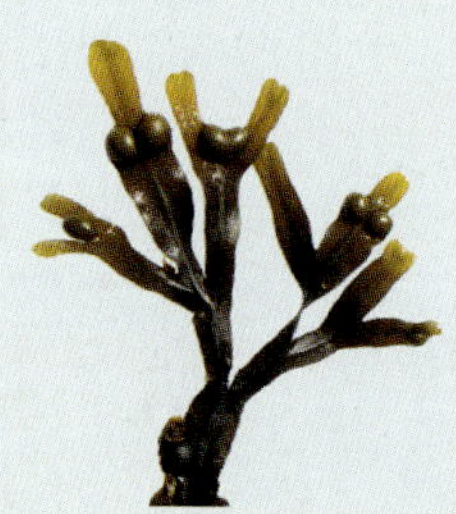

BLADDERWRACK
Fucus vesiculosus
An abundant seaweed on intertidal rocky shores throughout the northern hemisphere, it has distinctive vesicles or "bladders". As a source of iodine, it was once used to treat goitre.

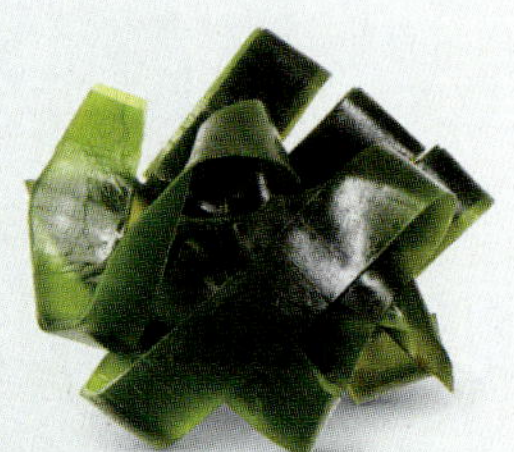

KOMBU OR HAIDAI
Saccharina japonica
An edible kelp that is widely consumed in East Asia, this herb is usually sold dried or pickled in vinegar. In Japan it is also eaten fresh with sashimi.

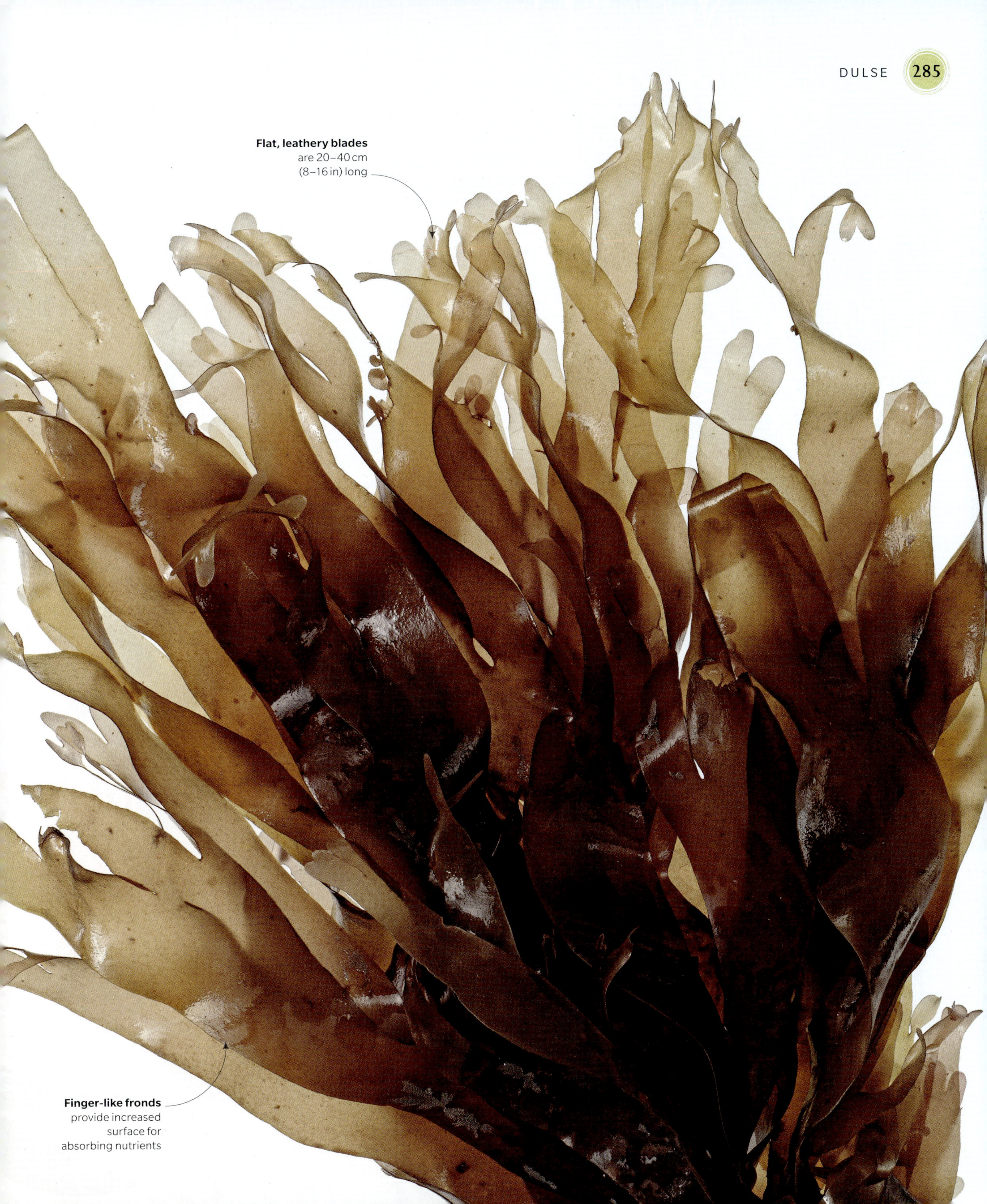
Flat, leathery blades are 20–40 cm (8–16 in) long
Finger-like fronds provide increased surface for absorbing nutrients

Uses Medicines

Parts used Entire body of fungus, including parasitized caterpillar

Active ingredients Adenosine and its derivative cordycepin, guanosine, cordymin, lovastatin

Habitat Grasslands at 3,000–5,000 m (9,800–16,400 ft) elevations that are covered in snow in winter

> “ In 2017... high quality pieces sold for as much as $140,000 per kilogram. ”
>
> DAVID ANDERSON and CHIA-YI HOU, *BusinessInsider.com*, 2021

Caterpillar Fungus

Ophiocordyceps sinensis

The “winter-worm, summer-grass” fungus known as *dong chong xia cao* in Chinese is highly sought after throughout Asia and is a major income source for rural communities wherever it occurs.

A dead caterpillar with an attached parasitic mushroom (*Ophiocordyceps sinensis*) may not seem an obvious source of herbal medicine, especially as it is inconspicuous and restricted to alpine grasslands in parts of the remote Himalayas and surrounds. However, wherever it occurs, it is hand picked by eagle-eyed locals as it emerges in the summer grass. It has a certain cachet as one of the most costly *materia medica* – only those of status can treat themselves with this fungus.

Life cycle of a miracle cure

Caterpillar fungus feeds on caterpillars of several moth species that live as larvae underground, feeding on plant roots. The invading fungus spreads through the caterpillar's body, eventually killing it and producing a single fruiting body. Recorded since the late-17th century in traditional Chinese medicine, the fungus has been used to treat ailments of the lungs and sexual problems. Modern research suggests it may be effective against some cancers, diabetes, and liver and kidney diseases. The fungus may absorb arsenic and heavy metals such as lead and mercury from the soil; these can build up in the body with heavy consumption of the fungus.

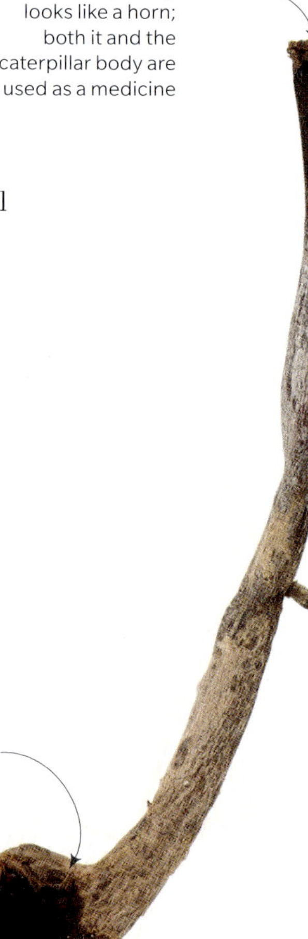

▼ Infested caterpillar
The fungus first spreads as a mass of filaments, called a mycelium; then its fruiting body pushes up through the soil to release its spores into the air.

Fruiting body looks like a horn; both it and the caterpillar body are used as a medicine

Fruiting body of the fungus emerges from head of dead caterpillar

Red Rice Fungus

Monascus purpureus

Normally, mould on food is considered unhealthy, but during its long coexistence with people, red rice fungus has acquired numerous culinary and medicinal uses, notably in the production of life-saving drugs – statins.

Uses Medicines; cooking

Parts used Entire organism, extracts

Active ingredients Monacolin K (in lactone form, identical to lovastatin)

Habitat Grows as a mould on cereal grains in damp conditions at temperatures of 25–32°C (77–90°F)

As do plants, many fungi produce chemicals that are medicinally valuable and red rice fungus, called *hong qu mei* in Chinese and known as a corn silage mould in the West, has a long history of use. In China, records of its medicinal application go back to the 16th century, and it remains popular in eastern Asia as a culinary ingredient and traditional medicine.

Traditional use and modern methods

Red yeast rice is produced by mixing steamed white rice with *Monascus purpureus* mould and allowing it to ferment for 4–6 days. The rice grains turn bright red and once dehydrated, can be powdered, stored, or used. Red yeast rice is used to dye dishes such as fermented bean curd, Peking duck, red rice vinegar, some Japanese *sake* and Chinese wines, and more. In traditional medicine, red rice fungus treats indigestion, diarrhoea, and limb weakness, but its role in battling cardiovascular disease is most significant. It creates a natural statin that reduces production and levels in the body of "bad" cholesterols.

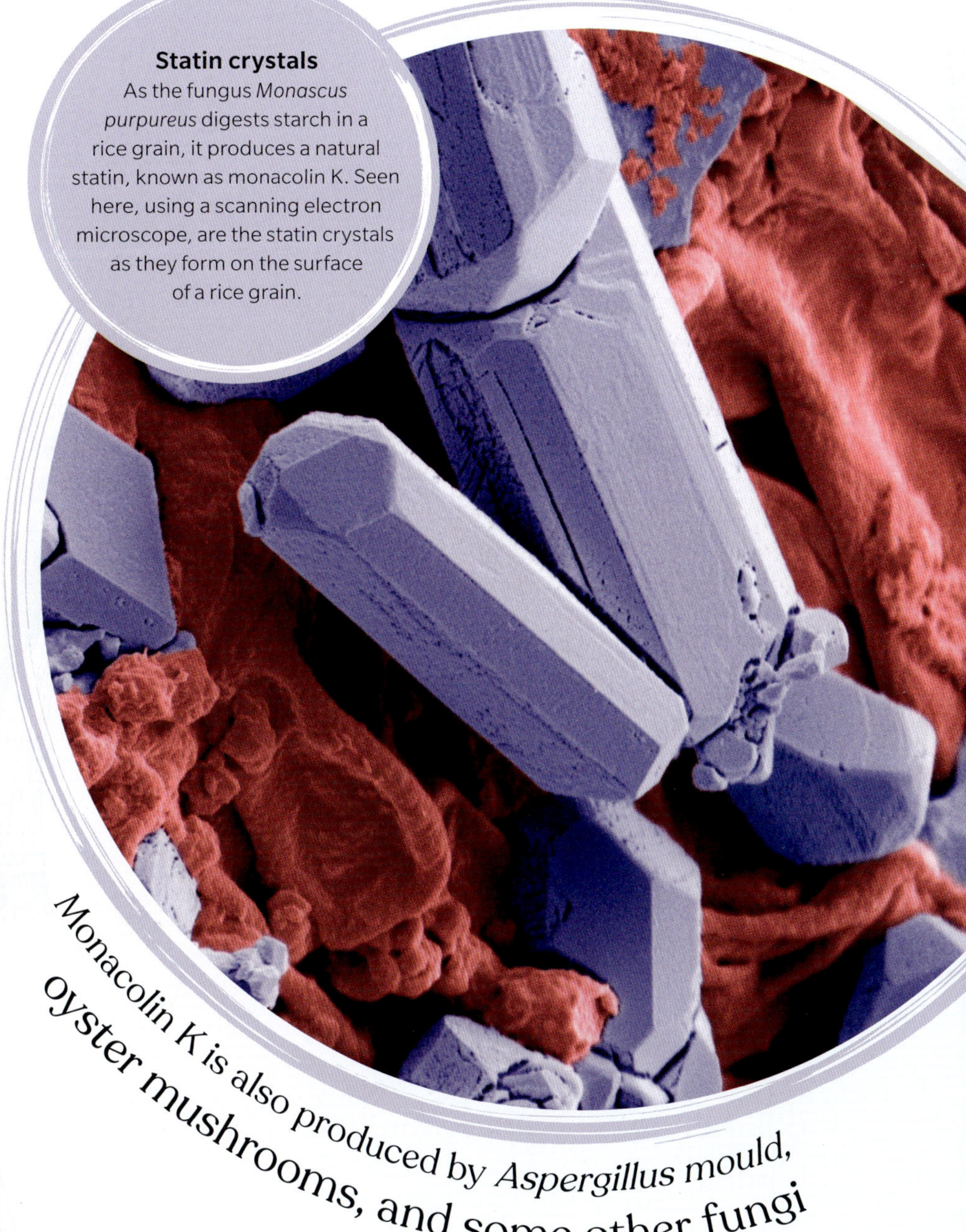

Statin crystals
As the fungus *Monascus purpureus* digests starch in a rice grain, it produces a natural statin, known as monacolin K. Seen here, using a scanning electron microscope, are the statin crystals as they form on the surface of a rice grain.

Monacolin K is also produced by *Aspergillus* mould, oyster mushrooms, and some other fungi

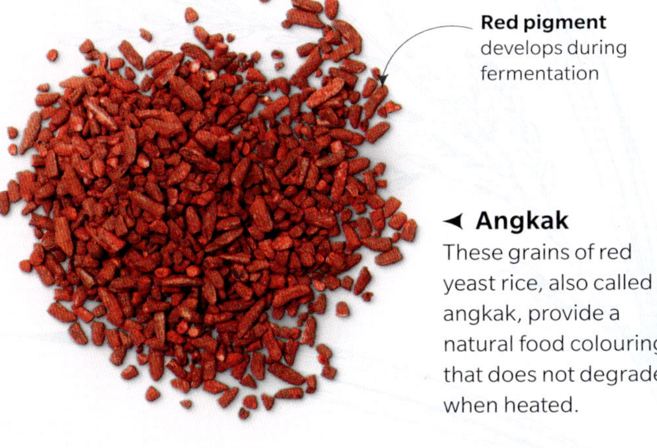

Red pigment develops during fermentation

◄ **Angkak**
These grains of red yeast rice, also called angkak, provide a natural food colouring that does not degrade when heated.

Uses Medicines; construction

Parts used Fruiting bodies, mycelia

Active ingredients Lucidenic acid, ganoderic acid, ergosterol, glucans

Habitat Temperate deciduous woodland

Pale growing tips of the fruiting bodies continue to elongate

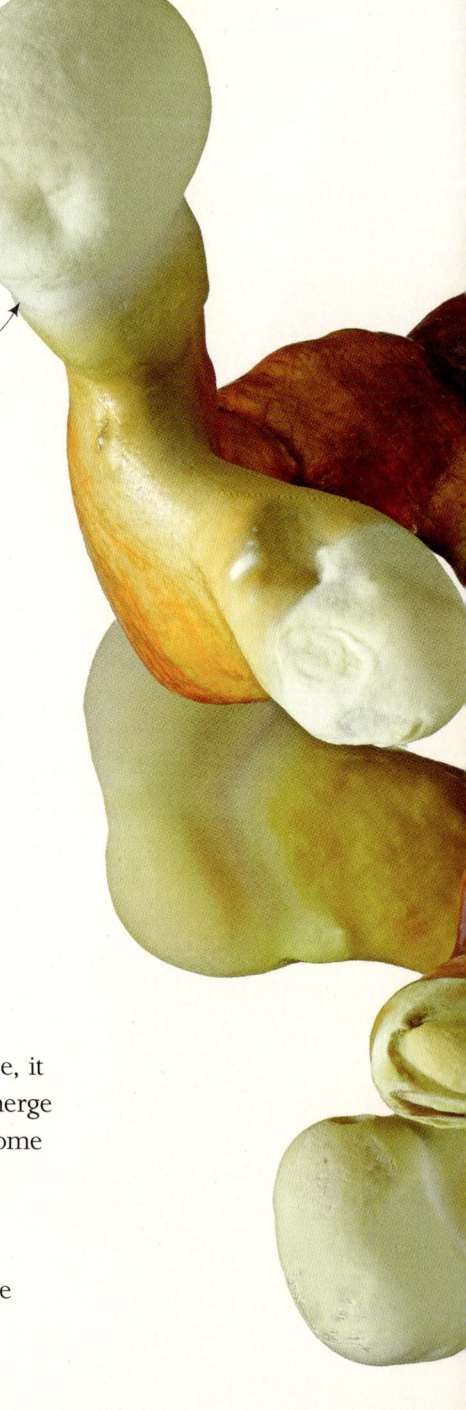

➤ Fungal forms
Fruiting bodies develop in different shapes depending on environmental conditions. The "antler" form (seen here growing on sawdust) develops when cultivated with low light and high carbon dioxide levels.

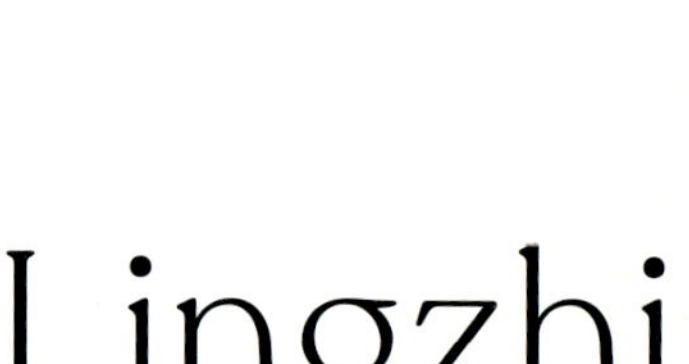

Lingzhi

Ganoderma lingzhi

This bracket fungus has a long history of use as a medicinal herb and is venerated across Asia, but its leathery texture and bitter flavour mean it is not widely consumed as a food.

Referred to as the "mushroom of immortality", *lingzhi* (known as *reishi* in Japan) has been used for its various healing abilities for more than 2,000 years. Despite this long history, there is still confusion over the identity of *lingzhi* fungus. Many herbal products list it as *Ganoderma lucidum*, but the fungus most widely utilized is *G. lingzhi*.

The mushroom is saprophytic (feeds from decaying organic matter), and spreads its branching mycelia (root-like structures) through the dead wood of deciduous trees, including maples (*Acer*). It will occasionally act as a parasite, weakening living trees by feeding upon them. When ready to reproduce, it forms bracket-shaped fruiting bodies that emerge from the tree trunk, usually near the base. Some of these fruiting bodies have stalks.

Favoured fungi

Lingzhi is hugely significant in Chinese culture and features commonly in its art. Among adherents of Daoist tradition, consuming *lingzhi* is a way to seek immortality, through the transcendence of time and space. While the mushroom's age-defying properties are likely

◄ Symbolic landscape
This Chinese embroidered silk landscape, created during the Qianlong period (1736–95), includes a rabbit (a symbol of longevity) and pair of *lingzhi* mushrooms growing at the base of a tree.

" If eaten customarily, it makes your body light and young. "

SHENNONG, *Classic of the Materia Medica,* 206 BCE to 220 CE

***Lingzhi* stems** darken with age, to a mahogany brown

exaggerated, *lingzhi* has been used traditionally to treat a variety of ailments, including viral infections, lung conditions, insomnia, diabetes, and liver diseases. Scientific research has documented anti-inflammatory, immunomodulatory, and antioxidant properties. Although *lingzhi* is not an effective primary treatment for cancer, it has been used to reduce side effects from other cancer treatments.

Wild *lingzhi* is increasingly rare, and most commercially available fungi are cultivated. Fungus farms grow the mycelia on buried rotten logs outside, or on compacted blocks of sawdust or grain indoors. The mushrooms are harvested and dried, after which they are simmered in hot water or ground into powder and made into tablets or capsules. In recent years, fungal mycelium has been used to produce building materials. It binds together organic matter, which can then be formed into any shape, including bricks. Despite its low environmental impact, the material is yet to be widely adopted by builders.

➤ ***Lingzhi* conks**
In light, well-aerated conditions, *lingzhi* develops flattened brackets known as conks. They emerge from the tree trunk or growing medium to release their spores.

Similar herbs

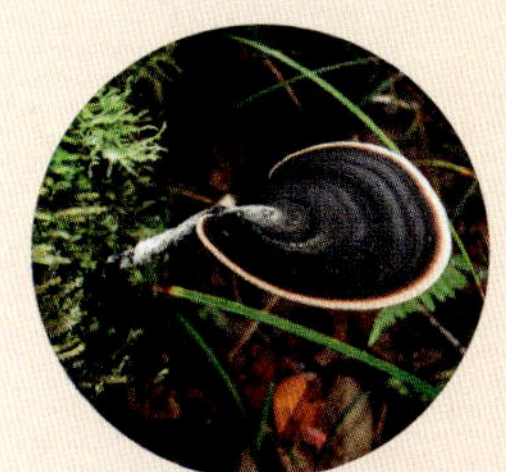

PURPLE REISHI
Ganoderma sinense
Used in traditional Chinese medicine, this native of China and Japan is thought to strengthen the immune system and protect the liver.

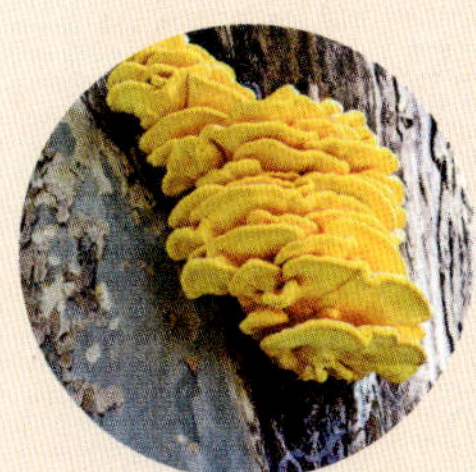

YELLOW REISHI
Laetiporus sulphureus
Occurring in Europe and North America, this edible mushroom tastes like chicken. It is used medicinally to treat diabetes.

Glossary

In this glossary, words in italics have a separate entry.

ADAPTOGEN A substance that improves the body's resistance to stress.

ALLELOCHEMICAL A chemical produced by a living organism that exerts a detrimental physiological effect on individuals of another species when released into the environment.

ALKALOID A compound containing nitrogen that can have various effects on body function.

ANALGESIC A medication that relieves various types of pain.

ANTHER The part of a *stamen* that produces *pollen* in the male reproductive organs of a flower.

ANTIOXIDANTS Molecules that fight free radicals in the body. Free radicals are compounds that can cause harm at high levels and are linked to illnesses such as diabetes, heart disease, and cancer.

ANTI-INFLAMMATORY Any drug used to reduce inflammation in the body.

ANTHELMINTIC Destroying or expelling intestinal worms.

ANTHROPOSOPHIC Pertaining to a formal educational, therapeutic, and creative system established by the Austrian spiritualist Rudolf Steiner (1861–1925). The system relies on mainly natural means to optimize physical and mental health and well-being.

ASTRINGENT Causing skin cells and other body tissues to contract; forming a protective coating and reducing bleeding and discharge.

AXIL The upper angle between a leaf and a stem, between a main stem and a side branch, or between a stem and a *bract*.

BILABIATE Possessing two lips; used to describe the *calyx* or the corolla (the whorl of fused or separate petals) of some flowers.

BIOREMEDIATION A process that uses mainly micro-organisms, plants, or microbial or plant *enzymes* to detoxify contaminants in the soil and other environments.

BITTER A digestive aid that stimulates secretion of digestive juices and improves the appetite.

BRACT A modified leaf at the base of a flower or flower cluster; a bract may resemble a normal leaf or be smaller and scale-like in appearance; in some cases, a bract may be large and brightly coloured.

CALYPTRA In flowering plants, a hood or cap-like structure; in mosses and other bryophytes, a protective structure that sheaths the growing embryo.

CALYX The outer part of a flower, usually small and green but sometimes brightly coloured; comprising the *sepals*, it encloses the petals in bud.

CAMPHOR A chemical formerly made by distilling the bark and wood of the camphor tree (*Cinnamomum camphora*) though now usually made from turpentine oil; with a very distinct smell, it stimulates respiration and circulation, and is a counter-irritant.

CARMINATIVE Relieves flatulence, colic, and digestive discomfort.

CHANNEL In traditional Chinese medicine, a channel is a pathway through which the life-energy known as *qi* (or ch'i) flows; channels are sometimes also known as meridians.

CHLOROPHYLL The green pigment in plants that is mainly responsible for light absorption to provide energy for growth.

CHINESE FIVE SPICE A mixture of spices used predominantly in Chinese cuisine; the five flavours of the spices allude to the five traditional Chinese elements (wood, fire, earth, metal, and water).

COLLOIDAL A mixture in which one substance (consisting of particles substantially larger than atoms or ordinary molecules but too small to be visible to the naked eye) is dispersed in another substance, usually liquid.

CORM An underground storage organ of a plant, including a swollen stem base that may be encased in a papery tunic.

DECOCTION A liquid medicinal preparation produced by simmering or boiling a herbal substance, and then straining.

DEMULCENT An agent that soothes and softens damaged, irritated, or inflamed tissues, for instance of the digestive tract.

DIAPHORETIC An agent that causes sweating in a patient, thus eliminating toxins from the body and lowering fever.

DIASCORDIUM In pre-modern medicine, usually a powder made from dried herbs and used to treat malignant fevers, plague, worms, colic, to promote sleep, and guard against putrefaction.

DICOT A flowering plant that has two seed leaves; short for dicotyledon.

DIOECIOUS Bearing male and female reproductive parts on separate plants.

DISC FLORET Any of the small tubular flowers at the centre of the flower head of certain Asteraceae species, such as the daisy; the central disc is usually surrounded by *ray florets*.

DIURETIC A chemical that can increase urine production.

EMETIC A substance that induces nausea and vomiting.

EMMENAGOGUE A drug or agent that increases menstrual flow.

EMULSIFIER Usually a thickening agent that helps combine ingredients such as oil and water that normally will not mix.

ENZYME A complex protein produced by cells that acts as a catalyst, speeding biological reactions without itself being used up in the reaction.

ESSENTIAL OIL A *volatile oil* (or oils) extracted from a plant, which has the plant's characteristic aroma or flavour.

EXPECTORANT An agent that encourages the expulsion of phlegm from the respiratory tract.

FLAVONOID A plant compound with a *phenolic* structure, including some plant pigments.

FLORET A single flower in a head of many flowers, including *disc florets* and *ray florets*.

FLORIOGRAPHY The language of flowers, widely used in traditional culture, allowing coded messages to be sent via floral arrangements or gifts of flowers.

FRUITING BODY The part of a fungus or slime mould that produces spores; mushrooms and toadstools are terms used for fungal fruiting bodies.

GALACTOGENOGUE Stimulating the production and flow of milk.

GLYCOSIDE A plant compound containing a sugar part (glycone) and a non-sugar part (aglycone).

HALLUCINOGENIC Producing altered states of consciousness, promoting a change in thought, mood, and perception.

HEAVY METALS (abbrev. HMs) Metals with relatively high densities, atomic weights, or atomic numbers. Essential HMs are necessary for such processes as growth, metabolism, and development in plants and animals; non-essential HMs are not required and may be toxic.

HERBES DE PROVENCE A mixture of dried herbs widely used in Mediterranean cuisines in meat, fish, and vegetable dishes, salads, and tomato-based soups. The herbs that are commonly used include basil, rosemary, tarragon, bay, and thyme.

HYDROSOL A water-based product made during the distillation of fresh flowers, leaves, fruits, and other plant material.

HYPERICIN A chemical found in the common St John's wort (*Hypericum perforatum*) that has traditionally been used to improve moods.

INFUSION A liquid preparation obtained by steeping plant material in either cold water (cold infusion) or hot water (hot infusion or tea).

LABELLUM A lip, especially an enlarged or otherwise distinctive petal. It attracts insects that pollinate the flower and acts as a landing platform for them, or may be modified as a pouch.

LIPIDS Organic compounds that are insoluble in water, such as oils.

MITOCHONDRION (pl. MITOCHONDRIA) Membrane-bound cell *organelles* that generate most of the chemical energy needed to power the cell's biochemical reactions.

MONOCOT A flowering plant that has only one seed leaf; short for monocotyledon.

MYCELIUM A network of tubular filaments produced by a fungus, usually underground but also sometimes in other places, such as rotting tree trunks.

NARCOTIC A drug that causes stupor and insensibility; historically it was often used to relieve pain. The term is widely applied to addictive drugs that are currently illegal in use.

NERVINE A type of herb intended to nourish and support the central nervous system and calm the nerves.

NOSEGAY BOUQUET A small bunch of scented flowers and herbs, typically given as a gift.

NEUROTRANSMITTER A chemical messenger in the body that transmits signals between nerve cells or from nerve cells to target cells.

OLIBANUM Also commonly known as frankincense, an aromatic resin used in incense and perfumes.

OPIATES A group of pain-relieving drugs from the opium poppy (*Papaver somniferum*), such as morphine, that work by interacting with opioid receptors in nerve cells around the body, especially in the brain and spinal cord.

ORGANELLES Small structures within cells that are surrounded by a membrane and have a specific function.

PALMATE A leaf with four or more leaflets that arise from a single point; can also be applied to palmately lobed leaves.

PERENNIAL A plant that persists for at least three years. Tropical perennials are usually evergreen but in temperate areas they usually die back in winter.

PHENOLIC COMPOUND Plant compounds with one or more hydrocarbon rings and hydroxyl groups; some function as *antioxidants* and have a beneficial impact on human health.

PHOTOSYNTHESIS In green plants, the synthesis of carbohydrates from carbon dioxide and water, using light energy absorbed by *chlorophyll*.

PHYTOCHEMICALS All chemicals produced by plants; the term is often restricted to those that may affect health but are not essential nutrients.

PHYTOESTROGEN A plant compound with oestrogen-like effects.

PINNATE A leaf with a central axis and two or more lateral leaflets (pinnae).

PINNULE A secondary division of a *pinnate* (feather-like) leaf, especially of a fern.

POLLEN Spores or grains containing male sex cells and carried on an *anther* in a flowering plant.

POLLINATION The transfer of *pollen* from the *anthers* to the *stigma* of either the same or different flowers, resulting in the fertilization of an egg cell in the ovary, and the development of a seed; this transfer may be aided by insects, animals, or the wind.

PROSTAGLANDINS Compounds, made in the body from fatty acids, that have physiological effects. They control processes such as inflammation and the induction of labour.

PSYCHOACTIVE CHEMICALS Substances that alter perception, mood, consciousness, cognition, or behaviour. Common examples of psychoactive substances include caffeine, anaesthetics, marijuana, and cocaine.

RACEME An unbranched flower cluster with several or many stalked flowers carried singly along a main axis, the youngest flower at the tip.

RAY FLORET Any of the small strap-shaped flowers in the flower head of certain Asteraceae species, such as the daisy, in which they surround the central *disc florets*, and the dandelion in which *disc florets* are absent.

RHIZOME A branched underground stem that grows horizontally and bears leafy shoots.

ROSETTE A group of leaves radiating from approximately the same point, often at ground level on a very short stem.

SAPONIN A soap-like *glycoside*, found widely in plants, that can have complex effects in herbal medicine; some saponins are used in the manufacture of steroid hormone drugs.

SCAPE An upright, leafless stalk, arising from the ground, with an inflorescence or flower at its tip.

SCANNING ELECTRON MICROSCOPE A type of microscope that produces images by scanning the surface of a sample with a focused beam of electrons.

SCHIZOCARP A fruit which splits into individual carpels, each with a single seed.

SEPAL Part of a *calyx*, the outer whorl of floral organs that protects the petals and reproductive parts when in bud. Sepals are usually green and may often appear insignificant but are in some cases showy.

SORUS (pl. SORI) A cluster of spore-producing structures typically on the underside of fertile fern fronds.

SPADIX A spike-like flower cluster, typical of the Aroid family (Araceae), that is usually fleshy and bears numerous small flowers.

SPORANGIUM (pl. SPORANGIA) A sac or body that contains or produces spores, used especially of cryptogams (flowerless and seedless plants that nevertheless increase by means of sexual fusion).

STAMEN The male reproductive organ of a flower, which consists of a filament bearing an *anther* that produces *pollen*.

STATIN A type of medicine that can help lower the level of low-density lipoprotein (LDL) cholesterol (commonly known as "bad cholesterol") in the blood.

STIGMA Part of the female reproductive organ of a flower, which receives *pollen*; often carried at the tip of a style.

STYLE The stem-like part of a flower's female reproductive organ on which the *stigma* is borne.

TINCTURE An extract of plant material, made using ethanol.

UMBEL A usually flat-topped or rounded flower cluster in which the individual flower stalks arise from a central point; such flower heads are characteristic of the carrot family (Apiaceae) umbels.

VASOCONSTRICTOR An agent that causes narrowing of the walls of blood vessels, typically by making the muscles of the blood vessel walls constrict.

VOLATILE ORGANIC COMPOUND (abbrev. VOC) Plant compound that evaporates at ambient temperatures; also applied to gases emitted from some solids and liquids such as paint.

VOLATILE OILS Complex, aromatic plant constituents that evaporate easily and may be extracted to produce *essential oils*, or isolated constituents, such as linalool (found in many flowers and spice plants).

Index

Page numbers in **bold** navigate to the main information for individual herbs, those in *italics* indicate photographs and illustrations.

A

D

Q R

Acknowledgments

DK would like to thank the following:

Additional text: Andrew Mikolajski

Proofreading: Joy Evatt

Indexing: Elizabeth Wise

Editorial assistance: Aashline R. Avarachan, Dharini Ganesh

Design assistance: Aarushi Dhawan, Rupanki Kaushik, Mahua Mandal, Pooja Pipil, Roohi Rais, Mitravinda V K

Technical assistance: Nand Kishore Acharya, Ashok Kumar, Mrinmoy Mazumdar, Syed Md Farhan

Picture research: Kate Sayer, Amy Moss, Martin Copeland

Colour retouching: Steve Crozier

Original photography: Gary Ombler

DISCLAIMER: The information in this book has been compiled as general guidance on the specific subjects addressed. It is not a substitute and should not be relied upon for medical, healthcare, or pharmaceutical professional advice. Please consult your healthcare provider before undertaking any of the nutrition, techniques, natural remedies, and alternative therapies set out in this book, and consult your GP before changing, stopping, or starting any medical treatment. So far as the author is aware the information given is correct and up to date as at November 2022. Practice, laws, and regulations all change and the reader should obtain up-to-date professional advice on any such issues. The author and publishers disclaim, as far as the law allows, any liability arising directly or indirectly from the use or misuse of the information contained in this book.

The publisher would like to thank the following for their kind permission to reproduce their photographs:

(Key: a-above; b-below/bottom; c-centre; f-far; l-left; r-right; t-top)

1 © Mary Jo Hoffman. **2-3 Dreamstime.com:** Marilyn Barbone (6); Sergei Chaiko (7); Marina Lohrbach (8). **Getty Images/iStock:** Marina Lohrbach (10); marilyna (9). **© Mary Jo Hoffman. 4-5 Dreamstime.com:** Olgasha. **6-7 Dreamstime.com:** Patrick Guenette (background). **8-9 Dreamstime.com:** Patrick Guenette (background). **10-11 Shutterstock.com:** LiliGraphie (t). **10 Bridgeman Images:** Heinrich Zinram Photography Archive (br). **Dreamstime.com:** Steve Allen (cr). **11 Shutterstock.com:** Seth Aronstam (bl). **12 Dreamstime.com:** Milosk50 (ftr); Mprozogo (tc); TasFoto (bl); Simona Pavan (br). **Shutterstock.com:** Starikov Pavel (fbr). **13 Alamy Stock Photo:** Nature Picture Library (tl); Zoonar GmbH (br). **Shutterstock.com:** Irina Borsuchenko (tc); Nick Pecker (tr). **14 Alamy Stock Photo:** Hamza Khan (clb). **Dreamstime.com:** Sadik Gulec (cr); TasFoto (tr); Yaroslav Zhak (bc); Olesia Sarycheva (cb). **15 123RF.com:** klevo (cl). **Dreamstime.com:** Cristina Dini (tl); Emanuele Ravecca (fcra); Julian Popov (ca); Jinfeng Zhan (cb); Alla Sravani (bc). **Getty Images/iStock:** Daniel Balakov (fbr). **Getty Images:** Universal Images Group (clb). **16 Alamy Stock Photo:** FionasMoments (cra). **Dreamstime.com:** Cristina Dini (cb); Irinayeryomina (bc); Mirzamlk (br). **17 Shutterstock.com:** George Chernilevsky (br). **18 Alamy Stock Photo:** Science History Images (cl); Vespasian (fcr). **Bridgeman Images:** Christie's Images (cb). **Getty Images:** Corbis historical/Photo Josse/Leemage (fcla). **Wellcome Images CC4 License:** Public Domain (ca). **19 Alamy Stock Photo:** Niday Picture Library (cl); World History Archive (ca). **Dreamstime.com:** Natalya Dralova (ftl). **Getty Images:** Leemage/Corbis (fcrb). **International Institute of Social History (Amsterdam):** chineseposters.net (bl). **Shutterstock.com:** Wirestock Creators (fbr). **Wellcome Images CC4 License:** (cla); Science Museum, London (cb). **20 Alamy Stock Photo:** agefotostock (bl). **21 Shutterstock.com:** Marilyn Barbone (tl). **22 Getty Images:** Siegfried Layda (bc). **23 123RF.com:** coboflupi (crb). **Alamy Stock Photo:** Pramote Polyamate (bc); SBS Eclectic Images (cr); Stephanie Jackson - gardens and flowes collection (br). **Science Photo Library:** Ted Kinsman (tc). **24 123RF.com:** baibaz (clb); lculig (br). **AF Fotografie:** (fcla). **Alamy Stock Photo:** Heritage Image Partnership Ltd (fcrb). **Getty Images/iStock:** SongSpeckels (cr). **25 Alamy Stock Photo:** Manfred Ruckszio (fcrb). **Bridgeman Images:** Look and Learn/Barbara Loe Collection (bl); Pictures from History (cla); Photo Josse (fcra). **Dreamstime.com:** Alfio Scisetti | Dreamstime.co (crb). **Getty Images/iStock:** kaanates (br). **Shutterstock.com:** azadjain1 (tc); Sucharut Chounyoo (fcl). **27 Alamy Stock Photo:** Asar Studios (tr). **Shutterstock.com:** ArtCookStudio (br). **28 Bridgeman Images:** British Library Board. All Rights Reserve (bl). **30 Alamy Stock Photo:** North Wind Picture Archives (br). **Exotic India. 31 Alamy Stock Photo:** IanDagnall Computing (tr). **32-33 Dreamstime.com:** Patrick Guenette (background). **34-35 Dreamstime.com:** Mariia Sultnova (crb/background). **34 Alamy Stock Photo:** Artokoloro (br). **Getty Images:** Science & Society Picture Library (tr). **35 © Board of Trustees of the Royal Botanic Gardens, Kew:** (l). **Shutterstock.com:** Coulanges (cr); Likit Supasai (br). **36 Dreamstime.com:** Mariia Sultnova (tc, bl). **Getty Images:** Universal Images Group (ftr). **Wellcome Collection:** Chinese Materia medica, C17: Plant drugs/Public Domai (br). **36-37 Dreamstime.com:** Kateryna Danylyuk (background). **37 Dreamstime.com:** Vishakha Shah (cr). **Getty Images:** Heritage Images (cb). **38 Dreamstime.com:** Potysiev Denis (cl, cr, bl). **© Board of Trustees of the Royal Botanic Gardens, Kew. 39 Alamy Stock Photo:** Sunny Celeste (tr); Tetiana Troichenko (bc). **Dreamstime.com:** Potysiev Denis (clb, bl, ca, tc, fcr, br). **40 Alamy Stock Photo:** Marcus Harrison - botanicals (tc, cb). **41 Alamy Stock Photo:** Marcus Harrison - botanicals (r); Met/Bot (bc). **Bridgeman Images:** Prismatic Pictures (tr). **Dreamstime.com:** Sunnychicka (cr). **Getty Images/iStock:** Pamela D Mcadams (clb). **42 Wellcome Collection:** (bl). **43 Dreamstime.com:** Irina Iarovaia (tr, crb, bl). **Getty Images:** Jamie Lamb/Elusive Images (bc). **44 Alamy Stock Photo:** Florilegius. **Dreamstime.com:** Irina Iarovaia (tr, bl). **45 Alamy Stock Photo:** Wildlife Gmbh (cr). **Dreamstime.com:** Irina Iarovaia (r). **Getty Images:** (bc). **46 Alamy Stock Photo:** Quagga Media (bc). **Biodiversity Heritage Library:** (tr). **47 Alamy Stock Photo:** Florilegius (tr). **Biodiversity Heritage Library. Wellcome Images CC4 License:** Public Domain (cla). **48 Dreamstime.com:** Patrick Guenette (ca). **Getty Images/iStock:** Sadasiba Behera (cra); im a photographer and an artist (bc). **49 Dreamstime.com:** Patrick Guenette (cl). **Getty Images:** Heritage Images (bc). **Getty Images/iStock:** Libin Jose. **50 Dreamstime.com:** Ekaterina Arkhangelskaia (tc). **Shutterstock.com:** Cosmicanna (b). **51 Dreamstime.com:** Ekaterina Arkhangelskaia (cra, cb); Ericaimama (tr); Friedemeier (cr). **State Library of New South Wales:** (tc). **52 Getty Images/iStock:** Ievgeniia Lytvynovych (tr, ca, clb, br). **Getty Images:** Burcu Atalay Tankut (cb). **52-53 Dreamstime.com:** Ims721940 (c). **53 Dreamstime.com:** Phichet Udomkaew (crb). **Getty Images/iStock:** Ievgeniia Lytvynovych (tr, cb). **Mary Evans Picture Library:** (br). **54-55 Dreamstime.com:** Labemax. **54 Dreamstime.com:** Patrick Guenette (tl). **55 Dreamstime.com:** Patrick Guenette (r). **Photo Scala, Florence:** Princeton University Art Museum/Art Resource N (br). **56 Dreamstime.com:** Patrick Guenette (bl); Luo Ming Zheng (tr). **Getty Images/iStock:** Tane-Mahuta (bc). **57 akg-images:** Sotheby's (br). **Dreamstime.com:** Foxyliam (tc, crb); Patrick Guenette (r). **Getty Images:** Buyenlarge (tr). **58 Alamy Stock Photo:** Valentyn Volkov (tc). **58-59 123RF.com:** alhontes (background). **59 Bridgeman Images:** British Library Board. **60 Alamy Stock Photo:** Florilegius (bc). **Biodiversity Heritage Library. 61 Biodiversity Heritage Library. 62 Dreamstime.com:** Patrick Guenette (clb, cr); Zetaty (bl); Björn Wylezich (fbl). **63 Alamy Stock Photo:** Stig Alenäs (cr). **Dreamstime.com:** Patrick Guenette (br). **64 Alamy Stock Photo:** imageBROKER/Horst Mahr (cla); Panther Media GmbH/Watzmann (clb). **Bridgeman Images:** Look and Learn (r). **Dreamstime.com:** Jochenschneider (bl). **65 Dreamstime.com:** Patrick Guenette (tc, br). **Getty Images:** Westend61 (bl). **66 Alamy Stock Photo:** Artepics (b). **Dreamstime.com:** Patrick Guenette (tl, crb). **67 Dreamstime.com:** Patrick Guenette (cra, br). **Gary Ombler:** (t). **68 Bridgeman Images:** Arni Magnusson Institute (tr). **Dreamstime.com:** Patrick Guenette (tl, fbl); Valeriy Kirsanov (bl). **69 Alamy Stock Photo:** Kumar Sriskandan (tc). **Dreamstime.com;** Patrick Guenette (fbr). **Getty Images/iStock:** Ivan-96 (br). **70-71 Getty Images:** Pierce Archive LLC/Buyenlarge (tr). **Shutterstock.com:** Morphart Creation (background). **70 Alamy Stock Photo:** WILDLIFE GmbH (bl). **71 Getty Images:** Popperfoto (br). **72 Bridgeman Images. Dreamstime.com:** Eskymaks (tr). **72-73 Shutterstock.com:** Morphart Creation (background). **73 Getty Images/iStock:** Kanjana Wattanakungchai (tr). **NMKonline:** (bc). **74 Alamy Stock Photo:** Inga Spence (t). **© The Trustees of the British Museum. All rights reserved:** (br). **Dreamstime.com:** Marina Vorontsova (tc, tr). **75 Alexander Turnbull Library, National Library Of New Zealand, Te Puna Matauranga o Aotearoa:** Alexander Turnbull Library (br). **Dreamstime.com:** Marina Vorontsova (fbl, fbr). **StockFood:** TH Foto (tr). **76 Dreamstime.com:** Maart (tc, br). **Wellcome Collection:** Chinese Materia Dietetica, Ming: Alcoholic beverages/Public Domai (bl). **76-77 Getty Images/iStock:** Emilio100. **77 Alamy Stock Photo:** agefotostock/J M Barnes (cr).

Dreamstime.com: Maart (tr). **Getty Images/iStock:** White_Caty (bc). **Shutterstock.com:** Archaeopteryx Tours (br). **78 Alamy Stock Photo:** Interfoto (bl); Wildlife Gmbh (br). **Dreamstime.com:** Foxyliam (tr). **Emily Yuko Hallett. 79 Alamy Stock Photo:** agefotostock, Javier Larrea (tr). **Dreamstime.com:** Foxyliam (ftr, fclb); Tetiana Kovalenko (clb). **Emily Yuko Hallett, Ph.D. 80 Alamy Stock Photo:** Album (br); Florilegius (clb). **Biodiversity Heritage Library. Wikipedia:** Rezergua (bc). **81 Alamy Stock Photo:** Florilegius (c); Marcus Harrison - botanicals (tr); Florilegius (cr). **Biodiversity Heritage Library. 82 123RF.com:** Eshved (cl). **Dreamstime.com:** Jurate Buiviene (br); Cristina Dini (bc). **Getty Images/iStock:** Arijeet Bannerjee (cb); Hans Joachim (cra). **Science Photo Library:** Jerry Mason (bl). **83 123RF.com:** Eshved (t, l, r). **Bridgeman Images:** (br). **Photo Scala, Florence:** The British Library Board (tl). **84 akg-images:** Roland and Sabrina Michaud (t). **Getty Images/iStock:** Ilbusca (tr). **84-85 Getty Images/iStock:** Ilbusca (b). **85 Alamy Stock Photo:** Album (bc). **Shutterstock.com:** Lippert Photography (tr). **86 Alamy Stock Photo:** Wildlife Gmbh (tr). **Dreamstime.com:** Ziprashantzi (cr). **Getty Images/iStock:** Ilbusca (cra). **Photo Scala, Florence:** (l). **87 akg-images:** Joseph Martin (cra). **Biodiversity Heritage Library. Getty Images/iStock:** Ilbusca (crb). **Getty Images:** Science & Society Picture Library (bc). **88 Bridgeman Images:** Alinari (tl). **Dreamstime.com:** Patrick Guenette (r). **89 Dreamstime.com:** Patrick Guenette. **90 Bridgeman Images:** Christie's Images (b). **Dreamstime.com:** Patrick Guenette (l, r). **91 akg-images:** Roland and Sabrina Michaud (tr). **Dreamstime.com:** Patrick Guenette (b); RukiMedia (crb); Barbara Pheby (bl); Brita Seifert (br). **92 akg-images:** De Agostini/C. Balossini (bc). **Dreamstime.com:** Yulya Opalnitskaya (r). **93 akg-images:** (cra). **Alamy Stock Photo:** Mohamed Haddad (tc). **Dreamstime.com:** Yulya Opalnitskaya (b). **94-95 Getty Images:** fabiommmayer/500px. **95 Alamy Stock Photo:** Hamza Khan (tr). **Dreamstime.com:** Awispa (fbl, fclb, bl, clb, bc, crb, br). **Getty Images:** Heritage Images (fcrb). **96 Dreamstime.com:** Awispa (bl, bc, br, fbr). **Getty Images:** Heritage Images (tl). **97 Dreamstime.com:** Awispa (fclb, bl, cb, crb, br, cra). **Getty Images:** Carlos Sanchez Pereyra (r). **98 Alamy Stock Photo:** Chronicle (c). **Dreamstime.com:** Awispa (clb, bl, cb, bc, crb, br); Tamara Kulikova (tc); Juan Francisco Moreno Gámez (tr). **99 Dreamstime.com:** Awispa (fbl, bl, clb, br, crb). **Getty Images:** Matteo Colombo (b). **Science Photo Library:** Jeremy Burgess (tc). **100 Alamy Stock Photo:** Hemis (tl). **Dreamstime.com:** Kseniia Gorova (bc, crb). **101 Dreamstime.com:** Kseniia Gorova (cla, bl, crb). **102 Bridgeman Images:** A. Dagli Orti/© Npl - Dea Picture Library (c); Archives Charmet (bc). **Dreamstime.com:** Kseniia Gorova (tc, bl). **103 Dreamstime.com:** Kseniia Gorova (l, r). **Science Photo Library:** Power And Syred (c). **104-105 123RF.com:** morphart (background). **106-107 Alamy Stock Photo:** Media Drum World. **Dreamstime.com:** Patrick Guenette (background). **107 Dreamstime.com:** Valentyn75 (bc). **108-109 Dreamstime.com:** Patrick Guenett (background). **108 Dreamstime.com:** Maxim Tatarinov (tl, tc); Maxim Tatarinov (ftl). **Getty Images:** Heritage Art/Heritage Images (bc). **110-111 Alamy Stock Photo:** CPA Media Pte Ltd. **Dreamstime.com:** Patrick Guenett (background). **110 Alamy Stock Photo:** Nature Picture Library (bl). **111 Dreamstime.com:** Colourdream (crb). **Mary Evans Picture Library:** Onslow Auctions Limited (tr). **112-113 123RF.com:** channarongsds (background). **112 Wellcome Images CC4 License:** Public Domain (c). **113 Bridgeman Images:** Royal Collection Trust/© His Majesty King Charles III, 2022 (tl). **Dreamstime.com:** Kenishirotie (br); Povarov (crb). **114 Alamy Stock Photo:** Ittichai Anusarn (bc). **114-115 Getty Images:** Tuul & Bruno Morandi (t). **116 Biodiversity Heritage Library. 117 Biodiversity Heritage Library. Wikipedia:** Public Domain (tc). **118 Getty Images/iStock:** Channarongsds (bl, c). **119 Bridgeman Images:** Pictures from History (cla). **Dreamstime.com:** Manfred Ruckszio (cr). **Getty Images/iStock:** Channarongsds (tl, c). **120 Dreamstime.com:** Nadin333 (bl). **Getty Images/iStock:** Channarongsds (tl, c). **120-121 Getty Images:** 500px, Patrick Gerhardt (t). **121 Alamy Stock Photo:** Archive PL (br). **Getty Images/iStock:** Channarongsds (crb). **122-123 123RF.com:** awispa (background). **Getty Images/iStock:** Viperagp (b). **123 Getty Images:** De Agostini Picture Library (bc). **TopFoto:** Roger-Viollet (tr). **124 Dreamstime.com:** Valentyn75 (tr). **Shutterstock.com:** Morphart Creation (br). **125 123RF.com:** dizolator (tl). **Dreamstime.com:** Grobler Du Preez (cl). **Getty Images:** larigan - Patricia Hamilton (b); mikroman6 (tr). **126 Getty Images/iStock:** dionisvero (cb); ilbusca (cra, br). **127 Alamy Stock Photo:** INTERFOTO (crb). **Getty Images/iStock:** ilbusca (cr, cla). **128 Bridgeman Images:** JBP/AIC (tc). **Getty Images/iStock:** ilbusca (tr, cl, crb, br). **129 Biodiversity Heritage Library. 130 Alamy Stock Photo:** Florilegius (tr); The Natural History Museum (bc). **Biodiversity Heritage Library. Missouri Botanical Garden:** (cra). **131 Alamy Stock Photo:** Florilegius (fcr). **Biodiversity Heritage Library. 132 Shutterstock.com:** hjochen (c). **133 Bridgeman Images:** Bridgeman Images (tr). **Dreamstime.com:** Genkistock (br). **134 Alamy Stock Photo:** The Granger Collection (bl). **Getty Images:** De Agostini Editorial (tl). **135 Dreamstime.com:** Czuber (crb). **Getty Images/iStock:** emer1940 (cra). **136-137 123RF.com:** kosolga (background). **Alamy Stock Photo:** Florilegius (t). **137 Dreamstime.com:** Suradech Kongkiatpaiboon (tc). **Shutterstock.com:** Nittakij (br); Shansh23 (bc). **138-139 123RF.com:** channarongsds (background). **139 akg-images. Dreamstime.com:** Yulan (br). **140 123RF.com:** channarongsds (background). **Alamy Stock Photo:** AztecBlue (bc). **Wellcome Images CC4 License:** Public Domain (cl). **141 Alamy Stock Photo:** imageBROKER (br). **Dreamstime.com:** Tristan Berlund (background). **Getty Images:** FlowerPhotos/Universal Images Group (c). **142 Alamy Stock Photo:** Florilegius (r). **Getty Images/iStock:** RukiMedia (fcla). **Shutterstock.com:** junjun (ftl). **142-143 Dreamstime.com:** Patrick Guenett (background). **143 Dreamstime.com:** Elena Elisseev (br). **Getty Images/iStock:** marilyna (bl). **144-145 Dreamstime.com:** Galina Sinelnikova (background). **144 akg-images:** Bergen, Kunstmuseum (c). **145 Getty Images/iStock:** Helin Loik-Tomson (fbr). **146 Alamy Stock Photo:** Album (bc); Florilegius (ftl). **Biodiversity Heritage Library. 147 Alamy Stock Photo:** Album (tr); Florilegius (cl). **Biodiversity Heritage Library. Naturalis Biodiversity Center:** Netherlands (cr). **148 Dreamstime.com:** Vivali (ftr, cr). **Getty Images:** Bettmann (br). **149 TfL from the London Transport Museum collection:** (l). **150 Dreamstime.com:** Ekaterina Arkhangelskaia (r). **Mary Evans Picture Library:** Mary Evans/J. Bedmar/Iberfoto (b). **151 Dreamstime.com:** Ekaterina Arkhangelskaia (bl, clb, tr). **Getty Images/iStock:** stsmhn (br). **152 Alamy Stock Photo:** Panther Media GmbH (tl). **Getty Images:** swim ink 2 llc (bl). **153 Biodiversity Heritage Library. Dreamstime.com:** Ekaterina Arkhangelskaia (bl, cb, ca, br). **Getty Images/iStock:** Gratysanna (crb). **Shutterstock.com:** Skyprayer2005 (cra). **154 Alamy Stock Photo:** Adam Eastland (br); PRISMA ARCHIVO (bl). **Dreamstime.com:** Bokasana (c); Tetiana Kovalenko (cr). **155 Dreamstime.com:** Bokasana (c). **156-157 Dreamstime.com:** Ekaterina Arkhangelskaia (background). **157 Alamy Stock Photo:** Florilegius (br); PhotoStock-Israel (tr). **158 Alamy Stock Photo:** Daybreak Imagery (bl); Frank Hecker (cl). **Getty Images:** Moment/Jacky Parker Photograph (r). **159 Alamy Stock Photo:** The Granger Collection (br). **Getty Images:** Digital Vision/Davies and Star (tr). **160 Getty Images:** Prisma/UIG (tl). **160-161 123RF.com:** morphart (background). **161 GAP Photos:** Geoff Kidd (cr). **162 The Bodleian Library, University of Oxford:** (t). **162-163 123RF.com:** morphart (background). **163 Alamy Stock Photo:** Valery Prokhozhy (br). **Shutterstock.com:** Kharbine-Tapabo (tc). **164 Getty Images:** Mondadori Portfoli (bl). **164-165 123RF.com:** arkadivna (background). **165 Alamy Stock Photo:** CPA Media Pte Ltd (br). **166 Alamy Stock Photo:** Album (cl); Florilegius (c); Hamza Khan (br). **Biodiversity Heritage Library. 167 Biodiversity Heritage Library. 168 Biodiversity Heritage Library. Dreamstime.com:** Pipa100 (cl); Plej92 (tl). **Shutterstock.com:** marilyn barbone. **169 123RF.com:** msokolyan (l, r). **Alamy Stock Photo:** WILDLIFE GmbH (br). **Shutterstock.com:** NIKCOA (tr). **170 123RF.com:** morphart (c). **Shutterstock.com:** anat chant (cl). **171 123RF.com:** morphart (bl, tr, c). **Alamy Stock Photo:** (br); BIOSPHOTO (tc). **172 Alamy Stock Photo:** INTERFOTO (b). **Dreamstime.com:** Svehlik21 (tr). **Shutterstock.com:** KAEDA9 (tc). **173 123RF.com:** morphart (c). **Shutterstock.com:** CMA/BOT (br). **174 Shutterstock.com:** Tiju AV (tl). **175 Alamy Stock Photo:** Boaz Rottem (cra). **Dreamstime.com:** Ziprashantzi (tr). **Getty Images/iStock:** Studio Light and Shade (bc). **StockFood:** Petr Gross (tc). **Wellcome Images CC4 License:** Public Domain (br). **176 Dreamstime.com:** Polelya (bl, br). **The Center for International Forestry Research (CIFOR):** Chandra Shekhar Karki (bc). **177 Dreamstime.com:** Polelya (bl, bc, br). **Science Photo Library:** Eye of Science (tr). **178-179 Depositphotos Inc:** msokolyan (background). **179 Alamy Stock Photo:** Artepics (tr); Premium Stock Photography GmbH (bl); bildagentur-online.com/th-fo (br). **Shutterstock.com:** Park_wncl (crb). **180 123RF.com:** phoenix28 (cl, br). **181 123RF.com:** phoenix28 (r). **Alamy Stock Photo:** Gibon Art (tr). **182 123RF.com:** Melinda Fawver (br); phoenix28 (c, cr). **Alamy Stock Photo:** Antiques & Collectables (tc). **Dreamstime.com:** Adam88x (bc). **183 123RF.com:** phoenix28 (tr, br). **Bridgeman Images:** Tarker (c). **184 123RF.com:** phoenix28 (tr, cl). **Alamy Stock Photo:** Florilegius (c). **185 123RF.com:** phoenix28 (ca). **Dreamstime.com:** Aleoks (cr). **Getty Images:** Hulton Deutsch (tl). **186 Getty Images/iStock:** Alla Koala (c, r, br). **187 Getty Images/iStock:** Alla Koala (tl, tr). **Shutterstock.com:** Kharbine-Tapabor (b); Halil ibrahim mescioglu (cra). **188 Alamy Stock Photo:** Archivah (bc). **188-189 123RF.com:** alekstaurus (background). **189 Dreamstime.com:** Onlyfabrizio (tr). **Nordiska museet:** (br). **190 Biodiversity Heritage Library. 191 Alamy Stock Photo:** Asar Studios (cb). **Biodiversity Heritage Library. 192 Getty Images/iStock:** ilbusca (b). **193 Getty Images/iStock:** ilbusca (ca). **Getty Images:** sommail (br). **Shutterstock.com:** dadalia (l). **194 Alamy Stock Photo:** ACTIVE MUSEUM/ACTIVE ART (tl). **Getty Images/iStock:** ilbusca (crb). **Getty Images:** scisettialfio (br). **195 Bridgeman Images:** British Library Board. (bl). **Getty Images/iStock:** ilbusca (tc, br). **Getty Images:** Madeleine_Steinbach (ca). **196 Getty Images/iStock:** Luchschen. **197 Alamy Stock Photo:** Rakesh Dhareshwar (c). **Dreamstime.com:** Mariia Sultanova (ftl, ftr, ca, cr, cb, bl, bc, br). **198 Dreamstime.com:** Mariia Sultanova (tr, cl, crb, bc). **Getty Images:** Heritage Images (c). **199 Alamy Stock Photo:** Nigel Cattlin (cb). **Dreamstime.com:** Lijam (bc); Björn Wylezich (bl); Mariia Sultanova (tc, cl, c, crb). **Science Photo Library:** Jean-Loup Charmet (tr). **200-201 Getty Images/iStock:** Epine_art (background). **201 Bridgeman Images:** Look and Learn (bc). **202-203 Getty Images/iStock:** Epine_art (background). **202 Alamy Stock Photo:** Lubo Ivanko (tr). **Getty Images/iStock:** clu (tl). **Shutterstock.com:** Alexander Shchukin (br). **203 Alamy Stock Photo:** Nature Photographers Ltd (tr). **Dreamstime.com:** Bert Folso (cr). **Science Photo Library:** Steve Gschmeissner (br). **204-205 Dreamstime.com:** Tristan Berlun (background). **206-207 Getty Images/iStock:** Nastasic (background). **206 Dreamstime.com:** Andrei Vasilev (cra). **Science & Society Picture Library:** National Railway Museum (bl). **Science Photo Library:** Power And Syred (br). **Shutterstock.com:** Arunsri Futemwong (crb). **207 Getty Images/iStock:** esolla. **208 Alamy Stock Photo:** Asar Studios (c). **Shutterstock.com:** Foxyliam (tr, l, cra, crb). **209 Alamy Stock Photo:** Hans Stuessi (bc). **Shutterstock.com:** Foxyliam (bl, cla, cra). **210 Alamy Stock Photo:** Maxim Tatarinov (cr). **Dreamstime.com:** Foxyliam (tl, cra, br). **211 Alamy Stock Photo:** The Picture Art Collection (tr). **© The Trustees of the British Museum. All rights reserved:** (bl). **Dreamstime.com:** Foxyliam (tl, br); Noraluca (crb). **212 Alamy Stock Photo:** UtCon Collection (fbl). **Biodiversity Heritage Library. 213 Alamy Stock Photo:** Florilegius (tc). **Biodiversity Heritage Library. 214 Science Photo Library:** SCIMAT (bl). **214-215 Dreamstime.com:** Tristan Berlun (background). **215 Bridgeman Images:** The Stapleton Collection (tr). **216 Alamy Stock Photo:** Heinz Tschanz-Hofmann (cl). **Bridgeman Images:** Florilegius (c). **Dreamstime.com:** Ekaterina Arkhangelskaia (cla, br, l); Maxim Tatarinov (bl). **217 Alamy Stock Photo:** Alain Guilleux (crb); Science Photo Library (br). **Wellcome Collection:** Yaohui tukao (Illustrated Congregation of Drugs) 193 (tr). **218 Getty Images/iStock:** Awispa (cl). **219 Dreamstime.com:** Bjorn Hovdal (tr); Olga Popova (cra). **Getty Images/iStock:** Awispa (crb, bl). **Getty Images:** Buyenlarge (tc); Universal Images Group/Hulton Fine Art (br). **220 Bridgeman Images:** Purix Verlag Volker Christen (tl). **220-221 Getty Images/iStock:** Elena. **221 Dreamstime.com:** (crb). **Getty Images:** DEA/G. DAGLI ORTI (bl). **222-223 Dreamstime.com:** Awispa (background). **223 Science Photo Library:** SCIMAT (tr). **224 © The Trustees of the British Museum. All rights reserved 224 Dreamstime.com:** Awispa (background); Wanida Larkjit (clb); Yutthasart Yanakornsir (bl). **Getty Images:** imageBROKER/Angela Serena Gilmour (bc). **225 123RF.com:** catarchangel (background). **akg-images:** Chicago, Art Institute © Aiden Lassell Ripley Estat (cr). **226 Alamy Stock Photo:** Florilegius (bl); Quagga Media (tl); The Natural History Museum (tr). **Biodiversity Heritage Library. 227 Alamy Stock Photo:** Florilegius (tr, fcr). **Biodiversity Heritage Library. 228-229 123RF.com:** robusta87 (background). **Alamy Stock Photo:** Heritage Image Partnership Ltd (tl). **229 Depositphotos Inc:** brozova (b). **230-231 123RF.com:** robusta87 (background). **Wolfoto/Wolfgang Rebhandl. 231 Alamy Stock Photo:** Contraband Collection (tr). **232 Getty Images:** Chris Hellier/Corbis. **232-233 123RF.com:** robusta87 (background). **233 Alamy Stock Photo:** Chronicle (tr); WILDLIFE GmbH (br). **Dreamstime.com:** Olivier Le Moal (bl). **Getty Images:** E+/tiborgartner (c). **Getty Images/iStock:** Narayana Murthy (fbl). **234 Getty Images/iStock:** GeorgePeters (br). **Science Photo Library:** Ted Kinsman (tl). **234-235 123RF.com:** bokasana (background). **Alamy Stock Photo:** Oleksandr Kovalchuk. **236-237 123RF.com:** bokasana (background). **236 AWL Images:** Karol Kozlowski (br). **Mary Evans Picture Library:** Ashmolean Museum (cl). **237 Getty Images:** Jan Woitas/DPA/AFP (bl). **Shutterstock.com:** Yonton7 (cr). **238 123RF.com:** morphart (clb, tr, br). **Alamy Stock Photo:** Historic Images (c). **239 123RF.com:** morphart (tr). **Alamy Stock Photo:** Tamer Adel (crb). **240 Getty Images:** Leemage (tr). **Science Photo Library:** Eye of Science (bc). **240-241 Getty Images:** DigitalVision Vectors/ibusc (background). **243 Alamy Stock Photo:** wsr (ca). **Getty Images/iStock:** Chushkin (tr); Chushkin (cr); sirichai_asawalapsakul (br). **244-245 123RF.com:** alekstaurus. **244 Shutterstock.com:** PeskyMonkey (bl). **245 Getty Images:** E+/Alina555 (br). **246-247 123RF.com:** alekstaurus (background). **246 Bibliothèque nationale de France, Paris:** (cr). **247 Getty Images:** Atelier Binder/ullstein bild (tr). **Shutterstock.com:** arun uppadhyay (br). **248 123RF.com:** logaryphmic (c). **249 Bridgeman Images:** Bridgeman Images (c). **250 123RF.com:** logaryphmic (tc, br). **Alamy Stock Photo:** blickwinkel (tl). **Dreamstime.com:** Artistas (cla); Iva Villi (clb). **251 AWL Images:** Hemis (br). **Bridgeman Images:** 2022 Museum of Fine Arts, Boston. All rights reserved./Gift of James Lawrence (tc). **252 Alamy Stock Photo:** Chronicle (cra). **Biodiversity Heritage Library. 253 Alamy Stock Photo:** Florilegius (bl). **Biodiversity Heritage Library. 254 Alamy Stock Photo:** agefotostock (l). **Dreamstime.com:** Miroslav Hlavko (cr). **256 Dreamstime.com:** EPhotocorp (bl). **257 Bridgeman Images:** Christie's Images (cra). **258 Exotic India. 259 Dreamstime.com:** Mohammed Anwarul Kabir Choudhury (br); Maxim Tatarinov (tc). **Shutterstock.com:** Nattika (tl); SOMMAI (tr). **260 Alamy Stock Photo:** Mohammed Anwarul Kabir Choudhury (br); Doukdouk (tl). **261 Alamy Stock Photo:** Steve Vidler (c). **262 123RF.com:** epine (tl, br). **Alamy Stock Photo:** agefotostock (c). **263 123RF.com:** epine (tr, br). **Getty Images/iStock:** bdspn (ca). **Getty Images:** ithinksky (bc). **264-265 Shutterstock.com:** Foxyliam (background). **266 Alamy Stock Photo:** De Luan (tr); flowerphotos (bc). **Getty Images/iStock:** ilbusca (tl). **267 Dreamstime.com:** Digitalimagined (tc). **Getty Images/iStock:** ilbusca (bl). **268 Getty Images/iStock:** rraya (l). **269 Getty Images/iStock:** chengyuzheng (b); rraya (l, tc, br). **Getty Images:** Sepia Times (tr). **270 Dreamstime.com:** Mohdoqba (bc); Onlyfabrizio (bl). **Getty Images/iStock:** rraya (cla). **Shutterstock.com:** Keith Hider (cl). **271 Getty Images/iStock:** mirzamlk (bl); rraya (br). **272 Biodiversity Heritage Library. 273 Biodiversity Heritage Library. The New York Public Library:** (ca). **Wikipedia:** Public Domain (ftl); Rezergua (fbr). **274 123RF.com:** morphart (tl, l, r). **Alamy Stock Photo:** incamerastock (crb). **275 123RF.com:** morphart (tr, crb). **276 123RF.com:** morphart (br). **Alamy Stock Photo:** agefotostock (t). **277 123RF.com:** morphart (cr). **Alamy Stock Photo:** blickwinkel (tr); GPNaturePhotos (tc). **Bridgeman Images:** British Library Board (br). **Shutterstock.com:** Sanskar hardaha (tl). **278-279 Getty Images/iStock:** Iamnee (background). **278 Getty Images/iStock:** bong hyunjung (ca). **Mereyama Mereco:** (bc). **279 Biodiversity Heritage Library. Bridgeman Images. 280 Bridgeman Images:** Purix Verlag Volker Christen (c). **Dreamstime.com:** Efesan (cl); Patrick Guenette (bl, cra). **281 Alamy Stock Photo:** Bill Gozansky (bl). **Dreamstime.com:** Patrick Guenette (tc, crb). **Getty Images:** Patrick Aventurier (br). **282 Alamy Stock Photo:** INTERFOTO (ca). **283 Alamy Stock Photo:** Nature Picture Library (tr); Madeleine Steinbach (bl). **Shutterstock.com:** Foxyliam (tl, r, b). **284 Alamy Stock Photo:** MJ Photography (tc). **Dreamstime.com:** Junyan Jiang (bl); Manfred Ruckszio (cb). **Getty Images/iStock:** YuanruLi (br). **285 Shutterstock.com:** Foxyliam (tl, tr, bl). **286 Getty Images/iStock:** Epine_art (background). **Getty Images:** Prot Tachapanit/EyeEm (bc). **287 Dreamstime.com:** Tristan Berlund (background). **Science Photo Library:** SCIMAT (br). **Shutterstock.com:** zhengchengbao (bl). **288 Alamy Stock Photo:** MET/BOT (bl). **288-289 Getty Images/iStock:** Epine_art (background). **289 Dreamstime.com:** Silvia Ganora (br). **Getty Images/iStock:** geargodz (bc). **Shutterstock.com:** KAISARMUDA (crb).

All other images © Dorling Kindersley

DK would especially like to thank:

Oxford Botanic Garden & Arboretum
www.obga.ox.ac.uk
Thank you to Mark Brent for supplying the rare maidenhair fern.

The National Herb Centre, Banbury
www.herbcentre.co.uk
A special thanks to the Directors, Sam and Nick Turner and to Jane Zammett and Shirley Cole.

Geoffrey Cooper
www.plantheritage.org.uk
Grower of exotic plants: cacti, succulents and trees. Plant Heritage, National Eucalyptus Reference Collection, Cote, Oxfordshire

Oxfordshire Chilli Garden
www.oxfordshirechilligarden.co.uk
Thank you for allowing us to photograph the Cayenne pepper.

Green & Gorgeous flower farm in Oxfordshire.
www.greenandgorgeousflowers.co.uk
Thank you to Rachel Siegfried for supplying the angelica.

Hebden Bridge Botanics via Etsy for young tea tree plants.